Head Direction Cells and the Neural Mechanisms of Spatial Orientation

Head Direction Cells and the Neural Mechanisms of Spatial Orientation

edited by Sidney I. Wiener and Jeffrey S. Taube

A Bradford Book
The MIT Press
Cambridge, Massachusetts
London, England

MIT Press books may be purchased at special quantity discounts for business or sales promotional use. For information, please email special_sales@mitpress.mit.edu or write to Special Sales Department, The MIT Press, 5 Cambridge Center, Cambridge, MA 02142.

This book was set in Times Roman by SNP Best-set Typesetter Ltd., Hong Kong.
Printed and bound in the United States of America.

Library of Congress Cataloging-in-Publication Data

Head direction cells and the neural mechanisms of spatial orientation / edited by Sidney I. Wiener and Jeffrey S. Taube.
  p. cm.
"A Bradford book."
Includes bibliographical references and index.
ISBN 0-262-23241-3 (alk. paper)
1. Space perception. 2. Neurons. 3. Head. I. Wiener, Sidney I. II. Taube, Jeffrey S.

QP491.H385   2005
152.14′2—dc22

                                                                            2004058791

10 9 8 7 6 5 4 3 2 1

To our parents

Contents

Foreword: History of the Discovery of Head Direction Cells

James B. Ranck Jr.

In January of 1984 I implanted some rats with electrodes intended for the subiculum. I had earlier recorded from what I thought was the subiculum and thought I had found neurons that had characteristics that, in retrospect, were all wrong. On Sunday, January 15, 1984, I lowered the electrode and recorded from the first of the rats. I was astounded to find a head direction cell. It was so clear that I felt confident about its characteristics within a few minutes: the firing was in absolute direction in the horizontal plane (yaw), independent of pitch, roll, and location; it was independent of the few behaviors observed that afternoon; and all the firing occurred within about 90°. That Sunday afternoon I made a TV tape of the cell and the rat; that is the tape that I have often used since. No one else was in the laboratory that afternoon. That evening, I went to a party and floated on air. I told at least one friend at the party that I had recorded from a very exciting cell that afternoon. She did not have the slightest idea what I was talking about, but at least she was the first person I told about the finding. (My wife was traveling at the time, so I did not have a chance to tell her how excited I was.)

The next day, I told Steve Fox, John Kubie, Bob Muller, and Greg Quirk. John Kubie remembered that someone—I do not remember who—had recorded from a neuron with similar properties and had made a TV tape of it. I had no recollection of the cell, but when we played the tape, lo and behold, it was a head direction cell, unappreciated at the time. This cell was in stratum oriens of CA1. If we had picked up on it, we would not have gotten anywhere (since such cells have only rarely been found there since). I guess we were lucky to let it slip by. Over the next few weeks I found more head direction cells on the same electrode as I lowered it through brain, and still more in the other rats. All these studies were nonquantitative, but they showed the same characteristics as the first head direction cell I saw. I brought a magnet into the room without effect, to check that the effect was not magnetic. I put one rat on a 20-foot cable and carried him around the room and into a new room, and the direction was maintained. The firing was correlated with absolute direction, independent of location. In an environment where a rat can move in many directions, hippocampal place cell firing is independent of direction. In this sense, head direction cells are the complement of O'Keefe's hippocampal place cells. Information about absolute location and absolute direction is adequate for navigation.

When the histology was done, it turned out that I had not been in subiculum at all, but rather in postsubiculum in all the rats. (At least my stereotaxic work had been consistent.) By April I had collected enough cells to write an abstract for the Neuroscience meetings.

I had read reviews of tests conducted from about 1900 to 1960 with rats running mazes. None of the authors even suggested that a sense of absolute direction was used in running these mazes. However, in the bird migration literature, the sense of direction is extensively discussed. Much of neuroscience tries to explain a behavior or behavioral mechanism that we already know about. This seemed to be a case where the neural mechanisms suggested a behavior or behavioral mechanism that was not adequately appreciated.

In the summer of 1984 John Kubie and Mark Stewart trained rats on an eight-arm radial maze placed at different sites in a large room. Some of the rats were trained with the food always on the arm pointing toward a single light, independent of location of the maze in the room. Other rats were trained with the food always on the arm pointing the same absolute direction, independent of location of the maze in the room. The rats learned to go to the arm pointing to the light fairly easily. Rats could learn to go to the arm in the same absolute direction, but it took them three times as much training. Kubic and Stewart reported this work at the spring 1985 meeting of the Eastern Psychological Association. I presented the finding on single neuron firing at a meeting in Pecs, Hungry in the summer of 1984. I had made a movie out of the January TV tape, but stupidly had not checked for compatibility with Hungarian projectors, so the talk was all words and still pictures, with the most dramatic part left out. The first publication (other than the 1984 abstract) is a chapter in the proceeding of this meeting.

When I presented the poster at the Society for Neuroscience meetings at Anaheim in 1984, I set up a TV show of the rat and head direction cell (using the TV tape from January). It was a big hit. A lot of people came to see it and many said "Wow" or the equivalent. I was especially pleased that one of the guards at the convention center spent most of his time watching the tape. You don't have to be a neuroscientist to be struck and entertained by the firing of these cells.

After the spring of 1984 I did not try to record any more head direction neurons, but worked with Bob Muller on getting a quantitative recording system to work, using an overhead TV camera and two different colored LEDs on the rat's head and using the difference between the location of the two to compute yaw. Muller and Kubie had already worked out a system for quantitative recording of place cells, so I thought that we could get the system for head direction cells going within a year. However, it seemed as if everything went wrong. We thought the system was finally working in the summer of 1986, just when Jeffrey Taube arrived from the University of Washington as a postdoctoral fellow.

However, the first quantitative recordings Jeff made of a head direction cell showed that it had a peak firing rate of only about 3 spikes/s, which seemed far too low compared with the way the cell spiking sounded over the audio system and how it looked on the oscilloscope. It took another few months to finally get the automatic tracking and cell recording system to function properly, and another year for Jeff and Bob to collect the data and analyze them. Another three years would pass before Jeff, Bob, and I published the first proper articles on these remarkable cells in *Journal of Neuroscience* (Taube et al., 1990a, 1990b).

Pat Sharp arrived in the summer of 1987 and was in the lab for two years. She did not work on head direction cells in Brooklyn, but has contributed many important articles since.

References

Ranck JB Jr (1986) Head direction cells in the deep cell layer of dorsal presubiculum in freely moving rats. In Electrical Activity of the Archicortex (G Buzsáki and CH Vanderwolf, eds), pp. 217–220. Budapest: Akademai Kiado.

Stewart M, Kubie J (1985) Can rats learn a compass direction? East Psychol Assn Abstr 56: 32.

Taube JS, Muller RU, Ranck JB Jr (1990a) Head-direction cells recorded from the postsubiculum in freely moving rats. I. Description and quantitative analysis. J Neurosci 10: 420–435.

Taube JS, Muller RU, Ranck JB Jr (1990b) Head-direction cells recorded from the postsubiculum in freely moving rats. II. Effects of environmental manipulations. J Neurosci 10: 436–447.

Preface

Sidney I. Wiener

Since the first publication of two full-length manuscripts on head direction cells by Jeffrey S. Taube, Robert U. Muller, and James B. Ranck Jr in 1990, there has been a rapidly accelerating growth in knowledge about and interest in these fascinating neurons. Like the place-selective hippocampal neurons, head direction cells serve as a particularly remarkable model of high-level cognitive processing at the level of single neurons. Found in about ten different brain areas, these cells fire action potentials only when the animal orients its head in a specific direction in space. Since different neurons are selective for different directions, those active at any given moment can provide an accurate spatial reference signal. These responses are strongly influenced by distal landmarks in the local environment (and thus are independent of the earth's magnetic field). However, they do not depend on these cues being viewed from a particular perspective or distance, and they persist in darkness or without any landmark cues. This stimulus invariance and robustness suggest that these responses can contribute information vital for spatial orientation behaviors such as navigation and can participate in brain representations of the head in space.

But how does the brain go about creating and maintaining these representations? When environmental cues are displaced, what are the neural mechanisms that permit the responses of the population of neurons to coherently follow them? What rules guide the anchoring of the cell responses to sensory inputs? How are the responses of the diverse brain structures in this network united? And how do head direction cells influence orienting behavior and navigation choices? This book will address such questions, and present the state of the art as well as directions for further research on issues that remain on the frontiers of our knowledge.

While this book is primarily intended for students and researchers in the cognitive sciences, neurosciences, computational sciences, and robotics, we hope that it may also prove useful to clinicians, philosophers, and all others who share our curiosity and passion to understand not only how spatial cognition works but, more generally, how the brain works.

Much of the work presented here is based upon presentations at a conference held at an estate in the Var region of France on September 14–18, 2002, under the sponsorship of the Treilles Foundation. This book, however, has been organized to provide a coherent, comprehensive, and didactic presentation of the topic in a manner accessible to nonspecialists, but comprehensive enough to serve as a reference for specialists as well. As much as possible, the actual researchers who made the scientific discoveries have been asked to explain their work, permitting a variety of viewpoints on several key issues.

We thank the National Science Foundation (US)-CNRS (France) for a collaboration grant awarded to the laboratories of Jeffrey Taube, Patricia Sharp, and Sidney Wiener. Thanks to Alain Berthoz for sparking and encouraging this collaboration and cochairing the Treilles Foundation meeting. Thanks to the chapter authors and other anonymous reviewers of the chapters. Thanks to the NIMH for support of an Independent Scientist Award to Jeffrey Taube and to France Maloumian for help with figures.

Overview

Sidney I. Wiener and Jeffrey S. Taube

Recent scientific discoveries provide a better understanding of how the human brain, while relatively modest in size, is capable of providing each of us with awareness, personality, emotion, memory, and comprehension. In the history of neuroscience research, this enigma of how consciousness can be embedded in matter has proved to be extremely challenging since the brain, in order to carry out all of these functions, has miniaturized hundreds of trillions of connections among its numerous neurons. The question of how nervous system anatomy and electrical activity are related to psychological function is readily addressed in studies of sensory and motor functions. However, the high level of interconnectivity and integration of circuits makes it somewhat more difficult to identify the brain basis of cognitive functions. Observations in neurology patients have demonstrated localization of functions such as the speech modules and areas specific for recognition of distinct categories of visual objects. The development of experimental animal models permits complementary examinations of the neurophysiological bases of cognitive functions at a single cell level. Examples include studies in the monkey that demonstrate the presence of "mirror cells" (cells that respond when the animal views another animal making a given movement) and "face recognition cells" (cells that respond to the view of specific faces, in some cases oriented in certain directions).

Rodents such as rats and mice also serve as useful experimental models for studying the brain basis of specific cognitive functions. Perhaps because of the necessity for efficient memory and recall mechanisms, as well as resourceful capacities for spatial orientation, evolution has led to the conservation of brain areas with comparable anatomy and physiology among a variety of mammals, including man. In fact, both mnemonic and spatial cognitive functions are attributed to the same circuits in the limbic system, centered on a brain structure known as the hippocampus. This pairing of mnemonic and spatial functions is particularly valuable since it is often useful for memories to be associated with, and recalled at, particular places, and conversely, that the means for navigating toward important locations be well memorized.

Two important models for studying the neurophysiological basis for spatial cognition at the single cell level are the place responses of neurons of the hippocampus ("place cells") and the head direction cells (found in many structures of the brain's limbic system). Hippocampal place cells discharge action potentials when the animal occupies a small location within its environment. In open fields, these responses are often independent of the direction the animal is facing, although the responses can become directional when the animal performs stereotypic behaviors on a linear track. Complementing this, head direction cells discharge when the animal is facing a particular direction, independent of the position it occupies. In both cases the responses are independent of what the animal is viewing and they persist even in darkness or in the absence of prominent landmarks. Furthermore, different neurons are selective for different head orientations, or locations in the case of place cells, providing a fairly comprehensive representation by as few as a dozen or so neurons.

These properties suggest (but do not prove) that these neurons play an important role in signaling these types of information and could hence participate in fundamental mechanisms involved in determining orientation and in navigation. One clue that these properties are associated with high-level functions is that the activity of head direction cells is *stimulus-invariant*; that is, it does not depend upon any particular sensory stimulus, such as viewing a particular cue from a certain angle. Rather, the cell will fire, for example, whether the animal stands facing directly into a corner, or is scanning from the other end of (or even outside) the room, as long as it is oriented in the same direction. The responses depend only upon the topographic relation between the position of the head and the external environment. The neuronal discharges are not simply dependent on a single sensory modality like vision; rather, it is *supramodal* (i.e., drawing upon many modalities, but independent of each of them). Several chapters will elaborate on the essential roles of different sensory modalities, emphasizing the vestibular sense, which are utilized interchangeably in the elaboration of these responses. Furthermore, head direction cells depend upon movement-related signals. Another indication of the importance of the head direction signal is that it is *pervasive*. It has been reported that up to 10 different brain structures contain neurons selective for head direction. This finding is commensurate with the importance of orientation information for the planning and execution of many types of goal-oriented movements. The place and head direction signals are *stable*. Individual neurons maintain the same selectivity when the animal is placed in the same environment over the course of weeks or even months. Head direction cell firing shows little adaptation, and these neurons continue to discharge indefinitely as long as the animal maintains its head oriented in the same direction. This combination of properties indicates that these cells are viable candidates as reliable sources of highly processed, robust information concerning the head direction.

This book aims to help better understand how this type of signal arises, its properties, and how it may be used for elaborating orienting and navigation behaviors. The book is divided into five parts, whose subjects are, respectively: (1) representations of directional orientation: head direction cell properties and anatomy, (2) the influence of vestibular and motor cues on head direction cells and place cells, (3) relations between the head direction system, spatial orientation, and behavior, (4) neural mechanisms of spatial orientation in nonhuman primates and humans, and (5) theoretical studies and computational approaches to modeling head direction cell firing and navigation. The book may be read in order, or individual chapters may be selected for more rapid responses to burning questions. Although the chapters have been written so that they can also be read separately, themes introduced in the first three chapters are returned to many times.

The first chapter by Sharp provides an overview of the basic properties of head direction cells and introduces some fundamental concepts. The chapter is based on the anatomical framework discussed in further detail in the next chapter, and it provides a comparison of the properties of the head direction neurons in the respective structures. The second chapter by Hopkins presents the anatomical infrastructure of the head direction system. These brain structures are the basis of the functional circuitry that gives rise to the properties of these neurons, and they are taken into account in most discussions of head direction cells. This chapter also provides information that will be indispensable for computational neuroscientists to understand the circuit dynamics as the basis for internal representations of direction in models of the head direction system. For those not yet familiar with the anatomical substrates of the head direction system, this chapter is an excellent place to start, and the reader's attention here will be amply rewarded. Toward this end, the chapter is didactically presented in the framework of establishing general organizing principles. Many details have necessarily been left out, but interested readers will appreciate the extensive bibliography that serves as a springboard to the technical and specialized literature.

The next two chapters explore the influence of visual cues on head direction cell activity. Taube begins by providing a two-part discussion. The first part is concerned with how landmarks exert control over the directional tuning of head direction cells. We can immediately discard the idea that head direction cells encode direction in "absolute space," since rotation of stable distal visual cues in the absence of the animal (and often in its presence) leads to similar shifts in the cells' preferred direction of firing. The second part is concerned with how head direction cells respond when the animal locomotes in planes other than earth horizontal—specifically, in the vertical plane and upside down on the ceiling. The findings from these studies lead to important constraints on how the brain evolved to process spatial information efficiently. In fact, the insensitivity of the head direction system to linear translations and distances relative to cues demonstrates an anatomical division of function every bit as revealing as the separation of color, motion, and form processing in the primate visual system. Similarly, head direction cells are principally selective for the orientation of the head in the horizontal plane (in other words, about the yaw axis, or the azimuthal direction). If the head is pointed upward or downward (i.e., along the pitch axis) the directional firing concerns the projection of the head orientation onto the horizontal plane. Similarly, there is no evidence for modulation by rotations along the roll axis (leaning over to the left or right). Two mysteries that will not be resolved in this and following chapters are why head direction cells are selective only for the head direction in the horizontal plane, and where in the brain one finds representations of head direction in roll or pitch planes (although some clues are provided in the chapters by Duffy et al., and Taube). After Taube's explanation of visual cue control over head direction cells, Zugaro and Wiener delve into the issue of characterizing the nature of, and mechanisms by which, visual cues control head direction cells (and most likely place cells as well).

To understand the head direction system, it is necessary to consider how the signals originate and are updated through analysis of information processing in various nuclei. The first section, therefore, concludes with a chapter by Bassett and Taube that discusses how the head direction signal is generated, most likely by areas within the brainstem that are associated with the vestibular system. The authors describe an ascending flow of information that propagates rostrally and culminates in the projection of the head direction signal into the entorhinal cortex, the major gateway into the hippocampus. The authors also discuss a descending stream of information that contains information about visual landmarks and how the two information streams are integrated to form a stable representation of one's perceived directional heading.

The next section characterizes the types of sensory and motor information that control head direction cell firing. The stimulus invariance referred to above derives from the particularly intriguing capacity of head direction cells to integrate signals concerning the environment, in particular, visual cues with other information generated by self-movements (referred to as *idiothetic*; Mittelstaedt and Mittelstaedt, 1980; cited in chapter 7). These often ignored sensory modalities, including vestibular, proprioceptive, and optic field flow inputs, will prove to be crucial. This convergence and integration raises several theoretical issues. For example, how are these diverse types of information calibrated so that the motor signals concerning a particular rotation are coherent with the resulting shift in angular heading of a visual cue in the environment? First, Glasauer describes the brain's infrastructure for processing vestibular input signals that enter into the head direction system. Stackman and Zugaro then discuss the impact of this information on head direction cells, emphasizing the studies that show their critical role in generating the head direction signal, since vestibular lesions suppress them. They also review the many studies that examine how head direction cells respond under conditions of cue conflict, where the spatial information from one sensory or motor source differs from that of a second source.

The next chapter extends these themes in discussions of areas associated with the principal circuit that carries head direction signals between brainstem, thalamus, and cortex. Knierim describes studies comparing head direction cell and hippocampal place responses. The coherence of these two representations after cue manipulations is shown to be related to the familiarity of the animal with the environment, and a conceptual model is proposed to account for the findings. Continuing with the theme of hippocampal place responses, Muller and Brunel discuss the issue of the extent to which place cells contain secondary firing correlates that are related to the directional heading of the animal. They review and provide a theoretical basis for understanding studies that show that place cell activity is directionally modulated when behavior is stereotypically oriented, such as when an animal shuttles back and forth on a linear track.

The next section concerns the relationship between head direction cell activity and an animal's spatial behavior. Mizumori and colleagues show how sensory control of directional responses varies in structures outside the core limbic system pathways, with some exciting new data on a cortical zone that may be involved in the expression of directional navigation behaviors. The next chapter by Wiener and Schenk reviews the directional discrimination capacities in rodents, as well as studies of their ontogenesis. Dudchenko and colleagues then review the current state of knowledge on the relation between head direction cell responses and orientation behaviors. While the former data are derived primarily from rats, behavioral and physiological observations in monkeys and the presence of homologous underlying neuroanatomical pathways among mammalian species studied leads us to suppose that similar functions are present in humans. The final chapter in this section by Aggleton reviews the literature concerning behavior and learning deficits associated with lesions to various structures of the head direction cell system, and compares results from studies in man and rodent.

The next section is concerned with spatial and directional orientation in non-human primates as well as humans. The chapter by Rolls reviews the various types of directional and view responses found in monkeys, and proposes several computational frameworks by which this activity could participate in spatial learning. Duffy et al. then review brain systems in the monkey that process other types of orienting information, in particular the heading-related activity in the posterior parietal cortical area MSTd with special emphasis on the importance of optic flow signals. The next two chapters focus on psychophysical studies of directional orientation in man. First, Israël and Warren study how perception of static and dynamic orientation is informed by visual and self-movement signals in humans. Then, Hicheur and colleagues deal with anticipatory processes in the control of head orientation during locomotion in man and provide evidence for distinct processing of angular and linear displacements.

Computational studies are an effective way to consolidate the existing knowledge about head direction cells and to test the feasibility of theories concerning the functional organization of these millions of neurons, as well as their applicability for navigation problem solving. In the last section of the book, Touretzky first presents a tutorial demonstrating how to implement a popular model of head direction cells, the continuous attractor network. Arleo and Gerstner then apply this approach for guiding the navigational system for mobile robots.

The fact that as many as ten different brain structures show head direction responses reinforces the notion that this signal has proved useful over the course of evolution. Thus, nature has provided us with a robust message that this signal is important and hence can serve as a vital key for understanding brain function. The prominence, strength, and clarity of this signal is the rationale for assembling our knowledge on these fascinating cells and how they may underlie mechanisms of spatial orientation and our sense of direction. Unfortunately, because of space limitations, related issues such as angular direction processing for gaze orientation or pointing are not dealt with. Nonetheless, head direction processing is carried on in parallel (and sometimes overlapping) circuits with these other functions, and important general concepts will undoubtedly be arrived at by comparative studies. We hope the present volume will facilitate this endeavor.

I REPRESENTATIONS OF DIRECTIONAL ORIENTATION: HEAD DIRECTION CELL PROPERTIES AND ANATOMY

1 Regional Distribution and Variation in the Firing Properties of Head Direction Cells

Patricia E. Sharp

Head Direction Cells Were Discovered in a Brain Region Known as the Postsubiculum (Dorsal Presubiculum)

Head direction (HD) cells were first discovered in rats in a part of the subicular complex known as the postsubiculum (Ranck, 1984). Any one HD cell fires whenever the rat's head is pointed in a particular direction in the horizontal plane (over an approximately 90° range), and is nearly silent any other time. Within the range of the cell's preferred direction, the firing rate makes a triangular or Gaussian tuning curve (figure 1.1), so that the firing rate is highest in the middle of the range, and falls off symmetrically around that center (Taube et al., 1990a). Different HD cells have different preferred directions, so that for any direction the rat faces, certain corresponding members of the HD cell population are active.

At the time that HD cells were discovered, the investigation of hippocampal place cells (O'Keefe and Nadel, 1978) was already well under way. These hippocampal cells fired when the rat was in a particular location, so that the entire set of hippocampal place cells appeared to form a "map" of the environment (O'Keefe and Nadel, 1978). The discovery of these place cells opened an important new area of investigation. It offered the opportunity to gain insight into how the brain orchestrates the complex cognitive task of navigation.

This hippocampal place cell discovery also fueled the tendency to focus experimental activity solely on the hippocampus proper, to the exclusion of other, anatomically related, areas. Thus, the investigation of spatial memory and cognition was very pointedly "hippocampocentric."

An important step toward breaking this tendency was initiated by Jim Ranck in the 1980s. Ranck reasoned that the hippocampal spatial signals must be part of a larger spatial information processing circuit, so he began the novel investigation of the spatial firing

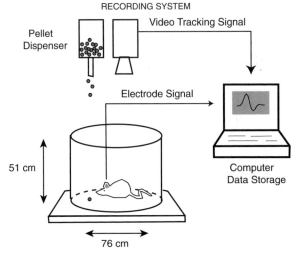

RECORDING SYSTEM

Pellet Dispenser

Video Tracking Signal

Electrode Signal

Computer Data Storage

51 cm

76 cm

OVERHEAD VIEW OF CYLINDRICAL RECORDING CHAMBER

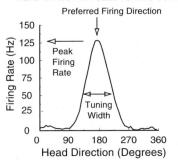

0,360

270

90

180

0,360

270

90

180

HEAD DIRECTION CELL TUNING CURVE

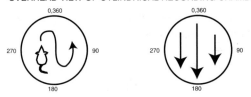

Preferred Firing Direction

Peak Firing Rate

Tuning Width

Firing Rate (Hz)

150

125

100

75

50

25

0

0   90   180   270   360

Head Direction (Degrees)

Figure 1.1

(Top) The recording paradigm (Muller et al., 1987) used for most of the work reviewed here. Hungry rats constantly search for food pellets that are dropped periodically into the recording chamber throughout the recording session. The rats use a series of seemingly random trajectories with which they traverse each portion of the cylinder many times, and from all possible directions. Throughout each session continuous recordings are made of the animal's position and directional heading, as well as the activity of the cell under study. (Middle) Overhead view of the cylindrical recording chamber. The right-hand drawing indicates that the HD cell depicted in the lower panel fired any time that the rat's head was aligned approximately with the arrows shown there. (Bottom) Directional tuning curve for a typical HD cell recorded from the postsubiculum. For this, the video tracker data (indicating the rat's moment-to-moment directional heading) from a recording session are divided into 60 equal directional bins, from 0° to 360°. Then, the average firing rate of the cell is calculated for each bin. The result is the cell's average firing rate over the session for each possible directional heading. The preferred firing direction is calculated as the mean of this distribution, and is 180° for the cell shown here. The peak firing rate is the average rate of the cell when the rat is facing the preferred direction (128 Hz for the cell shown here). The tuning width is twice the standard deviation of the tuning function, and is 80° for the cell shown here.

patterns in the nearby subicular complex which is, of course, closely interconnected with the hippocampus proper. This work led to the discovery of the HD cells in the postsubicular region.

As outlined in the following pages the initial discovery of the postsubicular HD cells has prompted investigations of navigation-related activity in numerous additional portions of the rat limbic system. One surprising finding from this work is that HD cells similar to those in the postsubiculum also exist in numerous additional brain regions. Indeed, the findings reviewed later lead to the suggestion that much of the rat limbic system is involved in directional information processing.

Detailed Investigations of the HD Cells Provided Insight into the Mechanism for Generation of the Directional Signal

Detailed investigations of the HD cells (Taube et al., 1990a,b) revealed the fundamental principles that govern the behavior of these cells. As described elsewhere in this volume, this behavior seems to be generated through two basic mechanisms.

One of these is a process known as angular path integration. In this, the angular movements of the animal serve to update the HD cell-firing pattern. For example, if cells that code for "north" are firing at one point in time, and the animal subsequently turns 90° clockwise, then this angular motion itself will somehow cause the north HD cells to stop firing, and the "east" HD cells to begin firing. In this way, the HD cell population correctly signals that (as a result of the head turn) the directional heading of the animal has changed from north to east.

The second major factor that controls HD cells is the presence of environmental landmarks. In a familiar environment, the HD cells become "attached" to stimuli in the environment, meaning that the preferred direction of the cells can be controlled by the position of salient, stable landmarks (e.g., Taube et al., 1990b).

HD Cells Have Been Found Throughout a Limbic System Circuit Similar to That Described by Papez (1937)

The postsubicular cortex is part of a set of interconnected brain regions that form a loop around the limbic region (figure 1.2; see also chapter 2 of this volume). This loop begins with the lateral mammillary nucleus (LMN), which sends its major ascending output to the anterodorsal nucleus (ADN) of the anterior thalamus (Seki and Zyo, 1984; Shibata, 1992). The ADN, in turn, sends projections to several limbic cortical areas, including the postsubiculum and retrosplenial cortex (Shibata, 1993; Thompson and Robertson, 1987; van Groen and Wyss, 1990). The postsubiculum, in turn, sends a major projection back down to the LMN to complete the loop (Allen and Hopkins, 1989). Each of these areas has been shown to contain HD cells.

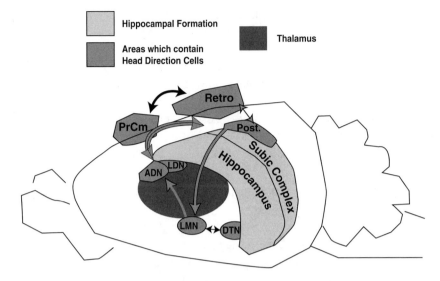

Figure 1.2
Schematic diagram of most of the regions of the rat brain in which HD cells have been observed (lateral cutaway view). It should be noted that although a small number of HD cells have been reported in the hippocampus (see text), the hippocampus is not indicated as being a HD cell-containing region here, because the great majority of cells recorded in this region do not fit the definition of HD cells. (The striatum, which also contains HD cells, has been omitted here for clarity.)

The laterodorsal thalamic nucleus also contains HD cells (Mizumori and Williams, 1993), and, anatomically it forms a subcomponent of the loop previously described. Specifically, the lateral dorsal nucleus (LDN) is reciprocally connected to a set of limbic cortical structures similar to those for ADN (Thompson and Robertson, 1987).

In addition to its ADN projection, the LMN is also strongly and reciprocally connected to the dorsal tegmental nucleus (DTN) of Gudden (Ban and Zyo, 1963; Hayakawa and Zyo, 1984, 1985). HD cells have also been discovered in this nucleus, and, as further discussed in the following pages, it appears that this may be the site at which angular head velocity information (critical for path integration) might enter the HD cell system.

HD Cells Have Also Been Discovered in Areas Outside of the Limbic System

Head direction cells have also been discovered in regions outside of this limbic circuit, including the medial precentral nucleus (anterior cingulate cortex; Mizumori et al., 2002), and the striatum (not shown in figure 1.2, for clarity; Wiener, 1993; Mizumori et al., 2000; Ragozzino et al., 2001). In addition, a small population of HD cells has been discovered in the hippocampus proper (Leutgeb et al., 2000).

HD Cells Throughout the Limbic System Have the Same General Directional Firing Characteristics, but Also Show Subtle Differences from One Region to the Next

All HD cells in each region previously mentioned show the same general characteristics (see figure 1.1). Specifically, by definition, an HD cell must (1) show a single triangular or Gaussian peak in its directional tuning curve, (2) have a firing rate that falls off around the center of this distribution in a reasonably symmetric fashion, and (3) have firing rates outside of the preferred firing direction that are zero or near zero.

Within these limits, however, there are subtle differences in the directional firing properties of the HD cells from one region to the next, and these can provide clues about how and where the directional signal is initially constructed.

Examination of these subtle properties requires a detailed analysis of the directional tuning curves for the population of HD cells in each region. The brain regions for which these kinds of analyses are available are (1) postsubicular cortex, (2) retrosplenial cortex, (3) ADN, (4) LMN, and (5) DTN. All further discussion will be restricted to the properties of HD cells in these regions.

HD Cells in Many Regions Display Effects of Momentary Angular Head Velocity, and the Nature of This Effect Varies across Regions

Effects of Angular Head Velocity on HD Cell *Firing Rate*
Recall that one mechanism through which the HD cells track directional heading is a process involving angular path integration. This suggests that angular head velocity information (such as might be provided by the vestibular system, optic flow, motor command signals, etc.) must enter the HD cell circuit at some point. Indeed, cells that have angular head velocity as a primary correlate have been found in some of the same regions as the HD cells themselves, including the LMN (Stackman and Taube, 1998), DTN (Bassett and Taube, 2001; Sharp et al., 2001b), and postsubiculum (Sharp, 1996). One likely input pathway for this information is through the DTN, which is possibly in a position to receive both vestibular (via the nucleus prepositus hypoglossis) and motor command (via the habenula) input (Hayakawa and Zyo, 1985; Liu et al., 1984).

Theoretical models of the HD cell system (e.g. Redish et al., 1996; Zhang, 1996; Skaggs et al., 1995) predict the existence of a cell type that fires in relation to both angular velocity and head direction. That is, these models predict a type of HD cell that would fire at higher rates for turns in one direction (clockwise versus counterclockwise) than the other. This type of cell is critical to the theoretical path integration circuit, because the combined directional and angular motion information is essential for updating the distribution of activity of the HD cell population. For example, a cell that fires optimally when the head is facing north *and* turning clockwise would signal that the head is about to be facing east.

These predicted angular velocity (AV)-by-HD cells have been observed in the LMN by Stackman and Taube (1998). Specifically, these authors reported that LMN HD cells tended to show differential rates during clockwise versus counterclockwise head turning. Also, laterality was a significant influence on this differential rate, so that cells in the right LMN tended to have higher rates during clockwise turns, while those in the left LMN tended to prefer counterclockwise turns.

It should be noted that a similar study conducted by Blair, Cho, and Sharp (1998) did not observe any HD cells that showed a significant influence of clockwise versus counterclockwise head turning on firing rate. Rather, as described later in this chapter, these authors found an influence of angular head velocity on both the directional tuning width and the preferred direction. It is not clear how to explain the different findings between these two laboratories. One possibility is that there were slight differences in the exact subregions of LMN sampled across the two laboratories. Another possibility (discussed later) is that in the two laboratories, recording sessions were of different lengths.

The predicted AV-by-HD cells have also been observed in the DTN (Bassett and Taube, 2001; Sharp et al., 2001a). Specifically, a fraction of the HD cells in this region also show an effect of momentary angular head velocity. An example of this is shown in figure 1.3 (middle row, right column) for a DTN HD cell. Here, samples from the recording session have been separated into those which took place when the rat happened to be turning its head clockwise (at >120°/s) and those when the rat was turning counterclockwise (at >120°/s). Separate directional tuning functions have been constructed for each of these turn conditions. For the DTN cell recorded here, firing rates were slightly, but significantly, higher during counterclockwise, as opposed to clockwise, head motion (at least over the central portion of the preferred directional range).

Thus, that portion of the LMN and DTN cells that shows a joint influence of direction and angular velocity on firing rate is well suited to playing a critical role in angular path integration, as discussed previously.

Effects of Angular Head Velocity on HD Cell *Preferred Firing Direction*
Interestingly, HD cells in several regions display an effect of angular head velocity on preferred firing direction, rather than (or in addition to) firing rate. This is true for cells in LMN (Blair et al., 1998; Stackman and Taube, 1998), ADN (Blair and Sharp, 1995; Taube and Muller, 1998), and retrosplenial cortex (Cho and Sharp, 2001). Examples of this for cells in each of these regions are shown in figure 1.3. Note, in each case, the tuning curve constructed from clockwise turn samples appears to be shifted to the left, relative to the tuning function for counterclockwise turns.

One way to interpret this angular velocity-related shift is to suggest that these HD cells actually anticipate the animal's future head direction, as if the path integration mechanism gets a bit ahead of itself. To see this, imagine an HD cell that has an overall preferred direction of north. If the rat is turning into the north direction from the west, it must use

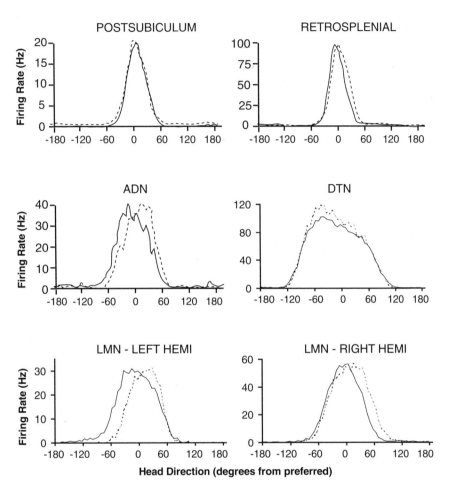

Figure 1.3
Turn-specific directional tuning curves for a typical HD cell from each region discussed in the text. These tuning functions were constructed as described for figure 1.1, except that separate tuning functions were made for all samples taken during clockwise head turns (solid lines) and all samples taken during counterclockwise head turns (dashed lines). HEMI, hemisphere.

a clockwise motion. If the cell anticipates arrival at a northward heading, then the cell will fire optimally when the head direction is slightly to the left (west) of exact north. In contrast, when the animal turns into the north heading from the east, it will necessarily use a counterclockwise motion, and will anticipate by showing optimal firing slightly to the east of its preferred direction. Thus, the overall tuning curves will be shifted in relation to each other.

If we accept this interpretation, then it is possible to use the clockwise and counterclockwise tuning curves to determine the exact amount of time by which each HD cell predicts the future direction. The method used for this involves a "time slide" analysis (Blair and Sharp, 1995; Taube and Muller, 1998). In this type of analysis, the data for the time when spikes occur is shifted in relation to the samples of directional heading. The shifting is done over a series of 16.6 ms time bins, both backward and forward in time. It is reasoned that the amount of time by which a cell anticipates the actual directional heading is the time slide value at which the tuning curve is most narrow (Blair and Sharp, 1995; Taube and Muller, 1998) and at which the peak rate and directional information content are highest (Taube and Muller, 1998). A somewhat different approach is to do this same time slide analysis but divide the data into samples collected when the rat happens to be turning clockwise versus those when it happens to be turning counterclockwise (Blair and Sharp, 1995). It is reasoned that the time slide value at which the clockwise and counterclockwise tuning curves overlap represents the interval by which the cell anticipates future directional heading (see Blair and Sharp, 1995, for the details of this reasoning).

This latter analysis has been done for the HD cells in each region for data collected in my own laboratory, using precisely the same recording and analysis methods for the cells in each area (Blair and Sharp, 1995; Blair et al., 1998; Cho and Sharp, 2001; Sharp et al., 2001b). The average anticipatory time interval for the HD cells in each region is shown in table 1.1.

Note that the cells in LMN anticipate by the largest interval (approx. 38 ms), while those in ADN and retrosplenial cortex anticipate by only about 25 ms. One possible interpretation of this result is that the LMN is closer to the source of the actual HD signal generation (the path integrator circuit) than are the ADN and retrosplenial regions.

Table 1.1
Average directional firing properties for head direction cells in various parts of the head direction cell circuit

Region	Tuning Width (degrees)	Peak Rate (Hz)	Antic. Time Int. (msec)	N
Retrosplenial cortex	44.6 (2.7)	32.3 (10.7)	25.05 (3.3)	12
Postsubiculum	65.3 (3.6)	26.7 (3.2)	−7.70 (5.6)	18
ADN	57.4 (2.4)	50.3 (6.0)	23.2 (3.4)	19
LMN	79.9 (3.5)	37.2 (5.5)	38.5 (3.2)	23
DTN	109.4 (6.8)	47.0 (15.6)	~0.0	6

Note that postsubicular HD cells show an anticipatory time interval that is close to zero, suggesting that they code for the exact, momentary directional heading.

It should be noted that the anticipatory intervals reported from the Taube laboratory are in reasonably good agreement with those presented here, in that they also report the longest anticipatory intervals for the LMN, with medium values for ADN, and values close to zero for postsubiculum (see Stackman and Taube, 2003). However, they report somewhat larger anticipatory values for both LMN and ADN than those shown in table 1.1. Specifically, using the time slide analysis for ADN cells, they found that the directional tuning curves showed the highest peak firing rate values at a time slide value of 49.60 ms. The optimal slide value for the tuning width measure was 38.09 ms, while that for information content was 45.24 ms. Thus, the values reported by Stackman and Taube (2003) suggest that ADN cells anticipate by about twice as long as reported here (table 1.1). Similarly, the values reported by Stackman and Taube (2003) for their LMN data suggest that the LMN HD cells anticipate directional heading by about 70 ms.

It is not clear how to explain these quantitative differences between the two laboratories in estimates of the amount by which LMN and ADN cells anticipate future directional heading. However, one methodological difference between the two laboratories involves the length of the recording sessions. The data recorded in table 1.1 were obtained from pellet-chasing sessions that were always at least 15 minutes long and, in most cases lasted 30 minutes or more (Blair and Sharp, 1995; Blair et al., 1998). In contrast, values reported in Stackman and Taube (2003) were based on sessions that were only 8 minutes long (Taube and Muller, 1998; Stackman and Taube, 1998). It could be argued that the 8-minute session times used in the Taube laboratory are too short to obtain reliable values when performing the sort of detailed analysis required for these anticipatory time interval estimates. One relevant consideration for this is the fact that any one HD cell fires only over a limited portion of the entire 0°–360° directional range (indeed, as mentioned previously, this is a critical part of the definition of HD cells). In contrast, during the pellet-chasing session, the rat usually distributes its heading evenly, over time, across the full directional range. This means that, for an HD cell whose tuning curve is 90° in width, the rat will be facing a direction outside of this range about three-fourths of the time. Thus, only about one-fourth of the session time (2 minutes out of an 8-minute session) is of use for examination of that cell's tuning curve. Within that limited range, each individual data point that goes into the tuning curve is based on an even more limited sample. Specifically, each data point consists of the average rate over a 6° directional bin. This means that for an 8-minute session any one data point is based on approximately 8 seconds of session time. In addition, it is typically the case that 5% to 10% of the total data is lost due to accidental occlusion of one of the rat's headlights during the session. Thus, it seems that any one data point from an 8-minute session would be quite susceptible to any nondirectional (possibly random) influences on the firing rate. Accordingly, it seems there could be considerable sampling error in the determination of the exact peak rate, minimum width, etc. across a series of time slides.

It is not clear whether this session time difference accounts for the differences across the two laboratories. In particular, it is not clear why the estimates in table 1.1 would be smaller for both ADN and LMN than those from the Taube laboratory, since any sampling error would be expected to be equally likely to produce an underestimate versus an overestimate.

The anticipatory time interval data are not available for cells in the DTN, since this analysis has not been conducted for the small sample of HD cells collected in this region (Sharp et al., 2001b). However, it appears that the anticipatory interval for the DTN HD cells is probably close to zero, since there was no consistent shift in the preferred direction as a function of angular velocity for these cells.

Effects of Angular Head Velocity on *Tuning Curve Width*

Cells in the LMN showed an effect of angular head velocity on tuning curve width, as well as preferred direction (Blair et al., 1998). Interestingly, the nature of this effect was dependent on which hemisphere each HD cell was located in. For LMN HD cells in the right hemisphere, the tuning curve was more narrow during clockwise turns, while for HD cells in the left hemisphere, the tuning curve was more narrow for counterclockwise samples. Thus, LMN HD cells show relatively narrow tuning functions during head turns in the ipsiversive direction. The average ipsi- versus contraversive tuning curve width difference was 5°.

This hemisphere-specific pattern suggests a somewhat lateralized influence from angular velocity signals, and this is compatible with hemispheric segregation often observed for clockwise, versus counterclockwise, angular velocity signals in the vestibular system.

The combined influence of angular head velocity on both preferred direction and tuning width can be seen by careful examination of the examples of LMN HD cells in the lower two panels of figure 1.3. These combined influences result in a somewhat complex hemisphere-specific pattern. For example, for the LMN HD cell in the right hemisphere, the clockwise and counterclockwise tuning functions are very closely aligned (almost overlapping) along the left portion of their tuning curves. In contrast, the right-hand portion of the counterclockwise tuning function is shifted considerably to the right of that for clockwise turns. To understand this pattern, consider that first, as discussed previously, the entire tuning function for clockwise turns is shifted to the left of that for counterclockwise functions. At the same time, the clockwise tuning function is more narrow, so that the left-hand side of that curve shifts inward to the right, and the right-hand side of the curve shifts inward to the left. This means that, for this clockwise curve, the left-hand side of the curve is pushed to the left, due to the anticipatory shift of preferred direction, but it is pushed to the right by narrowing. These two influences apparently cancel each other, so that the left portion of the clockwise tuning curve winds up aligned with the counterclockwise function. In contrast, the right side of the clockwise curve is pushed to the left both by the anticipatory shift in preferred direction, and by the narrowing. Thus, this right-hand portion of the clockwise turn function winds up considerably more to the left than the corresponding portion of the counterclockwise tuning curve.

It should be noted that Stackman and Taube (1998) did not report any evidence for this kind of effect of angular velocity on tuning curve width. It seems that a likely explanation for this has to do with the short (8-minute) session times used in that study. As discussed at length earlier, it may be that this session duration does not provide adequate sampling for certain types of detailed analysis. Indeed, we have examined 8-minute-long segments of our own LMN data to see whether we observe the effect discussed here of angular velocity on tuning width. This effect does not show up in these brief samples, and, thus, it would likely have been missed in the Stackman and Taube (1998) data.

Very modest effects of angular velocity on contra-versus ipsilateral tuning curve width have also been observed for HD cells in both the DTN (Sharp et al., 2001b) and retrosplenial cortex (Cho and Sharp, 2001). These will not be discussed further here.

Peak Firing Rate Generally Does Not Show Significant Differences from One Region to the Next

Table 1.1 shows the average peak firing rates for HD cells in each limbic region. In general, there is considerable variability in the peak rates of HD cells within any one area. For example, the range of peak rates was 5.94–115.3 ms in postsubiculum (Taube et al., 1990a), 9.2–112.8 ms in LMN (Blair et al., 1998), and 10.2–117.3 ms in ATN (Blair and Sharp, 1995). In general, when direct comparisons have been made on cells reported in the same study, there are usually no significant differences between regions (e.g., Blair et al., 1998; Taube, 1995), although Stackman and Taube (1998) did report significantly higher rates for LMN, as compared to either ADN or postsubicular HD cells.

HD Cell Tuning Width Shows Regional Variation

There are consistent regional variations in average tuning curve width from one region to the next (e.g., Stackman and Taube, 1998; Sharp et al., 2001b). In general, HD cells in both LMN and DTN are more broadly tuned than those in other regions. The functional significance of these differences is not clear.

Summary

The data reviewed above demonstrate that the HD cell signal is found in numerous brain regions, both inside and outside of the limbic system. It will not be surprising if future investigations reveal yet more regions containing this signal.

The HD cells in most areas show an influence of momentary angular head velocity, and this is generally compatible with the fact that the cells are partly controlled through a process of angular path integration.

The functional significance of the overall pattern of regional variation in HD cell properties has yet to be fully understood. However, lesion studies beyond the scope of the present review, as well as the data previously reviewed have led to a proposed model for construction of the HD cell signal (see, e.g., Sharp et al., 2001b, and chapter 5 of this volume). According to this view, angular velocity information first enters the HD cell circuit via inputs to the DTN. The DTN combines this AV information with a representation of the current directional heading. The resulting AV-by-HD signal (see figure 1.3, middle row, right column) then serves to update the HD cell pattern in LMN, as described earlier. This results in an anticipatory prediction of future direction for HD cells in LMN. This anticipatory HD signal is then passed along to the more rostral areas, with some delay, so that these "downstream" areas show a smaller anticipatory time interval. Finally, in cortical areas such as the retrosplenial and postsubicular regions, the HD cell population receives visual input about environmental landmarks so that the current HD cell pattern can be corrected by the relative position of any familiar landmarks. Further work is needed to test this model.

References

Allen GV, Hopkins DA (1989) Mammillary body in the rat: topography and synaptology of projections from the subicular complex, prefrontal cortex, and midbrain tegmentum. J Comp Neurol 286: 311–336.

Ban T, Zyo K (1963) Experimental studies on the mammillary peduncle and mammillotegmental tracts in the rabbit. Med J Osaka Univ 13: 241–270.

Bassett JP, Taube JS (2001) Neural correlates for angular head velocity in the rat dorsal tegmental nucleus. J Neurosci 21: 5740–5751.

Blair HT, Cho J, Sharp PE (1998) Role of the lateral mammillary nucleus in the rat head direction circuit: A combined single unit recording and lesion study. Neuron 21: 1387–1397.

Blair HT, Sharp PE (1995) Anticipatory head-direction cells in anterior thalamus: Evidence for a thalamocortical circuit that integrates angular head motion to compute head direction. J Neurosci 15: 6260–6270.

Chen LL, Lin LH, Green EJ, Barnes CA, McNaughton BL (1994) Head-direction cells in the rat posterior cortex. I. Anatomical distribution and behavioral modulation. Exp Brain Res 101: 8–23.

Cho J, Sharp PE (2001) Head direction, place, and movement correlates for cells in the rat retrosplenial cortex. Behav Neurosci 115: 3–25.

Hayakawa T, Zyo K (1984) Comparative anatomical study of the tegmentomammillary projections in some mammals: A horseradish peroxidase study. Brain Res 300: 335–349.

Hayakawa T, Zyo K (1985) Afferent connections of Gudden's tegmental nuclei in the rabbit. J Comp Neurol 235: 169–181.

Leutgeb S, Ragozzino KE, Mizumori SJY (2000) Convergence of head direction and place information in the CA1 region of hippocampus. Neurosci 100: 11–19.

Liu R, Chang L, Wickern G (1984) The dorsal tegmental nucleus: An axoplasmic transport study. Brain Res 310: 123–132.

Mizumori SJY, Pratt WE, Cooper BG, Guazzelli A (2002) The behavioral implementation of hippocampal processing. In PE Sharp ed., The Neural Basis of Navigation: Evidence from Single Cell Recording. Kluwer, Boston.

Mizumori SJY, Ragozzino KE, Cooper BG (2000) Location and head direction representation in the dorsal striatum of rats. Psychobiol 28: 441–462.

Mizumori SJY, Williams JD (1993) Directionally selective mnemonic properties of neurons in the lateral dorsal nucleus of the thalamus of rats. J Neurosci 13: 4015–4028.

O'Keefe J, Nadel L (1978) The Hippocampus as a Cognitive Map. New York: Oxford University Press.

Papez JW (1937) A proposed mechanism of emotion. Arch Neurol Psychiatry 38: 725–744.

Ragozzino KE, Leutgeb S, Mizumori SJY (2001) Dorsal head direction and hippocampal place representations during spatial navigation. Exp Brain Res 139: 372–376.

Ranck JB, Jr. (1984) Head-direction cells in the deep layers of the dorsal presubiculum in freely-moving rats. Soc Neurosci Abstracts 10: 599.

Redish AD, Elga AN, Touretzky DS (1996) A coupled attractor model of the rodent head-direction system. Network 7: 671–685.

Seki M, Zyo K (1984) Anterior thalamic afferents from the mammillary body and the limbic cortex in the rat. J Comp Neurol 229: 242–256.

Sharp PE (1996) Multiple spatial/behavioral correlates for cells in the rat postsubiculum: Multiple regression analysis and comparison to other hippocampal areas. Cerebral Cortex 6: 238–259.

Sharp PE, Blair HT, Cho J (2001a) The anatomical and computational basis of the rat head-direction cell signal. Trends Neurosci 24: 289–294.

Sharp PE, Tinkelman A, Cho J (2001b) Angular velocity and head direction signals recorded from the dorsal tegmental nucleus of Gudden in the rat: Implications for path integration in the head direction cell circuit. Behav Neurosci 115: 571–588.

Shibata H (1992) Topographic organization of subcortical projections to the anterior thalamic nuclei in the rat. J Comp Neurol 323: 117–127.

Shibata H (1993) Direct projections from the anterior thalamic nucleus to the retrohippocampal region of the rat. J Comp Neurol 337: 431–445.

Skaggs WE, Knierim JJ, Kudrimoti HS, McNaughton BL (1995) A model of the neural basis of the rat's sense of direction. In G Tesauro, DS Touretzky, and TK Leen, eds., Advances in Neural Information Processing Systems 7, Cambridge, MA: MIT Press, pp. 173–180.

Stackman RW, Taube JS (1998) Firing properties of lateral mammillary single units: Head direction, head pitch, and angular head velocity. J Neurosci 18: 9020–9037.

Stackman RW, Taube JS (2003) Correction for Stackman and Taube, 1998. J Neurosci 23: 1555–1556.

Taube JS (1995) Head-direction cells recorded in the anterior thalamic nuclei of freely moving rats. J Neurosci 15: 70–86.

Taube JS, Muller RU (1998) Comparisons of head direction cell activity in the postsubiculum and anterior thalamus of freely moving rats. Hippocampus 8: 87–108.

Taube JS, Muller RU, Ranck JB Jr (1990a) Head-direction cells recorded from the postsubiculum in freely moving rats. I. Description and quantitative analysis. J Neurosci 10: 420–435.

Taube JS, Muller RU, Ranck JB Jr (1990b) Head-direction cells recorded from the postsubiculum in freely moving rats. II. Effects of environmental manipulations. J Neurosci 10: 436–447.

Thompson SM, Robertson RT (1987) Organization of subcortical pathways for sensory projections to the limbic cortex I. Subcortical projections to the medial limbic cortex in the rat. J Comp Neurol 265: 175–188.

Van Groen T, Wyss MJ (1990) The postsubicular cortex in the rat: characterization of the fourth region of the subicular cortex and its connections. Brain Res 529: 165–177.

Wiener SI (1993) Spatial and behavioral correlates of striatal neurons in rats performing a self-initiated navigation task. J Neurosci 13: 3802–3817.

Zhang K (1996) Representation of spatial orientation by the intrinsic dynamics of the head-direction cell ensemble: A theory. J Neurosci 16: 2112–2126.

2 Neuroanatomy of Head Direction Cell Circuits

David A. Hopkins

With the discovery of head direction (HD) cells in the postsubiculum (Ranck, 1985—cited by Muller et al., 1996; Taube et al., 1990; Muller et al., 1996), a succession of studies followed that explored the existence and characteristics of HD cells in related parts of the central nervous system (CNS) that were connected, directly and indirectly, with the postsubiculum (Sharp et al., 2001). Thus, HD cells have also been identified in the anterior thalamic nuclei (Taube, 1995), lateral mammillary nucleus (Blair et al., 1998; Stackman and Taube, 1998), dorsal tegmental nucleus of Gudden (Bassett and Taube, 2001), retrosplenial cortex (Chen et al., 1994; Cho and Sharp, 2001), lateral dorsal thalamic nucleus (Mizumori and Williams, 1993) and striatum (Wiener, 1993). The neuroanatomical literature that is essential to understanding the substrates of head direction cell circuits is relatively complex because of the many areas and levels of the CNS that have been identified as containing head direction cells (Sharp et al., 2001), and because of multiple sensory (vestibular, visual, idiothetic) inputs that might influence HD cells (Blair and Sharp, 1996; Brown et al., 2002; Wiener et al., 2002). This chapter will focus on the primary HD cell way stations and their connections. In a series of elegant studies, two groups of investigators (van Groen, Wyss and colleagues; Shibata) have delineated the efferent and afferent connectivity of the subicular and retrosplenial cortices and their relationships with the thalamus and other subcortical structures, including the hypothalamus and dorsal striatum. They have demonstrated that the connections among these areas are very specific and topographically organized, and that they differentially target specific cortical laminae and thalamic nuclei. There are also some bilateral connections from retrosplenial cortex to the anterior thalamus, and commissural connections are prominent.

For historical reasons, it is appropriate to begin a review of HD cell circuits by starting with the postsubiculum (Ranck, 1985; Taube et al., 1990). Therefore, I have opted to begin our journey with a description of the neuroanatomy of the subicular complex and work systematically through the retrosplenial cortex, thalamus, mammillary body (MB), and brainstem, reviewing their structure and interconnections. Finally, data on the neuro-chemistry and synaptology of HD cell circuits will be summarized, with emphasis on studies by Gonzalo-Ruiz, Lieberman, and coworkers.

Because of the strong connections between the postsubiculum and the anterior thalamus, many physiological investigations have concentrated on the MB, especially the lateral mammillary nucleus (LM) and associated circuits (Sharp et al., 2001). However, similarities in the connectivity of other parts of the MB that also form distinct, but parallel, circuits (Allen and Hopkins, 1989) suggest that the medial mammillary nucleus (MM) and its associated circuits could also be playing a role in the modulation of HD cell activity. In keeping with this, it is worth noting that neuronal activity recorded at several levels of the MB circuits to be described below has been correlated not only with head direction but also with angular head velocity, place, and hippocampal theta rhythm.

Thus, the present overview will consider the neuroanatomical organization of the post-subiculum, retrosplenial cortex, the thalamus, and the MB as a nodal or linking center with the midbrain and cerebellum. This summary will outline the major circuits, as well as the intrinsic organization and more local connections representing anatomical substrates that it is hoped will be relevant to neural models of head direction cell circuit functions, including not only head direction but also other aspects of behavior related to spatial navigation and memory (Vann and Aggleton, 2004).

Postsubiculum and Subicular Complex

Cytoarchitecture of the Postsubiculum

The subicular complex (figures 2.1, 2.2) is considered part of the hippocampal formation (Amaral and Witter, 1995) or parahippocampal region (van Groen and Wyss, 1990a,b). It has been variously divided into from three to five somewhat distinct subdivisions, depending on the authority, namely, the subiculum proper, presubiculum, postsubiculum, para-subiculum and prosubiculum. Some authors do not distinguish between the pre- and postsubiculum, interpreting the latter as a dorsal extension of the presubiculum (Amaral and Witter, 1995). However, the identification of HD cells within the postsubiculum (Ranck, 1985; Taube et al., 1990) as well as its distinct neurochemical organization and connections (van Groen and Wyss, 1990b,c) justify its recognition as a separate entity (figures 2.1, 2.2C). The prosubiculum, a poorly defined transitional area between the subiculum and hippocampal CA1 field (Amaral and Witter, 1995), does not see current use in the HD cell literature and is not well defined in the rodent brain (Slomianka and Geneser, 1991).

The postsubiculum has six layers grouped into external (layers I–III) and internal (layers IV–VI) laminae (van Groen and Wyss, 1990b). Layers II and III of the postsubiculum in Nissl-stained sections contain darkly stained clusters and parallel rows of cells, respectively, while in comparison the adjacent presubiculum lacks these distinct

Retrosplenial and Postsubicular Cortex

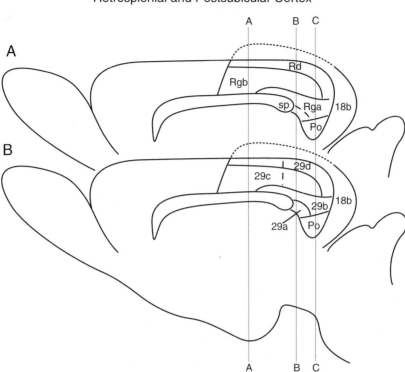

Figure 2.1
Diagrams of the rat cingulate cortex in the sagittal plane showing the cytoarchitectonic subdivisions of the retrosplenial cortex and the postsubiculum on the medial surface according to two different conventions. (A) Granular and dysgranular cortex (based on van Groen and Wyss and Sripanidkulchai). (B) Brodmann's areas (based on Vogt and Peters and Shibata). The vertical lines, labeled A, B, and C, show the levels of the coronal sections illustrated in figure 2.2. The visual association cortex (area 18b, Oc2M) is located on the dorsal (represented by a dotted line) and posterior surfaces of the cerebral cortex lateral to the retrosplenial cortex. The vertical dashed line in areas 29c and 29d in (B) demarcates rostral and caudal subdivisions. See list of abbreviations for all figures on page 39.

features. Furthermore, the postsubiculum has a dense fiber plexus in its superficial layers. In sections stained for acetylcholinesterase, the deep layers of the postsubiculum stand out and distinguish it from the presubiculum and retrosplenial cortex (van Groen and Wyss, 1990b).

Connectivity of the Postsubiculum
The postsubiculum has reciprocal connections primarily with the anterior dorsal (AD) (figure 2.3) and lateral dorsal/laterodorsal (LD) nuclei of the thalamus (van Groen and Wyss, 1990b). The LM also receives a very focused projection from the postsubiculum (Allen and Hopkins, 1989; van Groen and Wyss, 1990b). With respect to cortical

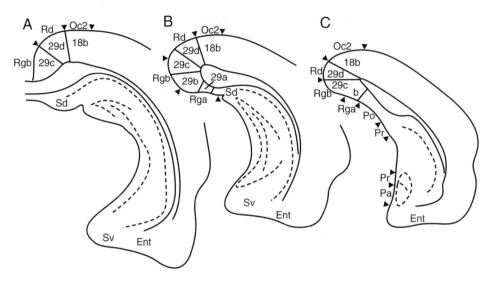

Figure 2.2
Diagrams of the cerebral cortex in the coronal plane showing the relationships between the cytoarchitectonic subdivisions of the retrosplenial cortex and the subicular complex. See figure 2.1 for locations of coronal sections defined by A, B, and C.

projections, the postsubiculum projects to other parts of the subicular complex, as well as to the perirhinal, entorhinal and retrosplenial cortex. In contrast to relatively light projections to the retrosplenial cortex, the postsubiculum receives projections from each of the major parts of the retrosplenial cortex (figure 2.3A), as will be summarized in detail in the section on the retrosplenial cortex. Thus, the postsubiculum is a nodal point in HD cell circuits and is a gateway into the hippocampus proper via its connections with the entorhinal cortex, which, in turn, projects via the perforant pathway directly and indirectly to the dentate gyrus and CA3 (Amaral and Witter, 1995). Other parts of the subicular complex are also intimately related to areas that contain HD cells. The complexity of these circuits may underlie observations that at different levels of the HD circuits, HD cells may be associated with properties such as angular velocity, head pitch angle, place or EEG theta rhythm, in addition to head direction.

Retrosplenial Cortex

The retrosplenial cortex (i.e., caudal or posterior cingulate cortex) contains HD cells (Chen et al., 1994; Cho and Sharp, 2001) and has abundant connections with other components of HD cell circuits. Because different authors who have made major contributions to the neuroanatomical study of these areas use different terminologies, comparisons among studies can be difficult. To facilitate this anatomical analysis, a synthesis of the compet-

A CORTICAL EFFERENTS

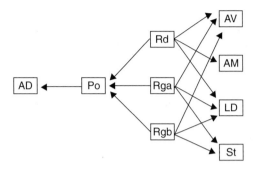

B CORTICAL AFFERENTS

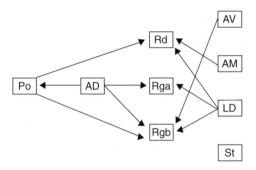

Figure 2.3
Diagrams highlighting major efferent (A) and afferent (B) connections of the retrosplenial cortex with the post-subiculum, thalamus, and striatum. Note that the retrosplenial cortex projects to the postsubiculum, which in turn projects to the AD. The AD is the only thalamic nucleus with a strong projection to the Po.

ing cytoarchitectonic descriptions is provided before the summary of connectivity as it relates to HD cell circuits.

Cytoarchitecture of the Retrosplenial Cortex

The retrosplenial cortex is situated in the caudal part of the cingulate cortex and derives its name from its position in relationship to the splenium of the corpus callosum (figure 2.1). On the basis of cytoarchitectonic criteria, the retrosplenial cortex has been subdivided into granular and agranular or dysgranular parts by Wyss and Sripanidkulchai (1984). In the present overview, retrosplenial dysgranular cortex is the preferred terminology because, although certainly less granular, this part of the retrosplenial cortex does have a recognizable granular layer IV (van Groen and Wyss, 1992a). The retrosplenial cortex in rats has also been subdivided according to the numbering convention of

Brodmann's areas in man (Vogt and Peters, 1981; Vogt and Miller, 1983; Shibata, 1998, 2000). Figures 2.1 and 2.2 show a synthesis of the two main parcellations of the retrosplenial cortex, based on published studies of the cytoarchitecture and connectivity. Following van Groen, Wyss, and colleagues (Wyss and Sripanidkulchai, 1984; Sripanidkulchai and Wyss, 1986, 1987; van Groen and Wyss, 1992a, 2003), the retrosplenial cortex can be divided into dorsal dysgranular and ventral granular parts (figure 2.1A). The granular part has been further subdivided into *a* and *b* parts, with the granular *b* part located in general more caudally and medially. In terms of Brodmann's areas, the retrosplenial granular "a" cortex corresponds roughly to area 29*a*, retrosplenial granular *b* to areas 29b/c and retrosplenial dysgranular to area 29d, respectively (figures 2.1B, 2.2). Visual area 18b or medial prestriate occipital cortex area 2 (Oc2M, Zilles, 1985), located on the dorsal surface of the posterior cortex, adjacent to the caudal, dysgranular retrosplenial cortex, also contains HD cells (Chen et al., 1994). The terminology used by van Groen and Wyss will be favored in the sections to follow, because of the substantial number of classic studies carried out by them.

Connections of the Retrosplenial Cortex and Subicular Complex
Efferent projections of the retrosplenial cortex (figure 2.3A) are characterized by being abundant to the postsubiculum (Po) and to the anteroventral (AV), anteromedial (AM), and lateral dorsal (LD) thalamic nuclei, while being sparse to the anterodorsal (AD) thalamic nucleus. The retrosplenial dysgranular (Rd) cortex projects strongly to the postsubicular cortex (van Groen and Wyss, 1992a) as well as to the LD and AV thalamic nuclei, and bilaterally to the AM thalamic nuclei (van Groen and Wyss, 1992a; Shibata, 1998). Projections to the AD thalamic nucleus are sparse. In addition, the retrosplenial dysgranular cortex also projects to the dorsomedial striatum (van Groen and Wyss, 1992a), a site from which HD cells have been recorded (Wiener, 1993).

The retrosplenial granular *a* and *b* cortical projections are similar to those from the dysgranular cortex in that they also terminate heavily in the postsubiculum and AV and LD thalamic nuclei (van Groen and Wyss, 1990a, 2003; Shibata, 2000). In summary, the three major subdivisions of the retrosplenial cortex have fairly similar projections to areas that contain HD cells. Surprisingly, the AD is not a major target of the retrosplenial cortex, but rather the retrosplenial cortex must exert its influence on the AD and HD cells therein via the postsubiculum.

In contrast to the efferent projections, afferent projections to the retrosplenial cortex (figure 2.3B) appear to be somewhat more selective in terms of which subregions they target. Thus, the retrosplenial cortex receives major afferent inputs from the postsubiculum and thalamic inputs from the AD, AM, and LD thalamic nuclei (van Groen and Wyss, 1992b, 2003). Finally, retrosplenial granular *a* cortex receives major inputs from the subiculum proper (but not the postsubiculum) and from the AD thalamic nucleus. However, there are no direct or monosynaptic, reciprocal connections between the retro-

splenial cortex and the AD thalamic nucleus, which is an exception to the norm of reciprocal connections between thalamus and cerebral cortex. Instead, these two major components of the HD cell circuits must communicate via the postsubiculum. Interestingly,
some HD cells in the retrosplenial dysgranular cortex show an association between direction and angular movement, but no such relationship was found in retrosplenial granular
cortex (Chen et al., 1994). On the other hand, Cho and Sharp (2001) report little correlation with angular head velocity, although some HD cells "are influenced by angular velocity" and direction of turning, perhaps confounded with high running speed.

The Thalamus

Cytoarchitecture of the Anterior and Lateral Dorsal Thalamic Nuclei
HD cells have been identified in the AD and LD thalamic nuclei. The AD nucleus is one
of three major anterior thalamic nuclei (Gurdjian, 1927), a group that also includes the
anteroventral (AV) and anteromedial (AM) nuclei (figure 2.4A). In Nissl-stained sections,
the AD is characterized by medium-sized cells measuring over 15 μm in long axis with
darkly staining cytoplasm that distinguishes the AD from the adjacent AV that contains
smaller cells measuring 10–12 μm in long axis with sparse Nissl substance (Dekker and
Kuypers, 1976; Oda et al., 2001). The lateral border of the AD contains a distinct row of
neurons that also sharply demarcates the AD from the AV. The AM is less well defined,
and in some planes is more or less continuous with the AV. Interestingly, the AM has
received little specific attention, and neuronal activity of its cells has not been correlated
with either head direction or theta.

The lateral dorsal nucleus is located lateral and dorsolateral to AD and AV and contains
mainly medium-sized cells in its dorsal lateral aspect and a mixture of cell sizes, including large cells ventromedially (Thompson and Robertson, 1987). Gurdjian (1927) speculated that the LD had commissural and internuclear connections with adjacent nuclei and
its partner on the opposite side, but there appear to be no recent data to confirm this point.

Neurochemistry of the Anterior, Lateral, and Reticular Thalamic Nuclei
Clear borders and distinctions among the nuclei of the anterior group are evident when
different neurochemical markers are used. These studies are important for a number of
reasons: (1) they aid in cytoarchitectonic delineations, (2) they provide additional information on connectivity, and (3) they provide information on the neurochemical and functional nature of the synaptic inputs to the anterior nuclei. Many markers have been used
that selectively or differentially stain the anterior thalamus. Among the first distinctive
markers were the esterases, acetylcholinesterase (AChE), the enzyme that catalyses the
hydrolysis of acetylcholine, and the related enzyme, butyrylcholinesterase (BuChE), a
coregulator of cholinergic neurotransmission (Darvesh et al., 2003). AChE is found in the
highest concentrations in axons in the AD and AV, while BuChE is highly concentrated in

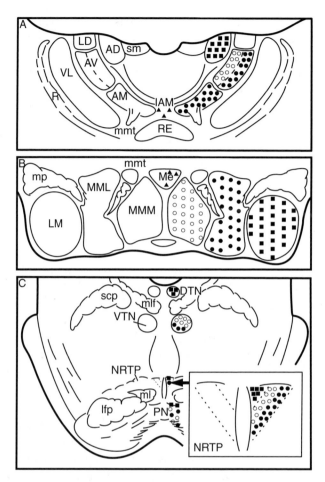

Figure 2.4
Diagrams of coronal sections of rat brain showing the topographical organization of efferent projections from the mammillary body. (A) Distribution of terminal fields of ascending axons in the thalamus. (B) Cells of origin in the MB. (C) Distribution of terminal fields of descending axons in the midbrain tegmentum. Inset in (C) represents the rostral, dorsomedial NRTP and shows the topography of descending projections from the MB. Squares represent projections of the LM; closed and open circles represent projections of MML and MMM, respectively; and triangles represent projections of Me.

neurons in AD and LD (Robertson et al., 1986; Tago et al., 1992). Interestingly, in the AD and LD, the two thalamic nuclei that harbour HD cells, AChE staining overlaps with zinc-rich terminals that originate in the post and presubiculum (Mengual et al., 2001), which is consistent with connectional studies (van Groen and Wyss, 1990a,b).

Intrinsic Organization and Local Circuits of the Anterior, Lateral Dorsal, and Reticular Thalamic Nuclei

Most authors agree that neurons of the AD and AV thalamic nuclei are relatively homogeneous in morphology and connections, and that there is little or no evidence for interneurons in these nuclei. Thus, Wang et al. (1999) were unable to confirm the presence of a small population of GABAergic neurons in AD and AV that they reported previously (Gonzalo-Ruiz et al., 1996), and it would appear that virtually all AD and AV neurons are projection neurons. In terms of models of HD cell activity that would invoke inhibition or disinhibition in the anterior thalamus, more complex information processing may be dependent on extrinsic circuits. Some recent studies of the relationship of the anterior and LD nuclei with the reticular nucleus of the thalamus point to possible local circuits that could influence activity in HD cell circuits. The anatomical substrates of local circuits are associated with the thalamic reticular nucleus, which provides a topographically organized GABAergic projection to the AD and AV (Gonzalo-Ruiz and Lieberman 1995a,b; Lozsádi, 1995). The synaptic relationship between the anterior thalamus and the reticular nucleus is such that the projection to the reticular nucleus is most likely excitatory, based on the observation that the synapses are formed by axon terminals with round synaptic vesicles making asymmetrical contacts (Lozsádi, 1995). In contrast, the reticular thalamic nucleus projection to the anterior thalamus forms GABAergic symmetrical synapses and has axon terminals with pleomorphic vesicles (Wang et al., 1999), which is consistent with an inhibitory function.

The notion that thalamic nuclei lacking interneurons can interact via the reticular nucleus is reinforced by the discovery of Crabtree et al. (1998), who demonstrated that intrathalamic pathways could link modality-related nuclei in the dorsal thalamus via the reticular nucleus. It is possible that comparable pathways could exist for AD and AV. To date, this has not been studied but it seems quite likely based on the results of Pinault and Deschênes (1998). They demonstrated that closely adjacent reticular nucleus neurons sometimes projected axons into separate nuclei with related functions and showed particularly dramatic examples of adjacent reticular neurons with extensive axonal arbors in AD and LD (Pinault and Deschênes, 1998; their figure 10). With the demonstration of local circuits such as these, inhibition and disinhibition within the anterior thalamic nuclei would not be dependent on the existence of interneurons.

Connections of the Anterior and Lateral Thalamic Nuclei

The connections of the anterior and lateral dorsal thalamus with the retrosplenial cortex have been described above and will be touched on again in the section on mammillary nuclei circuits. By way of summary, the principal thalamic nuclei related to HD cell circuits are the AD and LD (figures 2.3, 2.4A). The AD has the most notable projections to the retrosplenial granular cortex but does not receive significant reciprocal projections. This is in contrast to the reciprocal projections between AD and the postsubiculum. The LD projects most strongly to the retrosplenial dysgranular cortex as well as the pre- and parasubiculum, while receiving cortical projections from the entire retrosplenial cortex, and both post- and presubiculum. Interestingly, lesions of the LD do not appear to result in notable changes in the activity of HD cells in the postsubiculum (Golob et al., 1998). The lateral posterior (LP) thalamic nucleus has connections with the retrosplenial cortex and is, therefore, related to parts of the HD cell circuits but as yet no information is available regarding HD cells in the LP.

The Mammillary Body

Cytoarchitecture of the Mammillary Body

The caudal and ventral border of the hypothalamus in the rat and other species is marked by a pair of macroscopically visible protuberances on the ventral external surface of the brain. These protuberances are formed by an agglomeration of a number of small nuclei of variable prominence, known collectively as the mammillary body (from L. *mammilla*: diminutive for breast). The anatomical organization of the mammillary body has been studied for over 75 years (Gurdjian, 1927; Rose, 1939; Allen and Hopkins, 1988). The MB is made up of two main subdivisions: the lateral and medial nuclei. The lateral mammillary nucleus (LM) is a single, roughly spherical nucleus that has no apparent subdivisions. The medial nucleus is further subdivided into medial (MMM) and lateral (MML) subnuclei (figure 2.4B), in which three to six subnuclei have been identified.

On the basis of cytoarchitectonic and Golgi studies, Allen and Hopkins (1988) strived to consolidate the different MB parcellations, taking into account connectivity as well. This approach led to the conclusions that the cellular organization of the LM was rather uniform with distinct, large neurons, and the medial nucleus could be subdivided into five smaller subnuclei. On the basis of cell size, efferent connections and immunocytochemical staining, the posterior nucleus should simply be considered a caudal extension of the medial MB. Of course, at the present time, the subtlety of the anatomical parcellations, e.g., the LM and at least five subnuclei in the medial MB (Allen and Hopkins, 1988), exceeds the refinement that can be obtained in physiological recording or lesion studies. Consequently, the present review is a partially simplified picture of the organization of the nuclei and connections of the MB (figure 2.4) that shows the LM and three major subdivisions of the medial nuclei (figure 2.4B), namely, the pars lateralis (MML), pars medialis (MMM), and pars medianus (Me). With respect to the cytoarchitecture, the LM harbours the largest neurons in the MB, while the MML and Me have significantly smaller neurons, and those in the MMM are intermediate in size. MB neurons in each subnucleus have rather similar morphologies. It is of particular interest to modeling of HD circuits that there is no anatomical evidence for interneurons in the MB. In keeping with this, Guillery (1955) has estimated that the number of axons in the mammillothalamic tract, the main efferent tract of the MB, is approximately equal to the number of neurons in the nucleus. According to available evidence from Golgi-stained material, MB neurons in the rat do not appear to have recurrent axon collaterals (Veazey et al., 1982; Allen and Hopkins, 1988), although Cajal (1911) remarks that a very few axon collaterals of neurons in the MB appear to ramify within the nucleus after separating from their initial trajectory, although their destination could not be determined.

Neurochemistry of the Mammillary Body
Although many neurochemical mappings of the brain identify specific markers in the MB, a few studies have explicitly focused on the neurochemical organization of the mammillary body (Gonzalo-Ruiz et al., 1993, 1996, 1999; Wirtshafter and Stratford, 1993). In the present context, these studies establish that the ventral tegmental nucleus (VTN) and dorsal tegmental nucleus (DTN) contribute a substantial, topographically organized GABAergic projection to the MB. Electron microscopy demonstrates that GABAergic terminals contain pleomorphic vesicles and form axosomatic and axodendritic synapses in the MB (Gonzalo-Ruiz et al., 1993).

Efferent Connections of the Mammillary Body
MB projections and circuits have several characteristics that are likely to be important in modulating and integrating sensory and motor functions that determine HD cell activity. Some of these characteristics are (1) cortical and subcortical inputs, (2) ascending and descending projections, (3) highly topographically organized connections, (4) bilateral connections, (5) many divergent axon collaterals, and (6) reciprocal connections.

Neuroanatomical Tracing: Technical Considerations   Because MB neurons have widely divergent axon collaterals, it has been possible to apply a range of neuroanatomical tracing methods to reveal special features of MB connectivity, even though the MB consists of small, tightly packed nuclei at the base of the brain. While the MB was known to have substantial ascending and descending connections, the question arose about the degree of collateralization (Cajal described bifurcating axon collaterals of LM neurons) of individual neurons. Retrograde degeneration studies confirmed that MB neurons projected both to the thalamus and to the tegmentum (Fry, 1970; Fry and Cowan, 1972), but such methods are not very sensitive because retrograde changes and neuronal death vary depending on age and proximity of axon lesions to the cell body. As the terminal fields of some MB neuron axon collaterals are widely separated, it has been advantageous to utilize fluorescent retrograde tracers to elucidate the degree of collateralization and determine which cells send long ascending and descending collaterals from individual MB subnuclei (van der Kooy et al., 1978; Takeuchi et al., 1985; Hayakawa and Zyo, 1989). These experiments show that most MB neurons do have long axon collaterals that project to both the thalamus and brainstem (Takeuchi et al., 1985). In related studies, transnuclear transport (Takeuchi et al., 1985) has been used to identify descending MB neuron collaterals to the pons without confounding labeling caused by other projection neurons that are adjacent to the MB (de Olmos and Heimer, 1977; Takeuchi et al., 1985; Liu and Mihailoff, 1999). With this method, a neuroanatomical tracer such as wheat germ agglutinin-horseradish peroxidase conjugate (WGA-HRP) is transported retrogradely from one nucleus (e.g., the AD) to neurons in another nucleus (e.g., the LM), followed by anterograde transport via axon collaterals to a third nucleus (e.g., the DTN). Direct and collateral efferent MB projections have been distinguished, including projections from adjacent lateral, posterior and supramammillary regions (Liu and Mihailoff, 1999). This has permitted unambiguous interpretations of MB connectivity.

Ascending Projections   Ascending projections from the MB to the thalamus have been extensively studied, and a rich literature demonstrates that the MB provides a massive, topographically organized projection to the anterior thalamic nuclei (Powell and Cowan, 1954; Guillery, 1955; Cruce, 1975; Seki and Zyo, 1984; Shibata, 1992). Figure 2.4A shows a schematic diagram of ascending projections that emphasizes the bilateral LM projection to the anterodorsal (AD) thalamic nucleus and the ipsilateral projections from the medial and median mammillary nuclei to the anteroventral (AV) and anteromedial (AM) thalamic nuclei, respectively. The lateral dorsal (LD) thalamic nucleus is also depicted because it is a site containing HD cells (Mizumori and Williams, 1993), even though the MB does not project to the LD. As previously mentioned, bilateral lesions in the LD do not significantly affect the properties of HD cells in the postsubiculum (Golob et al., 1998). Nonetheless, lesions that include both the LD and AD nuclei impair spatial memory performance (Wilton et al., 2001).

Descending Projections   Descending projections from the MB (figures 2.4C and 2.5) terminate topographically in the tegmental nuclei of Gudden (Guillery, 1957; Cruce, 1977; Hayakawa and Zyo, 1984, 1989; Takeuchi et al., 1985; Torigoe et al., 1986; Allen and Hopkins, 1990; Liu and Mihailoff, 1999). The LM projects to the DTN, the MML and MMM project to the posterior ventral tegmental nucleus (VTNp), and the Me projects to the anterior VTN (VTNa). Figure 2.5 illustrates the distribution of descending projections after an injection of WGA-HRP in the medial and lateral mammillary nuclei (Allen and Hopkins, 1990). The widespread nature of descending MB projections is evident, including projections to medial parts of two precerebellar relay nuclei, the nucleus reticularis tegmenti pontis (NRTP) and the pontine nuclei (PN), first identified in the rat by Guillery (1957) and Cruce (1977). The projection to these precerebellar nuclei is so highly precise and topographically organized that the LM and MM have separate, but adjacent, terminal fields (figure 2.6). With large injections of tracer in the anterior thalamus, retrograde label-

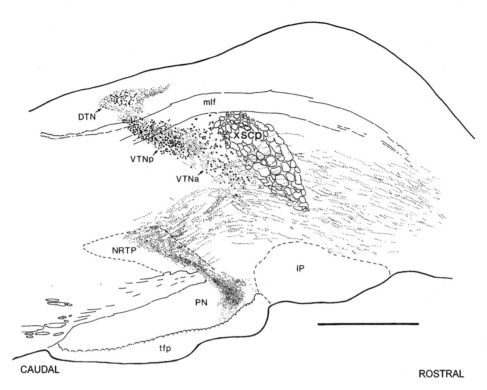

Figure 2.5
Camera lucida drawing of the distribution of anterograde and retrograde labeling in the midbrain tegmentum and pons after injection of WGA-HRP into the medial and lateral mammillary nuclei. The drawing is a composite based on four serial sagittal sections. Large, irregular dots indicate retrogradely labeled neurons and the fine stippling indicates anterograde axonal and terminal labeling. Scale bar: 1 mm.

ing of MB neurons, followed by anterograde transnuclear transport in descending axon collaterals (Takeuchi et al., 1985), confirms that the MB projections are not due to projections from nearby hypothalamic regions (Liu and Mihailoff, 1999). Moreover, small injections in the anterior thalamus or MB reveal that descending axon collaterals from each subnucleus of the MB give rise to highly topographically organized projections to the VTN (Takeuchi et al., 1985; Shibata, 1987).

Afferent Connections: Topography and Synaptic Organization
The MB receives afferent projections from many sources, but the primary ones of interest with respect to HD cells are those related to the cerebral cortex (figures 2.1 and 2.3) and the tegmental nuclei of Gudden (figure 2.7). Cortical afferents to the MB (figure 2.8) arise from the subicular complex (Allen and Hopkins, 1989; Shibata, 1989; Kishi et al., 2000) and the prefrontal/infralimbic cortex (Allen and Hopkins, 1989, 1998; Hurley et al., 1991). A strong projection to the LM originates in the postsubiculum, where HD cells were

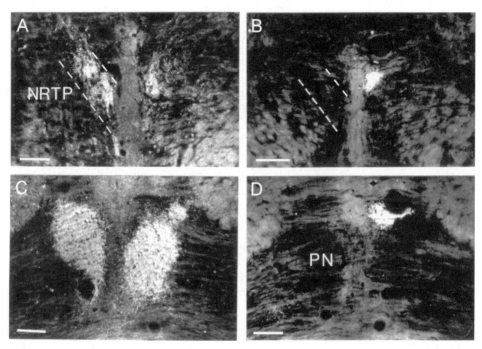

Figure 2.6
Dark-field photomicrographs of coronal sections showing topography of mammillary body projections to the pontine precerebellar relay nuclei after injections of WGA-HRP into the left medial (A,C) and right lateral (B,D) mammillary nuclei. Photomicrographs correspond to boxed area showing nucleus reticularis tegmenti pontis (NRTP) and pontine nuclei (PN) in figure 2.4C. (A, B) Anterograde labeling (bright, fine grains) in the NRTP. The dashed lines indicate the lateral border of the dorsomedial NRTP and the separation between terminal fields from the medial and lateral nuclei. (C,D) Anterograde labeling in the medial pontine nuclei. Labeling is bilateral in A and C because the injection in the left medial mammillary nucleus partially involved the right nucleus as well.

first discovered (Ranck, 1985). In contrast, efferents from the subicular cortex proper terminate in a topographically organized fashion in the medial mammillary nuclei (Meibach and Siegel, 1977; Allen and Hopkins, 1989; Shibata, 1989; Witter et al., 1990; Kishi et al., 2000). Subiculum projections terminate in horizontally oriented layers across the medial nuclei such that rostrodorsal subicular afferents terminate more dorsally in the MB than afferents from the caudoventral subiculum which terminate preferentially more ventrally. In addition, Kishi et al. (2000) have recently shown that parts of the medial (septal) subiculum have a topographically organized projection in which lateral-to-medial (temporal-to-septal) cells of origin terminate in a ventrolateral-to-dorsomedial pattern in the medial nuclei. The combination of the two patterns suggests a rather complicated three-dimensional matrix of subicular inputs to the MB.

    In contrast to projections from the subicular complex, those from the dorsal and ventral tegmental nuclei terminate topographically in a pattern that seems more to respect the

A   Distribution of Afferent Projections to the MB from Gudden's Tegmental Nuclei

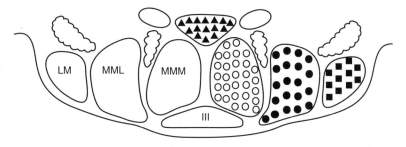

B   Cells of Origin of Tegmental Projections to MB

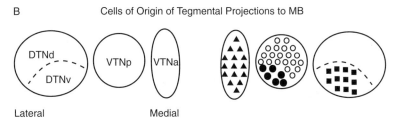

Lateral   Medial

Figure 2.7
Diagrams showing (A) the distribution of afferent projections from the tegmental nuclei of Gudden in the different subnuclei of the mammillary body and (B) the locations of the cells of origin of the projections from the midbrain tegmentum.

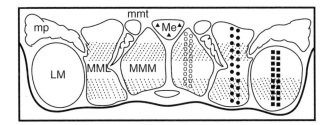

Figure 2.8
Diagram illustrating the distributions of afferents from the subicular complex (dashed lines), midbrain (open circles, closed circles and squares following the convention in figures 2.4 and 2.7) and prefrontal cortex (filled triangles) in the medial mammillary nucleus. Afferents from the subicular complex are distributed in a horizontal fashion across the medial mammillary nucleus, a pattern orthogonal to the distribution of midbrain afferent projections. Afferent projections from the midbrain and the prefrontal cortex converge in the midline in the pars medianus.

boundaries of the individual subnuclei in the medial and lateral mammillary body (Shibata, 1987; Allen and Hopkins, 1989). In other words, each of the tegmental nuclei targets a specific MB subnucleus as summarized in figure 2.7. If one compares the distribution of subicular complex afferents with the organization of MB efferents (figure 2.4) and brainstem afferents (figure 2.7), it is apparent that these two sources of afferents tend to be organized in patterns that are, at least in part, orthogonal to each other (figure 2.8). That is, the subicular complex terminates in horizontal layers that do not respect the borders of the medial nuclei, while the efferent ascending and descending projections and brainstem afferents of the MB are highly topographically organized and preserve point-to-point relationships that respect nuclear boundaries. Additional refined neuroanatomical tracing experiments will be required to further elucidate the manner in which descending and ascending afferents interdigitate in the MB.

The existence of complex patterns of afferent projections to the MB raises questions about the nature of the synaptic inputs to the MB. It turns out that there are notable differences with respect to the synaptic organization and inputs to the MB that are revealed by electron microscopic studies (Allen and Hopkins, 1988, 1989, 1998). Synapses in the MB and elsewhere can be classified morphologically into two main types on the basis of the synaptic vesicles (round or pleomorphic) in the axon terminal and the nature of the pre- and postsynaptic membranes (asymmetrical or symmetrical). Two main classes of axon terminals are found in the MB (figure 2.9; Allen and Hopkins, 1988). Axon terminals that contain mainly round vesicles and form asymmetric synaptic junctions (RA) are found in association with small dendrites and, rarely, on proximal dendrites and somata. In contrast, axon terminals with pleomorphic vesicles form symmetric synapses (PS) on neuronal somata and both proximal and distal dendrites, as well as dendritic spines. The LM contains a greater proportion of PS synapses than RA synapses while the two types are equally frequent in the medial nuclei.

RA and PS synapses are correlated with excitatory and inhibitory inputs, respectively (Uchizono, 1965; Hopkins and Allen, 1989; Gonzalo-Ruiz et al., 1993, 1999). Subicular (figure 2.9A) and prefrontal cortex afferents to the MB are predominantly of the RA type (Allen and Hopkins, 1989) while those from the tegmental nuclei (figure 2.9B) are virtually exclusively of the PS type (Allen and Hopkins, 1989; Hayakawa and Zyo, 1991, 1992), which is in keeping with the known GABAergic projections from the DTN and VTN (Wirtshafter and Stratford, 1993; Gonzalo-Ruiz et al., 1999). As previously noted, inhibitory inputs to the MB from the tegmentum could play a role in modulating ascending activity in the absence of MB inhibitory interneurons and, thereby, help give rise to a continuous attractor network (Sharp et al., 2001; see chapter 19, this volume).

Reciprocal Connections

The reciprocal nature of connections between the MB and tegmental nuclei can also be appreciated in figure 2.5, which shows the pattern of retrogradely labeled neurons in the

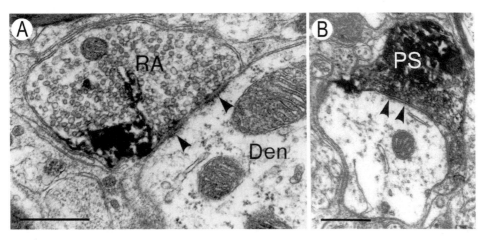

Figure 2.9
Electron micrographs of labeled axodendritic synapses in the lateral mammillary nucleus following injections of WGA-HRP into the caudoventral subicular complex (A) and the midbrain tegmentum (B). Note that the labeled axon terminal from the subicular complex (A) contains round synaptic vesicles and forms an asymmetric synaptic junction (RA) whereas the labeled axon terminal from the midbrain tegmentum (B) contains pleomorphic synaptic vesicles and forms a symmetric synaptic junction (PS) with a dendrite (Den). Scale bars: 0.5 μm.

DTN, VTNa and VTNp. Thus, each part of the MB is reciprocally and topographically connected with the tegmental nuclei of Gudden (Takeuchi et al., 1985; Shibata, 1987; Hopkins and Allen, 1989), as summarized in figure 2.7, which shows the relationship between the cells of origin in the tegmental nuclei (figure 2.7B) and the terminal fields of their projections to the MB (figure 2.7A). Just as the VTN receives a complex input from the medial mammillary nuclei, there is corresponding topography in the organization of the cells of origin of the ascending reciprocal projections.

Precerebellar Relay Nuclei and Head Direction Cell Circuits

The strikingly close anatomical relationships of the lateral and medial MB projections to the dorsomedial areas of the precerebellar relay nuclei (figure 2.6) lead one to speculate that, although they are distinct circuits, there would likely be some similarities in functions for the respective projections. Both of these precerebellar relay targets, i.e., the NRTP and PN, of the descending projections from the MB, project to the cerebellar cortex and, in turn, receive inputs from the medial and lateral deep cerebellar nuclei (Watt and Mihailoff, 1983). Although there is extensive literature on the efferent projections of these precerebellar relay nuclei showing that the dorsomedial NRTP and rostromedial PN are reciprocally connected with the cerebellum, this literature does not clearly indicate the precise cerebellar target of the precerebellar relay cells that receive the projection from the MB. However, the dorsomedial NRTP projects to the cerebellar flocculus (Blanks et al., 1983), paraflocculus (Osani et al., 1999), vermis lobules VI and VII (Azizi et al., 1981;

Hopkins et al., 1985; Serapide et al., 2002), paravermis (Torigoe et al., 1986) and crus I (Mihailoff et al., 1981; Serapide et al., 2002). The rostromedial PN project to the cerebellar paraflocculus (Burne et al., 1978; Aas and Brodal, 1989) and vermis lobules VI, VII and XI (Azizi et al., 1981). Double-labeling experiments in the cat (Aas and Brodal, 1989) demonstrated that projections from the medial mammillary nucleus overlapped with the cells of origin of projections to the paraflocculus, which is a component of the vestibulo-cerebellum (Barmack et al., 1992; Balaban et al., 2000). In the rat, rostral dorsomedial regions of the NRTP and PN that receive descending projections from the LM and MM project to the cerebellar vermis (Hopkins et al., 1985) and ventral paraflocculus (Osanai et al., 1999). These pathways could influence optokinetic responses (Cazin et al., 1980). After large lesions of the vermis and fastigial nucleus, rats are impaired in their ability to navigate toward a visible platform (Joyal et al., 1996). Unfortunately, no experiments in the rat so far have combined anterograde tracing from the MB with retrograde and antero-grade tracing from the cerebellar cortex and deep cerebellar nuclei. Nevertheless, it does appear that the corresponding areas of the NRTP and PN that receive MB afferents project to vestibular (flocculus and paraflocculus) and visual (parts of vermis) regions of the cerebellar cortex. In terms of functional considerations, it is important to note that secondary vestibular inputs have strong and direct access to the primary HD cell circuit via projections from the nucleus prepositus hypoglossi to the DTN (Liu et al., 1984; Hayakawa and Zyo, 1985), which in turn projects massively to the LM (Groenewegen and Van Dijk, 1984).

Functional Considerations

The organization of HD cell circuits outlined in the present review shows that they are made up of a subset of closely related circuits that include the retrosplenial cortex, subicular complex, anterior thalamus, mammillary bodies, tegmental nuclei of Gudden, and precerebellar relay nuclei. Even though the HD cell literature focuses on the postsubiculum, AD and LM, the original report on HD cells in the anterior thalamus by Taube (1995) leaves open the possibility that some of the cells that were recorded could have been in the AV. It is important to keep this consideration in mind for future studies of HD and related cells because of some of the parallels in the connectivity of the AD and AV nuclei and the topographical relationship of MB circuits to the cerebral cortex and precerebellar relay nuclei.

The finding that activity of HD cells in the AD is modulated by active locomotion (Taube, 1995; Zugaro et al., 2001), as is the activity of theta-related cells, confirms a functional relationship between these two types of cells and supports the idea that other MB circuits (i.e., medial mammillary nuclei circuits) as well as the LM circuit might also be involved in modulating head direction or HD cell activity. In this respect, Albo et al. (2003) examined the neuronal activity of neurons in the anterior thalamus in relation to theta in anesthetized rats and reported that 12% of AD cells were rhythmic and 47% were intermediate, i.e., cells fired rhythmically or showed phase locking to theta, for a total of 59%. This percentage is close to the estimates by Taube (1995) and Taube and Bassett (2003) that 60% of AD cells are HD cells, but it remains to be determined whether 60% of neurons in the AD exhibit modulation by both head direction and theta.

In addition to HD cells, angular velocity and pitch cells have also recently been identified in the DTN (Basset and Taube, 2001) as have theta-related cells (Kocsis et al., 2001). In the DTN, only 11% of recorded cells were modulated by head direction, while 75% were sensitive to angular head velocity, with 21% of this latter population also sensitive to pitch (Bassett and Taube, 2001). Interestingly, 45% of angular head velocity cells were also modulated by linear velocity (Bassett and Taube, 2001). Theta-related cells have also been identified in the DTN, as well as in the VTNa and VTNp, and in spite of the differences in connectivity of the three tegmental nuclei of Gudden, neurons in each of the nuclei had similar response characteristics (Kocsis et al., 2001). The findings that head direction, angular head velocity, and linear velocity are often positively correlated raises the question of the degree to which these variables may be confounded in some experimental situations (Cho and Sharp, 2001). These data suggest that parallels or similarities in the connections of distinct MB circuits might play a role in neuronal functions related to HD cell characteristics.

In addition to possible interactions of HD cells and theta-related cells that have recently been identified in the medial mammillary circuit, it was shown some time ago that large lesions in the medial pons that include all or part of the descending and reciprocal ascending pontine connections of the MB result in a shift in hippocampal activity to more or less constant rhythmical slow activity, i.e., theta activity that is correlated with the initiation and performance of certain types of voluntary movement (Kolb and Whishaw, 1977). Kolb and Whishaw suggested that this change might have been due to release of rostral systems, e.g., hippocampal formation and septal nuclei, from inhibition originating more caudally in the brainstem. Moreover, ascending reciprocal projections from the tegmental nuclei of Gudden are probably inhibitory to MB neurons (Allen and Hopkins, 1989; Gonzalo-Ruiz et al., 1999). In addition, the LM receives a particularly strong projection from the nucleus incertus (Goto et al., 2001; Olucha-Bordonau et al., 2003). This nucleus is in close proximity to the DTN, and it has been suggested that it is involved in behavioral activation and theta generation. Taken together, these findings raise the possibility of a role for the connections between the MB and midbrain/pons in the modulation of theta-related activity, as well as modulation of HD cell activity.

Because the proportions and activity of functional cell types (head direction, angular velocity, pitch) present in the AD, LM, and DTN differ (Muller et al., 1996; Sharp et al., 2001; Taube and Bassett, 2003), it is clear that the activity of cells in MB is being modified in ways that change the preferred or peak firing characteristics at different levels or way stations of the MB circuits. It is, as yet, unknown how and which inputs and pathways are performing these transformations. The basis for head direction responses, with silent periods interspersed with continuous firing for an indefinite period, is probably based on the particular membrane properties of these neurons. However, with respect to neuronal membrane properties, LM neurons are silent at resting potential but "switch from tonic repetitive firing to a low threshold bursting pattern in a voltage-dependent manner" (Llinás and Alonso, 1992), with bursting occurring in response to an EPSP when the neuron was hyperpolarized. Possible neuroanatomical substrates for this would be excitatory synaptic inputs from the subicular complex (Allen and Hopkins, 1989) and inhibitory inputs from the DTN forming an inhibitory feedback loop (Allen and Hopkins, 1989; Hayakawa and Zyo, 1992; Gonzalo-Ruiz et al., 1993, 1999).

   With regard to the function of MB projections to the precerebellar relay nuclei, it has been suggested that this pathway could represent an anatomical substrate for limbic system influences on cerebellar-mediated somatic and autonomic responses (Allen and Hopkins, 1990). However, in the present context, and with the discovery of HD and theta-related cells in the MB and tegmental nuclei of Gudden, it is also pertinent to consider the projections to the precerebellar nuclei in terms of possible modulation of visual and vestibular functions. It was reported as early as 1955 that electrical stimulation of the cat MB elicited contralateral turning of the eyes and head (Akert and Andy, 1955), a response perhaps mediated in part via descending mammillotegmental projections. Consistent with this, the medial NRTP, PN and flocculus play a role in vestibulo-ocular reflexes (Cazin et al., 1980; Miyashita et al., 1980; Miles and Lisberger, 1981; Hess et al., 1989). Whether pretectal or superior colliculus afferents to the dorsomedial NRTP and PN (Burne et al., 1981) converge on the same precerebellar relay neurons that receive MB afferents remains to be determined, but this would be one way in which visual information could interact with HD cell activity.

Three Main MB Circuits: Mammillary Nuclei at the Crossroads

Neuroanatomical studies strongly suggest that the MB is at the crossroads of not just one, but at least three distinct circuits (figure 2.10; Allen and Hopkins, 1989), with highly interconnected way stations involving the cerebral cortex (retrosplenial, postsubicular, medial prefrontal), thalamus, MB, midbrain tegmentum, and pons. In terms of the cortical inputs to these three circuits, it is notable that there are also converging inputs of cortical efferents in the pons. That is, areas of the cortex that project to the MB also send direct, partially overlapping, projections to pontine precerebellar relay nuclei (Aas and Brodal, 1989; Allen and Hopkins, 1998). In the present context, HD cells have been identified almost exclusively in the circuit that involves the LM (figure 2.10C). At different levels of this circuit, HD cells exhibit different properties or additional characteristics with respect to head direction, angular velocity, and head pitch (Goodridge and Taube, 1997; Blair et al., 1998; Stackman and Taube, 1998; Taube and Muller, 1998; Bassett and Taube, 2001). However, there are cells in at least parts of all three MB circuits whose firing activ-

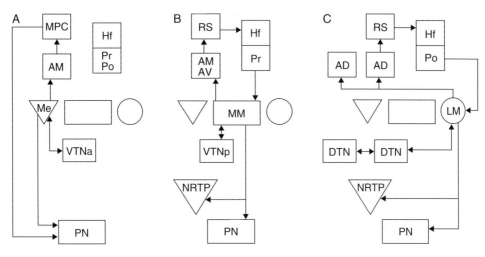

Figure 2.10
Three circuit diagrams (modified from Allen and Hopkins, 1989) indicating that each of three major subdivisions of the mammillary body (Me, MM and LM) receives relatively non-overlapping projections from the medial prefrontal cortex (A), subicular complex (B, C), or the dorsal (C) and ventral tegmental nuclei (A, B) and that the subnuclei of the mammillary body project topographically to the thalamus, midbrain tegmentum, and pons.

ity is synchronized with theta activity (Kocsis and Vertes, 1994; Kirk et al., 1996; Kocsis et al., 2001). Although HD cells and theta-related cells have been identified in different experimental paradigms, it seems likely that some cells in these circuits might show activity correlated with both, and it has been shown that active movement, a correlate of hippocampal theta activity (Vanderwolf, 1969), is associated with increased activity in AD HD cells (Zugaro et al., 2001).

Vann and Aggleton (2004) have also remarked on the parallels in connectivity of the LM and MM, while noting that the related circuits are more involved in head direction and theta, respectively. They speculate that the two systems may act synergistically in memory processes and that, in view of the precise topographical organization of MB circuits, other yet-to-be discovered functions may be associated with the medial MB and the prefrontal/anterior cingulate cortex. This is in keeping with Allen and Hopkins (1989, 1998), who have shown that the median MB is preferentially connected with the prefrontal cortex (figure 2.10A) and that circuits involving it are separate or distinct from those in the medial and lateral mammillary nuclei.

At the present time, researchers studying HD cells have focused on MB circuits associated with the LM (figure 2.10C), while those studying theta-related cells have focused on MB circuits associated with the medial nuclei (figure 2.10A,B). The anatomical organization of the MB suggests that these and other circuits associated with the mammillary nuclei deserve a closer look with respect to head direction cells and other functions related to spatial navigation and memory.

Summary and Conclusions

The neuroanatomy of HD cell circuits is characterized by the multiple levels of the central nervous system (CNS) that are involved. The nature of the hierarchical organization of these circuits has yet to be fully elucidated, but it is reasonable to assume that information processing starts with sensory information about head position, movement, and spatial navigation (Sharp et al., 2001; Brown et al., 2002; Wiener et al., 2002), with vestibular information being critical (Stackman and Taube, 1997; Brown et al., 2002). Sensory information ascends to the tegmentum and MB, way stations with prominent reciprocal and bilateral connections (figure 2.10). Similarly, reciprocal and bilateral connections are present between the thalamus and cerebral cortex. The MB is situated ideally at the crossroads between afferent connections from descending cortical pathways and ascending connections from the brainstem. The connections of three identified limbic circuits (figure 2.10) are such that ample substrates exist for sensory inputs, motor responses, as well as feedback (reciprocal and bilateral connections) to generate signals related to head position, spatial navigation, and locomotion (Stackman and Taube, 1997; Brown et al., 2002; Wiener et al., 2002). Sensory inputs (vestibular, visual, idiothetic) may gain access to the MB via projections from the nucleus prepositus hypoglossi that has primarily vestibular connections and projects to the DTN (Liu et al., 1984), which, in turn, projects to the LM (Groenewegen and Van Dijk, 1984). Once relayed to the MB, sensory information can be forwarded via the anterior nuclei of the thalamus to the cerebral cortex. However, not only is there an ascending flow of sensory information, but the MB projections descending to the precerebellar nuclei of the pons (NRTP, PN) also provide an anatomical substrate whereby cerebellar activity can potentially be modulated, given that the dorsomedial NRTP and pons have been implicated in the control of vestibulo-ocular reflexes. The MB is a complex, highly organized hypothalamic structure that links cortical, thalamic, brainstem, and cerebellar way stations associated with HD neurons. Future studies in this exciting field may reveal the extent to which the medial MB and its circuits are also involved in spatial navigation, locomotion, and learning.

In conclusion, at several levels of the CNS there are circuits that could enable comparisons of inputs from the body bilaterally and from the environment, and could also provide feedback loops. The complex pathways outlined above form a neuroanatomical substrate with excitatory and inhibitory connections that will provide the basis for neural models of how the brain computes the head direction signal.

Acknowledgments

I would like to thank Andrew Reid and Andrea LeBlanc for their assistance with the figures and manuscript preparation. This work was supported by MRC/CIHR of Canada.

Abbreviations

AD	anterodorsal thalamic nucleus	NRTP	nucleus reticularis tegmenti pontis
AM	anteromedial thalamic nucleus	Oc2M	medial prestriate occipital cortex area 2
AV	anteroventral thalamic nucleus	Pa	parasubiculum
cst	corticospinal tract	PN	pontine nuclei
DTN	dorsal tegmental nucleus of Gudden	Po	postsubiculum
Ent	entorhinal cortex	Pr	presubiculum
HD	head direction	R	reticular thalamic nucleus
Hf	hippocampal formation	Rd	retrosplenial dysgranular cortex
IAM	interanteromedial thalamic nucleus	RE	reuniens thalamic nucleus
III	third ventricle	Rga	retrospelenial granular a cortex
IP	interpeduncular nucleus	Rgb	retrosplenial granular b cortex
LD	laterodorsal thalamic nucleus	RS	retrosplenial cortex
lfp	longitudinal fasciculus pons	scp	superior cerebellar peduncle
LM	lateral mammillary nucleus	Sd	subiculum, dorsal
LP	lateral posterior thalamic nucleus	sm	stria medullaris
Me	medial mammillary nucleus, pars medianus	sp	splenium of the corpus callosum
ml	medial lemniscus	Sv	subiculum, ventral
mlf	medial longitudinal fasciculus	VL	ventral lateral thalamic nucleus
MML	medial mammillary nucleus, pars lateralis	VTN	ventral tegmental nucleus of Gudden
MMM	medial mammillary nucleus, pars medialis	VTNa	VTN pars anterior
mmt	mammillothalamic tract	VTNp	VTN pars posterior
mp	mammillary peduncle	xscp	decussation of superior cerebellar peduncle
MPC	medial prefrontal cortex		

References

Aas J-E, Brodal P (1989) Demonstration of a mamillo-ponto-cerebellar pathway. A multi-tracer study in the cat. Eur J Neurosci 1: 61–74.

Akert K, Andy OJ (1955) Experimental studies on corpus mammillare and tegmentomammillary system in the cat. Am J Physiol 183: 591.

Albo Z, Viana Di Prisco G, Vertes RP (2003) Anterior thalamic unit discharge profiles and coherence with hippocampal theta rhythm. Thal Rel Sys 2: 133–144.

Allen GV, Hopkins DA (1988) Mamillary body in the rat: a cytoarchitectonic, Golgi, and ultrastructural study. J Comp Neurol 275: 39–64.

Allen GV, Hopkins DA (1989) Mamillary body in the rat: topography and synaptology of projections from the subicular complex, prefrontal cortex, and midbrain tegmentum. J Comp Neurol 286: 311–336.

Allen GV, Hopkins DA (1990) Topography and synaptology of mamillary body projections to the mesencephalon and pons in the rat. J Comp Neurol 301: 214–231.

Allen GV, Hopkins DA (1998) Convergent prefrontal cortex and mammillary body projections to the medial pontine nuclei: a light and electron microscopic study in the rat. J Comp Neurol 398: 347–358.

Amaral DG, Witter MP (1995) Hippocampal formation. In G Paxinos, ed., The Rat Nervous System, 2nd ed. New York: Academic Press, pp. 443–493.

Azizi SA, Mihailoff GA, Burne RA, Woodward DJ (1981) The pontocerebellar system in the rat: an HRP study. I. Posterior vermis. J Comp Neurol 197: 543–558.

Balaban CD, Schuerger RJ, Porter JD (2000) Zonal organization of flocculo-vestibular connections in rats. Neuroscience 99: 669–682.

Barmack NH, Baughman RW, Eckenstein FP, Shojaku H (1992) Secondary vestibular cholinergic projection to the cerebellum of rabbit and rat as revealed by choline acetyltransferase immunohistochemistry, retrograde tracers, and orthograde tracers. J Comp Neurol 317: 250–270.

Bassett JP, Taube JS (2001) Neural correlates of angular head velocity in the rat dorsal tegmental nucleus. J Neurosci 21: 5740–5751.

Blair HT, Cho J, Sharp PE (1998) Role of the lateral mammillary nucleus in the rat head direction circuit: a combined single unit recording and lesion study. Neuron 21: 1387–1397.

Blair HT, Sharp PE (1996) Visual and vestibular influences on head-direction cells in the anterior thalamus of the rat. Behav Neurosci 110: 643–660.

Blanks RHI, Precht W, Torigoe Y (1983) Afferent projections to the cerebellar flocculus in the pigmented rat demonstrated by retrograde transport of horseradish peroxidase. Exp Brain Res 52: 293–306.

Brown JE, Yates BJ, Taube JS (2002) Does the vestibular system contribute to head direction cell activity in the rat? Physiol Behav 77: 743–748.

Burne RA, Mihailoff GA, Woodward DJ (1978) Visual corticopontine input to the paraflocculus: a combined autoradiographic and horseradish peroxidase study. Brain Res 143: 139–146.

Burne RA, Azizi SA, Mihailoff GA, Woodward DJ (1981) The tectopontine projection in the rat with comments on visual pathways to the basilar pons. J Comp Neurol 202: 287–307.

Cajal SR (1911) Histologie du Système Nerveux de L'Homme et des Vertébrés. Vol. II. Paris: Maloine; Madrid: Instituto Ramon Y Cajal, pp. 457–460.

Cazin L, Precht W, Lannou J (1980) Pathways mediating optokinetic responses of vestibular nucleus neurons in the rat. Pflüg Arch 384: 19–29.

Chen LL, Lin LH, Green EJ, Barnes CA, McNaughton BL (1994) Head-direction cells in the rat posterior cortex. I. Anatomical distribution and behavioral modulation. Exp Brain Res 101: 8–23.

Cho J, Sharp PE (2001) Head direction, place, and movement correlates for cells in the rat retrosplenial cortex. Behav Neurosci 115: 3–25.

Crabtree JW, Collingridge GL, Isaac JT (1998) A new intrathalamic pathway linking modality-related nuclei in the dorsal thalamus. Nat Neurosci 1: 389–394.

Cruce JAF (1975) An autoradiographic study of the projections of the mammillothalamic tract in the rat. Brain Res 85: 211–219.

Cruce JAF (1977) An autoradiographic study of the descending connection of the mammillary nuclei of the rat. J Comp Neurol 176: 631–644.

Darvesh S, Hopkins DA, Geula C (2003) Neurobiology of butyrylcholinesterase. Nat Rev Neurosci 4: 131–138.

Dekker JJ, Kuypers HG (1976) Morphology of rat's AV thalamic nucleus in light and electron microscopy. Brain Res 117: 387–398.

De Olmos J, Heimer L (1977) Mapping of collateral projections with the HRP-method. Neurosci Lett 6: 107–114.

Fry WJ (1970) Quantitative delineation of the efferent anatomy of the medial mammillary nucleus of the cat. J Comp Neurol 139: 321–336.

Fry FJ, Cowan WM (1972) A study of retrograde cell degeneration in the lateral mammillary nucleus of the cat, with special reference to the role of axonal branching in the preservation of the cell. J Comp Neurol 144: 1–24.

Golob EJ, Wolk DA, Taube JS (1998) Recordings of postsubiculum head direction cells following lesions of the laterodorsal thalamic nucleus. Brain Res 780: 9–19.

Gonzalo-Ruiz A, Lieberman AR (1995a) Topographic organization of projections from the thalamic reticular nucleus to the anterior thalamic nuclei in the rat. Brain Res Bull 37: 17–35.

Gonzalo-Ruiz A, Lieberman AR (1995b) GABAergic projections from the thalamic reticular nucleus to the anteroventral and anterodorsal thalamic nuclei of the rat. J Chem Neuroanat 9: 165–174.

Gonzalo-Ruiz A, Lieberman AR, Sanz-Anquela JM (1995) Organization of serotoninergic projections from the raphe nuclei to the anterior thalamic nuclei in the rat: a combined retrograde tracing and 5-HT immunohisto-chemical study. J Chem Neuroanat 8: 103–115.

Gonzalo-Ruiz A, Romero JC, Sanz JM, Morte L (1999) Localization of amino acids, neuropeptides and cholin-ergic neurotransmitter markers in identified projections from the mesencephalic tegmentum to the mammillary nuclei in the rat. J Chem Neuroanat 16: 117–133.

Gonzalo-Ruiz A, Sanz JM, Lieberman AR (1996) Immunohistochemical studies of localization and co-localization of glutamate, aspartate and GABA in the anterior thalamic nuclei, retrosplenial granular cortex, thalamic reticular nucleus and mammillary nuclei of the rat. J Chem Neuroanat 12: 77–84.

Gonzalo-Ruiz A, Sanz-Anquela MJ, Lieberman AR (1995) Cholinergic projections to the anterior thalamic nuclei in the rat: a combined retrograde tracing and choline acetyl transferase immunohistochemical study. Anat Embryol (Berl) 192: 335–349.

Gonzalo-Ruiz A, Sanz-Anquela JM, Spencer RF (1993) Immunohistochemical localization of GABA in the mammillary complex of the rat. Neuroscience 54: 143–156.

Goodridge JP, Taube JS (1997) Interaction between the postsubiculum and anterior thalamus in the generation of head direction cell activity. J Neurosci 17: 9315–9330.

Goto M, Swanson LW, Canteras NS (2001) Connections of the nucleus incertus. J Comp Neurol 438: 86–122.

Groenewegen HJ, Van Dijk CA (1984) Efferent connections of the dorsal tegmental region in the rat, studied by means of anterograde transport of the lectin *Phaseolus vulgaris*-leucoagglutinin (PHA-L). Brain Res 304: 367–371.

Guillery RW (1955) A quantitative study of the mamillary bodies and their connections. J Anat 89: 19–32.

Guillery RW (1957) Degeneration in the hypothalamic connections of the albino rat. J Anat 91: 91–115.

Gurdjian EJ (1927) The diencephalon of the albino rat. J Comp Neurol 43: 9–114.

Hayakawa T, Zyo K (1984) Comparative anatomical study of the tegmentomammillary projections in some mammals: a horseradish peroxidase study. Brain Res 300: 335–349.

Hayakawa T, Zyo K (1985) Afferent connections of Gudden's tegmental nuclei in the rabbit. J Comp Neurol 235: 169–181.

Hayakawa T, Zyo K (1989) Retrograde double-labeling study of the mammillothalamic and the mammil-lotegmental projections in the rat. J Comp Neurol 284: 1–11.

Hayakawa T, Zyo K (1991) Quantitative and ultrastructural study of ascending projections to the medial mammillary nucleus in the rat. Anat Embryol (Berl) 184: 611–622.

Hayakawa T, Zyo K (1992) Ultrastructural study of ascending projections to the lateral mammillary nucleus of the rat. Anat Embryol (Berl) 185: 547–557.

Hess BJM, Blanks RHI, Lannou J, Precht W (1989) Effects of kainic acid lesions of the nucleus reticularis tegmenti pontis on fast and slow phases of vestibulo-ocular and optokinetic reflexes in the pigmented rat. Exp Brain Res 74: 63–79.

Hopkins DA, Morrison MA, Allen GV (1985) Mamillary body projections to precerebellar relay nuclei in the rat. Anat Rec 211: 85A.

Hurley KM, Herbert H, Moga MM, Saper CB (1991) Efferent projections of the infralimbic cortex of the rat. J Comp Neurol 308: 249–276.

Joyal CC, Meyer C, Jacquart G, Mahler P, Caston J, Lalonde R (1996) Effects of midline and lateral cerebellar lesions on motor coordination and spatial orientation. Brain Res 739: 1–11.

Kirk IJ, Oddie SD, Konopacki J, Bland BH (1996) Evidence for differential control of posterior hypothalamic, supramammillary, and medial mammillary theta-related cellular discharge by ascending and descending path-ways. J Neurosci 16: 5547–5554.

Kishi Y, Tsumori T, Ono K, Yokota S, Ishino H, Yasui Y (2000) Topographical organization of projections from the subiculum to the hypothalamus in the rat. J Comp Neurol 419: 205–222.

Kocsis B, Vertes RP (1994) Characterization of neurons of the supramammillary nucleus and mammillary body that discharge rhythmically with the hippocampal theta rhythm in the rat. J Neurosci 14: 7040–7052.

Kocsis B, Viana Di Prisco G, Vertes RP (2001) Theta synchronization in the limbic system: the role of Gudden's tegmental nuclei. Eur J Neurosci 13: 381–388.

Kolb B, Whishaw IQ (1977) Effects of brain lesions and atropine on hippocampal and neocortical electroencephalograms in the rat. Exp Neurol 56: 1–22.

Liu H, Mihailoff GA (1999) Hypothalamopontine projections in the rat: anterograde axonal transport studies utilizing light and electron microscopy. Anat Rec 255: 428–451.

Liu R, Chang L, Wickern G (1984) The dorsal tegmental nucleus: an axoplasmic transport study. Brain Res 310: 123–132.

Llinás RR, Alonso A (1992) Electrophysiology of the mammillary complex in vitro. I. Tuberomammillary and lateral mammillary neurons. J Neurophysiol 68: 1307–1320.

Lozsàdi DA (1995) Organization of connections between the thalamic reticular and the anterior thalamic nuclei in the rat. J Comp Neurol 358: 233–246.

Meibach RC, Siegel A (1977) Efferent connections of the hippocampal formation in the rat. Brain Res 124: 197–224.

Mengual E, Casanovas-Aguilar C, Perez-Clausell J, Gimenez-Amaya JM (2001) Thalamic distribution of zinc-rich terminal fields and neurons of origin in the rat. Neuroscience 102: 863–884.

Mihailoff GA, Burne RA, Azizi SA, Norell G, Woodward DJ (1981) The pontocerebellar system in the rat: an HRP study. II. Hemispheral components. J Comp Neurol 197: 559–577.

Miles FA, Lisberger SG (1981) Plasticity in the vestibulo-ocular reflex: a new hypothesis. Annu Rev Neurosci 4: 273–299.

Miyashita Y, Ito M, Jastreboff PJ, Maekawa K, Nagao S (1980) Effect upon eye movements of rabbits induced by severance of mossy fiber visual pathway to the cerebellar flocculus. Brain Res 198: 210–215.

Mizumori SJY, Williams JD (1993) Directionally selective mnemonic properties of neurons in the lateral dorsal nucleus of the thalamus of rats. J Neurosci 13: 4015–4028.

Muller RU, Ranck JB Jr, Taube JS (1996) Head direction cells: properties and functional significance. Curr Opin Neurobiol 6: 196–206.

Oda S, Kuroda M, Kakuta S, Kishi K (2001) Differential immunolocalization of m2 and m3 muscarinic receptors in the anteroventral and anterodorsal thalamic nuclei of the rat. Brain Res 894: 109–120.

Olucha-Bordonau FE, Teruel V, Barcia-Gonzàlez J, Ruiz-Torner A, Valverde-Navarro AA, Martínez-Soriano F (2003) Cytoarchitecture and efferent projections of the nucleus incertus of the rat. J Comp Neurol 464: 62–97.

Osani R, Nagao S, Kitamura T, Kawabata I, Yamada J (1999) Differences in mossy and climbing afferent sources between flocculus and ventral and dorsal paraflocculus in the rat. Exp Brain Res 124: 248–264.

Pinault D, Deschênes M (1998) Projection and innervation patterns of individual thalamic reticular axons in the thalamus of the adult rat: a three-dimensional, graphic, and morphometric analysis. J Comp Neurol 391: 180–203.

Powell TPS, Cowan WM (1954) The origin of the mamillo-thalamic tract in the rat. J Anat 88: 489–497.

Ranck JB Jr (1985) Head direction cells in the deep cell layer of dorsal presubiculum in freely moving rats. In G Buzsàki and CH Vanderwolf, eds., Electrical Activity of Archicortex. Budapest: Akademai Kiado, pp. 217–220.

Robertson RT, Gorenstein C (1987) "Non-specific" cholinesterase-containing neurons of the dorsal thalamus project to medial limbic cortex. Brain Res 404: 282–292.

Robertson RT, Lieu CL, Lee K, Gorenstein C (1986) Distribution of "non-specific" cholinesterase-containing neurons in the dorsal thalamus of the rat. Brain Res 368: 116–124.

Rose J (1939) The cell structure of the mammillary body in the mammals and in man. J Comp Neurol 74: 91–115.

Ruggiero DA, Giuliano R, Anwar M, Stornetta R, Reis DJ (1990) Anatomical substrates of cholinergic-autonomic regulation in the rat. J Comp Neurol 292: 1–53.

Seki M, Zyo K (1984) Anterior thalamic afferents from the mammillary body and the limbic cortex in the rat. J Comp Neurol 229: 242–256.

Serapide MF, Parenti R, Pantò MR, Cicirata F (2002) Multiple zonal projections of the nucleus reticularis tegmenti pontis to the cerebellar cortex of the rat. Eur J Neurosci 15: 1854–1858.

Sharp PE, Blair HT, Cho J (2001) The anatomical and computational basis of the rat head-direction cell signal. Trends Neurosci 24: 289–294.

Shibata H (1987) Ascending projections to the mammillary nuclei in the rat: a study using retrograde and antero-grade transport of wheat germ agglutinin conjugated to horseradish peroxidase. J Comp Neurol 264: 205–215.

Shibata H (1989) Descending projections to the mammillary nuclei in the rat, as studied by retrograde and antero-grade transport of wheat germ agglutinin-horseradish peroxidase. J Comp Neurol 285: 436–452.

Shibata H (1992) Topographic organization of subcortical projections to the anterior thalamic nuclei in the rat. J Comp Neurol 323: 117–127.

Shibata H (1998) Organization of projections of rat retrosplenial cortex to the anterior thalamic nuclei. Eur J Neurosci 10: 3210–3219.

Shibata H (2000) Organization of retrosplenial cortical projections to the laterodorsal thalamic nucleus in the rat. Neurosci Res 38: 303–311.

Slomianka L, Geneser FA (1991) Distribution of acetylcholinesterase in the hippocampal region of the mouse: II. Subiculum and hippocampus. J Comp Neurol 312: 525–536.

Sripanidkulchai K, Wyss JM (1986) Thalamic projections to retrosplenial cortex in the rat. J Comp Neurol 254: 143–165.

Sripanidkulchai K, Wyss JM (1987) The laminar organization of efferent neuronal cell bodies in the retrosple-nial granular cortex. Brain Res 406: 255–269.

Stackman RW, Taube JS (1997) Firing properties of head direction cells in the rat anterior thalamic nucleus: dependence on vestibular input. J Neurosci 17: 4349–4358.

Stackman RW, Taube JS (1998) Firing properties of rat lateral mammillary single units: head direction, head pitch, and angular head velocity. J Neurosci 18: 9020–9037.

Tago H, Maeda T, McGeer PL, Kimura H (1992) Butyrylcholinesterase-rich neurons in rat brain demonstrated by a sensitive histochemical method. J Comp Neurol 325: 301–321.

Takeuchi Y, Allen GV, Hopkins DA (1985) Transnuclear transport and axon collateral projections of the mamil-lary nuclei in the rat. Brain Res Bull 14: 453–468.

Taube JS (1995) Head direction cells recorded in the anterior thalamic nuclei of freely moving rats. J Neurosci 15: 70–86.

Taube JS, Bassett, JP (2003) Persistent neural activity in head direction cells. Cerebral Cortex 13: 1162–1172.

Taube JS, Muller RU (1998) Comparisons of head direction cell activity in the postsubiculum and anterior thal-amus of freely moving rats. Hippocampus 8: 87–108.

Taube JS, Muller RU, Ranck JB Jr (1990) Head direction cells recorded from postsubiculum in freely moving rats. I. Description and quantitative analysis. J Neurosci 10: 420–435.

Thompson SM, Robertson RT (1987a) Organization of subcortical pathways for sensory projections to the limbic cortex. I. Subcortical projections to the medial limbic cortex in the rat. J Comp Neurol 265: 175–188.

Thompson SM, Robertson RT (1987b) Organization of subcortical pathways for sensory projections to the limbic cortex. II. Afferent projections to the thalamic lateral dorsal nucleus in the rat. J Comp Neurol 265: 189–202.

Torigoe Y, Blanks RHI, Precht W (1986) Anatomical studies on the nucleus reticularis tegmenti pontis in the pigmented rat. II. Subcortical afferents demonstrated by the retrograde transport of horseradish peroxidase. J Comp Neurol 243: 88–105.

Uchizono K (1965) Characteristics of excitatory and inhibitory synapses in the central nervous system of the cat. Nature 207: 642–643.

Van der Kooy D, Kuypers HGJM, Catsman-Berrevoets CE (1978) Single mammillary body cells with divergent axon collaterals. Demonstration by a simple, fluorescent retrograde double labeling technique in the rat. Brain Res 158: 189–196.

Vanderwolf CH (1969) Hippocampal electrical activity and voluntary movement in the rat. Electroenceph Clin Neurophysiol 26: 407–418.

Van Groen T, Kadish I, Wyss JM (1999) Efferent connections of the anteromedial nucleus of the thalamus of the rat. Brain Res Rev 30: 1–26.

Van Groen T, Wyss JM (1990a) The connections of presubiculum and parasubiculum in the rat. Brain Res 518: 227–243.

Van Groen T, Wyss JM (1990b) The postsubicular cortex in the rat: characterization of the fourth region of the subicular cortex and its connections. Brain Res 529: 165–177.

Van Groen T, Wyss JM (1990c) Connections of the retrosplenial granular a cortex in the rat. J Comp Neurol 300: 593–606.

Van Groen T, Wyss JM (1992a) Connections of the retrosplenial dysgranular cortex in the rat. J Comp Neurol 315: 200–216.

Van Groen T, Wyss JM (1992b) Projections from the laterodorsal nucleus of the thalamus to the limbic and visual cortices in the rat. J Comp Neurol 324: 427–448.

Van Groen T, Wyss JM (1995) Projections from the anterodorsal and anteroventral nucleus of the thalamus to the limbic cortex of the rat. J Comp Neurol 358: 584–604.

Van Groen T, Wyss JM (2003) Connections of the retrosplenial granular b cortex in the rat. J Comp Neurol 463: 249–263.

Vann SD, Aggleton JP (2004) The mammillary bodies: two memory systems in one? Nat Rev Neurosci 5: 35–44.

Veazey RB, Amaral DG, Cowan WM (1982) The morphology and connections of the posterior hypothalamus in the cynomolgus monkey (Macaca fascicularis). I. Cytoarchitectonic organization. J Comp Neurol 207: 114–134.

Vogt BA, Miller MW (1983) Cortical connections between rat cingulate cortex and visual, motor, and post-subicular cortices. J Comp Neurol 216: 192–210.

Vogt BA, Peters A (1981) Form and distribution of neurons in rat cingulate cortex: areas 32, 24, and 29. J Comp Neurol 195: 603–625.

Wang B, Gonzalo-Ruiz A, Morte L, Campbell G, Lieberman AR (1999a) Immunoelectron microscopic study of glutamate inputs from the retrosplenial granular cortex to identified thalamocortical projection neurons in the anterior thalamus of the rat. Brain Res Bull 50: 63–76.

Wang B, Gonzalo-Ruiz A, Sanz JM, Campbell G, Lieberman AR (1999b) Immunoelectron microscopic study of gamma-aminobutyric acid inputs to identified thalamocortical projection neurons in the anterior thalamus of the rat. Exp Brain Res 126: 369–382.

Watt CB, Mihailoff GA (1983) The cerebellopontine system in the rat. I. Autoradiographic studies. J Comp Neurol 215: 312–330.

Wiener SI (1993) Spatial and behavioral correlates of striatal neurons in rats performing a self-initiated navigation task. J Neurosci 13: 3802–3817.

Wiener SI, Berthoz A, Zugaro MB (2002) Multisensory processing in the elaboration of place and head direction responses by limbic system neurons. Brain Res Cogn Brain Res 14: 75–90.

Wilton LA, Baird AL, Muir JL, Honey RC, Aggleton JP (2001) Loss of the thalamic nuclei for "head direction" impairs performance on spatial memory tasks in rats. Behav Neurosci 115: 861–869.

Wirtshafter D, Stratford TR (1993) Evidence for GABAergic projections from the tegmental nuclei of Gudden to the mammillary body in the rat. Brain Res 630: 188–194.

Witter MP, Ostendorf RH, Groenewegen HJ (1990) Heterogeneity in the dorsal subiculum of the rat. Distinct neuronal zones project to different cortical and subcortical targets. Eur J Neurosci 2: 718–725.

Wyss JM, Sripanidkulchai K (1984) The topography of the mesencephalic and pontine projections from the cingulate cortex of the rat. Brain Res 293: 1–15.

Zilles K (1985) The Cortex of the Rat: a Stereotaxic Atlas. Berlin: Springer-Verlag.

Zugaro MB, Tabuchi E, Fouquier C, Berthoz A, Wiener SI (2001) Active locomotion increases peak firing rates of anterodorsal thalamic head direction cells. J Neurophysiol 86: 692–702.

3 Head Direction Cell Activity: Landmark Control and Responses in Three Dimensions

Jeffrey S. Taube

Navigation represents one of the most fundamental cognitive functions upon which mammals depend for survival. Two fundamental processes important for navigation are landmark navigation and path integration (Barlow, 1964; Gallistel, 1990; McNaughton et al., 1991; Taube, 1998). Landmark navigation involves the use of environmental cues (landmarks) and is sometimes referred to as piloting. The sensory information used by the animal can be derived from any of the sensory modalities (visual, auditory, olfactory) and is used in an episodic fashion. The second process is path integration (sometimes referred to as dead reckoning) and involves monitoring the sensory/motor cues that are generated during an animal's movements through the environment. The sensory/motor systems involved in path integration are often referred to as *idiothetic* cues and include vestibular, proprioceptive, and motor efference copy information. For idiothetic cues to provide accurate information about the organism's orientation, they must be used in a continuous manner. Under most circumstances, both processes are used simultaneously, but when information from one source of spatial cues is absent, the animal must rely on the other set of cues. The first section of this chapter focuses on the types of landmark cues that affect head direction (HD) cell activity, and the reader is referred to chapter 7 by Stackman and Zugaro for a description of how idiothetic cues affect HD cell firing. We first consider how cues external to the body can affect HD cells. We then discuss experiments that have explored the development of cue control and spatial orientation as it relates to HD cells. Because many animals function in a three-dimensional environment, in the second section we describe the response of HD cells when an animal is in different earth-centered planes, in particular, when the animal is locomoting in the vertical plane or is upside down. We conclude this section by describing HD cell responses in different planes under conditions of zero gravity (0–g).

Landmark Control of HD Cells

Cue Card Rotation

To investigate the control exerted by a salient visual landmark on HD cells, Taube et al. (1990b) rotated a prominent visual cue (a large white sheet of cardboard taped to the inside wall of a cylindrical enclosure 1 m in diameter) to various positions and monitored the response of HD cells. For these cue rotation sessions, the animal was removed from the cylinder between recording sessions and thus did not see the card being repositioned. The animal was placed in a small, opaque box, and before being reattached to the recording cable and returned to the cylinder, the experimenter walked around the room turning the box slowly back and forth. This procedure was designed to disorient the rat and encourage it to use landmark cues for updating its spatial orientation upon its return to the cylinder. Under these conditions, the preferred directions of HD cells shifted an amount nearly equal to the cue card rotation, and thus maintained the same relationship with the cue card as in the original recording session (figure 3.1A). Similarly, when the cue card was returned to its initial position, the cell's preferred direction shifted back to its original position. Rotation of the cue card had no effect on the cell's peak firing rate or directional firing range. Similar results have been obtained for HD cells in all brain areas where this manipulation has been conducted (ADN: Taube, 1995; LMN: Stackman and Taube, 1998;

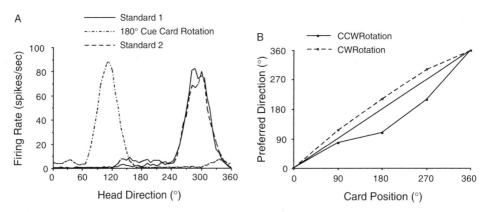

Figure 3.1
Cue card rotation sessions. (A) HD cell response following rotation of the cue card. For standard sessions 1 and 2 the cue card was positioned at a 3:00 bearing on the cylinder wall. In the cue card rotation session, the card was rotated 180° to the 9:00 position with the rat out of view. Note that the cell's preferred firing direction shifted about 180° during the card rotation session and then returned to its original position when the card was returned to its 3:00 position in the second standard session. There was little change in the cell's peak firing rate and directional firing range during the cue rotation session. (B) HD cell responses when the cue card is rotated in 90° steps in the presence of the rat. Whether the card was rotated in (clockwise) (CW) or (counterclockwise) (CCW) direction, the preferred firing direction generally shifted along with the cue card, although there were consistent under-rotations. The 45° line depicts a hypothetical perfect shift. (Reproduced with permission: A, copyright 2002 by Kluwer Press; B, copyright 1990 by the Society for Neuroscience.)

retrosplenial cortex: Chen et al., 1994). These findings indicate that, although vestibular information is believed critical for the *generation of the HD signal* (see chapter 7), a prominent visual landmark can exert control over a cell's preferred direction.

Experiments involving cue rotation commonly rotate the cue by 90°. Although the preferred firing direction usually shifts a similar amount, the shift is usually not exactly 90°, and there is a small deviation between the two amounts. The most common error is an underrotation of the preferred firing direction, where the preferred firing direction shifts less than 90°. Overrotations (shifts greater than 90°) are observed, but their frequency compared to underrotations is lower. For cue rotation experiments conducted on PoS and ADN HD cells, the mean amounts of deviation were underrotations of 18.9° and 13.2°, respectively (Taube et al., 1990b; Taube, 1995). These deviations, although small, are larger than the mean deviation of about 5° observed across two recording sessions when cues are kept constant and the rat is removed from the cylinder between sessions, and is then reattached to the recording cable (Taube et al., 1990b; Taube, 1995). This finding indicates that other cues in the environment are influencing the preferred firing direction. Moreover, the cue card rotation experiments indicate that spatial information obtained from the cue card overrode any potential spatial information obtained from either static background cues within the recording room or the earth's geomagnetic cues, which, in theory, could also provide allocentric directional information about the animal's orientation.

When the cue card is rotated 90° in the presence of the rat, a sensory conflict situation arises between spatial information from the visual landmark and spatial information derived from idiothetic sources. If prominent olfactory cues were present on the cylinder floor, such as urine spots or rat boli, there would also be a spatial information conflict between the olfactory marks and the cue card. Taube et al. (1990b) rotated the white cue card in four 90° counterclockwise (CCW) steps without removing the rat from the cylinder. The experiment was repeated the next day on the same cell, but the four 90° card rotations were in the clockwise (CW) direction. For each rotation of the card, the preferred firing direction of the PoS HD cells shifted a similar amount, although the shifts were always underrotations (figure 3.1B). These results demonstrate the strong influence a prominent visual landmark exerts over the preferred firing direction. This landmark spatial information can therefore override most of the information derived from idiothetic and olfactory sources.

Further discussion of how HD cells respond under cue conflict conditions is discussed in chapter 7 by Stackman and Zugaro. Similarly, the importance of whether the visual landmark cue is positioned in the foreground or in the background is addressed in chapter 4 by Zugaro and Wiener.

Landmark Removal and HD Cell Responses in the Dark

Although the visual cue can exert control of the preferred direction of HD cells, HD cell activity is not dependent on the presence of the visual reference cue, because PoS HD cells continue to show direction-specific discharge even when the visual cue is removed from the enclosure (figure 3.2). Furthermore, removal of the visual cue has no effect on the cell's peak firing rate or range of firing. The initial cue removal experiments occurred with the rat out of view when the cue card was removed, and without a reference landmark, a cell's preferred direction usually shifted (Taube et al., 1990b). Similar results were obtained for HD cells in the ADN and PoS when the room lights were turned off, or when an animal was blindfolded. Both manipulations had little effect on HD cell firing once the animal was in the environment, although over time (approx. 8 min) many cells shifted their preferred directions 20° to 30° (Goodridge et al., 1998). As expected, if the animal was introduced into the environment in the dark or with a blindfold on, then the preferred directions of HD cells usually shifted compared to the first session when the animal could view the landmark. Turning the room lights off and on had similar effects for HD cells in the retrosplenial cortex (Chen et al., 1994).

In contrast, Mizumori and Williams (1993) reported that lateral dorsal thalamic HD cells did *not* show direction-specific discharges when the animal was first placed on the apparatus in the dark. Once directional firing was established with the lights on, when the lights were turned off a second time, the preferred direction of lateral dorsal thalamic cells started to rotate systematically in one direction after 2 to 3 min. These results suggest that lateral dorsal thalamic cells may be fundamentally different from PoS and ADN HD cells in that they require visual inputs, because, in theory, idiothetic sensory information from internal sources should have been able to sustain HD cell firing in the absence of visual cues.

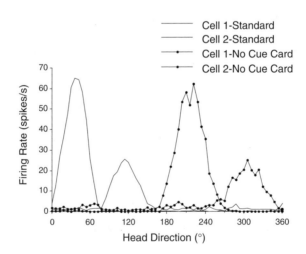

Figure 3.2
HD cell responses following removal of the cue card. Two HD cells were recorded during this series. Following an initial session in the cylinder with the cue card present (standard), the rat was removed from the cylinder and then returned after the card had been removed. During the card removal session, both HD cells shifted their preferred directions, about 168° counterclockwise. There was little change in the peak firing rates and directional firing ranges of the cells during the cue removal session. (Reproduced with permission: copyright 2002 by Kluwer Press.)

Establishment of Cue Control

Another question that arises is how long an animal must be exposed to a novel landmark before it develops control over the cell's preferred direction. Goodridge et al. (1998) trained and recorded rats in the cylinder without the cue card. All rats were consistently disoriented before being brought into the recording room. After identifying an HD cell, the cue card was introduced into the cylinder for different lengths of time—1, 3, or 8 minutes. A cue card rotation session was then conducted to determine whether the cue card had gained control over the cell's preferred direction. All 8-minute card exposure sessions resulted in a corresponding shift in the cell's preferred direction, while about half of the 1- and 3-minute exposure sessions led to a shift. Thus, only a single exposure to a novel cue for a few minutes was usually sufficient time to enable the cue to acquire stimulus control over HD cell responses.

A related issue is the manner in which a familiar landmark controls the cell's preferred firing direction when an animal is confronted with an inconsistency and perceives its directional heading to be in error. When the animal reorients using the familiar landmarks, does the preferred firing direction of the HD cell shift through all the intermediate head angles between the initial direction and the final direction? Or is activity reduced at one head direction while increasing simultaneously at another direction? In the cue card rotation experiments in which the rat remained in the cylinder during the cue rotations, the preferred firing direction shifted quickly to realign itself with the cue card. The shift was usually evident by the time the animal made its first pass through the cell's preferred firing direction. But this amount of time varies, of course, and is dependent on the behavior of the rat. To address this issue, using a finer temporal resolution, Zugaro et al. (2003) recorded ADN HD cells in a task that enabled them to determine how fast a familiar landmark cue could update the animal's perceived directional heading. They reported that the visual cue could shift the preferred firing direction as rapidly as 80 ms after changes in the visual scene. The data was more consistent with a network that shifted the preferred firing direction abruptly without passing through intermediate angles, than one that changed in a gradual progressive manner. These experiments are discussed further in chapter 4 by Zugaro and Wiener.

The control that the cue card can exert over the cell's preferred direction is sometimes remarkable. Goodridge and Taube (1995) recorded HD cells first in the cylinder with the cue card present. The animal was then removed from the cylinder, and the cue card was detached from the wall and removed from the cylinder. The animal then underwent the disorientation procedure previously described, in which the experimenter walked the animal around the room in an opaque box while rotating the box slowly back and forth. A second recording session was conducted without the cue card and, as predicted, the preferred firing direction usually shifted significantly from its previous value. Then, with the rat still in the cylinder, the cue card was returned to its original position along the inside wall of the cylinder after which a third recording session was conducted. Under these

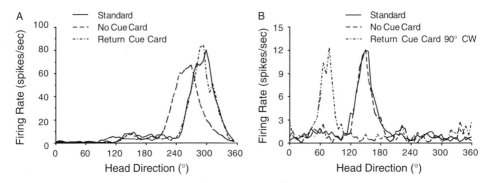

Figure 3.3
HD cell responses when the cue card is reintroduced into the cylinder in the presence of the rat following a cue card removal session. (A) During the No Cue Card session the preferred firing direction shifted about 30° clockwise. The cue card was then returned to the position it occupied in the Standard session, and the preferred direction shifted back to its original orientation. (B) This series was run similar to the series in (A) except that during the No Cue Card session the cell's preferred firing direction did *not* shift and remained similar to the Standard session. In the Return Cue Card session the card was attached to the wall in a 90° clockwise rotated position compared to the Standard session. Under these conditions, the preferred direction also shifted 90° clockwise. (Reproduced with permission: copyright 1995 by the American Psychological Association.)

conditions, the preferred firing direction usually shifted within 5 to 10 seconds to realign itself with the cue card in the same orientation as in the first recording session (figure 3.3). In a few instances, the preferred firing direction did not shift very much (<30°) between the baseline and the cue card removal sessions. When this occurred, the cue card was returned to the cylinder in a 90° rotated position while the rat was in the cylinder. In these situations, the preferred firing directions shifted approximately 90° rather rapidly to remain anchored to the cue card in the same relationship compared to the initial recording session. Both experimental manipulations demonstrate that, despite the spatial information from the animal's idiothetic cues, and despite the presence of olfactory markings on the floor, the preferred firing direction of the cell was controlled predominantly by the prominent visual landmark.

Auditory Landmarks
In another series of experiments Goodridge et al. (1998) tested the response of HD cells to rotation of a 1 Hz auditory click emanating from one of four audio speakers spaced uniformly around the inside cylinder wall. The clicks were generated from square waves passed through a sound amplifier and thus contained a mixture of sound frequencies. For these experiments, there was no cue card in the cylinder. Although previous studies have shown that rats can discriminate the localization of one click from a second click spaced 24° apart (Kelly and Glazier, 1978), rotation of the *auditory* cue did not lead to a corresponding shift in the cell's preferred direction. Thus, despite the fact that the animal was given extensive experience with the auditory click, it was not able to exert stimulus control

over the preferred direction of HD cells in the same manner as the cue card. It is possible, however, that if the auditory cue was made more salient, for example, by having the animal perform a task for which it had to utilize the spatial information about the cue to obtain a reward, then the cells might have shifted their preferred direction when the click was rotated.

Olfactory Cues

The responses of PoS and ADN HD cells following the rotation of a salient olfactory cue (a cotton-tipped swab soaked with peppermint extract) were also assessed in rats that were recorded in the cylinder without a cue card (Goodridge et al., 1998). Four swabs were spaced uniformly on the floor around the cylinder's perimeter. Only one of the swabs was soaked in peppermint. Following an initial recording session, the swab containing the peppermint odor was rotated to a new position, with the animal out of view. A second recording session showed that, in about half the cases, the cell's preferred direction shifted a similar amount. There were, however, several sizable underrotations, as well as a higher incidence of them, compared to cue card rotations. These results indicate that HD cells can be responsive to olfactory information, but visual landmark information exerts a greater influence over the cells' preferred firing directions than olfactory information.

Consistent with these results was the finding that when the floor paper of the apparatus was rotated, the preferred directions of HD cells in *blindfolded* rats frequently shifted in the same direction, although there were significant underrotations in all cases (Goodridge et al., 1998). Because the floor paper was not changed between recording sessions, this result suggests that the rats were using olfactory cues laid down on the floor paper to help them keep track of their directional orientation, although the results do not exclude the possibility that the rats were using tactile features from the urine and boli markings they had left on the floor.

Enclosure Shape

The geometric contour of the environment is an important determinant in the spatial references an animal selects for orientation. This conclusion is based on evidence that rats (Cheng, 1986; Margules and Gallistel, 1988), human toddlers (Hermer and Spelke, 1994), and, to a lesser extent, birds (Vallortigara et al., 1990) are unable to distinguish diagonally opposite corners inside a rectangular area after various forms of disorientation. This inability often occurs despite the presence of a salient visual cue that disambiguates the two corners. The animals and toddlers can, however, distinguish the two pairs of opposing diagonal corners by showing that they prefer one pair of diagonal corners over the other pair. This result suggests the geometry of the environment was being used as a landmark cue to distinguish the two pairs of corners.

The shape of an environment also plays an important role in determining how HD cells respond. When the shape of the animal's environment is changed, for example, from a cylinder to a rectangle, a cell's preferred direction frequently shifts to a new direction without affecting its peak firing rate or directional firing range (Taube et al., 1990b). Sometimes a cell's preferred direction will be unaffected by a change in the shape of one enclosure (e.g., going from a cylinder to a square), but will be affected when going to another shaped enclosure (e.g., rectangle) (Taube et al., 1990b).

Multiple HD Cell Recordings and Environmental Manipulations

On occasions when two or more HD cells are monitored simultaneously in the same animal, the effects of an environmental manipulation on the preferred direction for one cell are similar to the effects observed in other cells (Taube et al., 1990b; Taube, 1995) (see figure 3.2). This finding provides a strong demonstration that afferent input driving one HD cell similarly influences other HD cells within the same brain area, and indicates that HD cells within a particular brain area behave as a network, and their preferred directions remain a fixed angle apart (in register) from one other.

These findings can be compared with the effects of environmental manipulations on hippocampal place cells where the network of cells can also "remap," with some cells ceasing firing in the second environment, while other cells that were silent in the first environment start firing in the second environment (Kubie and Ranck, 1983). In contrast, HD cells have never been observed to cease firing under any environmental context and continue to discharge in some direction in all environments. These findings suggest that the animal's directional heading in any environment maps onto the entire neuronal network within a brain area. Thus, all the HD cells within a network are used for encoding directional headings in any given environment.

Development of Spatial Orientation and Cue Control in HD Cells

Several studies have explored the relationship between HD cell activity and the development of an animal's perceived spatial orientation. These studies have indicated that the extent to which an animal is disoriented when it is brought into an environment plays an important role in its ability to incorporate novel landmark cues into its spatial representation (Cheng, 1986; Margules and Gallistel, 1988). In addition, Biegler and Morris (1993) showed that the mere association between a reward and a landmark was insufficient to establish accurate performance; the landmark had to be perceived within a stable spatial framework before it could lead to correct behavior.

Knierim et al. (1995) extended these findings to the neural level by monitoring HD and place cells from two groups of rats in a cylinder containing a single salient visual cue attached to the wall. Rats from one group were hand carried from their cages and placed in the apparatus. Rats in the second group were disoriented on every trip into and out of the recording room (by placing them in an opaque box and gently spinning them back and forth when carried to the recording room), and thus were not allowed to form a stable spatial representation between the recording apparatus and the outside world. The authors found that the preferred directions of HD cells and the place fields of place cells recorded from disoriented animals frequently failed to establish a consistent relationship with the cue card, despite the fact that the cue card was the only intentionally introduced, stable reference point. Based on these findings, Knierim et al. postulated that visual landmarks exert control over orientation only after an animal has learned an association between the visual landmark information and its "internal sense" of directional heading as provided by idiothetic cues. When the rats are deprived of forming this link through disorientation, the cells will never form a stable spatial association with the cue card. It is only through active exploration that an animal will establish a consistent relationship between spatial information from landmarks and its own perceived spatial orientation (Poucet, 1993). These findings were consistent with the view that, in learning about the spatial relationships of an environment, animals first rely primarily on idiothetic cues, and that landmarks gain control of spatial behavior only after sufficient experience in linking information from idiothetic cues with spatial information from landmarks (Alyan and Jander, 1994).

If the preceding hypothesis is correct, then rats that are consistently disoriented at the start of an experiment should not be capable of learning to go to a particular location relative to a fixed landmark. Martin et al. (1997) and Dudchenko et al. (1997a) tested this hypothesis by examining the effects of disorientation on the acquisition of different spatial reference memory tasks. Both studies found that in an appetitively motivated radial-arm maze task, where one arm was consistently baited, animals that were disoriented before each trial were impaired in their ability to acquire the task relative to animals brought to the test apparatus in a clear container and not disoriented. Animals that were simply placed in an opaque container and carried into the testing room also had difficulty acquiring the task, which suggests that they needed to visually link the two environments in order to perform the task. However, disoriented animals were able to learn an aversively-motivated Morris water maze and a water version of the radial-arm maze under similar training conditions, which suggests that the effects of disorientation may interact with the quality or quantity of motivation involved in a given task. These results suggested that appetitive and aversive spatial tasks are dissociable, and that any impairment due to disorientation is specific to the appetitive radial-arm maze task. Under aversive training conditions, disoriented animals may be more motivated, and thereby quickly learn the spatial information concerning landmark cues.

To determine whether the behavioral impairment on the standard radial arm maze task was associated with a lack of landmark stimulus control over the preferred orientations of HD cells, following completion of the behavioral experiments, Dudchenko et al. (1997b) monitored HD and place cells in the same animals that showed significant acquisition deficits. This experiment assumes that HD cell activity at some level can guide the behavioral response of an animal (for further discussion of this issue see Muir and Taube, 2002 and chapter 11 by Dudchenko et al.). Landmark control in the radial-arm maze and in a cylinder was assessed by rotating the visual cue card with the animal out of view and then reexamining the cell's preferred direction when the rat was returned to the maze. Animals underwent disorientation treatment before and after each recording session. Despite the disorientation, rotation of either the cylinder's cue card or the curtain (for the radial-arm maze sessions) resulted in a corresponding shift in the cell's preferred direction. Similar findings were also reported for hippocampal cell place fields. These results suggest that the establishment of stimulus control of HD cells by a landmark does not require a learned association between that landmark and the linkage with idiothetic information. Thus, instability in the HD system is unlikely to account for the poor performance of the disoriented animals in the radial-arm maze. Rather, the impaired performance is more likely attributed to the animal's inability to utilize stable representations of the environment provided by HD and place cells.

HD Cell Responses in Three Dimensions

Hemitorus Model

In the first published reports, HD cell tuning curves were plotted using a two-dimensional graph that displayed firing rate versus head direction (Taube et al., 1990a). This convention is still commonly used. If, however, HD cell firing is represented in three-dimensional polar coordinates, the activity of the HD cell can be characterized as the surface of a hemitorus, shown in figure 3.4. In this figure, the positive y-axis represents the preferred direction of a two-dimensional HD cell response in polar coordinates. Under normal conditions, the z-axis is aligned with the gravitational vertical, and the x-y plane is horizontal. The length of the vector from the origin to the surface defines the magnitude of the HD cell response as a function of the animal's three-dimensional directional heading represented by the vector's direction. For example, consider an HD cell that responds maximally when the animal's head faces in the positive y axis direction. In general, HD cell responses are known to be independent of head pitch and roll, up to 90°. The model predicts that the cell will discharge at its peak rate when the rat's head is oriented anywhere along the y-z plane, as long as the animal's head orientation contains a positive y-axis component. Thus, the cell will continue to fire if the animal climbs the north wall (defined as the wall in the x-z plane by the positive y-axis), but not the south wall. If the animal climbs the West wall, the cell will respond whenever the animal's right side is down, but not the left, and, conversely, on the east wall. This model can be used to predict the two-dimensional response for any plane in the experiments described later in this chapter.

HD Cell Responses in the Vertical Plane

Many animals, including rats, spend part of their lives locomoting in planes outside the earth horizontal plane. To a first approximation, the pitch of the rat's head is not a strong determinant of HD cell firing. Thus, when the rat is locomoting on the floor, pitch or roll

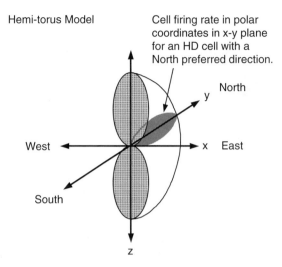

Hemi-torus Model

Cell firing rate in polar
coordinates in x-y plane
for an HD cell with a
North preferred direction.

Figure 3.4
Three-dimensional model of HD cell firing. The surface of the hemi-torus-shaped figure represents the maximum firing rate of a hypothetical cell as a function of azimuth and height. The cell's firing rate is plotted in three-dimensional polar coordinates and is tuned to 90° in the *x-y* plane. The firing rate of an HD cell when the animal points its head to various directions is represented by the distance away from the origin. Note that there are abrupt transitions from high firing rates to directions where the cell ceases responding. (Reproduced with permission: copyright 1998 by Elsevier Press.)

of the head to 45° does not appear to affect HD cell activity. However, how do HD cells respond when the animal is locomoting in an earth-vertical plane or when an animal is inverted and locomoting upside down on a ceiling surface? To address these questions and to better understand how an animal defines its horizontal reference frame, we conducted a series of experiments. In the first series, Stackman et al. (2000) monitored HD cell activity as a rat locomoted back and forth between a horizontal plane and a vertical plane, one that was 90° orthogonal to the floor of the recording cylinder. HD cell activity in the ADN and PoS was recorded in a tall cylinder that contained a wide rim (annulus) around the top with four equally spaced food wells (figure 3.5A). A vertical wire mesh "ladder" placed onto the inside cylinder wall allowed the rat to access the annulus. HD cells were monitored while rats climbed up and down the wire mesh to retrieve food pellets on the floor and annulus. The wire mesh was positioned at 0°, 90°, 180°, and 270° relative to the cell's preferred direction. Thus, this study also explored whether HD cell activity was affected when the rat was in a second horizontal plane that was significantly separated from, but still in sight of, the first horizontal plane.

    HD cell discharge properties were similar when the rat locomoted in either horizontal plane (floor or annulus). When the wire mesh position corresponded with the cell's preferred direction (0° position), HD cells continued to fire at peak rates *as the rat climbed up the wire mesh, but not when the rat climbed down* (figure 3.5B). If the rat turned its

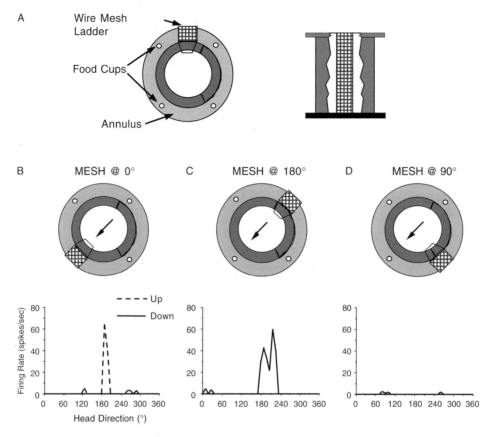

Figure 3.5
HD cell responses in the vertical plane. (A) Tall cylinder apparatus with annulus and food cups around top. The wire mesh allowed the rat to climb up and down the wall of the cylinder to reach the annulus. (B) HD cell responses when the mesh was positioned in the cell's preferred firing direction. (C) HD cell responses when the mesh was positioned opposite the cell's preferred firing direction. (D) HD cell responses when the mesh was positioned 90° clockwise relative to the cell's preferred firing direction. (Reproduced with permission: copyright 2000 by the American Physiological Society.)

head left or right when it was climbing the mesh, cell firing was reduced. With the mesh positioned 180° opposite the cell's preferred direction, cell firing continued when the rat ran down the mesh, but not when it ran up (figure 3.5C). Background firing rates were exhibited when the rat ran up or down the ladder when it was positioned 90° CW or CCW from the cell's preferred direction (90° and 270° positions) (figure 3.5D). These results indicate that cell discharge continued in the vertical plane if the rat approached and locomoted into this plane while facing the cell's preferred direction. These findings are therefore consistent with two hypotheses: (1) that the horizontal reference frame can be translated with the animal into an earth vertical plane, and (2) that HD cells define the horizontal reference frame as the animal's plane of locomotion.

Direction-specific firing remained intact when the animal was on the annulus, with little change in the cell's preferred direction. Interestingly, however, most HD cells had higher peak firing rates (approx. 10% to 30%) on the annulus compared to the cylinder floor. It is unclear whether this increased firing rate reflected additional encoding of height above the floor or some other factor, such as a heightened awareness of a need for proper coordination and balance so that the animal doesn't fall off the annulus.

In the tall cylinder experiments previously described, the rat ran up and down the vertical mesh more or less in a straight-ahead position, making few head turns to the left or right. Thus, the rat's directional headings were confined to a narrow range of angles, and a full 360° sampling in the vertical plane was not achieved. Although the vertical mesh was moved around the cylinder to different positions, the rats were not able to sample a full 360° in a single vertical plane. To address this issue in the second series of experiments, Kim et al. (2003) built a wire mesh track that was shaped in a spiral and attached to a wooden platform. The platform could be pitched at 0°, 30°, 45°, and 90° relative to horizontal (figure 3.6A). Rats were first trained to forage for food pellets in a cylinder, and then to run on the spiral track, starting at the outside portion of the spiral. The spiral track ended at the center of the platform, where there was a hole that the rat could go through to retrieve a food reward. As the rats learned to traverse the track, the platform was raised to greater inclinations over several days until the rats performed the task well when the platform was completely in the vertical position (i.e., 90°). Rats then underwent surgery for implantation of recording electrodes and, following recovery, were screened for the presence of HD cells in the ADN.

When HD cells were identified, they were then recorded in the sequence depicted in figure 3.6B: (1) in a cylinder that was 0.5 m high, (2) on the spiral platform positioned horizontally, (3) on the spiral platform after it had been rotated 90° or 180° in the horizontal plane, and (4) on the spiral platform when it was positioned in a vertical plane facing each of the four cardinal directions within the room (numbers 4–7 in figure 3.6B). Results were generally consistent across cells and animals. When the platform was rotated 90° or 180° in the azimuthal plane, only one of seven HD cells shifted their preferred firing direction by more than 30°, suggesting that these cells usually stayed with the room reference frame when the apparatus was in the horizontal plane. When the platform was pitched into the vertical plane, most HD cells "remapped" their preferred firing directions and appeared to use a platform reference frame rather than the room reference frame (figure 3.6C). This switch of reference frames to the platform was then maintained as the vertical platform was moved around the room to the four cardinal positions. Thus, all HD cells maintained the same preferred firing direction relative to the platform when it was in the vertical orientation, regardless of the cardinal position of the platform in the room (figure

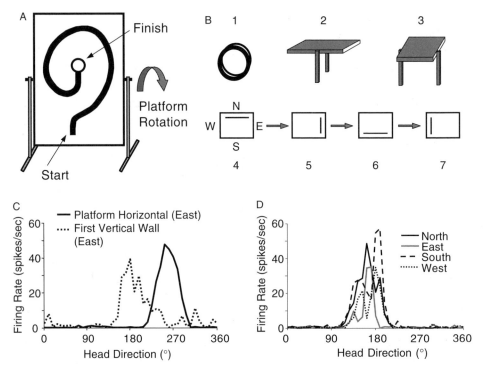

Figure 3.6
HD cell responses in the vertical plane. (A) Spiral track apparatus. The rat was placed at the bottom of the track and had to locomote around the spiral track to the center in order to retrieve food reward. (B) Experimental sequence. The cell was recorded in the cylinder (1), on the platform positioned horizontally (2), the platform positioned horizontally, but rotated by 90° (3), and then with the platform in the vertical orientation while facing each of the four cardinal directions within the room (4–7). Numbers 4 through 7 show an overhead view of the room with the position of the vertical platform shown as a solid line. (C) HD cell responses when the spiral track and platform were oriented in the horizontal plane with the start position along the East wall and when the track was positioned vertically along the East wall of the room. (D) HD cell responses on the spiral track in the vertical position when it was placed at the four cardinal positions within the room. Note that the preferred direction shifted between the horizontal and vertical planes, but was similar at all four cardinal positions when in the vertical plane.

3.6D). This preferred firing direction was unrelated to the cell's preferred firing direction when the platform was horizontal and positioned in the center of the room. These data suggest that the HD cells switched from a room reference frame when the board was in the horizontal position, to an apparatus reference frame when the board was in the vertical plane.

These results differ from those of Stackman et al. (2000) described previously, because the cells responded with the same preferred firing direction with respect to the platform in each of the cardinal wall positions. One hypothesis that would be consistent with the two experiments is that the animals in the tall cylinder experiments were using the room as a reference frame, while the animals in the spiral track task were using the platform/spiral as the reference frame. Using the platform/spiral as a reference frame, despite the fact that the entire landmark-filled room was still in view, was an unexpected result. It is possible that the difference between the two tasks is due to the rat locomoting itself from the floor to wall, in the tall cylinder task, whereas in the spiral track experiment, the rat was picked up from the floor and placed in the vertical plane and onto the spiral track by the experimenter. Future studies will test this hypothesis by repeating these experiments, win the rat locomoting from the floor onto the spiral track via a ramp.

Upside-Down, Inverted Locomotion

In the third series of experiments, we monitored HD cell activity when the animal was locomoting upside down on a ceiling (Calton and Taube, 2005). Food-restricted rats were trained to run around a 1.22 m × 1.22 m × 30.5 cm wide, square ring track that was oriented vertically (figure 3.7A). Each surface contained a wire mesh (25 cm wide) to allow the rats to grasp it and climb on. The floor surface was divided into two compartments. When the rat was in one floor compartment, the only way it could reach the other floor compartment was to climb up the wall, traverse the ceiling, then climb down the other wall. Food was available in only one floor compartment, and the rat started in the other floor compartment. The amount of food reward was limited so that once the rat reached the goal, it had to run back to the original compartment to get additional food. Thus, the rat learned to shuttle back and forth between the two floor compartments by traversing the walls and ceiling. The apparatus was centered in a white-colored square room in which a large black curtain hung from one wall. The purpose of the curtain was to provide a salient orienting cue for the rat. The apparatus could be rotated in the azimuthal plane so that we could examine HD cell responses, either when the preferred direction was aligned with the plane of the apparatus, or when the preferred direction was orthogonal to it. In addition to the ceiling-mounted video camera, three additional cameras were mounted alongside the apparatus to view the ceiling and the two vertical ladders.

A total of 24 HD cells in the ADN were recorded from five rats. Results showed two categories of responses. Some HD cells showed robust direction-specific firing while the animal locomoted upright on the floor and walls, but a loss of direction-specific firing when the animal was locomoting upside down on the ceiling (figure 3.7B). Although nondirectional, these cells displayed a general increase in their overall background firing rate when the rat was inverted on the ceiling. Whether this pattern of firing indicates that the animal lost its sense of orientation when on the ceiling is unclear, and it will be interesting to determine whether animals perform poorly on spatial tasks when HD cell discharge loses direction-specific firing. For a second class of cells, the directional tuning was maintained, albeit weaker and with a decreased peak firing rate and increased background firing level, in a room-centered reference frame when the animal locomoted upside down. Thus, these cells' preferred directions remained aligned with respect to the room,

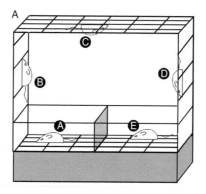

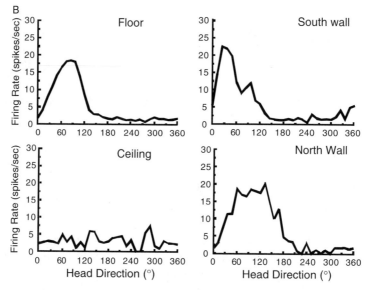

Figure 3.7
HD cell responses when the rat is inverted on the ceiling. (A) Square ring apparatus composed of wire mesh. The rat started in compartment A and proceeded to climb the vertical wall (B), then traversed the ceiling (C) and climbed down the opposite wall (D) in order to retrieve a food reward in compartment E. (B) Example of a HD cell response that lost direction-specific firing when the rat was inverted (Ceiling), but not on the two vertical walls (North and South). The tuning curve on the Floor is composed of time spent in compartments A and E.

as they discharged in the same direction as when the rat was on the floor. These results are consistent with the hemi-torus model. As with the first category of HD cell responses, cell activity on the walls was dependent on the direction from which the rat approached the wall when on the floor. If it approached the wall from the cell's preferred direction, then cell firing continued as the rat locomoted up the first wall and down the second wall. Conversely, if the rat approached the vertical surface from a head orientation that was not facing the cell's preferred direction, then the cell did not fire as the rat traversed both walls, up or down. Given that rats live in burrows and their natural habitat consequently involves three-dimensional space, it is surprising that so many HD cells lost their directional tuning when upside down. It is possible that, although they live in a three-dimensional world, they do not frequently invert themselves, and thus an upside-down orientation would be unfamiliar to them. It would be interesting to determine whether rats that frequently experience inverted orientations develop better directionally tuned HD cells over time.

As previously discussed, one model for how the HD system defines the horizontal reference frame is by using the plane in which the animal is currently locomoting. Thus, when the rat locomotes onto a vertical wall from the floor, it defines the vertical wall as its "azimuthal plane of locomotion," and HD tuning curves appear similar to tuning curves when the rat is on the floor. This model would then predict that when the rat locomotes onto the ceiling from the wall, it would translate the horizontal plane onto the ceiling surface, albeit inverted, and that directional cell firing should be maintained while it is on the inverted surface. However, our data showing that direction-specific activity was disrupted when the rat was upside down on the ceiling contradicts this prediction, and suggests that the model will need to be modified.

Sensing Up and Down

Closely related to one's sense of direction in the azimuthal plane is the sense of direction for up and down. Our sense of up/down (or static tilt) with respect to gravity results from the synthesis of available gravireceptor and visual cues, as demonstrated by the classic tilted room and rod-and-frame experiments of Witkin and Asch (1948a,b). Mittelstaedt (1982) proposed that three factors must be considered when determining the subjective sense of vertical: (1) the gravitational vector (**B**) as determined by information from the vestibular otoliths (although nonvestibular organs could also contribute, e.g., receptors within blood vessels as well as the kidney that detect fluid shifts in the body; (Mittlelstaedt, 1992); (2) the perceived longitudinal body axis, which is referred to as the idiotropic vector (**M**), and (3) the visual reference frame represented as a visual vector (**V**). Mittelstaedt postulated that the three factors or vectors summed in some weighted fashion (**B** + **M** + **V**) to yield an overall sense of up-down.

In turn, the visual polarity vector is determined by four components of the visual scene: (1) orientation of the main axes within the visual scene, (2) intrinsic polarity, (3) extrinsic polarity, and (4) visual motion (Howard and Childerson, 1994; Howard and Hu, 2001). Briefly, the orientation of the main axes within a visual scene is defined by the major orthogonal lines and surfaces in the room or environment, such as the orientation of the walls, floor, and ceiling. Intrinsic polarity refers to the orientation of objects within the visual scene that can be associated with tops and bottoms—examples include tables, chairs, trees, houses, and cars. Certain large-scale objects can also be included in this category, such as the ground, sky, and bodies of water (lakes). Extrinsic polarity refers to the spatial relationships between objects. Examples in this category include a lamp on a table, any small object being supported by the surface of a second (usually larger) object, a falling object, or an object hanging from the ceiling of the room. A sense of up/down can also be inferred from visual motion, where even a rotating scene lacking frame and polarity cues can induce perceived tilt (Held et al., 1975). The tilt illusion is stronger when the head is tilted away from the vertical or upside down (Young et al., 1975; Howard et al., 1988).

HD Cell Responses in Three Dimensions in Zero-g Parabolic Flight

Astronauts working in 0 g often experience a phenomenon known as visual reorientation illusions (VRIs). To understand this phenomenon, imagine the cabin of an orbiting spacecraft, where gravity receptor cues are absent and the notion of a "gravitational down" becomes meaningless. In this situation, astronauts usually speak of "visual down" by referencing the interior architecture of the spacecraft. When they float with their feet towards the spacecraft "floor," crew members rarely feel disoriented. However, Space Shuttle astronauts have reported that, when working upside down (relative to their normal 1-g orientation in training), or when right side up but viewing another crew member floating upside down, they frequently experience a sudden change in the direction of the perceived vertical (Oman et al., 1984). This perceptual change in the direction of "down" is referred to as a VRI (Oman et al., 1986, 1988). In this striking illusion, the surrounding walls, ceiling, and floors seem to exchange subjective identities. For example, crew members facing the ceiling or floor sometimes feel "upright." Spacewalking astronauts working upside down in the Space Shuttle payload bay have described looking up at the earth, experienced a VRI, and suddenly feared they would fall "down" to earth. The sudden change in perceived orientation (without concomitant vestibular motion cues) can trigger attacks of space motion sickness, cause reaching errors, and can make it more difficult for crew members to recognize landmark objects. VRIs often occur spontaneously, but are labile, and can be cognitively manipulated. VRIs happen because of the idiotropic tendency to assume that the surface beneath one's own feet is a floor, and because other people are normally seen in a gravitationally upright position. Headward fluid shift and gravireceptor unweighting are believed also to contribute to VRIs, and make some astronauts feel continuously inverted ("inversion illusion") (Matsnev et al., 1983; Oman et al., 1986; Lackner, 1992). VRIs can also occur on earth, such as when we exit the subway, and discover we are facing in an unexpected direction. The equivalent of a VRI is presumed to occur in rats when they return to a familiar environment after having locomoted from a novel environment, where the preferred firing direction of a recorded HD cell is shifted relative to the direction of the familiar environment (Taube and Burton, 1995). The shift in preferred firing direction usually occurs abruptly, and is suggested to be the neuro-physological correlate of the VRI (see chapter 7 by Stackman and Zugaro). In humans, VRIs are analogous to figure reversal illusions (e.g., Necker cube), except that it is the person's own subjective orientation that changes, rather than the perceived orientation or identity of the object.

Because VRIs are frequently debilitating in space and often lead to reaching errors, it is important to understand their underlying neural mechanisms, with the hope that this information will lead to the development of effective countermeasures. Thus, Taube and colleagues (Taube et al., 2004) were interested in determining how HD cells respond in 0 g when the rat locomotes in different three-dimensional planes. Specifically, do HD cells continue to respond in 0 g similarly the way they respond in 1 g? Do the three-dimensional response characteristics become more labile in 0 g, since the gravitational "down" reference is absent? Does the azimuthal response plane align with the plane of locomotion or with the visual reference frame? Finally, would HD cells occasionally shift their preferred direction 180° when the rat was upside down on the ceiling? This type of response would be consistent with the rat undergoing a VRI, and is similar to responses in astronauts who report perceiving themselves as upside down and their directional heading reversed by 180°.

To address these issues, the authors monitored HD cells during several periods of 0 g conditions during parabolic flight. Unrestrained rats locomoted in a clear rectangular, Plexiglas cage that had wire mesh covering the floor, ceiling, and one wall (figure 3.8A). The cage was visually up-down symmetrical, and surrounding environmental cues were arranged so that up-down visual cues were ambiguous. Because the 0-g conditions obtained in parabolic flight are brief (15–20 s), experiments had to be designed to get the rats to sample as many directions as possible within this short time period. The authors gently nudged the rats into different orientations within the cage. Seven HD cells were recorded from ADN across six rats, with generally consistent responses observed across all cells. Each HD cell was monitored across about 40 episodes of 0 g and the rats' movements were videotaped. All cells maintained their direction-specific discharge when a rat was on the cage floor during the 0 g and 1.8 g pull-out periods. However, direction-specific firing was usually disrupted when the rats were placed on the ceiling or wall, and there was no single direction at which the cells fired (figure 3.8B). There also appeared to be an increase in background firing. The loss of directional tuning upside down on the ceiling occurred whether the investigators were upright or inverted with respect to the aircraft. At least two cells consistently responded during some parabolas when the rat's head was oriented 180° opposite the preferred direction of the cell when the rat was on

A

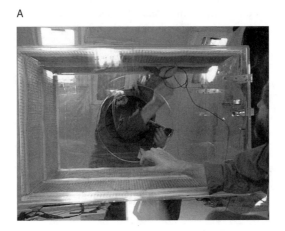

B

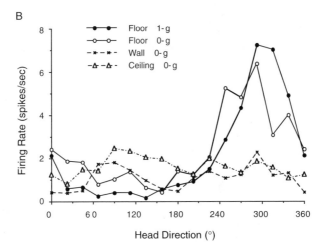

Figure 3.8
HD cell responses in 0-g parabolic flight. (A) Apparatus used for recording HD cells in parabolic flight. Wire
mesh covered the floor, one wall, and the ceiling. (B) HD cell responses when the rat locomoted on the floor in
1-g and when it locomoted on the floor, wall, or ceiling in 0-g. Note that the cell only maintained direction-
specific firing on the floor surface in 0-g. Cell activity on the wall and ceiling in 0-g was increased compared to
the floor but was not directional.

the floor. These responses suggest that during these particular parabolas the rats maintained a normal allocentric frame of reference in 0 g and 1 g when on the floor, but when placed on the ceiling or wall in 0 g, the rats appeared to be disoriented (as judged by the loss of directional specificity in HD cell firing). The occasional reversal of HD cell preferred direction across the cage axis of symmetry suggests that the rats may have experienced a VRI.

Were the rats disoriented when HD cells' activity lost their direction-specific responses on the wall and ceiling in 0 g? For that matter, were the rats in the vertical, square ring track experiments previously described disoriented on the ceiling when HD cell activity became non-directional and there was a general increase in background firing? In both conditions, HD cells increased their tonic background firing rate rather than becoming silent. This pattern of activity is similar to that observed when rats are spun blindfolded on a turntable for 1 min and are presumably disoriented during the rotations (for further discussion of HD cell responses when rats are disoriented, see chapter 11 by Dudchenko et al.). These results suggest that HD cells lost their direction-specific firing on the ceiling in both 0 g and 1 g, and on the wall in 0 g, because the animals were explicitly disoriented. Alternatively, perceptual disorientation may arise because of the loss of directional activity in HD cells.

Conclusions

HD cells receive and utilize information from both external landmark cues and internal cues concerned with their movements. The use of visual landmarks for controlling the directional tuning can occur quickly with brief exposures to the cue. Although salient visual landmark information usually overrides information from idiothetic sources, internal cues can predominate when the visual landmarks are perceived as unstable or there is a large disparity between information from the two cue sources. HD cells maintain their direction-specific firing when the animal is in a vertical plane, but usually lose their directional tuning when the animal is inverted.

Acknowledgments

This work was supported by National Institute of Mental Health grants MH48924 and MH01286, and a grant from the National Space Biomedical Research Institute through NASA Cooperative Agreement NCC 9-58. I would also like to thank the many colleagues and students who actually conducted all the experiments that are discussed here, including: Jeffrey Calton, Paul Dudchenko, Edward Golob, Jeremy Goodridge, Stanley Kim, Robert Muller, Charles Oman, Robert Stackman, Matthew Tullman, Kimberly Worboys, and of course James Ranck Jr, who discovered head direction cells.

References

Alyan SH, Jànder R (1994) Short-range homing in the house mouse, Mus musculus: stages in the learning of directions. Animal Behav 48: 285–298.

Barlow JS (1964) Inertial navigation as a basis for animal navigation. J Theoretical Biol 6: 76–117.

Biegler R, Morris RGM (1993) Landmark stability is a prerequisite for spatial but not discrimination learning. Nature 361: 631–633.

Calton JL, Taube JS (2005) Degradation of head direction cell activity during inverted locomotion. J Neurosci, in press.

Chen LL, Lin LH, Barnes CA, McNaughton BL (1994) Head direction cells in the rat posterior cortex. II. Contributions of visual and ideothetic information to the directional firing. Exp Brain Res 101: 24–34.

Cheng K (1986) A purely geometric module in the rat's spatial representation. Cognition 23: 149–178.

Dudchenko PA, Goodridge JP, Seiterle DA, Taube JS (1997a) Effects of repeated disorientation on the acquisition of two spatial reference memory tasks in rats: dissociation between the radial arm maze and the Morris water maze. J Exp Psych: Animal Behav Processes 23: 194–210.

Dudchenko PA, Goodridge JP, Taube JS (1997b) The effects of disorientation on visual landmark control of head direction cell orientation. Exp Brain Res 115: 375–380.

Etienne AS, Lambert SJ, Reverdin B, Teroni E (1993) Learning to recalibrate the role of dead reckoning and visual cues in spatial navigation. Animal Learn Beh 21: 266–280.

Gallistel CR (1990) The Organization of Learning. Cambridge, MA: MIT Press.

Goodridge JP, Dudchenko PA, Worboys KA, Golob EJ, Taube JS (1998) Cue control and head direction cells. Beh Neurosci 112: 749–761.

Goodridge JP, Taube JS (1995) Preferential use of the landmark navigational system by head direction cells. Behav Neurosci 109: 49–61.

Held R, Dichgans J, Bauer J (1975) Characteristics of moving visual areas influencing spatial orientation. Science 141: 722–723.

Hermer L, Spelke E (1994) A geometric process for reorientation in children. Nature 370: 57–59.

Howard IP, Cheung BSK, Landolt J (1988) Influence of vection axis and body posture on visually-induced self rotation. Advisory Group for Aerospace Research and Development 433: 15-1–15-8.

Howard IP, Childerson L (1994) The contribution of motion, the visual frame, and visual polarity to sensation of body tilt. Perception 23: 753–762.

Howard IP, Hu G (2001) Visually induced reorientation illusions. Perception 30: 583–600.

Kelly JB, Glazier SJ (1978) Auditory cortex lesions and discrimination of spatial location by the rat. Brain Res 145: 315–321.

Kim SY, Frohardt RJ, Taube JS (2003) Head direction cells shift reference frames in the vertical plane. Program No. 519.19. 2003 Abstract Viewer/Itinerary Planner. Washington DC: Society for Neuroscience.

Knierim JJ, Kudrimoti HS, McNaughton BL (1995) Place cells, head direction cells, and the learning of landmark stability. J Neurosci 15: 1648–1659.

Kubie JL, Ranck JB Jr (1983) Sensory-behavioral correlates in individual hippocampus neurons in three situations: space and context. In: Neurobiology of the Hippocampus, W Seifert (Ed) Academic Press: New York, NY, pp. 433–447.

Lackner JR (1992) Spatial orientation in weightless environments. Perception 21: 803–812.

Margules J, Gallistel CR (1988) Heading in the rat: determination by environmental shape. Animal Learn Behav 16: 404–410.

Martin GM, Harley CW, Smith AR, Hoyles ES, Hynes CA (1997) Opaque transportation with rotation blocks reliable goal location on a plus maze but does not prevent goal location in the Morris maze. J Exp Psych: Animal Behav Processes 23: 183–193.

Matsnev EI, Yakovleva IY, Tarasov IK, Alekseev VN, Kornilova LN, Mateev AD, Gorgiladze GI (1983) Space motion sickness: phenomenology, countermeasures, and mechanisms. Aviat Space Environ Med 54: 312–317.

McNaughton BL, Chen LL, Markus EJ (1991) "Dead reckoning," landmark learning, and the sense of direction: a neurophysiological and computational hypothesis. J Cog Neurosci 3: 190–202.

Mittelstaedt H (1982) A new solution to the problem of the subjective vertical. Naturwissenschaften 70: 272–281.

Mittelstaedt H (1992) Somatic versus vestibular gravity reception in man. In Sensing and Controlling Motion, Ann NY Acad Sci 656: 124–139.

Mizumori SJY, Williams JD (1993) Directionally-selective mnemonic properties of neurons in the lateral dorsal nucleus of the thalamus of rats. J Neurosci 13: 4015–4028.

Muir GM, Taube JS (2002) The neural correlates of spatial navigation and performance: Do head direction and place cells guide behavior? Behav Cog Neurosci Rev 1: 297–317.

Oman CM, Lichtenberg BK, Money KE (1984) Space motion sickness monitoring experiment: spacelab 1, paper 35, NATO AGARD symposium on motion sickness: mechanisms, prediction, prevention, and treatment Williamsburg, VA, 3 May, 1984.

Oman CM, Lichtenberg BK, Money KE, McCoy RK (1986) M.I.T./Canadian vestibular experiments on the Spacelab-1 mission: 4. Space motion sickness: symptoms, stimuli, and predictability. Exp Brain Res 64: 316–334.

Oman CM, Young LR, Watt DGD, Money KE, Lichtenberg BK, Kenyon RV, Arrott AP (1988) MIT/Canadian Spacelab experiments on vestibular adaptation and space motion sickness. In JC Huang, NG Daunton and VJ Wilson, eds., Basic and Applied Aspects of Vestibular Function. Hong Kong: Hong Kong University Press, pp. 183–192.

Poucet B (1993) Spatial cognitive maps in animals: new hypotheses on their structure and neural mechanisms. Psych Rev 100: 163–182.

Redish AD, Touretzky DS (1997) Cognitive maps beyond the hippocampus. Hippocampus 7: 15–35.

Stackman RW, Taube JS (1998) Firing properties of rat lateral mammillary nuclei single units: head direction, head pitch, and angular head velocity. J Neurosci 18: 9020–9037.

Stackman RW, Tullman ML, Taube JS (2000) Maintenance of rat head direction cell firing during locomotion in the vertical plane. J Neurophysiol 83: 393–405.

Taube JS (1995) Head direction cells recorded in the anterior thalamic nuclei of freely moving rats. J Neurosci 15: 70–86.

Taube JS (1998) Head direction cells and the neurophysiological basis for a sense of direction. Prog Neurobiol 55: 225–256.

Taube JS, Burton HL (1995) Head direction cell activity monitored in a novel environment and during a cue conflict situation. J Neurophysiol 74: 1953–1971.

Taube JS, Goodridge JP, Golob EJ, Dudchenko PA, Stackman RW (1996) Processing the head direction cell signal: a review and commentary. Brain Res Bull 40: 477–486.

Taube JS, Muller RU, Ranck JB Jr (1990a) Head-direction cells recorded from the postsubiculum in freely moving rats. I. Description and quantitative analysis. J Neurosci 10: 420–435.

Taube JS, Muller RU, Ranck JB Jr (1990b) Head-direction cells recorded from the postsubiculum in freely moving rats. II. Effects of environmental manipulations. J Neurosci 10: 436–447.

Taube JS, Stackman RW, Calton JL, Oman CM (2004) Rat head direction cell responses in 0-G parabolic flight. J Neurophysiol 92: 2887–2997.

Valloritigara G, Zanforlin M, Pasti G (1990) Geometric modules in animal's spatial representations: A test with chick (*Gallus gallus domesticus*). J Comp Psych 104: 248–254.

Witkin HA, Asch SE (1948a) Studies in space orientation. II. Perception of the upright with displaced visual fields and with body tilt. J Exp Psych 38: 455–477.

Witkin HA, Asch SE (1948b) Studies in space orientation. III. Perception of the upright in the absence of a visual field. J Exp Psych 38: 603–614.

Young LR, Oman CM, Dichgans JM (1975) Influence of head orientation on visually induced pitch and roll sensation. Aviation, Space, Env Med 46: 264–269.

Zugaro MB, Arleo A, Berthoz A, Wiener SI (2003) Rapid spatial reorientation and head direction cells. J Neurosci 23: 3478–3482.

Zugaro MB, Berthoz A, Wiener SI (2001) Background, but not foreground, spatial cues are taken as reference for head direction responses by rat anterodorsal thalamus neurons. J Neurosci 21: RC154 (1–5).

4 How Visual Cues Control Preferred Directions in Head Direction Cells

Michaël B. Zugaro and Sidney I. Wiener

Head direction neuronal activity and hippocampal place responses are dominantly anchored on visual cues. These cues can influence the directional firing in two different ways. First, familiar visual landmarks can directly inform the head direction system where the head is oriented in space, the same way a photograph of a familiar place reveals in which direction the camera faced when the shot was taken. The information thus provided by the visual landmarks is akin to a head direction (an angle) and can be used to correct or reset whatever the head direction was estimated to be before this information arrived. In the head direction cell system, this corresponds to modifying the preferred directions of the cells relative to the static landmarks, and is thus referred to here as *static cue-based updating* of the preferred directions. Although it may appear from the foregoing discussion that updating takes place at specific times, e.g., when a familiar environment is entered, it is not necessarily so, as such a process could occur regularly—and even almost continuously—as the animal moves about, thus preventing the loss of orientation bearings.

On the other hand, a quite different process occurs when the apparent movement of the surrounding visual scene is used to track self-movement. This is the second way visual cues can influence the head direction system. Under normal circumstances, when a subject moves about, turning the head in one direction produces a shift of the image of the visual scene in the opposite direction. Conversely, rotations of the visual scene convey information about rotations of the head in space. In a similar way, when one watches a film, one can deduce the speed and direction in which the camera shifted and turned when the shot was taken. The information thus provided by these optic flow signals concerns a head movement, that is, angular velocities and accelerations, as opposed to a head direction angle as described in the previous paragraph. This information can be used to keep track of one's orientation during self-movements. In the head direction cell system, this corresponds to updating the active population of cells according to changes in orientation that are signaled by the flow of the visual scene during movements. This belongs to the category of *dynamic cue-based updating* of the estimated, or represented, head direction (see also chapter 15 by Duffy et al.).

The present chapter focuses on the first issue, and will describe recent efforts to better understand the neuronal processes involved in static cue-based updating of the preferred directions of head direction cells on the basis of visual information. The issues include what types of visual cues best anchor head direction cells, what mechanisms are used to select and detect such cues, and what are the neuronal circuit dynamics of the establishment and disappearance of directional activity when the subject reorients in a familiar environment. The second issue is dealt with in the chapters 7 by Stackman and Zugaro and 15 by Duffy, et al., in this volume.

Historically, the characterization of those visual cues that influence spatial responses has been most studied in hippocampal neurons. This is, of course, quite relevant to the question at hand, since the head direction neuron system is intimately linked with hippocampus anatomically and functionally (Knierim et al., 1998). Indeed, the retrosplenial cortex and postsubiculum, which are both part of the head direction system, are among the principal sources of visual inputs to the hippocampus. In recordings in which rats forage for food in cylindrical enclosures, rotation of a contrasted card along the wall induces similar rotations of firing fields and of preferred directions (Muller and Kubie, 1987; Taube et al., 1990; Taube, 1995; Zugaro et al., 2000; also see chapter 3 by Taube in this volume). Possible criteria for selection of visual cues by the hippocampus include relative distance, salience, proximity to the firing field, and configurational properties of multiple cues.

But what are the necessary and sufficient conditions to define a visual cue for these neural orienting systems? Single contrasted cards have served as useful and simple experimental tools suitable for comparing the influences of visual cues and, for instance, vestibular cues. However, outside of the laboratory the visual environment often includes numerous visual items that do not necessarily provide coherent or stable spatial information. Which visual elements are relevant for head direction cells? More precisely, what sensory features (contrast, size, distance, etc.) characterize an effective static visual cue for anchoring spatial responses? And how do the head direction cells select those visual cues that will update their preferred directions? The present chapter will summarize some recent efforts toward answering these questions.

Preferred Directions Are Anchored to Background Visual Cues

Studies in Hippocampal Neurons

In experiments in which proximal and distal cues are displaced independently, place cells show a variety of responses: their firing fields can stay fixed relative to either the distal cues, or the proximal cues, or the room; some place cells simply stop discharging (O'Keefe and Speakman, 1987; Wiener et al., 1995; Gothard et al., 1996; Tanila et al., 1997). Cressant et al. (1997) compared the responses of hippocampal place cells before and after rotation of a group of three-dimensional objects arranged in a triangular configuration within an experimental cylinder. First, each object in the array was positioned against the enclosure wall. Hippocampal place responses were recorded, then the animal was removed and disoriented while the objects were rotated by 120° along the wall. In recordings after the animal was returned, the firing fields rotated together with the objects. However, when the experiment was repeated with the group of objects placed near the center of the platform, the firing fields shifted randomly and were not bound to the objects. To account for this difference, the authors proposed that the centrally placed objects were ignored because they did not provide reliable spatial information. For example, an object could be seen either to the right or to the left of another object, depending on the position of the rat.

Studies in Head Direction Cells   This inspired us to characterize the types of visual cues that anchor anterodorsal thalamic head direction cells (Zugaro et al., 2001). We modified the experimental protocol from that of Cressant et al. (1997) to test our working hypothesis that the critical factor for cue selection is whether the cues are in the foreground or in the background. In the baseline condition, the directional responses were (as in the latter study) recorded as the rat foraged for food morsels on a circular platform bordered by a tall, black cylinder. Three-dimensional objects with distinct profiles were placed in an equilateral triangular configuration along the wall (figure 4.1). In this case, the objects were considered to be in the visual background since no room landmarks were available above the cylinder walls. Then, the rat was removed from the platform and secluded in a small, opaque container. The objects were rotated by 120°, and the floor paper was changed. To disorient the rat, all lights were turned off, and an experimenter rotated the opaque container in an erratic manner while wandering around the room. The rat was then replaced on the platform, the lights were turned back on, and a second recording session was started.

This protocol was then repeated after the cylindrical enclosure was removed. In this condition, the objects still occupied the same positions on the platform. However, the visual background now consisted of four walls of pleated black curtains at a distance of about 1 m from the edge of the circular platform.

The results were remarkably different in the two conditions. In the proximal background condition, the preferred directions in all 30 recordings shifted by the same angle as the objects (figure 4.2). However, in the distal background condition they always remained fixed relative to the room, independent of the new positions of the objects. Note that the objects remained equally salient since, in the two conditions, the rats spent the same amount of time contacting the objects. Furthermore, the olfactory and tactile cues they provided remained the same. Thus, in both conditions, the preferred directions followed the cues lying in the background. These consisted of the objects in the proximal

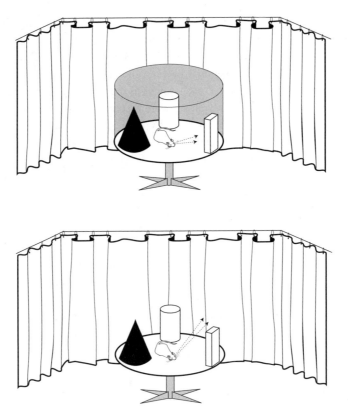

Figure 4.1
Experimental set-up. The elevated circular platform was at the center of a 3-m by 3-m room with black curtains
along the four walls. Three-dimensional objects with distinctive profiles were placed in a triangular configuration along the edge of the platform. Recordings took place in the presence and absence of a large black opaque
cylinder, which, when present, blocked the view of the room. (Top) The three-dimensional cues were in the background when the cylinder was present, but (bottom) in the foreground when the cylinder was removed. The
arrows schematically indicate the rat's view toward the background. (Adapted from Zugaro et al., 2001 with permission copyright 2001 by the Society for Neuroscience.)

background condition, and the curtains in the distal background condition. While no polarizing cues were intentionally placed on the curtains, the head direction system was apparently capable of anchoring onto the irregular pattern of alternating pleats or to some other
uncontrolled source of contrasts to which the rat visual system is sensitive. These factors
are better controlled for in the experiment described in the next section.

   The difference in efficacy of the same objects in controlling the preferred directions in
the two experimental conditions is interpreted as being due to the change in their relative
distance to the background. This criterion is functionally adaptive because stimuli that are
farthest in the background will, in general, remain more stable as the animal moves around,

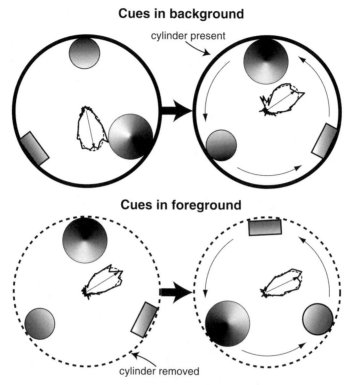

Cues in background

Cues in foreground

Figure 4.2
The cues controlled the preferred directions when in the background but not when in the foreground. Typical directional response curves (represented as polar plots) are superimposed on overhead views of the experimental apparatus. (Top) Comparisons of responses prior to and after object rotation, in the presence of the cylinder, show that the preferred direction followed these cues. (Bottom) When the cylinder was removed, the cues no longer controlled the directional responses. (Adapted from Zugaro et al., 2001 with permission copyright 2001 by the Society for Neuroscience.)

and thus will be more reliable as spatial references. This would be efficient, as well as parsimonious, since neurobiological mechanisms have been identified that automatically detect the distance of objects. The psychophysical literature (e.g., Foley, 1978) shows that relative depth in the visual field can be detected on the basis of several different stimulus attributes, including occlusion (objects blocked by others are more distant), parallax (during active displacements more distant objects appear to move less rapidly), texture contrast, shadows, vergence, accommodation, etc. Brain systems for detecting optic field flow could provide this sensitivity to the head direction system because, for example, the optokinetic system is more sensitive to optic flow at low, rather than high, velocities (Hess et al., 1989). An anatomical pathway that could convey optokinetic information to head direction cells passes via the vestibular nuclei to the dorsal tegmental nucleus of Gudden, then through the lateral mammillary nuclei, before arriving at the anterodorsal thalamic nucleus, where we recorded these responses.

Background Visual Cues Are Selected Based on Visual Motion Signals   Following up on these findings, the next experiment tested the hypothesis that anterodorsal thalamic head direction cells select background cues on the basis of visual motion signals, such as optic field flow or motion parallax (Zugaro et al., 2004). The previous experimental room was modified so that the far wall was now a smooth (unpleated) 3 m diameter cylindrical black curtain, and the rat was placed on a small 22 cm diameter elevated platform at the center. The experimental cues were two freely standing cues: a foreground card (height 60 cm, distance 36 cm), and a background card (height 240 cm, distance 144 cm) (figure 4.3). The cards were identically marked, proportionally dimensioned and subtended identical (nonoverlapping) visual angles from the central viewpoint. (Note that the foreground card, unlike proximal cues in experiments previously described, could not provide tactile or olfactory cues.) After baseline recordings, the rat was disoriented in darkness while the cards were rotated by 90° in opposite directions about the center (thus providing

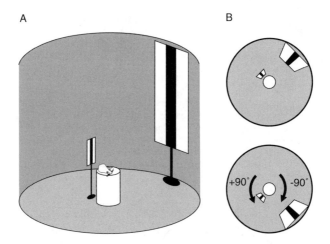

Figure 4.3
Experimental set-up and protocol. (a) The rats freely foraged for food pellets on an elevated platform (diameter 22 cm) located in the center of a room enclosed by a cylindrical black curtain (diameter 3 m). A foreground card (height 60 cm, distance 36 cm) and a background card (height 240 cm, distance 144 cm), each bearing two vertical white stripes, served as principal orienting cues. The cards' respective sizes and distances to the platform center were proportioned so that they occupied the same visual angles. (b) After an initial recording (top panel), the animal was removed from the platform, and the two cards were rotated in opposite directions (bottom panel). The rat was then disoriented in complete darkness and returned to the platform, and the light was turned back on, and a second recording began. Recording sessions including baseline and double cue rotations were conducted in continuous or stroboscopic light (flashes at 1.5 Hz). The equivalence of the intensity of reflected light from the two cards was controlled regularly with a luminance meter. (Reproduced from Zugaro et al., 2004 with permission.)

conflicting orienting cues); then the rat was returned. The preferred directions of the head direction cells were tested again to determine if they had anchored to the card in the foreground or the background. Several responses were possible. If the preferred directions were anchored (1) to the background card, they would rotate by −90°; (2) to the foreground card, they would rotate by +90°; (3) to the configuration of both cards, they would rotate by 180°, following the barycenter of the cards (i.e., if the cards were indistinguishable and an imaginary point lying between the two of them had anchored the directional response); or (4) to uncontrolled cues in the room, they would remain unchanged. Alternatively, if no environmental cue controlled the preferred directions, these would rotate by a random angle from session to session. Here, the preferred directions followed the background cue in 30 (of 53) cases, but followed the foreground cue in only five cases. (In thirteen other cases the system had an ambiguous response and was unable to distinguish between the two cards, responding as if these constituted but a single configurational orienting cue. In the remaining five cases, there was no shift relative to uncontrolled room cues.) In summary, under normal lighting conditions, the preferred directions of the head direction cells stayed anchored to the background card in the majority of the recording sessions, but only rarely followed the foreground card. Also, in a number of cases, the preferred directions followed the configuration of the two cards. This confirmed that the preferred directions of head direction cells are principally anchored to background, rather than foreground visual cues.

In the second phase of the experiment, the same baseline recording and cue shift protocol was repeated under stroboscopic lighting (flashes at 1.5 Hz). Stroboscopic lighting was intended to disrupt continuous visual inputs and block the processing of fine time-scale spatial changes in retinal stimulation triggered by self-motion, such as the relative shifts of images of the respective cards. The continuous movements of the two images across the retina could no longer be detected during head movements, and their relative distances could not be computed. As a result, this would prevent the rat's use of visual motion signals, such as motion parallax, to help distinguish background from foreground cues. Thus, under these conditions, the preferred directions of the head direction cells were expected to no longer be controlled by the background card. The results clearly corroborated this hypothesis: in this condition none of the cues dominated (Watson $U^2n = 0.11703$, $N = 51$, $p > 0.1$). Indeed, the preferred directions were equally likely to follow the background card (33%; 17 out of 51 sessions), the foreground card (27%; 14 sessions), or the configuration of both, as if the two cards were but a single cue (17 sessions) while in 3 sessions the uncontrolled room cues dominated. This indicates that visual motion inputs play a critical role in selection of anchoring cues by head direction cells. Such inputs include motion parallax signals conveying information about the relative apparent speed of movement, and hence distance, of surrounding objects during self-motion. An alternative, but related, mechanism is that head direction cells could receive critical information from the visual pathways specialized for detecting optic field flow in the extrafoveal periphery; these are most sensitive to slow movements of large areas of the visual field, which would be provided by the image of background cues on the retina. This also implies that there are interactions between systems that process static visual cues and those concerned with optic flow.

The Temporal Dynamics of Establishing Head Direction Responses

In order to better understand the functional dynamics of neuronal circuits, sensory neurophysiologists have classically employed stimulus-response latency measures. We applied this approach to head direction cells, by testing how rapidly preferred directions are updated after orienting visual cues are suddenly revealed as having rotated in the environment. Previous studies have attempted to address this question (Taube and Burton, 1995; Knierim et al., 1998; Zugaro et al., 2000; see chapter 3 by Taube). It appeared that, at least in pigmented rats (which have better vision than albino strains), the preferred directions were updated almost instantly. However, this qualitative observation could not be reliably quantified, because the experimental protocols did not permit updates occurring faster than 15 s to be reliably measured. (The experimenters had to wait for the foraging rat to orient in the preferred direction, which could take from a few to a few dozen seconds.) However, neural network simulations had predicted that preferred direction updates could be as rapid as a few hundred milliseconds (Zhang, 1996; Redish, 1999).

Our new protocol allowed this prediction to be tested (Zugaro et al., 2003; figure 4.4). The rats were trained to remain stationary while receiving small droplets of water delivered at a small reservoir at the center of the circular platform. This was done because the rats could not simply be held immobile, since physical constraint disrupts normal firing of head direction cells (see Taube et al., 1990; Knierim et al., 1995; Taube, 1995). Careful timing of the initiation of water delivery (via behavioral shaping) ensured that the animals approached the reservoir oriented in the preferred direction of the head direction cell that was being recorded. (This had been determined in a previous baseline foraging session.) From then on, the rats would remain immobile throughout the recording session, oriented in the preferred direction of the neuron. This protocol did not permit construction of the complete response curve of the head direction cell, since this would require sampling neuronal responses for each possible head direction. However, the advantage was that any changes in instantaneous firing rates that resulted from preferred direction updates could be monitored with a precision of a few milliseconds.

The apparatus was the now-classic 76 cm diameter opaque cylinder developed by Bob Muller. In order to trigger updates of directional responses in the head direction neurons, all room lights were turned off, and the contrasted card that served as the principal orienting visual cue was rotated by 90° from its reference position. (As in all of our experiments, the rats were tracked with infrared, light-emitting diodes, which did not permit the

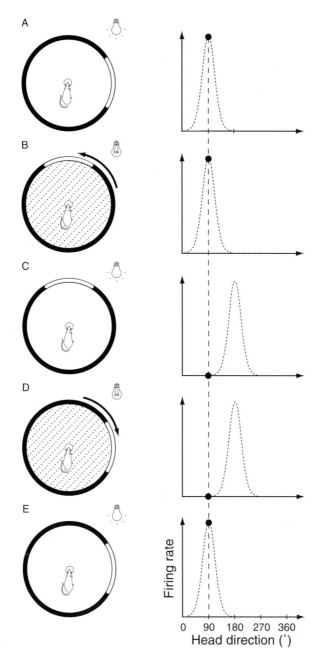

Figure 4.4
Experimental setup and protocol for testing the latency of head direction responses. (A) Because water was provided at a central reservoir, the rat remained immobile, oriented in the (previously determined) preferred direction of the neuron being recorded. A schematic of the neuron's response is shown at right; only the peak of the directional response curve is measured. (B) The lights are turned off and the cue card is rotated by +90°. The cell continues firing because this shift is not yet detected. (C) The lights are turned back on. The active cells stop firing and a new subpopulation corresponding to the new orientation relative to the card becomes active. (D) and (E) The protocol is repeated in the opposite sense, reactivating the neurons corresponding to the initial state. The protocol is then repeated until satiation occurs. (Adapted with permission from Zugaro et al., 2004.)

rats to see that this rotation was taking place.) The head direction cell continued to fire in darkness while the rat's head remained immobile. After the light was turned back on, firing rate changes were monitored as the cells responded to the new position of the card. Then, the lights were turned off again, the card was rotated back to its reference position, and firing rate changes were monitored after the lights were turned back on (see figure 4.3). The protocol was then repeated until the satiated rat moved away from the reservoir.

In order to analyze the latency of firing rate changes, two complementary approaches were used. The first method pooled all the action potentials emitted by all the head direction cells just before and just after light onset, i.e., during a small time interval when preferred direction updates were expected to occur. Assuming that all the cells respond in a similar manner, summing all responses smooths out variability in individual spike trains and makes the firing rate transition more readily visible (figure 4.5). This method yielded the following surprising result: The new preferred directions are established as rapidly as 80 ms after the contrasted card appears in its new orientation. Cells firing for the previous orientation become silent slightly more slowly, in 140 ms. The second approach consisted of examining the time course of firing rate changes on a trial-by-trial basis. This case-by-case analysis (in contrast with the first population sum analysis) showed that update latencies were indeed reproducible across cells, sessions, and animals, and confirmed the former results.

These results show that preferred-direction updates benefit from very rapid processing of visual signals in this familiar environment. This is consistent with the fact that the anterodorsal thalamic nucleus receives direct projections from the retina (Itaya et al., 1981; Ahmed et al., 1996), as well as indirect projections from the visual cortex via the postsubiculum (Vogt and Miller, 1983) and the retrosplenial cortex (Reep et al., 1994), and that visual stimulation of the retina evokes field potentials in the primary visual cortex with delays as brief as 40 ms (Galambos et al., 2000). Although rapid preferred-direction updates were predicted by neural network simulations (e.g., Zhang, 1996), the latencies found here were an order of magnitude briefer than expected from these predictions. This may be explained by the observation that, at the time of the experiments, all existing models of head direction cells used neurons whose activity was coded as a continuous value of the firing rate (rate coding), rather than neurons simulating actual action potentials that provide more veridical simulations of the dynamical properties of biological neural circuits.

This type of experiment could shed light on the question of how activity is propagated in the head direction cell circuit following shifts between one head orientation and another. Is there a simple extinction of activity of one group of neurons and activation of another group, or is there a wave of activation of neurons selective for directions intermediate between the initial and final states? Recently, Degris et al. (2004) developed a new model of the head direction system using integrate-and-fire formal neurons. In this model, state transitions could occur as rapidly as was demonstrated experimentally in AD thalamic

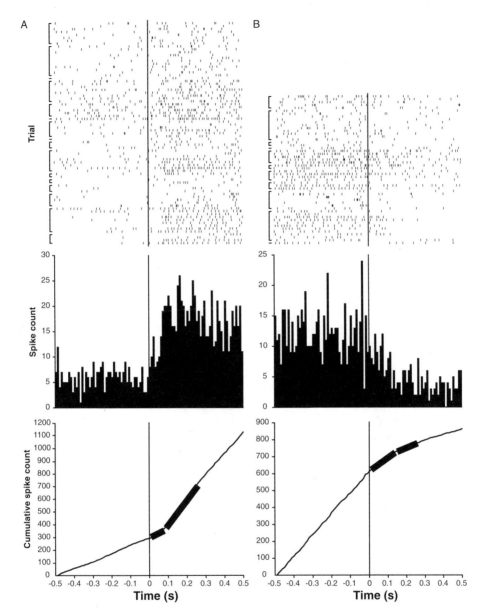

Figure 4.5

Latency of preferred direction updates in HD cells. Raster plots (top), peri-event histograms (middle), and cumulative histograms (bottom) (binwidth: 10 ms) of action potentials recorded from all of the HD cells analysed. Time zero indicates when the lights were turned on again. After light onset, the preferred directions return to their initial orientations (A), or shift to the rotated (nonpreferred) orientations (B). In order to determine the average latency of the preferred direction update, least squares estimates were computed from the cumulative histograms using the first 250 ms of data after light onset (thick curves). Transition points are at 80 ± 10 ms (A) for returns to the preferred orientation and 140 ± 10 ms (B) for shifts to the nonpreferred orientation. Brackets indicate trials from the same cell within a given session; the variations in spike density among the rows of rasters reflect differences in peak and background firing rates among the neurons. (Adapted with permission from Zugaro et al., 2003 copyright 2003 by the Society for Neuroscience.)

head direction cells. The model also predicts that the dynamics of these transitions should change, depending on the angle of rotation of the orienting visual cues: for rotations smaller than 70°, the activity profile is expected to briefly activate cells selective for the intermediate heading angles before arriving at the final state, while for larger rotations it should jump abruptly to the state corresponding to the new orientation. Further experimental studies will be required to determine if this dichotomy is present in real head direction cells.

While all of these studies provide some initial insights into how visual signals are processed in the head direction system, they also provoke new questions for future investigations. Can we track where the different types of visual information enter the head direction system and how they are transmitted to the respective structures in the network? Do these results concerning cue selection also apply to hippocampal place cell activity and if so, what are the respective roles of the hippocampal and the head direction cells in this process? Are neural mechanisms of distinguishing background from foreground, other than motion parallax, also employed for selecting anchoring visual cues? What precisely are the neural pathways that transmit these signals to the head direction system?

Acknowledgments

Thanks to our colleagues for their valuable participation in these studies: A. Arleo, C. Dejean, and A. Berthoz. This work was supported by the CNRS-NSF cooperation program, CNRS, ACI du Ministère de la Recherche, GIS. Thanks to Drs. N. Brunel, J. Droulez, and A. Reber for helpful discussions, F. Maloumian for illustrations, M.-A. Thomas and S. Doutremer for histology. M.B.Z. received a grant from the Fondation pour la Recherche Médicale.

References

Ahmed AK, Guison NG, Yamadori T (1996) A retrograde fluorescent-labeling study of direct relationship between the limbic (anterodorsal and anteroventral thalamic nuclei) and the visual system in the albino rat. Brain Res 729: 119–123.

Cressant A, Muller RU, Poucet B (1997) Failure of centrally placed objects to control the firing fields of hippocampal place cells. J Neurosci 17: 2531–2542.

Degris T, Brunel N, Wiener SI, Arleo A (2004) Rapid response of head direction cells to reorienting visual cues: A computational model. Neurocomputing 58–60c: 675–682.

Foley JM (1978) Primary distance perception, in R Held, HW Leibowitz and H-L Teuber eds., Handbook of Sensory Physiology, Vol. VIII, chap 6, Perception, Berlin: Springer-Verlag, pp. 181–213.

Galambos R, Szabo-Salfay O, Barabas P, Palhalmi J, Szilagyi N, Juhasz G (2000) Temporal distribution of the ganglion cell volleys in the normal rat optic nerve. Proc Nat Acad Sci (USA) 97: 13454–13459.

Gothard KM, Skaggs WE, Moore KM, McNaughton BL (1996) Binding of hippocampal CA1 neural activity to multiple reference frames in a landmark-based navigation task. J Neurosci 16: 825–835.

Hess BJM, Blanks RHI, Lannou J, Precht W (1989) Effects of kainic acid lesions of the nucleus reticularis tegmenti pontis on fast and slow phases of vestibulo-ocular and optokinetic reflexes in the pigmented rat. Exp Brain Res 74: 63–80.

Itaya SK, Van Hoesen GW, Jenq CB (1981) Direct retinal input to the limbic system of the rat. Brain Res 226: 33–42.

Knierim JJ, Kudrimoti H, McNaughton BL (1995) Hippocampal place fields, the internal compass, and the learning of landmark stability. J Neurosci 15: 1648–1659.

Knierim JJ, Kudrimoti H, McNaughton BL (1998) Interaction between idiothetic cues and external landmarks in the control of place cells and head direction cells. J Neurophys 80: 425–446.

Muller RU, Kubie JL (1987) The effects of changes in the environment on the spatial firing of hippocampal complex-spike cells. J Neurosci 7: 1951–1968.

O'Keefe J, Speakman A (1987) Single unit activity in the rat hippocampus during a spatial memory task. Exp Brain Res 68: 1–27.

Redish AD (1999) Beyond the Cognitive Map, from Place Cells to Episodic Memory, London: MIT Press-Bradford Books.

Reep RL, Chandler HC, King V, Corwin JV (1994) Rat posterior parietal cortex: topography of corticocortical and thalamic connections. Exp Brain Res 100: 67–84.

Tanila H, Shapiro ML, Eichenbaum H (1997) Discordance of spatial representation in ensembles of hippocampal place cells. Hippocampus 7: 613–623.

Taube JS (1995) Head direction cells recorded in the anterior thalamic nuclei of freely moving rats. J Neurosci 15: 70–86.

Taube JS, Burton HL (1995) Head direction cell activity monitored in a novel environment and during a cue conflict situation. J Neurophysiol 74: 1953–1971.

Taube JS, Muller RU, Ranck JB Jr (1990) Head-direction cells recorded from the postsubiculum in freely moving rats. II. Effects of environmental manipulations. J Neurosci 10: 436–447.

Vogt BA, Miller MW (1983) Cortical connections between rat cingulate cortex and visual, motor, and postsubicular cortices. J Comp Neurol 216: 192–210.

Wiener SI, Korshunov VA, Garcia R, Berthoz A (1995) Inertial, substratal and landmark cue control of hippocampal CA1 place cell activity. Eur J Neurosci 7: 2206–2219.

Zhang K (1996) Representation of spatial orientation by the intrinsic dynamics of the head-direction ensemble: a theory. J Neurosci 16: 2112–2126.

Zugaro MB, Arleo A, Berthoz A, Wiener SI (2003) Rapid spatial reorientation and head direction cells. J Neurosci 23: 3478–3482.

Zugaro MB, Arleo A, Dejean C, Burguière E, Khamassi M, Wiener SI (2004) Rat anterodorsal thalamic head direction neurons depend on dynamic visual signals to select anchoring distal cues. Eur J Neuro Sci 20: 530–536.

Zugaro MB, Berthoz A, Wiener SI (2001) Background, but not foreground, spatial cues are taken as references for head direction responses by rat anterodorsal thalamus neurons. J Neurosci 21: RC154, 1–5.

Zugaro MB, Tabuchi E, Wiener SI (2000) Influence of conflicting visual, inertial and substratal cues on head direction cell activity. Exp Brain Res 133: 198–208.

5 Head Direction Signal Generation: Ascending and Descending Information Streams

Joshua P. Bassett and Jeffrey S. Taube

Head direction cells hold considerable appeal as a neurobiological model system because they appear to represent a nexus between sensory and cognitive representations in the brain. Characteristic HD cell behavior requires integration of diverse sensory information, yet is sustainable in conditions of impoverished or conflicting cues. For instance, early studies of HD cells demonstrated that, while the HD signal was responsive to cues in the visual environment, it could maintain directional stability without them (Taube et al., 1990b). Two categories of sensory cues—stable environmental features (allothetic) versus self-generated motion (ideothetic)—broadly correspond to the kinds of information hypothesized to be necessary for spatial orientation, and to distinct neural pathways proposed to subserve that information. In this chapter we adopt a basic framework along these same lines. There is now considerable evidence that the HD signal arises from an ascending pathway originating in the vestibular end organs that continuously contributes information about self-generated movement in the environment. This ascending stream of ideothetic information converges with a descending stream of highly processed visual, multimodal, and mnemonic signals about objects, landmarks, and scenes in the environment. This descending stream of allothetic information may follow several possible anatomical pathways. By integrating one stream with the other, the HD system can update the organism's directional heading relative to stable environmental cues.

This chapter will review the experimental evidence for viewing HD cell activity as the result of a confluence of ascending ideothetic and descending allothetic information streams, including relevant anatomical data that suggests a physical segregation of the streams, and physiological and lesion studies that reveal the kind of information processed by these two streams. It is important to note that the concept of ascending and descending streams is illustrative, and only approximates the complex anatomical and computational reality. For example, like all sensory cues, visual environmental cues must first ascend from peripheral sense organs. For present purposes, we start with the descending stream only after elaborate higher-order processing has transformed visual input into signals corresponding to objects, scenes, and memories.

The Ascending Stream

A series of combined recording and lesion studies has supported the view that the HD signal arises in several connected structures as a "stream," or a roughly sequential iteration of HD information that can be interrupted by lesions made presynaptically to the recording site. Current evidence supports a framework for this ascending stream that ultimately begins at the peripheral vestibular organs and associated brainstem nuclei (i.e., medial vestibular nucleus and nucleus prepositus hypoglossi), and projects rostrally in the brain toward limbic structures associated with spatial cognition. Because HD cells signal head orientation in the yaw plane, the semicircular canals and medial vestibular nucleus (MVN) are the main focus at the origin of the stream, although it is unlikely that they act in complete isolation from the otoliths and other vestibular nuclei. The MVN projects to a closely associated adjacent structure, the nucleus prepositus hypoglossi (NPH), and this structure in turn projects to the dorsal tegmental nucleus of Gudden (DTN) in the midbrain. The DTN is the first site in the hypothesized processing sequence where directional firing has been identified, and it is the caudal node in a prominent reciprocal loop between DTN and the lateral mammillary nuclei (LMN). HD cell firing is present in the LMN and the anterodoral thalamic nucleus (ADN) to which it projects, and the ADN in turn is thought to project HD information to the postsubiculum (PoS) and retrosplenial cortex. In brief, then, the ascending stream follows approximately the following sequence: semicircular canals → medial vestibular nucleus → nucleus prepositus hypoglossi → dorsal tegmental nucleus of Gudden → lateral mammillary nuclei → anterodorsal thalamic nucleus → postsubiculum → entorhinal cortex. The retrosplenial cortex receives inputs from both the ADN and PoS and sends reciprocal connections back to these same structures. This circuit is outlined schematically with reference to anatomical landmarks in figure 5.1A.

While we emphasize here the rostral projection of the system from the periphery and brainstem, historically speaking, the circuit was traced backwards along this path. Head direction cells were first discovered in the postsubiculum (PoS) (Ranck, 1984; Taube et al., 1990a). Since then, investigators have been guided by the anatomical literature to discover HD cells in the laterodorsal thalamic nucleus (LDN) (Mizumori and Williams, 1993), the anterodorsal thalamic nucleus (ADN) (Taube, 1995), and the lateral mammillary nucleus (LMN) (Blair et al., 1998; Stackman and Taube, 1998) (see chapter 2 by Hopkins in this volume for a detailed discussion of the anatomy of this HD circuit). The PoS is anatomically situated at an important point with regard to afferent information entering the hippocampus, a structure that is critical for both mnemonic and spatial

A. Ascending Stream

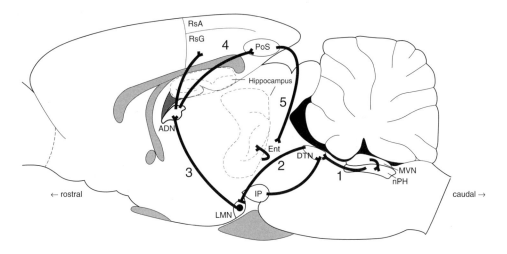

B. Descending Stream

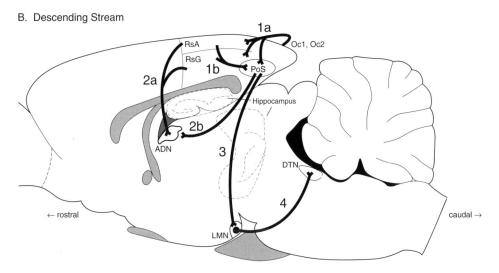

Figure 5.1
Anatomical pathways for the ascending and descending streams shown in a mid-sagital view of rat brain. (A) The ascending stream: (1)Velocity information enters the stream from the vestibular end organs and flows from the medial vestibular nucleus (MVN) to the nucleus prepositus hypoglossi (NPH), which projects to the dorsal tegmental nucleus of Gudden (DTN). Other subcortical structures, such as the interpeduncular nucleus (IP), project to the DTN as well, although their contribution to HD cell activity is unknown. (2) The lateral mammillary nuclei (LMN) are major targets for DTN projections, which are largely inhibitory. (3) The LMN project bilaterally to ADN. (4) ADN projects to the granular (RsG), but not the agranular (RsA) retrosplenial cortex, and to the postsubiculm (PoS). (5) PoS projects to the superficial layers of entorhinal cortex (Ent), which is the major source of input to the hippocampus. (B) The descending stream: (1) Cortical inputs enter PoS from visual (a) and retrosplenial cortex (b). (2) Cortically processed information descends to ADN from PoS (2a) and directly from retrosplenial cortex (2b). (3) PoS also projects to LMN, which does not receive afferents from ADN. (4) LMN neurons project back to DTN; some of these also send collaterals to ADN cells. Other abbreviations: Oc1, Oc2: occipital cortex (visual) areas 1 and 2. (Modified from Paxinos and Watson 1998.)

information processing (O'Keefe and Nadel, 1978). The PoS sends major projections to the superficial layers of entorhinal cortex, which in turn is a principal source of input to the hippocampus proper via the perforant and alveolar pathways (Amaral and Witter, 1995). In addition to the hippocampus, place cells have been identified in the superficial layers of the entorhinal cortex (Quirk et al., 1992).

Anatomical studies show that the PoS has reciprocal connections with the ADN and LDN (van Groen and Wyss, 1990a; Thompson and Robertson, 1987a,b). Goodridge and Taube (1997) demonstrated with complementary lesion and recording experiments that HD cell firing in the PoS depends on an intact ADN. In animals with complete bilateral lesions of ADN, no directional activity was encountered among 348 cells isolated in the PoS. One HD cell recorded in an animal with incomplete lesions had an atypically broad directional firing range. On the other hand, ADN HD cell firing persisted following lesions to the PoS, albeit with some abnormal features: moderately wider directional firing range, intrasession drift in some instances, and poor control by landmark cues. In contrast, Golob et al. (1998) demonstrated that a similar relationship did not exist between PoS and LDN. Electrolytic and neurotoxic lesions of LDN produced no marked effects on PoS HD cell firing, such as changes in peak firing rates, directional firing ranges, stability, or cue control. Because the LDN does not receive projections from LMN or ADN, it is presumed that HD cell activity in LDN is driven by projections from either PoS or retrosplenial cortex. For more discussion of LDN HD cell properties and their hypothesized role in spatial behavior, see chapter 10 by Mizumori, et al.

Another important issue that these lesion experiments address is the origin of the anticipatory firing properties observed for ADN HD cells (Blair and Sharp, 1995; Taube and Muller, 1998; see chapter 1 by Sharp). Temporal analyses of ADN, LMN, and retrosplenial HD cells, but not PoS HD cells, reveal that the cell's peak firing rate is reached before the head passes through the preferred firing direction. Thus, the cell's activity appears to anticipate where the head will be in the near future. For example, for a cell with a preferred firing direction at 50°, cell firing is highest at directions slightly less than 50° for counterclockwise (CCW) head turns and slightly more than 50° for clockwise (CW) head turns. The amount of time by which peak firing leads head direction, referred to as the anticipatory time interval (ATI), is about 25 ms for HD cells in the ADN. Lesions of either the PoS or hippocampus do not abolish or significantly reduce the ATI in ADN HD cells (Goodridge and Taube, 1997; Golob et al., 1998), indicating that neither the PoS, nor the hippocampus, is required for generating the anticipatory properties of ADN HD cells. In fact, ATI values were a little higher in ADN HD cells following PoS lesions, suggesting that this descending pathway constrains anticipation in intact animals.

Following these initial lesion studies, ADN HD cell activity was shown to depend on an intact LMN (Blair et al., 1998; Tullman and Taube, 1998), with Blair et al. (1999) demonstrating, in addition, some lateralized specificity in ADN directional responses following unilateral lesions. Blair et al. (1998) had previously reported LMN HD cells firing in a narrower directional range during head turns in the direction of the recording-site hemisphere (ipsiversive) than during head turns in the direction opposite to the recording-site hemisphere (contraversive). Following unilateral lesions to LMN, HD cells in ADN exhibited this same tendency, which was absent in intact animals. From this result, they concluded that the midline-crossing projections from LMN to ADN were essential to the symmetrical firing rate versus HD tuning curves found for normal ADN HD cells.

The complementary experiment, recording HD cells in LMN after ADN lesions, has not yet been performed, but given the anatomy of the system, one would predict that ADN lesions would be no more disruptive to LMN HD cell firing than PoS lesions are to ADN, that is, directional firing should persist with possible changes in cue control and anticipatory firing. However, because the LMN receives projections from the PoS, this pathway could influence HD cell activity in as-yet-undetermined ways.

Once investigators had demonstrated the importance of the LMN to the HD cell network, they turned their attention to the dorsal tegmental nucleus of Gudden (DTN), origin of a major projection to LMN via the mammillary peduncle. Modern tract-tracing studies reveal a prominent pattern of reciprocal connection between the LMN and the DTN (see chapter 2 by Hopkins for references). Besides the DTN and PoS, LMN has few other clearly demonstrated sources of input and none are of comparable volume (Amaral, 1987). Furthermore, the prominent reciprocal connections between the two structures are consistent with the attractor network models of HD signal generation that were being proposed around the time the recording and lesion studies of LMN were first being conducted (Skaggs et al., 1995; Redish et al., 1996; Zhang, 1996; Sharp et al., 1996). DTN has thus become a target of much interest in the effort to understand the origin of the HD signal.

In preliminary experiments, Bassett and Taube (2001b) demonstrated the importance of the DTN in the generation of the HD cell signal. HD cell activity was monitored in the ADN of rats that had received bilateral electrolytic lesions of the DTN. In general, direction-specific firing was absent. Surprisingly, however, directional activity was evident in a few instances. It remains to be determined whether this finding was the result of some tissue sparing or an alternate HD circuit.

By this point, Stackman and colleagues had already identified the vestibular end organs as critical contributors to HD signal generation by inactivating vestibular hair cells with neurotoxins, either permanently with sodium arsanilate (Stackman and Taube, 1997) or temporarily with tetrodotoxin (Stackman et al., 2002). In both cases, direction-specific firing within the ADN ceased throughout the time course of the neurotoxins' efficacy. Cells that had previously shown direction-specific firing exhibited nearly constant rates of firing across all directional headings (see chapter 7 by Stackman and Zugaro). Furthermore, previous studies had shown that ADN HD cell discharge is modulated by the animal's angular head velocity (Taube, 1995), and the vestibular lesions also disrupted the influence of angular head velocity on cells' firing rates.

Although direction-specific firing was not identified in any labyrinthectomized animals for up to three months postlesion, it is important to note that compensatory mechanisms usually occur within days to weeks of the lesion. At the physiological level, tonic firing returns to secondary neurons in the vestibular nuclei, reaching 50% of normal rates within 24 hours and recovering to prelesion rates by one week following the labyrinthectomies (Ris and Godaux, 1998). Although it is not clear what mechanisms contribute to the return of the resting discharge rate in vestibular neurons, these observations clearly indicate that the generation of the directional activity is not due to the tonic firing of vestibular neurons. Interestingly, humans with labyrinthectomies are capable of accurate navigation in familiar environments as long as vision is available (Brookes et al., 1993; Glasauer et al., 2002), which suggests that either some form of directional heading representation is present or the subjects use alternative, non-directional heading strategies for navigation.

Given the importance of the vestibular signal to the generation of HD cell activity, Taube et al. (1996) postulated that vestibular information reached limbic structures via the direct route previously described through the DTN and LMN. Evidence supporting this view has been demonstrated in two recent studies involving transynaptic tracers (Graf et al., 2002; Brown et al., 2004), which are discussed in further detail later in this chapter. In addition, Reti et al. (2002) conducted immunohistochemical studies involving the expression of the activity-dependent, immediate-early-gene product Narp. Secreted by excitatory presynaptic terminals, Narp is believed to be associated with changes in synaptic strength by regulating AMPA receptors at postsynaptic terminals. Among other places, Reti and colleagues found robust Narp expression in ADN. However, only in ADN was Narp expression suppressed following experimental labyrinth ablations. The authors concluded that plasticity of some connections in ADN is directly dependent on vestibular activity, a conclusion consistent with HD cell activity driven by the vestibular system.

Table 5.1 provides a summary of the effects of experimental lesions on components of the HD cell circuit.

Angular Head Velocity

A guiding assumption in understanding the mechanisms underlying the HD cell signal has been that a neural signal corresponding to directional heading is derivable from angular head velocity (AHV) information by way of two mathematical integrations over time: acceleration to velocity and velocity to angular displacement, as has been demonstrated in the associated oculomotor pathways (Robinson, 1989). The angular head displacement would then undergo a vector summation with the animal's previous directional heading to yield its current directional heading. The first integration is accomplished by the mechanical properties within the semicircular canals (friction of the endolymph along the walls of the semicircular canals, and the elastic properties of the cupola) in such a way that the

Table 5.1
HD cell activity following experimental lesions

	Recording Sites		
Lesion Sites	ADN	Postsubiculum	Hippocampus
Vestib	Directional activity absent (Stackman et al., 1997)	Directional activity absent (Stackman et al., 2002)	Place fields lost or severely degraded (Stackman et al., 2002)
DTN	Directional activity absent or altered (Bassett and Taube, 2000)*		
LMN	Directional activity absent (Blair et al., 1999; Tullman and Taube, 1998; see text for unilateral effects)		
ADN		Directional activity absent (Goodridge and Taube, 1997)	Incidence of directional place cells increases (Calton et al., 2003)
LDN		Directional activity unaffected (Golob and Taube, 1999)	
PoS	Cue control effects; intratrial drift (Goodridge and Taube, 1998)		Place cells lose landmark stability (Calton et al., 2003)
Retro	Cue control/path integration effects; intratrial drift (Bassett and Taube, 1999)*		
PPC	Path integration effects (Calton and Taube, 2001)		
Hippo	Path integration effects (Golob and Taube, 1999)	Path integration effects (Golob and Taube, 1999)	

Note: Shaded cells indicate loss of directional activity and therefore dependence on lesioned site.
Key: *, preliminary results; Vestib, vestibular hair cells; DTN, dorsal tegmental nucleus of Gudden; LMN, lateral mammillary nuclei; ADN, anterodorsal thalamic nucleus; LDN, laterodorsal thalamic nucleus; PoS, postsubiculum; Retro, retrosplenial cortex; PPC, posterior parietal cortex; Hippo, hippocampus.

signal entering the central nervous system via the VIIIth nerve reflects angular head velocity (Young, 2003). Therefore, investigators expected to encounter somewhere along the ascending stream a point at which there would be a transformation of angular head velocity information to angular head displacement, and hence to head direction. Two groups published, in short succession, recordings from DTN that were consistent with such a scheme of signal transformation, although neither group found a signal that encoded for the amount of angular head displacement (Bassett and Taube, 2001a; Sharp et al., 2001). It should be noted, however, that current network models of HD signal generation do not require a discrete angular head displacement signal; rather, the directional signal arises directly from integrating angular head velocity within the intrinsic circuitry (see chapter 20 by Touretzky for more discussion of HD cell network models).

Although these two published reports differ on some points, the principal type of neural correlate that was identified in the DTN was cells that discharged in relation to the animal's AHV. The firing of 75% of the cells in DTN correlated with the animal's AHV. Bassett and Taube (2001a) encountered two types of AHV modulated cells, referred to as "symmetric" and "asymmetric." Symmetric cells exhibited positive correlations between firing rate and AHV during head turns in either direction, and the firing rate by angular velocity functions tended to be very similar in either head-turn direction. Asymmetric cell activity was positively correlated with velocity in one head-turn direction (the "preferred" direction), but not in the other (the "nonpreferred" direction). Firing in the nonpreferred direction could be either negatively correlated with velocity, or show no velocity modulation (figure 5.2B).

For many cells of both types, symmetric and asymmetric, the response profiles showed steep rates of modulation at low velocities that tended to flatten out at some higher velocity. Because the response profiles reflect mean firing rates at instantaneous AHVs, there is a confound in interpreting these changes in modulation over the velocity range. The vestibular signal is dynamic and changes over the duration of a head turn, but a given point on the firing rate by velocity function can contain samples from anywhere along this response continuum, both from high-frequency (short duration) and low-frequency (long duration) components of a head turn. If the modulation rate is higher at low-velocity head turns, then on first examination these cells might appear to be most sensitive to low-frequency head movements, since low-frequency turns at high velocities would tend to result in very large movements. But low-frequency movements represent a minority in the overall range of natural head movements. Low instantaneous head velocities, however, always occur at the beginning and end of any head turn. Thus, no matter what the peak velocity of a given head turn is, it must always begin and end at zero and accelerate and decelerate through the range of low velocities. Therefore, the steep rate of modulation at low angular velocities may be adapted to movements at the beginning and end of each head turn. While Bassett and Taube identified twice as many symmetric as asymmetric cells (47.7% versus 27.3% of the DTN cell population), Sharp et al. reported only asymmetric cells (83.3% of the DTN cell population). The Sharp et al. finding was, in fact, somewhat more consistent with existing models of HD signal generation and, at present, symmetric AHV cells would seem to represent an interpretive challenge for investigators attempting to model the generation of the HD cell signal. Specifically, if HD cell signals can be accurately derived from asymmetric AHV signals alone, then what function do symmetric AHV cells serve?

In addition to AHV cells, Sharp et al. identified a small number of "traditional" HD cells within the DTN (14.3% of DTN cells). These HD cells resembled LMN HD cells somewhat in that most were modulated a small amount by head-turn direction, reaching higher peak rates or showing some tuning function asymmetry between different turn directions (i.e., CW versus CCW). In contrast, Bassett and Taube did not find any classic HD cells in their recordings, but did isolate a similarly small number of cells (11% of the

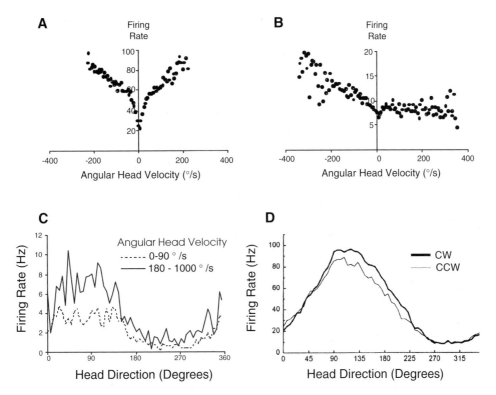

Figure 5.2
Firing characteristics of DTN neurons. (A) A symmetrical AHV cell that fires as a function of angular head velocity during CW (>0°/sec) or CCW (<0°/sec) head turns. (B) An asymmetrical AHV cell that fires as a function of angular head velocity during CW head turns, but is not velocity-modulated during CCW head turns. (C) A cell modulated by both HD and AHV. Firing rate by head direction functions were plotted for head movements with velocities of 0–90°/sec, 90–180°/sec, and 180–1000°/sec. The 90–180° function is omitted for clarity, but falls approximately in between the 0–90°/sec and 180–1000°/sec functions. (D) A DTN HD cell. Firing rate by HD functions are plotted for CW and CCW head turns. Note that the peak firing rate for CW head turns is higher. (Reproduced with permission from Bassett and Taube 2001a. A–C, copyright 2001 by the Society for Neuroscience and Sharp et al. 2001. D, copyright 2001 by the American Psychological Association.)

AHV cells) that were modulated by both angular head velocity and coarse head direction (figure 5.2C). The difference in results reported by the two groups raises the interesting possibility of regional specificity in cell response characteristics. The DTN is divisible into at least two subnuclei that have somewhat different connections (Petrovicky, 1971; Hayakawa and Zyo, 1990). The two DTN recording studies discussed above did not distinguish between subregions, but future studies that are able to make this distinction may provide more detail on early HD signal processing.

AHV cells have also been observed in the LMN, where they constituted about 43.7% of the cell population (Stackman and Taube, 1998). Both symmetric and asymmetric cells were found within the LMN (termed "fast" angular head velocity cells), in addition to a third type of AHV cell, referred to as "slow" AHV cells. The firing rate of slow AHV cells was negatively correlated with the speed of head turn for both turn directions. The cells accounted for 47.5% of the AHV cells within LMN, and were not observed in the DTN. The remaining velocity-modulated cells were fast AHV cells. In general, the properties of fast LMN AHV cells are similar to those in the DTN, although the correlation to angular head velocity is weaker and the sensitivity lower in the LMN, compared to the DTN.

Although no AHV cells have been reported in ADN, angular head velocity information is projected downstream from LMN. Taube (1995) reported a small but significant correlation between HD cell activity in ADN and angular head velocity. Thus, although the activity of ADN HD cells was primarily correlated with the animal's head direction, the cells' activity was modulated a small amount (1% of the firing rate variance) by the animal's angular head velocity, where HD cells fired at slightly higher firing rates with fast head turns through the cell's preferred firing direction, compared to slow head turns. This modulation of firing by angular head velocity is not observed in PoS HD cells (Taube and Muller, 1998), although Sharp (1996) reported that the activity of about 10% of the entire cell population in PoS was modulated by the animal's angular head velocity. The activity of these PoS cells was asymmetric and they were not modulated by head direction. Finally, it should also be noted that the linear speed of the animal also exerts a small influence over HD cell firing rates in PoS, ADN, and LMN, with faster speeds being correlated with higher firing (Taube et al., 1990a; Taube, 1995; Stackman and Taube, 1998).

In sum, the presence of activity modulated by angular head velocity, HD, and combinations of these signals in the DTN and LMN, along with the strong reciprocal connections between the two sites, has led investigators to hypothesize that the angular head velocity-to-directional displacement integration occurs within a network distributed across these two structures.

Angular head velocity information can be derived from several possible sensory sources, but the results of Stackman and colleagues' vestibular lesions strongly implicate the vestibular system as the origin of the velocity signals observed in DTN (Stackman and Taube, 1997; Stackman et al., 2002). Anatomically, there is a prominent pathway between the vestibular system and the DTN, by way of the nucleus prepositus hypoglossi (NPH). The NPH is adjacent to the medial vestibular nucleus, which primarily encodes information concerning angular head velocity in the horizontal plane, and is heavily innervated by its secondary afferents (McCrea and Baker, 1985). Functionally, the NPH has come to be viewed as the site of the putative neural integrator for eye movements (see chapter 6 by Glasauer for a more detailed discussion of the NPH). It is also a major contributor of afferent projections to the DTN (Liu et al., 1984).

Direct connections from the medial vestibular nucleus to the DTN have also been suggested as a route of velocity information to the DTN. This route, as opposed to the pathway through NPH, is attractive because it avoids the requirement of reconciling a hypothesized angular head velocity signal with the experimental studies associating NPH cell activity with eye movements in rats (Lannou et al., 1984). Eye movements and HD cell activity have not been simultaneously recorded in rats; but in monkeys, HD cells recorded in the presubiculum were independent of the eyes' position in the head (see chapter 14 by Rolls). Several tract-tracing studies have indeed found projections from both NPH and medial vestibular nucleus (Liu et al., 1984; Hayakawa and Zyo, 1985), allowing for a hypothetical scenario in which angular head velocity information from the medial vestibular nucleus drives the velocity-to-directional displacement integrator in the HD cell network. The NPH might then contribute an eye-velocity or position signal as an indication of error between the movement of the head and reflexive movements of the eyes during gaze correction (vestibular ocular reflex/optokinetic nystagmus), allowing head direction to be updated without visual conflict during small head movements in which the visual scene does not change.

Anatomical studies that target the DTN and could verify this scenario are complicated, however, by the possibility of tracer or lesion spread to the medial longitudinal fasciculus, which lies immediately ventral to the DTN. In two retrograde tracer studies that reported labeling in medial vestibular nucleus following injections in DTN, the injection sites appeared to overlap with the medial longitudinal fasciculus, and the authors therefore tended to discount their evidence for a direct medial vestibular nucleus → DTN pathway (Liu et al., 1984; Hayakawa and Zyo, 1985). In an early degeneration study by Morest (1961), a control lesion affecting the medial vestibular nucleus produced no labeling in DTN (although negative results in degeneration studies should not be viewed as conclusive).

Recent studies using new transsynaptic tracers do not clarify the issue very much. Brown et al. (2005) have recently injected pseudorabies virus into rat LMN. Visualization at two time points, 60 and 72 hours postinjection, revealed labeling at many of the expected sites, including DTN and NPH, and in the expected order. Concerning the question whether there is a direct medial vestibular nucleus → DTN pathway, however, the authors report that in no instance did medial vestibular nucleus labeling occur before, or without, NPH labeling. Of six animals showing DTN labeling at 60 hours postinjection, one animal showed NPH labeling and none showed medial vestibular nucleus labeling. At 72 hours postinjection, four animals showed NPH labeling, with three of these animals also showing medial vestibular nucleus labeling. Since the NPH is adjacent to the medial vestibular nucleus and is reciprocally connected with it, these data cannot distinguish between dual projections to the DTN from both medial vestibular nucleus and NPH, and projections to the DTN from the medial vestibular nucleus by way of NPH.

In another study, Graf et al. (2002) injected rabies virus into the medial rectus muscle in guinea pigs to map the oculomotor system. Labeling appeared in the medial vestibular nucleus and NPH at 60 hours postinjection. To the surprise of the authors, however, at 96 hours postinjection, significant labeling appeared in DTN and two of its afferent connections: LMN and the interpeduncular nucleus. As rabies virus is known to travel across synapses only in a retrograde direction, these results implied that NPH or medial vestibular nucleus, or both, receive projections from the DTN. This finding is somewhat in conflict with Liu et al. (1984), who found no terminal labeling in NPH, but it would confirm Morest's (1961) degeneration studies showing DTN projections to NPH (and to a lesser extent, medial vestibular nucleus). Confirmation of a DTN → NPH pathway is again complicated by a nearby structure, the laterodorsal tegmental nucleus, which has been shown independently to project to NPH (Cornwall et al., 1990). Two earlier studies of DTN efferents, for example, show projections to NPH, but the lesion sites in these studies either involve both the DTN and the laterodorsal tegmental nucleus (Briggs and Kaelber, 1971), or fail to make any distinction between structures in the region (Groenewegen and Van Dijk, 1984).

While vestibular signals are clearly critical for the generation of HD cell activity, other influences are also important. For example, it is noteworthy that HD cell firing is commonly observed to decline or cease when the rat is restrained and turned passively through the cell's preferred firing direction (Taube et al., 1990b; Taube, 1995; Knierim et al., 1995), a finding that also extends to velocity-modulated cells in the DTN (Sharp et al., 2001). Zugaro et al. (2002) found that passively moved rats exhibited greater velocity modulation of HD cell firing rates, with significantly lower peak firing rates during slow passive movements relative to active movements at the same velocity. These observations, along with the observation that HD cells in the LMN and ADN anticipate future head direction by a few tens of milliseconds (see chapter 1 by Sharp), suggest that motor and/or proprioceptive information can influence HD cell firing. A particularly compelling piece of evidence in support of this notion is the finding that, when rats are passively transported from a familiar environment to a novel one, the preferred firing directions of HD cells exhibit significantly more shift than when the rats are allowed to walk the same path between the two environments. The effect is equally robust in light and dark. Thus, even when optic flow and vestibular information are available, the animal's spatial representation of its environment is not as accurate as when the animal can move through the environment of its own volition (Stackman et al., 2003).

Direct evidence of motor inputs to HD cells is scarce, but there are at least three possible pathways that might provide motor information to the HD cell network. The laterodorsal tegmental nucleus is distinct from the DTN, but also projects to the LMN (Satoh and Fibiger, 1986). The medial reticular formation, which contains locomotor circuits, projects to the laterodorsal tegmental nucleus and could be the origin of a motor signal that reaches the HD circuit in the LMN. Alternatively (or additionally), the striatum, an area associated with the initiation of movement, projects to the ventral tegmental nucleus (Heimer et al., 1995), a major source of afferent input to the medial mammillary nuclei. The medial mammillary nuclei, in turn, project to all the anterior thalamic nuclei, including the ADN (Shibata, 1992). The third possibility is a cortical pathway from area 8 (the medial agranular field of Donoghue and Wise, 1982) to area 29d of retrosplenial cortex (Vogt and Miller, 1983), which in turn projects to the ADN and PoS (van Groen and Wyss, 1990a; Vogt and Miller, 1983). Area 8 includes the putative frontal eye fields in the rat, as well as motor or premotor representations of the vibrissae and neck (Neafsey et al., 1986). Neck movements would, of course, be relevant for updating head turns.

The search for anatomical evidence of nonvestibular influences on HD cell generation is complicated by the functional obscurity of the other major sources of afferents to DTN. If the DTN is a critical point in the HD system ascending stream, then these other inputs will likely be a focus of future investigations. For this reason, we review in the following pages the available anatomical and functional data of the major afferent inputs to the DTN.

Of particular interest may be the interpeduncular nucleus, because of its relative contribution and a reciprocal relationship with DTN that mirrors its connections with LMN. Hayakawa and Zyo (1984) subdivided the DTN into ventral and dorsal parts, which correspond approximately to pars centralis and pericentralis, respectively, of the rat brain atlas by Paxinos and Watson (1998). Interestingly, it is primarily the ventral subdivision that returns projections to LMN, while the dorsal subdivision projects to interpeduncular nucleus (Hayakawa and Zyo, 1990). Connections between the ventral and dorsal subdivisions are unknown, although Hayakawa and Zyo (1988) infer interneuron projections from the dorsal to ventral subdivisions, based on the preponderance of small neurons in the dorsal subdivision that resemble motor cranial nuclei interneurons and cannot support long or numerous axons. The ventral subdivision is richly connected with its contralateral counterpart (Liu et al., 1984). If the reciprocal connections between LMN and DTN form part of the velocity-to-angular displacement neural integrator, then the reciprocal DTN → interpeduncular nucleus connections may prove to be important to HD signal generation as well, with the DTN representing an intervening node in an LMN-interpeduncular nucleus loop. Previous reports, however, offer few hints as to what role the interpeduncular nucleus serves in regard to HD cell activity (for review, see Morley, 1986).

Another major source of afferent information to both subdivisions of DTN is the lateral habenular nucleus, which also projects to the interpeduncular nucleus (Contestabile and Flumerfelt, 1981; Hayakawa and Zyo, 1985). Like the interpeduncular nucleus, the function of the lateral habenular nucleus with respect to HD cells is unknown. The lateral habenular nucleus has been associated with an array of behaviors, too wide to provide clear information about its contribution. In a broad sense, the interpeduncular nucleus can be thought of as linking the limbic forebrain with midbrain regions involved in behavioral regulation and motivation (Andres et al., 1999).

Another DTN afferent of potential interest is the supragenual nucleus. Although its functions are also largely unknown, the supragenual nucleus has connections to circuits involved in eye movement (Ohtsuki et al., 1992; Stanton et al., 1988), and in contrast to the NPH, projects most of its DTN contacts to the contralateral side (Hayakawa and Zyo, 1985; Liu et al., 1984). Thus, this could be another instance where eye velocity or position information may influence the HD signal circuit.

The contributions of these various structures must ultimately be considered with the synaptology and neuropharmacology of their projections to DTN. Based on synapse morphology (Hayakawa and Zyo, 1988), the ventral division of the DTN receives primarily inhibitory contacts, even though the LMN projection there is excitatory (Hayakawa and Zyo, 1990). In contrast, the dorsal subdivision receives a majority of excitatory contacts. Thus, at least one of the major projections to DTN must be inhibitory to account for the inhibitory terminals that dominate the ventral subdivision. The projections from the rostral area of the interpeduncular nucleus, from which most of interpeduncular nucleus → DTN fibers project, are believed to be enkephalinergic, and are thus probably excitatory (Huitinga et al., 1985). Unlike the DTN → LMN projection, the DTN dorsal subdivision projection to the interpeduncular nucleus is also probably enkephalinergic (Hamill and Jacobowitz, 1984; Yamano and Tohyama, 1987). Moreover, the DTN was found to have a high concentration of glycine receptors (Araki et al., 1998), making the NPH—known to use glycine as an inhibitory neurotransmitter—a potential source of inhibitory afferents onto DTN (Spencer et al., 1989; Rampon et al., 1996). The neuropharmacology of the supragenual and lateral habenular projections to DTN is presently unknown.

Although it seems clear that vestibular information is essential to the HD signal, little is known about how the angular head velocity signal is transformed between the VIIIth nerve and the DTN. The horizontal semicircular canals are emphasized as the origin of HD cell activity, because they are most sensitive to yaw rotations of the head when the animal is upright in the horizontal plane. They are also activated when the rat is in a vertical plane or inverted upside down whenever the rat rotates its head from side-to-side, although a different overall otolith signal would be present. Nonetheless, naturalistic motions of a freely moving animal will rarely consist of pure horizontal angular head movements. For instance, a rat will often pitch its head up or down while foraging, which would lead to simultaneous activation of the horizontal and anterior (vertical) canals, as well as an alteration in the otolith signal. These considerations raise the question of whether inputs from all three semicircular canals are involved in processing the signal, and whether the otoliths contribute any information to the signal. In the monkey, secondary vestibular neurons fall into several classes, based on their firing behaviors, e.g., vestibular-only and position-vestibular-pause neurons (Scudder and Fuchs, 1992; Boyle et al., 1996). Do vestibular projections to the HD system specifically involve one of these classes of neuron? The cerebellum is intimately involved in many aspects of vestibular function; does it play a role in the HD signal? Finally, vestibular nucleus neurons are often classified as having one of two patterns of activity: regular or irregular (Goldberg and Fernandez, 1971). Do both types of neurons contribute to processing the HD cell signal, or is input from one cell type preferentially involved? In DTN AHV cells, there is no evidence of regular tonic firing (Bassett and Taube, 2001a); HD cell firing, when the head is still and pointing continuously in the cell's preferred firing direction, is irregular as well (i.e., the interspike interval varies considerably when the head is pointed within a small arc of the cell's preferred firing direction; Taube, 2004).

In summary, the serial processing of the HD signal in the ascending stream has already revealed much about the signal's transformation. The vestibular end organs provide crucial signals for the generation of HD cell activity. Angular head velocity information emanating from the vestibular system gives rise to a signal that encodes the animal's perceived directional heading. The directional signal appears first in the DTN and LMN, and is then projected rostrally to the ADN and then to the PoS. The PoS is connected to several sites, one of which is the superficial layers of the entorhinal cortex, the same layers that contain neurons that project into the hippocampus. Thus, head directional information can influence spatial representations in the hippocampus that encode information about the animal's location within the environment. Nonetheless, the significance of having somewhat similar HD signals in three or four nuclei that are connected in series remains unclear, and future experiments will undoubtedly attempt to address this issue.

The Descending Stream

A circuitry and sensorium sufficient for generating the HD signal appears complete within subcortical structures served by ideothetic movement information. Yet self-movement information is not sufficient by itself to allow directional orientation to be accurately maintained over long periods of time. A mechanism for taking a "fix" on stable environmental features is necessary to correct for accrued error in a representation based on integrated movement signals.

In most terrestrial mammals, the visual system is typically the richest source of spatial information, where rapid sampling of landmarks can provide relatively stable information concerning the animal's spatial orientation and location. Knowledge about visual landmark cues must be seen as the result of multistage cognitive processes involving many areas of visual cortex. Rats tested on several specific tasks involved in the broader task of navigation (orienting, locating large visual targets, and navigating to an invisible target) suffered little performance decrement following lesions to primary visual cortex, Oc1. Lesions that include extrastriate areas lead to far more significant deficits on these tasks, as do lesions to the superior colliculus, which lies along the major pathway from the retina to these secondary visual cortical areas (reviewed in Dean, 1990). Thus, visual information following the retinotectal pathway to the parietal and temporal visual areas (Oc2, Te1 and Te2) is assumed to be the origin of highly processed information about spatial cues to the descending stream, and PoS and retrosplenial cortex are both known to receive direct projections from visual cortex area 18a (lateral Oc2) (Vogt and Miller, 1983). Notably, Chen et al., (1994) found directional activity in the medial portion of Oc2.

It has also been suggested that the posterior parietal cortex (areas Par1, Par2 in the rat) plays an important role in processing environmental cues. Animals with posterior parietal cortex lesions exhibit some deficits in spatial behaviors (Kolb et al., 1994; for review, see Poucet and Benhamou, 1997), and anatomical connections exist to indirectly link posterior parietal cortex with sites containing HD cells (Vogt and Miller, 1983; Reep et al., 1994). HD cells in ADN, however, differed little from controls in animals with aspiration lesions of posterior parietal cortex (Calton and Taube, 2001). Firing parameters were unchanged and cells' preferred firing directions shifted, along with rotation of a prominent visual cue. Only when rats walked from a familiar environment into a novel one was directional stability affected, which suggests that the posterior parietal cortex may be involved in integrating self-movement signals with visual cues, but not necessarily in processing or retaining those visual cues. This latter finding is consistent with previous reports showing that animals with posterior parietal cortex lesions are impaired on spatial tasks involving path integration (Save and Moghaddam, 1996).

Studies of parietal cortex also remind us that a distinction between two segregated paths of descending visual signals and ascending vestibular signals is overly simplified. Visual and vestibular signals are integrated at many sites in the brain, aside from the limbic circuits discussed here. The conventional pathway described in primates entails vestibular information conveyed from the brainstem to a vestibular cortex (the parietal insular vestibular cortex, or PIVC) via the ventral posterior thalamus (Abraham et al., 1977; Grüsser et al., 1990a, Lang et al., 1979). This vestibular cortex projects to area 7 of the parietal cortex (Guldin et al., 1992; Olson and Musil, 1992). Grüsser et al. (1990b) postulated that the parietal insular vestibular cortex serves to recognize and control head and body position in space, suggesting that a vestibular signal may be integrated with visual information at the cortical level in a route that is independent of the ascending stream of information discussed in the previous section.

A constant stream of visual information is not necessary for stable HD cell firing, however, because HD cells can retain their directional responses for extended periods in the dark. Indeed, one of the remarkable features of HD cell behavior is that apparently the memory of environmental cues and self-movement information are sufficient to stabilize the rat's spatial representation. Thus, we next turn our focus to those areas thought to contribute mnemonic information about the environment to the descending stream.

The contribution of PoS HD cells to the representation of direction was revealed by the lesion study of Goodridge and Taube (1997). Following bilateral PoS lesions, ADN HD cell firing remained intact, but there was a significant decrease in the control of visual cues over HD cell preferred firing direction. HD cell preferred firing directions failed to follow a prominent visual cue during cue-rotation trials (figure 5.3), shifted more often and in larger amounts when rats locomoted between familiar and novel environments. In some instances, the preferred firing directions drifted during the course of single recording sessions, when the visual cue was left in place (for methods and more details of cue control data, see chapter 3 by Taube). Interestingly, another effect of PoS lesions was a moderate, but significant, increase of the directional firing range of ADN HD cells. This effect, together with the loss of cue control, suggests that there was a loss of spatial resolution encoded by HD cells following the lesions, as if information descending from PoS enabled a finer resolution than provided by the ascending stream alone.

The subiculum is considered to be the primary site of output by the hippocampus, and it also projects to the PoS (van Groen and Wyss, 1990a). With the close association of the

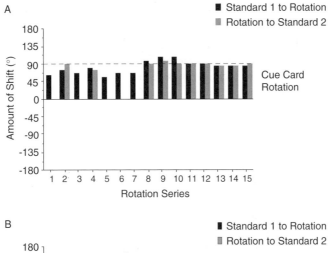

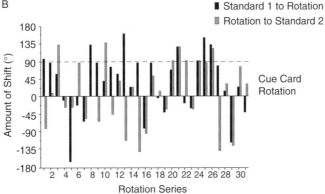

Figure 5.3
Cue control of ADN directional activity following PoS lesions. (A) Distribution of shifts in the preferred firing direction from intact animals and from (B) PoS-lesioned animals. Each rotation series (black and white bars) consists of a session recorded following a 90° rotation of a white cue card along the wall of the cylindrical recording arena (rotation), and a session recorded after restoring the cue card back to its original position (standard 2). Complete cue control would yield values of 90° for standard 1 to rotation and rotation to standard 2. The abscissa plots the number of each rotation series, and the ordinate plots the extent of shift that the rotation produced in the preferred firing direction of the cell. In (A) standard 2 sessions were not performed in rotation series 1, 3, 5, 6, and 7. Each number shown on the abscissa represents a different rotation series. (Reproduced with permission from Goodridge and Taube 1997; copyright 1997 by the Society for Neuroscience.)

hippocampus with memory in general, and spatial memory in particular, the hippocampus potentially represents a major contributor of mnemonic information to the directional signal. Golob and Taube recorded HD cells in the ADN following hippocampal lesions under several different experimental conditions. In the first experiment, HD cells were initially recorded in a novel environment, then recorded the next day in the same environment (Golob and Taube, 1997). On the second day, animals with hippocampal lesions would be expected to be unable to recall the environmental context from the first day. Previous studies reported that when an animal is placed into a novel context or environment, HD cells maintained their directional firing properties, but the preferred firing direction frequently shifted. If the animals were reintroduced into that environment at a later time, the HD cell's preferred firing direction returned to its former direction for that particular context (Taube et al., 1990a,b). Thus, under these conditions one might expect the preferred firing directions of HD cells from animals with hippocampal lesions to shift when they are placed in the enclosure on the second day, because they would lack a mnemonic trace of their experience from the first day. Contrary to these predictions, Golob and Taube reported that the preferred firing direction of each HD cell remained stable across days. This result occurred even when the animal was disoriented, to remove path integration cues, and then reintroduced into what was a novel environment the previous day (figure 5.4), and suggests that extrahippocampal structures are capable of creating and maintaining a representation of the animal's environmental context.

In the second experiment, rats walked from a familiar environment through a narrow passage into a novel environment (Golob and Taube, 1999). In control animals, the preferred firing direction of HD cells typically remains stable (i.e., shifts less than 30°), even

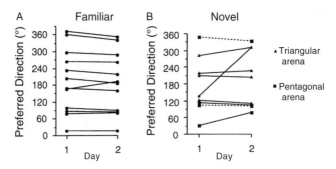

Figure 5.4
HD cell stability in familiar and novel enclosures in rats with hippocampal lesions. (A) The preferred directions of HD cells are shown for two consecutive days recorded within the familiar cylindrical recording arena. Most cells had stable preferred directions across days in the familiar enclosure. (B) Graphs plotting the preferred directions of cells recorded across the first two days in one of two novel enclosures (triangle- or pentagon-shaped arenas). Except for one cell, the preferred directions in these novel enclosures were also generally stable across days. (Reproduced with permission from Golob and Taube 1997—copyright 1997 by National Academy of Sciences, USA.)

though the shape of the environment is different and visual cues are arranged differently (Taube and Burton, 1995). In animals with hippocampal lesions, there was a period of continuous drift in the preferred firing direction when the animal first entered the novel environment, after which the preferred firing direction stabilized at a new direction. The new preferred direction was shifted more than 30° in 11 out of 12 cells (figure 5.5), and the cell then retained the new direction through multiple visits to the novel environment. To test if the deficit lay in establishing cue control or responding to visual cues, the authors next recorded HD cells in environments from which the usual polarizing visual cue had been removed during training, then added the cue at a later time. Under these conditions, the newly introduced cue did not alter the preferred firing directions that had been previously established in the cue's absence. Furthermore, rotations of this visual cue led to comparable shifts in each cell's preferred firing direction. When recorded in the dark, however, preferred firing directions drifted significantly and continuously. The results of this experiment show that hippocampal lesions produce some effects expected by the loss of memories for the visual cues in the environment or their configural relationships to one another. Directional drift, both in the dark and during the first moments in a new environment, is consistent with the loss of an environmental absolute against which to compare ongoing movements. But if the trace of environmental visual cues were completely gone, we would expect a new preferred firing direction for the same cell each time the rat entered the recording arena, and this was not the case. As with the posterior parietal cortex lesions, the underlying deficit appeared to be one of integrating information about self-movement when visual cues are unavailable, and the authors characterized the deficit as a failure in path-integration processes. The notion of the hippocampus as a site of path integration is supported by behavioral studies as well (McNaughton et al., 1996; Maaswinkel et al., 1999; Whishaw et al., 2001; cf., Alyan and McNaughton, 1999).

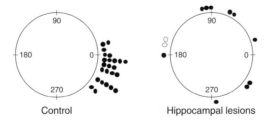

Figure 5.5
HD cell stability and path integration following hippocampal lesions. Polar plots showing the angular shifts in preferred direction during the first visit to a novel environment by active displacement along a passage leading from a familiar environment. Each dot on the periphery represents the magnitude of shift in the preferred direction for one HD cell. Each HD cell was recorded from a different animal. In general, HD cells in the sham-lesioned group maintained their preferred direction between the familiar and novel areas, with a small CW shift bias. HD cells in rats with hippocampal lesions had larger directional shifts than the control group, and the directional shifts were distributed randomly. The two open circles in the lesioned group denote cells that drifted <180° in the CW direction. (Modified from Golob and Taube 1999; reproduced with permission. Copyright 1999 by the Society for Neuroscience.)

Closely associated with the hippocampus, the retrosplenial cortex (posterior cingulate), another limbic system site where HD cells have been found, may contribute mnemonic information about the environment to the descending stream. It has long been known that the retrosplenial cortex is important for accurate performance on spatial tasks (see chapter 13 by Aggleton), following a few reports of "topographical amnesia" after damage that involved the retrosplenial cortex in humans (Maguire, 2001). Beginning in the 1970s Gabriel and colleagues have conducted studies mapping out a limbic circuit for discriminatory learning, in which the retrosplenial cortex plays the role of long-term storage of memories against which newly acquired information is compared (for review, see Gabriel, 1990). In 1994, Chen et al. recorded HD cells in rat retrosplenial cortex that had comparable firing properties as HD cells in PoS and ADN, and subsequently, the retrosplenial cortex became a focus for a number of behavioral experiments indicating its importance to spatial memory (see chapter 10 by Mizumori et al.).

Cho and Sharp (2001) further characterized HD cells in retrosplenial cortex, identifying them in both granular and dysgranular subdivisions of retrosplenial cortex. This result is noteworthy because the ADN projects only to the granular cortex (van Groen and Wyss, 1990b; Shibata, 1993), suggesting that HD cell activity in the retrosplenial cortex may not be merely a passive iteration of ADN HD activity. It should also be noted that the retrosplenial cortex receives input from the frontal eye fields in the medial prefrontal area (Guandalini, 1998), and single units in rabbit dysgranular retrosplenial cortex respond to quick-phase eye movements during vestibular or optokinetic nystagmus (Sikes et al., 1988). While direct vestibular projections to retrosplenial cortex are unknown, an imaging study in humans revealed activation of retrosplenial cortex during caloric vestibular stimulation (Vitte et al., 1996), suggesting that vestibular information is represented there (and highlighting again the difficulty of distinguishing between vestibular and eye-movement information). Thus, it is possible that the HD cell activity in retrosplenial cortex does not depend on HD cell activity in ADN. Among the cells recorded in retrosplenial cortex there was (1) little or no lateralization or turn-direction dependency of firing patterns, (2) little or no modulation by angular velocity, and (3) the magnitude of anticipatory firing was similar to ADN HD cells. Thus, there is no evidence for the kinds of signal transformation in the HD cell signal from ADN to retrosplenial cortex that are seen at other points in the ascending stream. On the other hand, Cho and Sharp described some non-HD cell types that contained other spatial patterns of firing, such as directionally dependent place cells, and cells whose activity was modulated by turn direction (CW versus CCW) or speed of movement.

To test the dependence between ADN and retrosplenial cortex on HD cell firing will require a complementary lesion study of the type Goodridge and Taube conducted on ADN and PoS. Preliminary data has shown that following electrolytic retrosplenial cortex lesions, HD activity was still intact in ADN (Bassett and Taube, 1999). As with PoS lesions, the primary effect appeared to be on the stability of the cell's preferred firing direction. Rotations of the visual cue did not always lead to an equal shift in each cell's preferred firing direction. Unlike what is true in intact animals, the preferred firing direction was not stable from one recording session to the next. Finally, there were large shifts in the preferred firing directions when rats locomoted between familiar and novel environments in the dark. The last finding is consistent with studies that inactivated the retrosplenial cortex while rats performed a radial-arm-maze task in the dark. Cooper and Mizumori reported that inactivation of retrosplenial cortex with lidocaine resulted both in impaired performance (Cooper and Mizumori, 1999) and in "remapping" of recorded hippocampal place cells (Cooper and Mizumori, 2001). Both effects were specific to dark conditions.

In summary, studies of lesion effects on HD cell responses to rotation of a prominent visual cue have begun to clarify the neural circuitry underlying the processing of landmark information. Figure 5.6 summarizes preferred firing direction shifts following 90° rotations of a cue card, after experimental lesions to various structures. If the cue card exerts complete control over the cell's preferred firing direction, then shifts would group

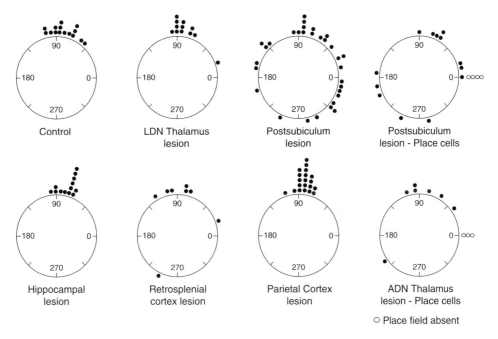

Figure 5.6
Summary of lesion effects on cue control of HD (three left columns) and hippocampal place cells (right column). Polar plots showing angular shifts in preferred firing direction or place field after white cue cards (initially centered on 0°) were rotated 90° CCW. Left columns: HD cells recorded in ADN after lesions to LDN, PoS, hippocampus, retrosplenial cortex, posterior parietal cortex, and in controls. Right column: place field shift in rats with lesions to PoS and ADN.

around 90°, as found in the control group. Note that lesions in the lateral dorsal thalamus, posterior parietal cortex, and hippocampus did not affect cue control over the preferred firing direction, while lesions of either the PoS or retrosplenial cortex did. These results are consistent with findings from hippocampal place cell recordings where lesions of the PoS, but not the ADN, led to poor cue control (Calton et al., 2003) (figure 5.6, right column). Taken together, these results indicate that for rats spatial information concerning landmarks proceeds either directly in the visual cortex → PoS pathway or in the visual cortex → retrosplenial cortex → PoS pathway. The two pathways, of course, are not mutually exclusive, and landmark information could enter the HD system via both pathways simultaneously.

Conclusion

One important issue concerning navigation is the question of where in the brain landmark information is integrated with ideothetic information concerning the animal's movements through space. In other words, where do the ascending and descending streams of information discussed in this chapter converge? Given the reciprocal connections between so many of the structures containing HD cells, it cannot be strictly accurate to view a single structure as the point of convergence. For instance, even neurons in the DTN could be affected by cortically processed information, by way of the PoS projection to LMN, and the LMN projection to DTN. Thus, while allothetic and ideothetic information streams must meet in order for successful orientation and navigation to occur, anatomical convergence is only figurative; in reality, it probably occurs across several structures: the LMN, ADN, PoS, and retrosplenial cortex. However, ADN HD cells seem, both by anatomy and firing characteristics, to reflect the features of both information streams. On one hand, the ADN is the principal target of the ascending output from the LMN-DTN circuit, and, on the other hand, is also heavily innervated by descending projections from both PoS and retrosplenial cortex. In their velocity modulation and anticipatory firing, ADN HD cells maintain traces of the velocity and motor signals that we presume are the origin of their activity, but they are as sensitive to experimental manipulation of environmental cues as HD cells in any structure.

References

Abraham L, Copack PB, Gilman S (1977) Brainstem pathways for vestibular projections to cerebral cortex in cat. Exp Neurol 55: 436–448.

Alyan SH, McNaughton BL (1999) Hippocampectomized rats are capable of homing by path integration. Behav Neurosci 113: 19–31.

Amaral DG (1987) Memory: anatomical organization of candidate brain regions. In: VB Mountcastle, F Plum F eds, Handbook of Physiology. Sec. 1, Vol. 5, Pt 1. Bethesda, MD: American Physiological Society, pp. 211–294.

Amaral DG, Witter MP (1995) Hippocampal formation. In G Paxinos, ed., The Rat Nervous System. 2nd Ed. San Diego, CA: Academic Press, pp. 443–493.

Andres KH, von During M, Veh RW (1999) Subnuclear organization of the rat habenular complexes. J Comp Neurol 407: 130–150.

Araki T, Yamano M, Murakami T, Wanaka A, Betz H, Tohyama M (1988) Localization of glycine receptors in the rat central nervous system: an immunocytochemical analysis using monoclonal antibody. Neurosci 25: 613–624.

Bassett JP, Taube JS (1999) Retrosplenial cortex lesions disrupt stability of head direction cell activity. Soc Neurosci Abstr 25: 1383.

Bassett JP, Taube JS (2001a) Neural correlates for angular head velocity in the rat dorsal tegmental nucleus. J Neurosci 21: 5740–5751.

Bassett JP, Taube JS (2001b) Lesions of the dorsal tegmental nucleus of the rat disrupt head direction cell activity in the anterior thalamus. Soc Neurosci Abstr 27: 852.29.

Blair HT, Sharp PE (1995) Anticipatory head direction signals in anterior thalamus: evidence for a thalamocortical circuit that integrates angular head motion to compute head direction. J Neurosci 15: 6260–6270.

Blair HT, Cho J, Sharp PE (1998) Role of the lateral mammillary nucleus in the rat head direction circuit: a combined single unit recording and lesion study. Neuron 21: 1387–1397. Erratum in: Neuron 1999, 22: 199.

Blair HT, Cho J, Sharp PE (1999) the anterior thalamic head-direction signal is abolished by bilateral but not unilateral lesions of the lateral mammillary nucleus. J Neurosci 19: 6673–6683.

Blanks RH, Precht W, Torigoe Y (1983) Afferent projections to the cerebellar flocculus in the pigmented rat demonstrated by retrograde transport of horseradish peroxidase. Exp Brain Res 52: 293–306.

Boyle R, Belton T, McCrea RA (1996) Responses of identified vestibulospinal neurons to voluntary eye and head movements in the squirrel monkey. Ann NY Acad Sci 781: 244–263.

Brandt T, Dieterich M (1999) The vestibular cortex. Its locations, functions, and disorders. Ann NY Acad Sci 871: 293–312.

Briggs TL, Kaelber WW (1971) Efferent fiber connections of the dorsal and deep tegmental nuclei of Gudden. An experimental study in the cat. Brain Res 29: 17–29.

Brookes GB, Gresty MA, Nakamura T, Metcalfe T (1993) Sensing and controlling rotational orientation in normal subjects and patients with loss of labyrinthine function. Amer J Otol 14: 349–351.

Brown JE, Card JP, Yates BJ (2005) Polysynaptic pathways from the vestibular nuclei to the lateral mammillary nucleus of the rat: substrates for vestibular input to head direction cells. Exp Brain Res 161: 47–61.

Calton JL, Stackman RW, Goodridge JP, Archey WB, Dudchenko PA, Taube JS (2003) Hippocampal place cell instability after lesions of the head direction cell network. J Neurosci 23: 9719–9731.

Calton JL, Taube JS (2001) Head direction cell activity following bilateral lesions of posterior parietal cortex. Soc. Neurosci. Abstr, Vol. 27, Program No. 537.30.

Chen LL, Lin LH, Green EJ, Barnes CA, McNaughton BL (1994) Head-direction cells in the rat posterior cortex. I. Anatomical distribution and behavioral modulation. Exp Brain Res 101: 8–23.

Cho J, Sharp PE (2001) Head direction, place, and movement correlates for cells in the rat retrosplenial cortex. Behav Neurosci 115: 3–25.

Contestabile A, Flumerfelt BA (1981) Afferent connections of the interpeduncular nucleus and the topographic organization of the habenulo-interpeduncular pathway: an HRP study in the rat. J Comp Neurol 196: 253–270.

Cooper BG, Mizumori SJ (1999) Retrosplenial cortex inactivation selectively impairs navigation in darkness. Neuroreport 10: 625–630.

Cooper BG, Mizumori SJ (2001) Temporary inactivation of the retrosplenial cortex causes a transient reorganization of spatial coding in the hippocampus. J Neurosci 21: 3986–4001.

Cornwall J, Cooper JD, Phillipson OT (1990) Afferent and efferent connections of the laterodorsal tegmental nucleus in the rat. Brain Res Bull 25: 271–284.

Dean P (1990) Sensory cortex: visual perceptual functions. In B Kold and RC Tees eds., The Cerebral Cortex of the Rat, Cambridge, MA: MIT Press.

Donoghue JP, Wise SP (1982) The motor cortex of the rat: cytoarchitecture and microstimulation mapping. J Comp Neurol 212: 76–88.

Gabriel M (1990) Functions of anterior and posterior cingulate cortex during avoidance learning in rabbits. Prog Brain Res 85: 467–483.

Gabriel M, Miller JD, Saltwick SE (1977) Unit activity in cingulate cortex and anteroventral thalamus of the rabbit during differential conditioning and reversal. J Comp Physiol Psych 91: 423–433.

Glasauer S, Amorim MA, Viaud Delmon I, Berthoz A (2002) Differential effects of labyrinthine dysfunction on distance and direction during blindfolded walking of a triangular path. Exp Brain Res 145: 489–497.

Goldberg JM, Fernandez C (1971) Physiology of peripheral neurons innervating semicircular canals of the squirrel monkey. III. Variations among units in their discharge properties. J Neurophysiol 34: 676–684.

Golob EJ, Taube JS (1997) Head direction cells and episodic spatial information in rats without a hippocampus. Proc Natl Acad Sci 94: 7645–7650.

Golob EJ, Taube JS (1999) Head direction cells in rats with hippocampal or overlying neocortical lesions: evidence for impaired angular path integration. J Neurosci 19: 7198–7211.

Golob EJ, Wolk DA, Taube JS (1998) Recordings of postsubiculum head direction cells following lesions of the laterodorsal thalamic nucleus. Brain Res 780: 9–19.

Goodridge JP, Taube JS (1997) Interaction between the postsubiculum and anterior thalamus in the generation of head direction cell activity. J Neurosci 17: 9315–9330.

Graf W, Gerrits N, Yatim-Dhiba N, Ugolini G (2002) Mapping the oculomotor system: the power of transneuronal labeling with rabies virus. Eur J Neurosci 15: 1557–1562.

Groenewegen HJ, Van Dijk CA (1984) Efferent connections of the dorsal tegmental region in the rat, studied by means of anterograde transport of the lectin Phaseolus vulgaris-leucoagglutinin (PHA-L). Brain Res 304: 367–371.

Grüsser OJ, Pause M, Schreiter U (1990a) Localisation and responses of neurones in the parieto-insular vestibular cortex of awake monkeys (*Macaca fascicularis*). J Physiol 430: 537–557.

Grüsser OJ, Pause M, Schreiter U (1990b) Vestibular neurons in the parieto-insular cortex of monkeys (*Macaca fascicularis*): visual and neck receptor responses. J Physiol 430: 559–583.

Guandalini P (1998) The corticocortical projections of the physiologically defined eye field in the rat medial frontal cortex. Brain Res Bul 47: 377–385.

Guldin W, Akbarian S, Grüsser OJ (1992) Cortico-cortical connections and cytoarchitechtonics of the primate vestibular cortex: a study in squirrel monkeys (*Saimiri sciureus*). J Comp Neurol 326: 375–401.

Guldin WO, Grüsser OJ (1998) Is there a vestibular cortex? Trends Neurosci 21: 254–259.

Hamill GS, Jacobowitz DM (1984) A study of afferent projections to the rat interpeduncular nucleus. Brain Res Bull 13: 527–539.

Hayakawa T, Zyo K (1984) Comparative anatomical study of the tegmentomammillary projections in some mammals: a horseradish peroxidase study. Brain Res 300: 335–349.

Hayakawa T, Zyo K (1985) Afferent connections of Gudden's tegmental nuclei in the rabbit. J Comp Neurol 235: 169–181.

Hayakawa T, Zyo K (1988) Fine structural survey of Gudden's tegmental nuclei in the rat: cytology and axosomatic synapses. Anat Embryol 177: 485–493.

Hayakawa T, Zyo K (1990) Fine structure of the lateral mammillary projection to the dorsal tegmental nucleus of Gudden in the rat. J Comp Neurol 298: 224–236.

Heimer L, Zahm DS, Alheid GF (1995) Basal ganglia. In G Paxinos ed., The Rat Nervous System. 2nd ed. San Diego, CA: Academic Press, pp. 579–628.

Huitinga I, Van Dijk CA, Groenewegen HJ (1985) Substance P- and enkephalin-containing projections from the interpeduncular nucleus to the dorsal tegmental region in the rat. Neurosci Lett 62: 311–316.

Kolb B (1984) Functions of the frontal cortex of the rat: a comparative review. Brain Res Rev 8: 65–98.

Kolb B, Buhrmann K, McDonald R, Sutherland RJ (1994) Dissociation of the medial prefrontal, posterior parietal, and posterior temporal cortex for spatial navigation and recognition memory in the rat. Cerebral Cortex 4: 664–680.

Knierim JJ, Kudrimoti HS, McNaughton BL (1995) Place cells, head direction cells, and the learning of landmark stability. J Neurosci 15: 1648–1659.

Lang W, Buttner-Ennever JA, Buttner U (1979) Vestibular projection to the monkey thalamus: an autoradiographic study. Brain Res 177: 3–17.

Lannou J, Cazin L, Precht W, Letaillanter M (1984) Responses of prepositus hypoglossi neurons to optokinetic and vestibular stimulations in the rat. Brain Res 301: 39–45.

Leigh RJ, Zee DS (1999) The Neurology of Eye Movements. 3rd ed. Oxford: Oxford Univ Press.

Liu R, Chang L, Wickern G (1984) The dorsal tegmental nucleus: an axoplasmic transport study. Brain Res 310: 123–132.

Maaswinkel H, Jarrard LE, Whishaw IQ (1999) Hippocampectomized rats are impaired in homing by path integration. Hippocampus 9: 553–561.

Maguire EA (2001) The retrosplenial contribution to human navigation: a review of lesion and neuroimaging findings. Scand J Psychol 42: 225–238.

McCrea RA, Baker R (1985) Anatomical connections of the nucleus prepositus of the cat. J Comp Neurol 237: 377–407.

McNaughton BL, Barnes CA, Gerrard JL, Gothard K, Jung MW, Knierim JJ, Kudrimoti H, Qin Y, Skaggs WE, Suster M, Weaver KL (1996) Deciphering the hippocampal polyglot: the hippocampus as path integration system. J Exp Biol 199: 173–185.

Mizumori SJ, Williams JD (1993) Directionally selective mnemonic properties of neurons in the lateral dorsal nucleus of the thalamus of rats. J Neurosci 13: 4015–4028.

Morest DK (1961) Connexions of the dorsal tegmental nucleus in rat and rabbit. J Anat 95: 229–249.

Morley BJ (1986) The interpeduncular nucleus. Int Rev Neurobiol 28: 157–182.

Neafsey EJ, Bold EL, Haas G, Hurley-Gius KM, Quirk G, Sievert CF, Terreberry RR (1986) The organization of the rat motor cortex: a microstimulation mapping study. Brain Res Rev 11: 77–96.

Ohtsuki H, Tokunaga A, Ono K, Hasebe S, Tadokoro Y (1992) Distribution of efferent neurons projecting to the tectum and cerebellum in the rat prepositus hypoglossi nucleus. Invest Ophthalmol Vis Sci 33: 2567–2574.

O'Keefe J, Nadel L (1978) The Hippocampus as a Cognitive Map. Oxford: Clarendon Press.

Olson CR, Musil SY (1992) Topographic organization of cortical and subcortical projections to posterior cingulate cortex in the cat: Evidence for somatic, ocular and complex subregions. J Comp Neurol 323: 1–24.

Paxinos G, Watson C (1998) The rat brain in stereotaxic coordinates, 3rd ed. San Diego: Academic Press.

Petrovicky P (1971) Structure and incidence of Gudden's tegmental nuclei in some mammals. Acta Anat (Basel). 80: 273–286.

Poucet B, Benhamou S (1997) The neuropsychology of spatial cognition in the rat. Crit Rev Neurobiol 11: 101–120.

Quirk GJ, Muller RU, Kubie, JL, Ranck, JB Jr (1992) The positional firing properties of medial entorhinal neurons: description and comparison with hippocampal place cells. J Neurosci 12: 1945–1963.

Rampon C, Luppi PH, Fort P, Peyron C, Jouvet M (1996) Distribution of glycine-immunoreactive cell bodies and fibers in the rat brain. Neurosci 75: 737–755.

Ranck JB Jr (1984) Head direction cells in the deep layer of dorsal presubiculum in freely moving rats. Soc Neurosci Abstr 10: 599.

Redish AD, Elga AN, Touretzky DS (1996) A coupled attractor model of the rodent head direction system. Network: Comput Neural Syst 7: 671–685.

Reep RL, Chandler HC, King V, Corwin JV (1994) Rat posterior parietal cortex: topography of corticocortical and thalamic connections. Exp Brain Res 100: 67–84.

Reti IM, Minor LB, Baraban JM (2002) Prominent expression of Narp in central vestibular pathways: selective effect of labyrinth ablation. Eur J Neurosci 16: 1949–1958.

Ris L, Godaux E (1998) Neuronal activity in the vestibular nuclei after contralateral or bilateral labyrinthectomy in the alert guinea pig. J Neurophysiol 80: 2352–2367.

Robinson DA (1989) Integrating with neurons. Ann Rev Neurosci 12: 33–45.

Save E, Moghaddam M (1996) Effects of lesions of the associative parietal cortex on the acquisition and use of spatial memory in egocentric and allocentric navigation tasks in the rat. Behav Neurosci 110: 74–85.

Satoh K, Fibiger HC (1986) Cholinergic neurons of the laterodorsal tegmental nucleus: efferent and afferent connections. J Comp Neurol 253: 277–302.

Scudder CA, Fuchs AF (1992) Physiological and behavioral identification of vestibular nucleus neurons mediating the horizontal vestibuloocular reflex in trained rhesus monkeys. J Neurophysiol 68: 244–264.

Sharp PE (1996) Multiple spatial/behavioral correlates for cells in the rat postsubiculum: multiple regression analysis and comparison to other hippocampal areas. Cerebral Cortex 6: 238–259.

Sharp PE, Blair HT, Brown M (1996) Neural network modeling of the hippocampal formation spatial signals and their possible role in navigation: a modular approach. Hippocampus 6: 720–734.

Sharp PE, Tinkelman A, Cho J (2001) Angular velocity and head direction signals recorded from the dorsal tegmental nucleus of Gudden in the rat: implications for path integration in the head direction cell circuit. Behav Neurosci 115: 571–588.

Shibata H (1992) Topographic organization of subcortical projections to the anterior thalamic nuclei in the rat. J Comp Neurol 323: 117–127.

Shibata H (1993) Efferent projections from the anterior thalamic nuclei to the cingulate cortex in the rat. J Comp Neurol 330: 533–542.

Sikes RW, Vogt BA, Swadlow HA (1988) Neuronal responses in rabbit cingulate cortex linked to quick-phase eye movements during nystagmus. J Neurophysiol 59: 922–936.

Skaggs WE, Knierim JJ, Kudrimoti HS, McNaughton BL (1995) A model of the neural basis of the rat's sense of direction. In G Tesauro, DS Touretsky, and TK Leen eds., Advances in Neural Information Processing Systems. Vol 7. Cambridge, MA: MIT Press, pp. 173–180.

Spencer RF, Wenthold RJ, Baker R (1989) Evidence for glycine as an inhibitory neurotransmitter of vestibular, reticular, and prepositus hypoglossi neurons that project to the cat abducens nucleus. J Neurosci 9: 2718–2736.

Stackman RW, Taube JS (1997) Firing properties of head direction cells in the rat anterior thalamic nucleus: dependence on vestibular input. J Neurosci 17: 4349–4358.

Stackman RW, Taube JS (1998) Firing properties of rat lateral mammillary single units: head direction, head pitch, and angular head velocity. J Neurosci 18: 9020–9037.

Stackman RW, Clark AS, Taube JS (2002) Hippocampal spatial representations require vestibular input. Hippocampus 12: 291–303.

Stackman RW, Golob EJ, Bassett JP, Taube JS (2003) Passive transport disrupts directional path integration by rat head direction cells. J Neurophysiol. 90: 2862–2874.

Stanton GB, Goldberg ME, Bruce CJ (1988) Frontal eye field efferents in the macaque monkey: II. Topography of terminal fields in midbrain and pons. J Comp Neurol. 271: 493–506.

Taube JS (1995) Head direction cells recorded in the anterior thalamic nuclei of freely moving rats. J Neurosci 15: 70–86.

Taube JS (2004) Interspike interval analyses on anterior dorsal thalamic head direction cells. Program No. 868.12 2004 Abstract Viewer/Itinerary Planner. Washington D.C.: Society for Neuroscience. Online.

Taube JS, Burton HL (1995) Head direction cell activity monitored in a novel environment and during a cue conflict situation. J Neurophysiol 74: 1953–1971.

Taube JS, Muller RU (1998) Comparison of head direction cell activity in the postsubiculum and anterior thalamus of freely moving rats. Hippocampus 8: 87–108.

Taube, JS, Muller RU, Ranck JB Jr (1990a) Head-direction cells recorded from the postsubiculum in freely moving rats. I . Description and quantitative analysis. J Neurosci 10: 420–435.

Taube JS, Muller RU, Ranck JB Jr (1990b) Head-direction cells recorded from the postsubiculum in freely moving rats. II. Effects of environmental manipulations. J Neurosci 10: 436–447.

Tullman ML, Taube JS (1998) Lesions of the lateral mammillary nuclei abolish head direction cell acivity in the anterior dorsal thalamus. Soc Neurosci Abstr 24: 1912.

Thompson SM, Robertson RT (1987a) Organization of subcortical pathways for sensory projections to the limbic cortex. I. Subcortical projections to the medial limbic cortex in the rat. J Comp Neurol 265: 175–188.

Thompson SM, Robertson RT (1987b) Organization of subcortical pathways for sensory projections to the limbic cortex. II. Afferent projections to the thalamic laterodorsal nucleus in the rat. J Comp Neurol 265: 189–202.

Van Groen T, Wyss JM (1990a) The postsubicular cortex in the rat: characterization of the fourth region of the subicular cortex and its connections. Brain Res 529: 165–177.

Van Groen T, Wyss JM (1990b) Connections of the retrosplenial granular a cortex in the rat. J Comp Neurol 300: 593–606.

Vitte E, Derosier C, Caritu Y, Berthoz A, Hasboun D, Soulie D (1996) Activation of the hippocampal formation by vestibular stimulation: a functional magnetic resonance imaging study. Exp Brain Res 112: 523–526.

Vogt BA, Miller MW (1983) Cortical connections between rat cingulate cortex and visual, motor, and post-subicular cortices. J Comp Neurol 216: 192–210.

Whishaw IQ, Hines DJ, Wallace DG (2001) Dead reckoning (path integration) requires the hippocampal formation: evidence from spontaneous exploration and spatial learning tasks in light (allothetic) and dark (ideothetic) tests. Behav Brain Res 127: 49–69.

Yamano M, Tohyama M (1987) Afferent and efferent enkephalinergic systems of the tegmental nuclei of Gudden in the rat: an immunocytochemical study. Brain Res 408: 22–30.

Young LR (2003) Spatial Orientation. In Pamela S Tsang and Michael A Vidulick eds., Principles and Practice of Aviation Psychology, Mahwah, NJ: Lawrence Erlbaum Associates.

Zhang K (1996) representation of spatial orientation by the intrinsic dynamics of the head direction cell ensemble: a theory. J Neurosci 16: 2112–2126.

Zugaro MB, Berthoz A, Wiener SI (2002) Peak firing rates of rat anterodorsal thalamic head direction cells are higher during faster passive rotations. Hippocampus 12: 481–486.

II INFLUENCE OF VESTIBULAR AND MOTOR CUES ON HEAD DIRECTION CELLS AND PLACE CELLS

6 Vestibular and Motor Processing for Head Direction Signals

Stefan Glasauer

Vestibular information serves a variety of functions, from spatial orientation to postural control and balance, from stabilization of gaze to regulation of autonomic function. It appears to be crucial for the generation of head direction signals as revealed by lesion studies (see chapter 7 by Stackman and Zugaro, this volume). Accordingly, vestibular lesions severely impair navigational abilities in the rat (Wallace et al., 2002). A possible anatomical pathway for transmission of vestibular signals is a projection from the medial vestibular nucleus (mVN) via the nucleus prepositus hypoglossi (NPH), and also directly from the mVN to the dorsal tegmental nucleus of Gudden (Liu et al., 1984), which contains neurons carrying head direction signals, but also information about angular head velocity (see chapter 5 by Bassett and Taube, this volume).

The mVN and NPH are part of the gaze-stabilization system for rotations in the horizontal plane. Neurons in both structures project directly onto extraocular motorneurons. In the following, processing of head angular velocity information from the semicircular canals to the NPH is reviewed, with special emphasis on findings in the rat. The role of cerebellar structures and interactions with other sensory inputs such as optic flow, and information about active head movements is considered.

The Vestibular End Organ

The vestibular end organ consists of semicircular canals and otoliths located in the inner ear, which detect angular and linear head acceleration, respectively. Head acceleration deflects sensory hair bundles, which in turn causes changes in the discharge rates of vestibular neurons. The otolith organs, utricle and saccule in mammals, detect linear acceleration of the head, including gravity in three dimensions. The saccule is oriented so that it mainly detects acceleration in the vertical direction, while the utricle measures linear acceleration in the horizontal plane. The semicircular canals consist of three pairs of membranous ducts filled with endolymph. Rotation of the head causes flow of the endolymph, which deflects hair cells connected to the cupula, a membrane within the canal. The horizontal canals are approximately oriented to measure rotation of the head in the horizontal plane (yaw rotation), while the two pairs of vertical canals detect torsional and vertical head rotation (roll and pitch). Left and right canals operate synergistically in a push-pull fashion: for example, for leftward horizontal head rotation, the left horizontal canal neurons increase their firing rate, while the discharge rate of right horizontal canal neurons decreases. In the rat, but also in other species, including humans, canal planes are orthogonal within 4–8 deg, and pairs of canals are essentially coplanar (see figure 6.1; Daunicht and Pellionisz, 1987; Blanks and Torigoe, 1989). The horizontal canals are usually inclined upwards; in the rat, by about 35° according to Blanks and Torigoe (1989).

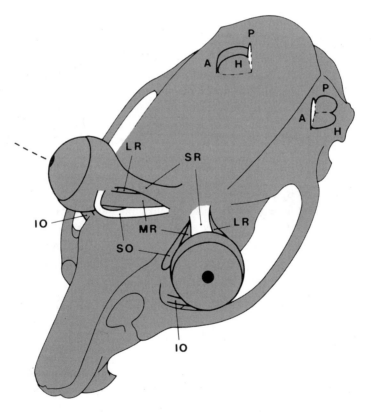

Figure 6.1
Semicircular canals (A, anterior; P, posterior; H, horizontal) and extraocular eye muscles (IO, SO, inferior and superior oblique; SR and IR, superior and inferior rectus; LR and MR, lateral and medial rectus) in the rat. The dashed line extending from the right eye indicates gaze direction. Left anterior and right posterior canal planes, shown in white, are roughly coplanar and almost coincide with the pulling directions of the left superior rectus and right superior oblique muscles. (Modified from Daunicht and Pellionisz, 1987.)

Vidal et al. (1986) reported that rats hold their heads so that the horizontal canals are parallel to the earth horizontal plane, except when the animals are at rest, and then are inclined by 5°.

The dynamics of canal responses to head rotation shows a characteristic frequency dependence. During sustained rotation, the afferent canal response declines exponentially. The time constant of this decay is 2.3–4 s in the rat (Curthoys, 1982), and around 6 s in humans. This high-pass characteristic is due to the mechanical properties of the system, which is tuned so that, in the physiologically relevant frequency range of head rotations, the semicircular canal response is approximately proportional to head angular velocity (Goldberg and Fernandez, 1971).

The primary vestibular neurons, situated in Scarpa's ganglion, send projections to multiple areas in the brainstem and cerebellum (for review, see Newlands and Perachio, 2003). The most prominent projections terminate in the vestibular nuclei (VN) and the vestibulocerebellum (see following pages.)

The Direct Pathway of the Vestibulo-ocular Reflex

One of the best examined sensory-to-motor systems is that of the vestibulo-ocular reflex (VOR). The VOR helps to stabilize gaze in response to head rotations and translations, thereby ensuring that the retinal image remains stable during external perturbations. (In the following, the term "gaze direction" is used to indicate the direction of the eye in spatial coordinates, while "eye position" denotes the angular position of the eye in head coordinates. Correspondingly, gaze velocity is the angular velocity of gaze direction, and eye velocity is the angular velocity of eye position.) This is achieved by brainstem circuits appropriately and rapidly processing head velocity information to yield compensatory counterrotation of the eye within the head. In afoveate animals with low visual acuity (Artal et al., 1998) such as the rat, the VOR is as good or even better than in foveate species such as humans or other higher primates. However, stabilization of the retinal image not only helps to maintain visual acuity, but also maintains the ability to distinguish object motion from self-induced retinal image motion. For example, while walking or running, it is important to distinguish whether optic flow is produced by self-motion or by an approaching predator.

The basic anatomic VOR pathway is the three-neuron arc from semicircular canals to extraocular eye muscles first described by Lorente de Nó (1933, see figure 6.2). The first neuron, located in the vestibular ganglion, transmits angular head velocity information from the sensory hair cells to the second neuron in the vestibular nuclei in the brainstem. These secondary vestibular neurons directly contact the third set of neurons, the motor neurons in the ocular motor nuclei. This reflex pathway is very fast, with latencies of only 5 ms to 10 ms (Huterer and Cullen, 2002). If visual stabilization would be exclusively achieved using visual feedback, then latencies would be larger than 50 ms, due to the

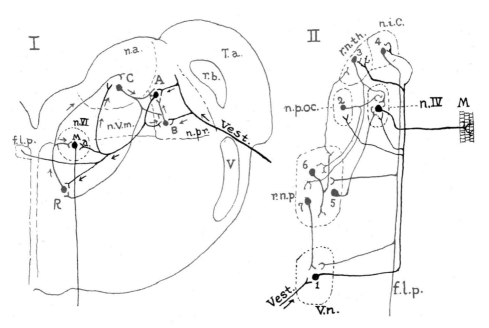

Figure 6.2
Schematic diagram of the basic three-neuron arc of the vestibulo-ocular reflex. Each cell in the drawing is meant to represent groups of neurons having similar connections. The three-neuron arc is highlighted in black, additional pathways in gray. (Diagram modified from Lorente de Nó, 1933.) All pathways and abbreviations are shown as drawn by Lorente de Nó. I. Horizontal VOR, connections in the medulla oblongata (transverse section, probably mouse). Sensory input is relayed from the horizontal semicircular canal via the primary vestibular neuron in the vestibular ganglion (not shown), which sends the vestibular afferent (Vest.) to the vestibular nuclei (n.pr.: nucleus proper of the descending vestibular root). The secondary neuron projects an axon collateral to the abducens nucleus (n.VI) and to various other brainstem sites. The motorneuron (M) in the abducens nucleus contracts the ipsilateral lateral rectus eye muscle. The pathway shown thus involves an inhibitory VN neuron. Rotation to the contralateral side inhibits the ipsilateral canal nerve, and leads to a contraction of the ipsilateral lateral rectus muscle. f.l.p, fasciculus longitudinalis posterior; n.v.m, nucleus ventromedialis; n.a., nucleus angularis; R, reticular nuclei; r.b., restiform body; T.a., tuberculum acusticum; V, fifth nerve. II. Pathway along the fasciculus longitudinalis posterior (f.l.p.) from the anterior semicircular canal via the vestibular nucleus (V.n.) to the trochlear nucleus (n.IV), which projects to the contralateral superior oblique eye muscle and the neural integrator for torsional and vertical eye movements, the interstitial nucleus of Cajal (n.i.C.). Again, this pathway is that of an inhibitory VOR interneuron. r.n.p., reticular nuclei in the pons; n.p.oc., nucleus para-ocularis; r.n.th., reticular nuclei in the thalamus.

complex processing chain from the retina to extraocular motor neurons (for review, see Takemura and Kawano, 2002). The semicircular canal system transmits three-dimensional angular velocity signals, and the eye can be rotated with three degrees of freedom (horizontal, vertical, and torsional rotations). The necessary sensory-to-motor transformation is largely facilitated by the fact that the coordinate systems of canals and extraocular eye muscles are almost coplanar, that is, one semicircular canal mainly excites one of the six extraocular muscles of each eye. For example, stimulation of the left horizontal canal will cause contraction of the lateral rectus eye muscle of the right eye and the medial rectus of the left eye, thereby leading to rotation of both eyes compensatory for the head rotation. In the rat, the misalignment between coordinate systems of eye muscles and canals amounts to 15.5°–34.2° (see figure 6.1; Daunicht and Pellionisz, 1987), which is relatively large compared to other species (Ezure and Graf, 1984).

Eye movements in response to vestibular stimulation are examined experimentally using a sinusoidal or steplike stimulus. For larger rotational amplitudes, slow phases of compensatory eye movements are interrupted by rapid saccadic changes in eye position, the fast phases of nystagmus. These rapid changes are necessary to keep the eye within the oculomotor range, which in rats is around 20° (Fuller, 1985).

Secondary neurons in the three-neuron arc have been examined in various animals including rabbits, cats, and monkeys. For the horizontal VOR, secondary neurons are located mainly in the medial vestibular nucleus (mVN). They consist of several types of neurons classified by their discharge properties. The most important class is the so-called position-vestibular-pause neurons (see figure 6.3), which discharge proportional to head angular velocity, but also carry eye (angular) position information and pause during saccades (Buettner et al., 1978; Scudder and Fuchs, 1992; Roy and Cullen, 1998, 2002; McCrea and Gdowski, 2003; Gdowski and McCrea, 2000). Thus, the direct pathway of the VOR is not exclusively dedicated to transmit head angular velocity signals to ocular motor neurons, but contributes significantly to other types of eye movements by carrying signals related to angular eye position and/or velocity. Consequently, the secondary neurons of the VOR must receive multiple inputs from other sources in brainstem and cerebellum. The inhibition of position-vestibular-pause neurons during saccades, probably caused by input from inhibitory saccadic burst neurons, is thought to mediate the suppression of the VOR during active combined eye and head movements (Roy and Cullen, 1998). Another class of secondary VOR neurons, the eye-head-velocity neurons (sometimes also called gaze-velocity neurons), have been identified to be floccular target neurons, i.e., to receive inhibitory input from Purkinje cells in the floccular lobe of the cerebellum.

Following a step in head velocity, the eye velocity response decays in a way similar to the afferent discharge of primary semicircular canal neurons. However, the time constant of the VOR response is not exclusively determined by that of the afferent canal response. In rats, the so-called velocity-storage mechanism (Raphan et al., 1979) increases the time constant to around 8s (Hess et al., 1989; Quinn et al., 1998; for review, see also Brettler et al., 2000). Velocity storage is a central neural process that enhances the VOR at low frequencies, and is mainly found for the horizontal VOR. Velocity storage not only prolongs the eye movement response to steps in head velocity, but also other behavioral responses as shown by psychophysical experiments in humans. It depends on intact commissural connections between the vestibular nuclei (Wearne et al., 1997), can be severely shortened by unilateral mVN inactivation (Straube et al., 1991), and is modulated by cerebellar influence (see following pages).

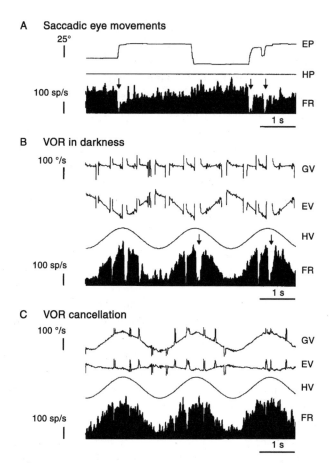

Figure 6.3
Responses of a secondary vestibular neuron in the VN (a position-vestibular-pause neuron) to eye movements and sinusoidal whole body rotations about a vertical axis of head-fixed monkeys (A) During ipsilateral saccadic eye movements, firing rate (FR) pauses (arrows) and is modulated with eye position (EP) even though the head (HP, head position) does not move. (B) Gaze velocity (GV, eye in space), eye in head velocity (EV), head velocity (HV), and firing rate (FR) of the same neuron during sinusoidal rotation in darkness. The neuron is clearly modulated with head velocity (HV) and pauses during ipsilateral quick phases of nystagmus (arrows). (C) Response of the same neuron while the monkey fixates a target that is rotating with the animal. Again, the firing rate is related to head velocity in space (HV), which, in this condition, is almost equal to gaze velocity (GV). (Modified from Roy and Cullen, 1998.)

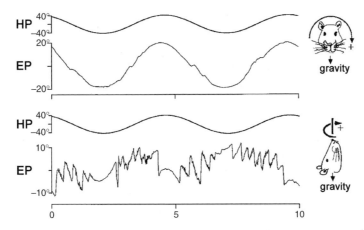

Figure 6.4
Eye movements (EP, eye position) in response to 0.2 Hz 20° roll rotation (HP, head position) over time (s). The orientation of the axis of rotation with respect to the head remained constant. In the upper traces, rotation was in a normal upright position with respect to gravity, which also caused otolith input. In the lower traces, the axis of rotation coincided with gravity, that is, the animal looked upward and only semicircular canal input was available, which decreased VOR gain and caused significantly more quick phases. (Modified from Brettler et al., 2000.)

For rotations around an axis which is not earth vertical, the otoliths contribute to the VOR response (rats: Brettler et al., 2000; figure 6.4). Consider a pitch rotation of the head around an earth horizontal axis; since the head changes its direction with respect to gravity, the otoliths are stimulated. This additional stimulation enhances the VOR response considerably. In the rat, this otolith-canal interaction leads to response gains for roll head rotations around unity even for frequencies lower than 0.1 Hz, while pure yaw VOR shows a marked gain decrease below this frequency (Brettler et al., 2000). Additionally, head tilt with respect to gravity results in compensatory changes in eye position. For example, in rats, constant lateral head tilt of 20° causes vertical eye deviation of about 6° (Hamann et al., 1998) with upward deviation of the ipsi- and downward deviation of the contralateral eye.

Otoliths also play an important role if the axis of rotation does not coincide with the center of the vestibular system, i.e., the midpoint between the labyrinths. In this case, head rotation is accompanied by head translation resulting in centrifugal or centripetal acceleration, which in turn stimulates the otoliths and modifies the VOR depending on the distance of the target. Behaviorally, the presence or absence of centrifugal acceleration sensed by the otoliths may also affect perception of rotation, as shown in humans (Mittelstaedt and Mittelstaedt, 1997). Pure linear translation also evokes compensatory eye movements mediated by the otoliths, the so-called linear or translational VOR (rats: Hess and Dieringer, 1991). Convergence of utricular and horizontal canal afferents onto secondary

VOR neurons in the mVN has been shown to be relatively rare (Zhang et al., 2001), suggesting that, for the horizontal VOR, otolith-canal convergence, if present, may be mediated via indirect cerebellar pathways.

Apart from neurons related to eye movements, the VN also contain non-eye-movement related neurons, which are influenced by active and passive head-on-trunk movements (see section on Non-Eye-Movement-Related neurons in the Vestibular Nuclei, later in this chapter).

Transforming Velocity to Position: the Oculomotor Integrator

The direct three-neuron pathway of the VOR alone only provides a signal about eye velocity. Velocity, however, is not suited as a command signal for ocular motorneurons. Rather, the velocity signal must be transformed to a signal proportional to eye position, which can then be used to hold the eye in a desired gaze direction (for review, see Robinson, 1989). This transformation, mathematically an integration, has been proposed by Robinson (1981) and was shown to be neurally realized in separate anatomical brainstem structures. The nucleus prepositus hypoglossi (NPH) and the adjacent mVN are crucial for transforming horizontal eye velocity signals to eye position signals (see figure 6.5), the interstitial nucleus of Cajal has been shown to integrate torsional and vertical eye velocity signals (for review, see Fukushima and Kaneko, 1995; Moschovakis, 1997). As shown by lesion studies, not only the neurons in these nuclei, but also the commissural fibers between the VN and NPH are an important part of the ocular motor velocity-to-position integrator (rat: Tham et al., 1989; monkey: Anastasio and Robinson, 1991). For the NPH, the commissural fibers have been shown to be predominantly inhibitory, contacting, in part, inhibitory GABAergic NPH neurons (Arts et al., 2000). This observation is compatible with the idea of velocity-to-position integration being achieved by a positive feedback loop achieved by reciprocal commissural inhibition (Robinson 1989; Sklavos and Moschovakis, 2002).

However, these brainstem structures, the so-called final oculomotor integrators, are responsible for only part of the integration process. The high-frequency portions of the eye velocity signal are integrated by the mechanics of the oculomotor plant. For this reason, the above-mentioned three-neuron arc of the VOR together with the mechanical properties of extraocular eye muscles, viscosity, and inertia of the eye ball can produce a change in gaze direction. Furthermore, the floccular lobe of the cerebellum contributes significantly to the integration process (see Cerebellar Contributions to Vestibular and Motor Processing, later in this chapter).

NPH, mVN, and the interstitial nucleus of Cajal not only integrate head velocity signals coming from the vestibular labyrinth, but also command signals from the saccadic burst generators. Saccades are rapid gaze shifts reorienting eye position in response to visual targets, during visual search, or as nystagmus quick phases during VOR. The burst

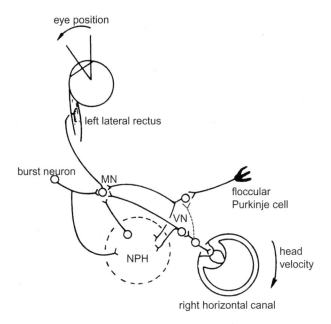

eye position

left lateral rectus

burst neuron

MN

floccular
Purkinje cell

VN

head
velocity

NPH

right horizontal canal

Figure 6.5
The basic circuitry of the neural velocity-to-position integrator for the VOR. For a head rotation to the right (lower right), the right horizontal canal transduces head velocity via the primary sensory neuron to the vestibular nuclei (VN). Secondary neurons in the VN project to the motorneurons (MN); some of them receive additional input from the floccular Purkinje cells (dashed connection, added by the author), and all project via collaterals to the neural integrator located in the prepositus hypoglossi (NPH) and medial VN. The NPH generates an eye position command and also projects to the motor neuron. The motor neuron commands the left lateral rectus eye muscles and produces a compensatory change in eye position. Motor neuron and neural integrator receive additional input from the burst neurons in the reticular formation to generate quick phases of nystagmus and saccadic eye movements. Additional inputs to the secondary vestibular neurons, for example from inhibitory burst neurons, are not shown for clarity. Also, the bilateral structure of the integrator with its necessary commissural connections between both ipsi- and contralateral NPH is omitted to emphasize the processing of afferent head velocity signals. (Modified from Robinson, 1989.)

generator for horizontal saccades is located in the paramedian pontine reticular formation and projects to the NPH (rats: Iwasaki et al., 1999). Quite often, saccades are accompanied by rapid changes in head direction, thus forming combined eye-head saccades. Spontaneous saccades in head-fixed rats are rare, mostly horizontal, usually less than 10° in amplitude, but can reach eye velocities up to 400° (Hikosaka and Sakamoto, 1987).

In the rat, velocity-to-position integration is far from perfect; in darkness, the eye drifts back to its zero position with a time constant of 1.6 to 4 s (Strata et al., 1990). Following lesions of the NPH and mVN in the monkey (Cannon and Robinson, 1987; Straube et al., 1991), the eye drifts with a time constant equal to the mechanical time constant of the eye plant (about 200 ms), i.e., neural integration is completely abolished. In monkeys, time constants for gaze-holding are above 20 s, and decrease to around 2 s following isolated

NPH lesions (Kaneko, 1997). Analysis of VOR responses in the same animals revealed that integration of eye velocity signals for VOR was equally affected by the NPH lesion (Goldman et al., 2002), thus confirming that the NPH is part of a common oculomotor integrator for gaze holding and VOR. However, in monkeys, the time constant after NPH lesions is still about 10 times higher than that of the oculomotor plant. Presumably, remaining function of the spared cerebellum and mVN is responsible for this finding.

Single cell recordings in the NPH revealed that neurons related to eye movements show various patterns of discharge, reaching from eye velocity signals to eye position signals (cat: Delgado-Garcia et al., 1989; Escudero et al., 1992; monkey: McFarland and Fuchs, 1992; Sylvestre et al., 2003). NPH neurons are usually classified with respect to their discharge properties during saccades. Burst-tonic neurons (see figure 6.6) discharge a burst of action potentials during saccades and show tonic eye position (in head) sensitivity. Tonic neurons, less frequently observed, exhibit only an eye position sensitivity such as one would expect from integration of a velocity signal. A third type is called eye-head velocity neurons. Their discharge rate is proportional to eye velocity during smooth pursuit eye movements, but to head velocity when eye movements are visually suppressed during passive head rotation by fixation of a target that moves with the head. Eye-head velocity neurons are also sensitive to eye position, and some also show bursts during saccades (McFarland and Fuchs, 1992). Most of these types of neurons are also found in the regions of the mVN adjacent to the NPH (McFarland and Fuchs, 1992). The eye-head velocity neurons in the mVN are floccular target neurons. Whether this is also the case in the NPH is not known to date.

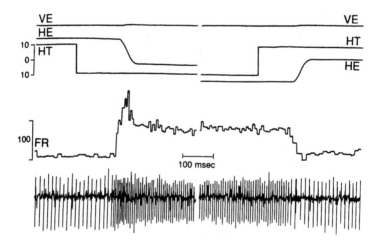

Figure 6.6
Neuronal response of a burst-tonic neuron in the NPH of the monkey. Upper traces show vertical (VE) and horizontal (HE) eye position together with horizontal target position (HT). Lower traces show firing rate (FR) and original neuron discharge. (Modified from McFarland and Fuchs, 1992.)

The NPH not only projects to the ocular motor nuclei—specifically, the contralateral abducens nucleus—but is part of a network for visual-vestibular interaction (McCrea, 1988), as shown by tracer studies (McCrea and Baker, 1985; Belknap and McCrea, 1988). Neurons projecting to the abducens nucleus usually send collaterals to the cerebellar flocculus (Escudero et al., 1996). In turn, the NPH receives direct inhibitory input from the floccular Purkinje cells (Yingcharoen and Rinvik, 1983). Inhibitory projections from the NPH to the dorsal cap of the inferior olive, which sends climbing fibers to the contralateral flocculus, are also involved in the NPH-cerebellar network (Arts et al., 2000). Burst-tonic neurons carrying signals similar to those observed in the ocular motor nuclei have been shown to project back to the superior colliculus (Hardy and Corvisier, 1996; Corvisier and Hardy, 1997), which is organized in a retinotopic map and codes the position of targets for saccadic eye movements (Bergeron et al., 2003). NPH neurons projecting to the contralateral abducens, which in turn projects to the lateral rectus eye muscle of the contralateral eye, are inhibitory; those projecting to the ipsilateral abducens are excitatory (Moreno-Lopez et al., 2002). Neural integration of an eye velocity signal by inhibitory NPH neurons may be achieved by collaterals and commissural projections to contralateral NPH neurons forming a positive feedback loop (for discussion and review see Robinson, 1989, and Moschovakis, 1997) formed by reciprocally connected inhibitory neurons (for neural network models of the integrator, see Sklavos and Moschovakis, 2002). As previously mentioned, the predominantly inhibitory, GABAergic nature of the commissural connections has been demonstrated anatomically (Arts et al., 2000).

The NPH and mVN also project back to the lateral mesencephalic tegmental region (Gerlach and Thier, 1995), which receives input from the superior colliculus. Reciprocal connections with the trigeminal nuclei, mainly to the VN, are supposed to supply proprioceptive information from the extraocular eye muscles (Buisseret-Delmas et al., 1999), even though the contribution of this information for eye movements is under debate (Lewis et al., 2001). Furthermore, the NPH is supposed to be implicated in control of REM sleep via its inhibitory connections to the locus coeruleus (Kaur et al., 2001), from which it also receives inputs that are supposed to regulate vestibulo-ocular responses during changes in alertness (Schuerger and Balaban, 1999). The projections from the NPH to the dorsal tegmental nucleus of Gudden (Liu et al., 1984; Hayakawa and Ziu, 1985) suggest that the NPH plays a major role in relaying vestibular signals to the head direction cell system (see chapter 5 by Bassett and Taube, this volume).

Although the NPH is usually considered to be the horizontal oculomotor integrator, several experimental findings and theoretical considerations support another, although related, view: that the NPH provides an efference copy or prediction of angular eye position and/or velocity in head (Belknap and McCrea, 1988). This view is supported by the projections of the NPH to the inferior olive (Arts et al., 2000) and to the superior colliculus (Corvisier and Hardy, 1997), both of which are thought to receive an efference copy signal. Consistent with this view, models of oculomotor integration not relying on feed-forward processing (Galiana and Guitton, 1992; Green and Galiana, 1998) propose that, rather than constituting the neural integrator, the NPH may implement an internal forward model of the dynamics of the eye in order to predict eye position, which, in turn, is used in a feedback loop for distributed integration.

There is not yet a detailed study in the rat that compares NPH neuron discharge to eye movements or combined eye and head movements. However, neurons in the NPH of the rat have been shown to respond to vestibular and optokinetic stimulation (Lannou et al., 1984), with their firing rate apparently also reflecting the fast phases of vestibular/opto-kinetic nystagmus. For a better understanding of how the NPH may be involved in trans-mitting vestibular signals to the head direction cell system, a detailed analysis of NPH neurons unrelated to eye movements (vestibular-only neurons, McFarland and Fuchs, 1992) would be desirable. These neurons may be comparable to vestibular-only neurons found in the mVN, some of which project to neck motor neurons (McCrea et al., 1999), but it has also been suggested that they participate in navigation (Roy and Cullen, 2001, 2004; see also below). Also, it is not known what information is coded in NPH during active head movements.

Visual-Vestibular Interactions

Optic flow, that is, motion of the whole visual field usually caused by self-displacement, evokes the so-called optokinetic nystagmus (OKN) and the ocular following response (for review, see Takemura and Kawano, 2002), compensatory eye movements that help stabi-lize the retinal image similar to the VOR. The OKN is most efficient for low-frequency stimuli, and thus complements the VOR, which is effective only for higher frequencies (see earlier paragraphs). Under natural stimulation, i.e., head rotation in light conditions, VOR and OKN are synergistic and together produce compensatory nystagmus over the whole frequency range. The compensatory responses mainly consist of eye movements even in rats with the head unrestrained (see figure 6.7; Hess et al., 1985; Dieringer and Meier, 1993). Conflicting vestibular and optokinetic stimulation consequently can cancel nystagmus (rat: Niklasson et al., 1990). OKN responses are also modified by otolith input. If the axis of a visual stimulus coincides with the direction of gravity, the OKN response is maximal, while it is otherwise reduced (Barmack, 2003).

Functionally, this effect, which is mediated by the cerebellum, is caused by a conflict between the rotation of the scene indicating changing orientation with respect to gravity and the static otolith input caused by the constant orientation of gravity with respect to the head.

One pathway for the horizontal OKN consists of direct connections from the pretectal nucleus of the optic tract to the NPH (Korp et al., 1989) and the vestibular nuclei. Lesion of the nucleus of the optic tract completely abolishes OKN in the rat (Cazin et al., 1980).

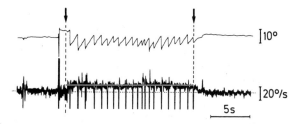

Figure 6.7
Optokinetic nystagmus in the head-restrained rat in response to a 10°/s horizontal visual motion stimulus (vertical stripes rotating around the animal at constant angular velocity). Upper trace shows horizontal eye position, lower trace shows horizontal eye velocity (gray horizontal line indicates stimulus velocity). Dashed vertical lines and arrows indicate onset and offset of visual stimulation. After a slow onset, compensatory eye velocity reaches a constant plateau of about 10°/s, i.e., the eye rotates with the stimulus. Quick phases of nystagmus, visible as downward vertical lines in the velocity trace, reset eye position (upper trace) to about the value before stimulus onset. (Modified from Hess et al., 1985.)

Probably more important are pathways from the nucleus of the optic tract through precerebellar nuclei, such as the nucleus reticularis tegmenti pontis, the dorsolateral pontine nuclei, and the inferior olive to the cerebellar flocular lobe, which are thought to be responsible for OKN (Büttner-Ennever et al., 1996). In primates, the visual medial superior temporal area (MST) of the cerebral cortex sends projections to the dorsolateral pontine nuclei, which project to the ventral paraflocculus of the cerebellum (for review, see Takemura and Kawano, 2002). The cerebellar flocular lobe directly projects to vestibular nucleus neurons and, in the rat, also to the NPH (see following section). Consistent with the connections to the NPH and the vestibular nuclei, optokinetic (Waespe and Henn, 1977; Boyle et al., 1985) or, in primates, smooth pursuit responses (e.g., Scudder and Fuchs, 1992; Roy and Cullen, 2003) are found in secondary vestibular neurons which are part of the direct VOR pathway, showing that visual-vestibular interaction takes place very early in the processing chain. In foveate animals, the OKN and ocular following response are enhanced by the smooth pursuit system, which uses similar anatomical pathways and also interacts with vestibular responses at the level of secondary vestibular neurons (for review, see Fukushima, 2004).

Cerebellar Contributions to Vestibular and Motor Processing

The cerebellum plays an important role in motor control and learning in general (for review, see Ito, 2002). It is also of major importance for processing of vestibular signals as revealed by lesion studies. The cerebellar cortex (for review, see Voogd and Glickstein, 1998) is built of four main groups of neurons: granule cells, Purkinje cells, and two types of inhibitory interneurons (Golgi cells and stellate/basket cells). Inputs to the cerebellar cortex are mainly supplied by mossy fibers terminating on granule cells, and climbing fibers from the inferior olive contacting Purkinje cells. The axons of the granule cells, the parallel fibers, are contacted by the dendritic trees of the Purkinje cells. Output from the cerebellar cortex is exclusively conveyed by the inhibitory Purkinje cells. Their axons terminate on the deep cerebellar nuclei and certain brainstem nuclei such as the vestibular nuclei and, in the rat, the NPH (Balaban et al., 2000).

The most caudal part of the cerebellum is called vestibulocerebellum; it consists of the floccular lobe (flocculus and paraflocculus) and the nodulus and uvula complex of the posterior vermis (lobules IX and X). Its parts are important for different functions related to vestibular and oculomotor processing (for review, see Barmack, 2003). Lesion of the cerebellar flocculus severely damages velocity-to-position integration. In the rat, lesion of the inferior olive also damages gaze holding, leading to time constants of 600–900 ms (Strata et al., 1990), but lesion of flocculus and paraflocculus reduces the time constant even more (Tempia et al., 1992). Mossy fiber input to the floccular lobe is supplied by the NPH and the vestibular nuclei (rat: Blanks et al., 1983; Roste, 1989; Barmack et al., 1992, 1993; Osanai et al., 1999) and visual structures such as the pontine nuclei, previously mentioned. Another input to the floccular lobe, perhaps even more important than the NPH and VN input, originates in the paramedian tract neurons, a brainstem structure that receives axon collaterals of all input to the extraocular motorneurons (Büttner-Ennever et al., 1989). Lesion of this cell group also severely damages gaze holding, as shown in the monkey (Nakamagoe et al., 2000). An important input for climbing fiber activity in the flocculus is supplied from the dorsal cap of the inferior olive, which receives input from inhibitory neurons in the NPH (Arts et al., 2000).

Lesions of the floccular lobe also damage the ability for adaptive adjustment of the VOR, that is, for VOR motor learning. The physiological basis of VOR adaptation is well examined (for review, see Lisberger, 1998; Ito 1982, 2002; see figure 6.8) and based on mossy and climbing fiber projections to the flocculus carrying semicircular canal afferent, retinal slip, and efferent copy information about eye movements. It is still debated whether adaptation occurs only in the flocculus (e.g., Babalian and Vidal, 2000), or whether it also modifies the synaptic strength of floccular target neurons in the vestibular nuclei (e.g., Highstein, 1998; Lisberger, 1998). The inhibitory influence by which the flocculus affects the VOR gain is exerted by a monosynaptic connection from PCs to secondary VOR neurons, the so-called floccular target neurons. For the horizontal VOR, the floccular target neurons are the eye-head-velocity neurons in the mVN (McCrea et al., 1987; Roy and Cullen, 2003). It is not known whether eye-head-velocity neurons in the NPH also receive direct floccular input.

Lesions of the cerebellar nodulus and uvula affect the velocity storage mechanism of the VOR (Waespe et al., 1985; Angelaki and Hess, 1994) and OKN (Hasegawa et al., 1994) and the otolith-mediated changes in VOR and OKN responses (Angelaki and Hess, 1995; Cohen et al., 2002), but do not significantly change the gain of the VOR or OKN (Barmack et al., 2002). Mossy fiber input to nodulus and uvula is supplied by primary vestibular

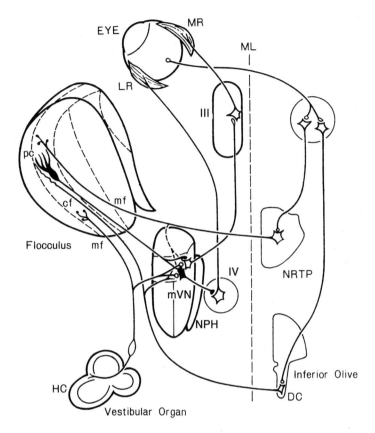

Figure 6.8
Pathways for the contribution of the cerebellar flocculus to the VOR. Purkinje cells (pc) in the flocculus project to the eye-head velocity cells in the mVN. They receive retinal slip information from mossy fiber (mf) input via the nucleus reticularis tegmenti pontis (NRTP) and from climbing fiber (cf) input via the dorsal cap (DC) of the inferior olive. Climbing fiber inputs are thought to act as a teaching signal to modify the PC contribution to the VOR. Vestibular information about head velocity is transmitted directly via mossy fibers from the horizontal semicircular canal (HC) and floccular projecting neurons in the mVN (not shown). Eye-head velocity cells project to the motorneurons in the ocular motor nuclei (III, VI) and to the NPH (not shown). PCs also receive input from the NPH and from the paramedian tract cell group (not shown) carrying efference copy information about eye velocity and position. Excitatory synapses are shown as open circles; inhibitory cells and synapses are shown filled. (Modified from Ito, 1982.)

afferents originating in the vestibular ganglion (Barmack et al., 1993) and from secondary vestibular neurons in the VN. In turn, nodulus and uvula project to the VN, possibly to vestibular-only neurons that transmit head angular velocity signals about passive head rotation (Roy and Cullen, 2004).

Both NPH and mVN also project to the oculomotor subnuclei of the inferior olive. However, olivary-projecting neurons do not project to the extraocular motorneurons and vice versa (Wentzel et al., 1995). The other major input to the inferior olive is supplied by the nucleus of the optic tract (see above) and is thought to convey retinal slip information used, for example, for VOR adaptation (for review, see Büttner-Ennever and Horn, 1997).

Theories of cerebellar function for motor control (Kawato and Gomi, 1992; Darlot, 1993; Miall et al., 1993; Wolpert et al., 1998) propose that the cerebellum enhances sensory and motor function by implementing internal forward or inverse models of sensors and actuators to predict the consequences of motor commands, to compare the prediction with the desired action, and to use the error between both to enhance the motor command. Considering the VOR, nodulus and uvula may implement an internal forward model of the vestibular system, thereby implementing parts of the velocity storage system and predicting canal input from otolith input and efferent copies of head motor commands and vice versa to enhance sensory information. The floccular lobe may implement a forward model of the dynamical properties of the eye to predict the eye movement resulting from canal afferent input to enhance velocity-to-position integration (Glasauer, 2003).

Gaze Orienting: Combined Eye-Head Movements

Combined eye-head movements usually do not contribute significantly to retinal image stabilization (rat: Dieringer and Meier, 1993). Rather, they are used to reorient or redirect gaze. Gaze reorientation is, under natural circumstances, composed of a saccadic eye movement, together with a head movement. Since the head cannot be moved at the same speed as the eye, head movement in combined eye-head saccades outlasts the eye movement. After the saccadic eye movement is finished and has reached its goal, the remaining head movement does not lead to a change in gaze direction; rather, gaze is stabilized in space, that is, the eye counterrotates within the moving head. As shown by several behavioral studies, the VOR during the saccadic eye movement is suppressed. A neural correlate of this suppression has been found in monkeys. The position-vestibular-pause neurons in the VN, which are VOR interneurons, pause during saccadic eye movements, and thus no longer contribute to the VOR (Roy and Cullen, 1998). This suppression is supposed to be mediated by inhibitory input from saccadic burst neurons.

In the period immediately after the eye saccades, when gaze has reached its goal, the active head movement still continues, but gaze is stabilized. Since the head moves actively with respect to the trunk, several signals could be responsible for gaze stabilization during this period: VOR signals from the semicircular canals, prorioceptive reafferent signals from the neck, or efference copy signals of neck motor commands. In the squirrel monkey, most secondary vestibular neurons receive proprioceptive input from the neck, either as head position or head velocity information. Consequently, the squirrel monkey shows a significant cervico-ocular reflex, i.e., a VOR-like eye movement response to passive trunk-under-head rotation (Gdowski and McCrea, 2000). In most other species, modulation of secondary vestibular neurons by neck proprioceptive input is negligible (e.g., rhesus monkey: Roy and Cullen, 2002). In the rat, proprioceptive projections from the neck to the VN and NPH have been shown to exist anatomically (Neuhuber and Zenker, 1989; Xiong and Matsushita, 2001). However, during active eye-head gaze shifts, gaze stabilization following the eye saccade is primarily achieved by VOR signals from the semicircular canals, modulated by efference copy of neck motor commands (rhesus monkey: Roy and Cullen, 2002; squirrel monkey: McCrea and Gdowski, 2003).

Non-Eye-Movement–Related Neurons in the Vestibular Nuclei

Active head movements cause major changes in the sensitivity of neurons in the VN that are not related to eye movements, the so-called vestibular-only (VO) neurons (Gdowski and McCrea, 1999). These neurons, which are also found in the mVN, faithfully encode head rotation in space independently of eye movements for passive whole-body rotation, but are mostly insensitive to active head-on-trunk motion (Roy and Cullen, 2001, 2004), even though active head movements on a stationary trunk cause semicircular canal afferent discharge. Some VO neurons are vestibulospinal neurons, i.e., they participate in head stabilization (McCrea et al. 1999); others may serve as relays to thalamocortical pathways mediating higher vestibular functions such as spatial orientation and navigation, including the head direction cell system (Roy and Cullen, 2001, 2004). Specifically, due to their insensitivity to active head movements mentioned earlier, some of them code trunk-in-space velocity rather than, as expected from vestibular neurons, head-in-space velocity (Gdowski and McCrea 1999, see fig. 6.9). It has been suggested that VO neurons are reciprocally connected to uvula and nodulus of the cerebellum, but they may also be target neurons of the rostral fastigial nuclei of the cerebellum, which show non-eye-movement–related vestibular activity, and apparently code trunk-in-space rather than head-in-space velocity (for review, see Büttner et al. 2003).

Summary

In this review, the processing from sensory vestibular afferent signals to motor output for gaze stabilization has been outlined. Already at the level of the secondary vestibular

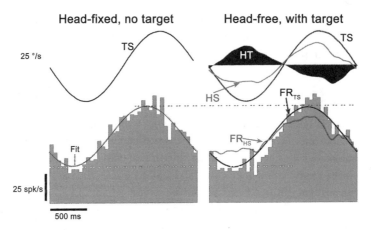

Figure 6.9
Discharge of a secondary vestibular-only neuron in the VN. (monkey). (Left) During head-fixed rotation of the whole animal in darkness, this neuron approximately encodes trunk-in-space (TS) velocity, which, in this condition, equals head-in-space velocity. The fit is shown as dashed line. (Right) In the head-free animal, which looked at a space fixed target and consequently made active head-on-trunk movements (HT), the same neuron still encoded trunk-in-space velocity rather than head-in-space velocity (HS, gray line) as would be expected from a secondary vestibular neuron receiving semicircular canal afferent input. The expected firing rates from head-in-space motion (Fit_{HS}) and trunk-in-space motion (Fit_{TS}) are shown for comparison. (Based on Gdowski and McCrea, 1999.)

neurons in the mVN, a convergence of vestibular afferents with visual and oculomotor signals from different sources—such as the cerebellum, the NPH, the saccadic burst generators, and reafferent and/or efference copies of active head motion—is found, i.e., a pure vestibular signal coding head velocity no longer exists (for review, see McCrea et al., 2001). Neurons in the mVN not only participate in the VOR and in head movement control as outlined previously, but also serve to mediate, e.g., autonomic function (Porter and Balaban, 1997), or participate in higher cognitive functions via projections from/to the cortex (for review, see Fukushima, 1997). Other parts of the VN can initiate the startle reflex via vestibulospinal pathways (Li et al., 2001) or contribute to posture and balance.

The NPH, playing a major role for oculomotor velocity-to-position integration, carries signals related to eye velocity and position. Given that the NPH is believed to constitute the predominant input of vestibular signals for the head direction system, this suggests that head direction cells, in fact, may code gaze direction, which, in the rat, is almost equivalent to head direction, considering that the rat achieves gaze shifts almost exclusively by combined eye-head movements. Alternatively, vestibular-only neurons found in the mVN, which often do not respond to active head-on-trunk movements, but only to passive rotation of the head (McCrea et al., 1999; Gdowski and McCrea, 1999; Roy and Cullen, 2001, 2004), may constitute the pathway for vestibular signals to the head direction system.

References

Anastasio TJ, Robinson DA (1991) Failure of the oculomotor neural integrator from a discrete midline lesion between the abducens nuclei in the monkey. Neurosci Lett 127: 82–86.

Angelaki DE, Hess BJM (1994) The cerebellar nodulus and ventral uvula control the torsional vestibulo-ocular reflex. J Neurophysiol 72: 1443–1447.

Angelaki DE, Hess BJM (1995) Inertial representation of angular motion in the vestibular system of rhesus monkeys. II. Otolith-controlled transformation that depends on an intact cerebellar nodulus. J Neurophysiol 73: 1729–1751.

Artal P, Herreros de Tejada P, Munoz Tedo C, Green DG (1998) Retinal image quality in the rodent eye. Vis Neurosci 15: 597–605.

Arts MP, De Zeeuw CI, Lips J, Rosbak E, Simpson JI (2000) Effects of nucleus prepositus hypoglossi lesions on visual climbing fiber activity in the rabbit flocculus. J Neurophysiol 84: 2552–2563.

Babalian AL, Vidal PP (2000) Floccular modulation of vestibulooocular pathways and cerebellum-related plasticity: An in vitro whole brain study. J Neurophysiol 84: 2514–2528.

Balaban CD, Schuerger RJ, Porter JD (2000) Zonal organization of flocculo-vestibular connections in rats. Neuroscience 99: 669–682.

Barmack NH (2003) Central vestibular system: vestibular nuclei and posterior cerebellum. Brain Res Bull 60: 511–541.

Barmack NH, Baughman RW, Eckenstein FP (1992) Cholinergic innervation of the cerebellum of the rat by secondary vestibular afferents. Ann N Y Acad Sci 656: 566–579.

Barmack NH, Baughman RW, Errico P, Shojaku H (1993) Vestibular primary afferent projection to the cerebellum of the rabbit. J Comp Neurol 327: 521–534.

Barmack NH, Errico P, Ferraresi A, Fushiki H, Pettorossi VE, Yakhnitsa V (2002) Cerebellar nodulectomy impairs spatial memory of vestibular and optokinetic stimulation in rabbits. J Neurophysiol 2002 87: 962–975.

Belknap DB, McCrea RA (1988) Anatomical connections of the prepositus and abducens nuclei in the squirrel monkey. J Comp Neurol 268: 13–28.

Blanks RH, Precht W, Torigoe Y (1983) Afferent projections to the cerebellar flocculus in the pigmented rat demonstrated by retrograde transport of horseradish peroxidase. Exp Brain Res 52: 293–306.

Blanks RH, Torigoe Y (1989) Orientation of the semicircular canals in rat. Brain Res. 487: 278–287.

Boyle R, Büttner U, Markert G (1985) Vestibular nuclei activity and eye movements in the alert monkey during sinusoidal optokinetic stimulation. Exp Brain Res 57: 362–369.

Brettler SC, Rude SA, Quinn KJ, Killian JE, Schweitzer EC, Baker JF (2000) The effect of gravity on the horizontal and vertical vestibulo-ocular reflex in the rat. Exp Brain Res 132: 434–444.

Buettner UW, Büttner U, Henn V (1978) Transfer characteristics of neurons in vestibular nuclei of the alert monkey. J Neurophysiol 41: 1614–1628.

Buisseret-Delmas C, Compoint C, Delfini C, Buisseret P (1999) Organisation of reciprocal connections between trigeminal and vestibular nuclei in the rat. J Comp Neurol 409: 153–168.

Büttner U, Glasauer S, Glonti L, Guan Y, Kipiani E, Kleine J, Siebold C, Tchelidze T, Wilden A (2003) Multimodal signal integration in vestibular neurons of the primate fastigial nucleus. Ann N Y Acad Sci 1004: 241–251.

Büttner-Ennever JA, Cohen B, Horn AK, Reisine H (1996) Efferent pathways of the nucleus of the optic tract in monkey and their role in eye movements. J Comp Neurol 373: 90–107.

Büttner-Ennever JA, Horn AK (1997) Anatomical substrates of oculomotor control. Curr Opin Neurobiol 7: 872–879.

Büttner-Ennever JA, Horn AK, Schmidtke K (1989) Cell groups of the medial longitudinal fasciculus and paramedian tracts. Rev Neurol (Paris) 145: 533–539.

Cannon SC, Robinson DA (1987) Loss of the neural integrator of the oculomotor system from brain stem lesions in monkey. J Neurophysiol 57: 1383–1409.

Cazin L, Magnin M, Lannou J (1982) Non-cerebellar visual afferents to the vestibular nuclei involving the prepositus hypoglossal complex: an autoradiographic study in the rat. Exp Brain Res 48: 309–313.

Cazin L, Precht W, Lannou J (1980) Pathways mediating optokinetic responses of vestibular nucleus neurons in the rat. Pflugers Arch 384: 19–29.

Cohen B, John P, Yakushin SB, Buettner-Ennever J, Raphan T (2002) The nodulus and uvula: source of cerebellar control of spatial orientation of the angular vestibulo-ocular reflex. Ann N Y Acad Sci 978: 28–45.

Corvisier J, Hardy O (1997) Topographical characteristics of preposito-collicular projections in the cat as revealed by *Phaseolus vulgaris-leucoagglutinin* technique. A possible organisation underlying temporal-to-spatial transformations. Exp Brain Res 114: 461–471.

Curthoys IS (1982) The response of primary horizontal semicircular canal neurons in the rat and guinea pig to angular acceleration. Exp Brain Res 47: 286–294.

Darlot C (1993) The cerebellum as a predictor of neural messages. I. The stable estimator hypothesis. Neuroscience 56: 617–646.

Daunicht WJ, Pellionisz AJ (1987) Spatial arrangement of the vestibular and the oculomotor system in the rat. Brain Res 435: 48–56.

Delgado-Garcia JM, Vidal PP, Gomez C, Berthoz A (1989) A neurophysiological study of prepositus hypoglossi neurons projecting to oculomotor and preoculomotor nuclei in the alert cat. Neuroscience 29: 291–307.

Dieringer N, Meier RK (1993) Evidence for separate eye and head position command signals in unrestrained rats. Neurosci Lett 162: 129–132.

Escudero M, Cheron G, Godaux E (1996) Discharge properties of brain stem neurons projecting to the flocculus in the alert cat. II. Prepositus hypoglossal nucleus. J Neurophysiol 76: 1775–1785.

Escudero M, de la Cruz RR, Delgado-Garcia JM (1992) A physiological study of vestibular and prepositus hypoglossi neurones projecting to the abducens nucleus in the alert cat. J Physiol 458: 539–560.

Ezure K, Graf W (1984) A quantitative analysis of the spatial organization of the vestibulo-ocular reflexes in lateral- and frontal-eyed animals—I. Orientation of semicircular canals and extraocular muscles. Neuroscience 12: 85–93.

Fuller JH (1985) Eye and head movements in the pigmented rat. Vision Res 25: 1121–1128.

Fukushima K (1997) Corticovestibular interactions: anatomy, electrophysiology, and functional considerations. Exp Brain Res 117: 1–16.

Fukushima K (2004) Roles of the cerebellum in pursuit-vestibular interactions. Cerebellum 2: 223–232.

Fukushima K, Kaneko CR (1995) Vestibular integrators in the oculomotor system. Neurosci Res 22: 249–258.

Galiana HL, Guitton D (1992) Central organization and modeling of eye-head coordination during orienting gaze shifts. Ann N Y Acad Sci 656: 452–471.

Gdowski GT, McCrea RA (1999) Integration of vestibular and head movement signals in the vestibular nuclei during whole-body rotation. J Neurophysiol 82: 436–449.

Gdowski GT, McCrea RA (2000) Neck proprioceptive inputs to primate vestibular nucleus neurons. Exp Brain Res 135: 511–526.

Gerlach I, Thier P (1995) Brainstem afferents to the lateral mesencephalic tegmental region of the cat. J Comp Neurol 358: 219–232.

Glasauer S (2003) Cerebellar contribution to saccades and gaze holding: a modelling approach. Ann N Y Acad Sci 1004: 206–219.

Goldberg JM, Fernandez C (1971) Physiology of peripheral neurons innervating semicircular canals of the squirrel monkey. I. Resting discharge and response to constant angular accelerations. J Neurophysiol 34: 635–660.

Goldman MS, Kaneko CR, Major G, Aksay E, Tank DW, Seung HS (2002) Linear regression of eye velocity on eye position and head velocity suggests a common oculomotor neural integrator. J Neurophysiol 88: 659–665.

Green AM, Galiana HL (1998) Hypothesis for shared central processing of canal and otolith signals. J Neurophysiol 80: 2222–2228.

Hamann KF, Reber A, Hess BJM, Dieringer N (1998) Long-term deficits in otolith, canal and optokinetic ocular reflexes of pigmented rats after unilateral vestibular nerve section. Exp Brain Res 118: 331–340.

Hardy O, Corvisier J (1996) Firing properties of preposito-collicular neurones related to horizontal eye movements in the alert cat. Exp Brain Res 110: 413–424.

Hasegawa T, Kato I, Harada K, Ikarashi T, Yoshida M, Koike Y (1994) The effect of uvulonodular lesions on horizontal optokinetic nystagmus and optokinetic after-nystagmus in cats. Acta Otolaryngol Suppl 511: 126–130.

Hayakawa T, Zyo K (1985) Afferent connections of Gudden's tegmental nuclei in the rabbit. J Comp Neurol 235: 169–181.

Hess BJM, Blanks RH, Lannou J, Precht W (1989) Effects of kainic acid lesions of the nucleus reticularis tegmenti pontis on fast and slow phases of vestibulo-ocular and optokinetic reflexes in the pigmented rat. Exp Brain Res 74: 63–79.

Hess BJM, Precht W, Reber A, Cazin L (1985) Horizontal optokinetic ocular nystagmus in the pigmented rat. Neuroscience 15: 97–107.

Hess BJM, Dieringer N (1991) Spatial organization of linear vestibuloocular reflexes of the rat: responses during horizontal and vertical linear acceleration. J Neurophysiol 66: 1805–1818.

Highstein SM (1998) Role of the flocculus of the cerebellum in motor learning of the vestibulo-ocular reflex. Otolaryngol Head Neck Surg 119: 212–220.

Hikosaka O, Sakamoto M (1987) Dynamic characteristics of saccadic eye movements in the albino rat. Neurosci Res 4: 304–308.

Huterer M, Cullen KE (2002) Vestibuloocular reflex dynamics during high-frequency and high-acceleration rotations of the head on body in rhesus monkey. J Neurophysiol 88: 13–28.

Ito M (1982) Cerebellar control of the vestibulo-ocular reflex–around the flocculus hypothesis. Annu Rev Neurosci 5: 275–296.

Ito M (2002) Historical review of the significance of the cerebellum and the role of Purkinje cells in motor learning. Ann N Y Acad Sci. 978: 273–288.

Iwasaki H, Kani K, Maeda T (1999) Neural connections of the pontine reticular formation, which connects reciprocally with the nucleus prepositus hypoglossi in the rat. Neuroscience 93: 195–208.

Kaneko CRS (1997) Eye movement deficits after ibotenic acid lesions of the nucleus prepositus hypoglossi in monkeys. I. Saccades and fixation. J Neurophysiol 78: 1753–1768.

Kaur S, Saxena RN, Mallick BN (2001) GABAergic neurons in prepositus hypoglossi regulate REM sleep by its action on locus coeruleus in freely moving rats. Synapse 42: 141–150.

Kawato M, Gomi H (1992) The cerebellum and VOR/OKR learning models. Trends Neurosci 15: 445–453.

Korp BG, Blanks RH, Torigoe Y (1989) Projections of the nucleus of the optic tract to the nucleus reticularis tegmenti pontis and prepositus hypoglossi nucleus in the pigmented rat as demonstrated by anterograde and retrograde transport methods. Vis Neurosci 2: 275–286.

Lannou J, Cazin L, Precht W, Le Taillanter M (1984) Responses of prepositus hypoglossi neurons to optokinetic and vestibular stimulations in the rat. Brain Res 301: 39–45.

Lewis RF, Zee DS, Hayman MR, Tamargo RJ (2001) Oculomotor function in the rhesus monkey after deafferentation of the extraocular muscles. Exp Brain Res 141: 349–358.

Li L, Steidl S, Yeomans JS (2001) Contributions of the vestibular nucleus and vestibulospinal tract to the startle reflex. Neuroscience 106: 811–821.

Lisberger SG (1998) Physiologic basis for motor learning in the vestibulo-ocular reflex. Otolaryngol Head Neck Surg 119: 43–48.

Liu R, Chang L, Wickern G. (1984) The dorsal tegmental nucleus: an axoplasmic transport study. Brain Res 310: 123–132.

Lorente de Nó R (1933) Vestibulo-ocular reflex arc. Arch Neurol Psychiatry 30: 245–291.

McCrea RA (1988) Neuroanatomy of the oculomotor system. The nucleus prepositus. Rev Oculomot Res 2: 203–223.

McCrea RA, Baker R (1985) Anatomical connections of the nucleus prepositus of the cat. J Comp Neurol 237: 377–407.

McCrea RA, Gdowski GT (2003) Firing behaviour of squirrel monkey eye movement-related vestibular nucleus neurons during gaze saccades. J Physiol 546: 207–224.

McCrea RA, Gdowski GT, Boyle R, Belton T (1999) Firing behavior of vestibular neurons during active and passive head movements: vestibulo-spinal and other non-eye-movement related neurons. J Neurophysiol 82: 416–428

McCrea R, Gdowski G, Luan H (2001) Current concepts of vestibular nucleus function: transformation of vestibular signals in the vestibular nuclei. Ann N Y Acad Sci 942: 328–344.

McCrea RA, Strassman A, May E, Highstein SM (1987) Anatomical and physiological characteristics of vestibular neurons mediating the horizontal vestibulo-ocular reflex of the squirrel monkey. J Comp Neurol 264: 547–570.

McFarland JL, Fuchs AF (1992) Discharge patterns in nucleus prepositus hypoglossi and adjacent medial vestibular nucleus during horizontal eye movement in behaving macaques. J Neurophysiol 68: 319–332.

Meier RK, Dieringer N (1993) The role of compensatory eye and head movements in the rat for image stabilization and gaze orientation. Exp Brain Res 96: 54–64.

Miall RC, Weir DJ, Wolpert DM, Stein JF. (1993) Is the cerebellum a smith predictor? J Mot Behav 25: 203–216.

Mittelstaedt ML, Mittelstaedt H (1997) The effect of centrifugal force on the perception of rotation about a vertical axis. Naturwissenschaften 84: 366–369.

Moreno-Lopez B, Escudero M, Estrada C (2002) Nitric oxide facilitates GABAergic neurotransmission in the cat oculomotor system: a physiological mechanism in eye movement control. J Physiol 540: 295–306.

Moschovakis AK (1997) The neural integrators of the mammalian saccadic system. Front Biosci 2: D552–D577.

Nakamagoe K, Iwamoto Y, Yoshida K (2000) Evidence for brainstem structures participating in oculomotor integration. Science 288: 857–859.

Neuhuber WL, Zenker W (1989) Central distribution of cervical primary afferents in the rat, with emphasis on proprioceptive projections to vestibular, perihypoglossal, and upper thoracic spinal nuclei. J Comp Neurol 280: 231–253.

Newlands SD, Perachio AA (2003) Central projections of the vestibular nerve: a review and single fiber study in the Mongolian gerbil. Brain Res Bull 60: 475–495.

Niklasson M, Tham R, Larsby B, Eriksson B (1990–91). The influence of visual and somatosensory input on the vestibulo-oculomotor reflex of pigmented rats. J Vestib Res 1: 251–262.

Osanai R, Nagao S, Kitamura T, Kawabata I, Yamada J (1999) Differences in mossy and climbing afferent sources between flocculus and ventral and dorsal paraflocculus in the rat. Exp Brain Res 124: 248–264.

Porter JD, Balaban CD (1997) Connections between the vestibular nuclei and brain stem regions that mediate autonomic function in the rat. J Vestib Res 7: 63–76.

Quinn KJ, Rude SA, Brettler SC, Baker JF (1998) Chronic recording of the vestibulo-ocular reflex in the restrained rat using a permanently implanted scleral search coil. J Neurosci Methods 80: 201–208.

Raphan T, Matsuo V, Cohen B (1979) Velocity storage in the vestibulo-ocular reflex arc (VOR). Exp Brain Res 35: 229–248.

Robinson DA (1981) The use of control systems analysis in the neurophysiology of eye movements. Annu Rev Neurosci 4: 463–503.

Robinson DA (1989) Integrating with neurons. Annu Rev Neurosci 12: 33–45.

Roste GK (1989) Observations on the projection from the perihypoglossal nuclei to the cerebellar cortex and nuclei in the cat. A retrograde WGA-HRP and fluorescent tracer study. Anat Embryol (Berl) 180: 521–533.

Roy JE, Cullen KE (1998) A neural correlate for vestibulo-ocular reflex suppression during voluntary eye-head gaze shifts. Nat Neurosci 1: 404–410.

Roy JE, Cullen KE (2001) Selective processing of vestibular reafference during self-generated head motion. J Neurosci 21: 2131–2142.

Roy JE, Cullen KE (2002) Vestibuloocular reflex signal modulation during voluntary and passive head movements. J Neurophysiol 87: 2337–2357.

Roy JE, Cullen KE (2003) Brain stem pursuit pathways: dissociating visual, vestibular, and proprioceptive inputs during combined eye-head gaze tracking. J Neurophysiol 90: 271–290.

Roy JE, Cullen KE (2004) Dissociating self-generated from passively applied head motion: neural mechanisms in the vestibular nuclei. J Neurosci 24: 2102–2111.

Schuerger RJ, Balaban CD (1999) Organization of the coeruleo-vestibular pathway in rats, rabbits, and monkeys. Brain Res Brain Res Rev 30: 189–217.

Scudder CA, Fuchs AF (1992) Physiological and behavioral identification of vestibular nucleus neurons mediating the horizontal vestibuloocular reflex in trained rhesus monkeys. J Neurophysiol 68: 244–264.

Sklavos SG, Moschovakis AK (2002) Neural network simulations of the primate oculomotor system IV. A distributed bilateral stochastic model of the neural integrator of the vertical saccadic system. Biol Cybern 86: 97–109.

Strata P, Chelazzi L, Ghirardi M, Rossi F, Tempia F (1990) Spontaneous saccades and gaze-holding ability in the pigmented rat. I. Effects of inferior olive lesion. Eur J Neurosci 2: 1074–1084.

Straube A, Kurzan R, Büttner U (1991) Differential effects of bicuculline and muscimol microinjections into the vestibular nuclei on simian eye movements. Exp Brain Res 86: 347–358.

Sylvestre PA, Choi JT, Cullen KE (2003) Discharge Dynamics of Oculomotor Neural Integrator Neurons During Conjugate and Disjunctive Saccades and Fixation. J Neurophysiol 90: 739–754.

Takemura A, Kawano K (2002) Sensory-to-motor processing of the ocular-following response. Neurosci Res 43: 201–206.

Tham R, Larsby B, Eriksson B, Odkvist LM (1989) Effects on the vestibulo- and opto-oculomotor system in rats by lesions of the commissural vestibular fibres. Acta Otolaryngol 108: 372–377.

Tempia F, Ghirardi M, Dotta M, Strata P (1992) Spontaneous gaze shifts in intact head-free rats and following inferior olive and cerebellar lesions. Eur J Neurosci 4: 1239–1248.

Vidal PP, Graf W, Berthoz A (1986) The orientation of the cervical vertebral column in unrestrained awake animals. I. Resting position. Exp Brain Res 61: 549–559.

Voogd J, Glickstein M (1998) The anatomy of the cerebellum. Trends Neurosci 21: 370–375.

Waespe W, Cohen B, Raphan T (1985) Dynamic modification of the vestibulo-ocular reflex by the nodulus and uvula. Science 228: 199–202.

Waespe W, Henn V (1977) Vestibular nuclei activity during optokinetic after-nystagmus (OKAN) in the alert monkey. Exp Brain Res 30: 323–330.

Wallace DG, Hines DJ, Pellis SM, Whishaw IQ (2002) Vestibular information is required for dead reckoning in the rat. J Neurosci 22: 10009–10017.

Wearne S, Raphan T, Cohen B (1997) Contribution of vestibular commissural pathways to spatial orientation of the angular vestibuloocular reflex. J Neurophysiol 78: 1193–1197.

Wentzel PR, Wylie DR, Ruigrok TJ, De Zeeuw CI (1995) Olivary projecting neurons in the nucleus prepositus hypoglossi, group y and ventral dentate nucleus do not project to the oculomotor complex in the rabbit and the rat. Neurosci Lett 190: 45–48.

Wolpert DM, Miall RC, Kawato M. (1998) Internal models in the cerebellum. Trends Cogn Sci 2: 338–347.

Xiong G, Matsushita M (2001) Ipsilateral and contralateral projections from upper cervical segments to the vestibular nuclei in the rat. Exp Brain Res 141: 204–217.

Yingcharoen K, Rinvik E (1983) Ultrastructural demonstration of a projection from the flocculus to the nucleus prepositus hypoglossi in the cat. Exp Brain Res 51: 192–198.

Zhang X, Zakir M, Meng H, Sato H, Uchino Y (2001) Convergence of the horizontal semicircular canal and otolith afferents on cat single vestibular neurons. Exp Brain Res 140: 1–11.

7 Self-Motion Cues and Resolving Intermodality Conflicts: Head Direction Cells, Place Cells, and Behavior

Robert W. Stackman and Michaël B. Zugaro

More than 130 years ago, Darwin suggested that animals might rely on internal or self-motion cues for navigation (Darwin, 1873). Recent studies have tried to define when and how self-motion cues are used for spatial memory and navigation. Most theories of navigation contend that animals exhibit a hierarchical use of external landmark cues over internal or self-motion cues. Here, we review literature regarding the influence of self-motion cues on head direction cell and place cell activity.

Self-Motion Cues

Overview

The presence of landmarks or extra-maze cues influences the performance of humans and laboratory animals on spatial memory and navigational tasks. Navigation is, however, often preserved *in the absence of external landmark cues, or in an unfamiliar environment*. Navigating based solely on information derived from self-motion cues is known as path integration (Barlow, 1964; Gallistel, 1990; Etienne et al., 1996). Self-motion cues are defined as those information sources that result from the animal's own movements and include vestibular, motor efference copy, proprioceptive, optic, and auditory flow. It is generally considered that intact navigation under conditions in which one of these self-motion cues has been eliminated reflects the fact that the remaining cues are sufficient to support navigation. *Place* and *head direction cell* (see chapter 1 by Sharp) activity remains stable in the absence of polarizing cues (often a large cue card) in darkness (Quirk et al., 1990; Goodridge and Taube, 1995), or when the rat is blinded (Hill and Best, 1981; Save et al., 1998) or blindfolded (Goodridge et al., 1998). A number of studies have been conducted to determine what cue sources support spatial firing in the absence of landmark cues. Taube and Burton (1995) found that when a rat walks from a familiar cylinder through a passageway into a distinct, novel environment that is out of view of the familiar one, preferred firing directions of head direction cells shifted by an average of only about 18° of their respective original orientations. Without familiar cues to maintain directional firing, the rat likely utilizes internal or self-motion cues during the initial journey into the novel environment. Recent studies have found that manipulations of single self-motion cues tend to produce dramatic effects on the spatial firing of head direction cells and place cells. These studies normally involve disrupting one particular cue by lesion (e.g., vestibular labyrinthectomy) or occlusion (e.g., extinguishing room lights), then examining the consequence on spatial cell firing under conditions that are believed to require self-motion cues. This last point is important to note. As previously mentioned, theoretical views of navigation suggest that landmark cues will be used preferentially over self-motion cues as references for spatial behavior. An arguable extension of this view has been that self-motion cues exert little, if any, influence on navigation during conditions where familiar landmarks are available.

Vestibular Stimulation by Passive Rotation

A commonly used protocol to provide vestibular stimulation in the yaw plane is to passively rotate the animals by turning the substrate on which they are standing or reposed (see Matthews et al., 1988; Gavrilov et al., 1998). If acceleration and velocity profiles are appropriately selected, the resulting vestibular stimulus is comparable to that arising during spontaneous, active movements. This intentionally excludes the usual accompanying motor command and feedback signals. In experiments studying vestibular influences, the manipulations must be performed in darkness to avoid possible interference from visual updating signals. However, one caveat with regard to interpreting such manipulations as vestibular is that the rotational forces also stimulate a variety of somatic receptors, which might provide some information about angular movement, albeit less precisely than that provided by the vestibular system.

Blair and Sharp (1996) directly tested the hypothesis that vestibular signals could update head direction responses. While rats were foraging for food pellets in a cylindrical apparatus, the apparatus was rotated by 90° either at high velocities—thus above vestibular detection threshold—or at very low velocities, thus preventing the vestibular system from detecting the rotation. The same procedure was repeated under lighting and in darkness. With the lights on, after rapid rotations, the preferred directions of the head direction cells were unchanged (in five out of eight neurons). But after slow rotations, they shifted by approximately 90°. Thus, only when the vestibular system could detect the rotations were the head direction responses updated appropriately, keeping the preferred directions stable in space. When the vestibular system could not detect the rotations, the same cells presumably continued to discharge, although the head orientation was changing, resulting in a shift of preferred directions. These results are compatible with earlier behavioral studies (e.g., Mittelstaedt and Mittelstaedt, 1980).

Somewhat surprisingly, though, in darkness the results were less clear-cut. Whether the apparatus was rotated at fast or slow velocities, the preferred directions were equally likely to remain stable, shift by 90°, or even shift by an intermediate angle, as if resulting from a compromise between stability and rotation. The reasons for this are not clear. One possibility is that in darkness olfactory or tactile cues may have exerted an increased influence upon directional responses, thus weakening the expected influence of vestibular signals.

In order to test whether the directional selectivity of head direction cells could be maintained for prolonged periods of time based on inertial signals only, rats were placed on small, elevated pedestals and passively rotated in darkness (Chen et al., 1994a; Knierim et al., 1998). How this protocol affected head direction cell responses depended on the actual characteristics of the rotations. At high constant velocities, the cells rapidly lost their directional selectivity. However, when the rotations were more chaotic, with velocities and directions changing at irregular intervals to mimic natural head movements, cell firings were directional, although the preferred directions drifted rapidly. In such conditions, preferred directions were maintained considerably longer (from 10 s to 3 min in 11 out of 15 cells in the study by Knierim et al.). Because the vestibular organs are sensitive to head accelerations and are only transiently stimulated by rotations at constant velocity, these findings are consistent with the hypothesis that vestibular signals are required to update head direction responses when no exteroceptive cues are present. As for otolithic vestibular signals, they do not seem to influence directional responses, as head direction cells are not sensitive to the vertical component of the head orientation (Stackman et al., 2000); see chapter 3 by Taube).

Since head direction cells are thought to receive angular velocity signals from vestibular inputs, several computational models predict that head direction cell discharges in the anterodorsal thalamus could be modulated by head angular velocity. This question was addressed in a number of experimental studies in which directional responses between high velocity and low velocity movements were compared (Taube, 1995; Blair and Sharp, 1995; Blair et al., 1997; Stackman and Taube, 1997; Blair et al., 1998). Most of these studies did find that discharge rates increased with angular velocity (but see Taube and Muller, 1998). However, because these results were obtained in freely moving animals, the effect could as well have been triggered by motor, rather than vestibular, signals. Also, the magnitude of the modulation was controversial, possibly because the results were not obtained with highly reliable methods. The analyses extracted and pooled many small discontinuous episodes from the recording sessions according to head angular velocity, ignoring that the ensemble of self-movement signals was most probably not consistent across such episodes. Zugaro et al. (2002) compared head direction cell responses in Long-Evans rats passively rotated at fast, versus slow, velocities. This paradigm minimized the potential influence of motor signals (since the rats were immobile) and provided consistent quasisinusoidal stimulation of the vestibular system. Because tight restraint drastically alters the firing rates of the head direction cells (Taube, 1995, and see section on Motor Efference later in this chapter), the rats were not restrained during passive rotations; instead, they were trained to remain immobile in order to receive water rewards from a small reservoir at the center of the rotating platform. Fourteen anterodorsal thalamic head direction cells were recorded from three rats. The peak firing rates were 36% higher on average during fast (approx. 150 deg/s) than slow (approx. 40 deg/s) rotations. No cells changed their peak firing rate by less than 10%, and three cells (21%) increased their peak firing rate by more than 50%. This shows that in passively rotated rats, the peak firing rates of the head direction cells are modulated by angular velocity signals, most probably of vestibular origin (optic field flow, another sensory signal possibly involved, also reaches the head direction system via the vestibular nucleus).

Vestibular Lesion

It has been suggested that vestibular input updates the spatial firing properties of limbic neurons *in the absence of landmarks* (McNaughton et al., 1995, 1996), or when such landmarks are unstable, unreliable, or unfamiliar. Specifically, the vestibular influence may have a more relevant influence on spatial firing when visual cues or landmarks are not available. Recent studies were designed to test this conditional dependence of head direction and place cells on vestibular input. The first experiment to directly test the influence of the vestibular system on HD cell activity that involved lesioning the vestibular apparatus did so by neurotoxic means.

Head Direction Cells   The objective of the following studies was to test the effect of vestibular lesions on head direction cell activity. The vestibular apparatus of female Long-Evans rats was lesioned by bilateral transtympanic injections of sodium arsanilate (Stackman and Taube, 1997). Sodium arsanilate causes a permanent vestibular lesion by inducing vestibular hair cell death and a progressive degeneration of the vestibular root of the VIIIth cranial nerve (Chen et al., 1986; Kaufman et al., 1992). Anterodorsal thalamic electrodes of lesioned rats were screened with the intent to record head direction cells under conditions thought to require self-motion cues, such as in the absence of the cue card, in darkness, or in an unfamiliar environment. However, no head direction cells were found in any of the vestibular-lesioned rats despite the fact that histological reconstructions revealed that electrodes did pass through the anterodorsal thalamic nuclei.

Next, head direction cells were recorded from intact rats, then recorded again after vestibular lesion with sodium arsanilate. The directional firing of anterodorsal thalamic neurons was abolished by vestibular lesion in all of the cases (see fig. 7.1 and plate 1) (Stackman and Taube, 1997). Head direction cell waveforms were consistent before and after the lesion; thus, cell isolation was maintained over the course of lesion onset. This experiment was repeated for eight head direction cells, all with similar results. Background

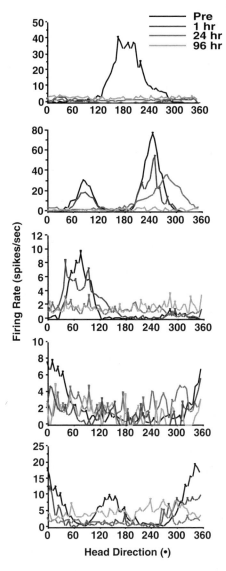

Figure 7.1
Lesion of the vestibular apparatus abolishes directional firing of anterior thalamic neurons. Five head direction cells were recorded before (Pre) and after (1–96 hr) transtympanic injection of the toxin sodium arsanilate. Rats displayed behaviors consistent with a loss of vestibular function within 24 hours of receiving sodium arsanilate, yet continued to move freely about the cylindrical arena during unit recording sessions. The isolation of each cell was maintained, and each cell's waveform was consistent over the entire course of each experiment. (Redrawn with permission from Stackman and Taube, 1997.) See plate 1 for color version.

firing rates increased postlesion, albeit not significantly, and there was no change in the mean overall firing rates. Electrodes were monitored for several days to weeks postlesion, but directional firing never returned in any of the rats. Electrodes were advanced further through the anterior thalamus to identify other directional cells, but none were ever found. Transtympanic control injections of saline had no effect on head direction cell activity. In many vestibular-lesioned rats, anterodorsal thalamic cells were recorded that discharged in a rhythmic burst-firing pattern. This burst-firing pattern was never observed in anterodorsal thalamic neurons recorded from intact rats, and none of the anterodorsal thalamic head direction cells recorded adopted a burst-firing pattern postlesion. These findings imply that the vestibular lesion altered the firing properties of thalamic neurons.

Rats exhibit a characteristic profile of transient changes in motor behavior after bilateral lesion of the vestibular system. These changes include head dorsiflexion (i.e., head pitch), a wide hindpaw and forepaw stance, increased tendency to circle and to walk backwards, and a complete failure to rear. Most of these lesion-induced changes in posture and movement tend to subside in the weeks following the lesion. The lesion-induced disruption of directional firing did not appear to be caused by aberrant motor behavior. Specifically, despite the recovery of motor behavior and the reduction in postural abnormalities, head direction cell activity did not return. Vestibular-lesioned rats continued to explore and to forage for randomly distributed food pellets in the recording cylinder. As previously mentioned, the firing rates of anterodorsal thalamic head direction cells are modulated by angular head velocity, and this modulation is also disrupted by vestibular lesion. It is interesting that the vestibular lesion abolished the directional firing of anterodorsal thalamic neurons even in a familiar environment in the presence of landmarks previously shown to influence head direction cells. These data indicate that vestibular input is critical for head direction cell activity, *independent of the presence of landmarks*. The lack of a conditional dependence of head direction cells upon vestibular input (i.e., only in the absence of landmarks) suggests that vestibular information is essential for the generation of the head direction cell signal.

Temporary inactivation of the vestibular apparatus by transtympanic injection of tetrodotoxin produced a similar disruption of directional firing of postsubicular head direction cells (Stackman et al., 2002). Transtympanic tetrodotoxin inactivates the vestibular apparatus for approximately 36 to 72 hrs, after which vestibular function fully recovers (Saxon et al., 2001). Directional firing of postsubicular neurons was observed to recover over a time course that matched the recovery of vestibular function.

Hippocampal Place Cells   Vestibular input is also essential for the location-specific firing properties of hippocampal CA1 neurons. Place cells ($n = 10$) were recently recorded from female Long-Evans rats before, during, and after tetrodotoxin-induced inactivation of the vestibular system. In all cases the location-specific firing was abolished by vestibular inactivation (see fig 7.2 and plate 2). CA1 neurons continued to discharge in their

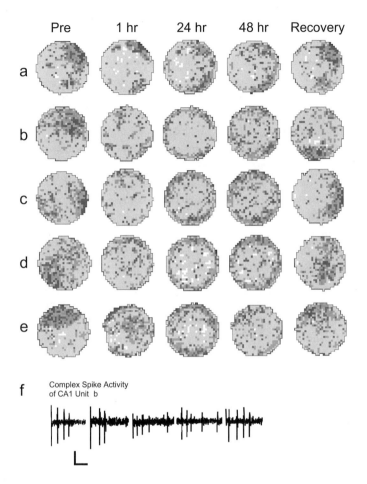

Figure 7.2
Temporary inactivation of the vestibular system disrupts location-specific firing of hippocampal neurons. Plot illustrates firing rate versus location maps for five (a–e) representative hippocampal place cells recorded before (Pre), during (1–48 hr), and after (Recovery) tetrodotoxin-induced inactivation of the vestibular apparatus. For each map, increasing firing rates are coded from yellow, orange, red, green, blue, and purple, with yellow pixels depicting locations where no spikes were fired. Within 1 hr after vestibular inactivation the location-specific firing was substantially attenuated or abolished. The recovery of place fields occurred concomitant with the recovery of vestibular function, which took between 48 and 96 hours post injection. These plots also provide examples of the types of changes in place field location evident after recovery from vestibular inactivation (b and d). Despite the loss of location-specific firing, hippocampal neurons continued to exhibit a complex-spike pattern of discharge (f). The isolation of each cell was maintained, and each cell's waveform was consistent over the entire course of each experiment. (Redrawn with permission from Stackman et al., 2002.) See plate 2 for color version.

characteristic complex-spike firing patterns, and waveforms were consistent, during vestibular inactivation (Stackman et al., 2002). These observations indicate that the interruption of location-specific firing caused by the vestibular lesion was not due to a loss of unit isolation.

As the rats recovered from the vestibular inactivation, location-specific firing recovered as well, consistent with similar head direction cell studies. While the place fields of four cells recovered to locations consistent with prelesion baseline recording sessions, the place fields of the six remaining cells shifted their locations upon vestibular recovery. It is possible that the repeated exposure of the rats to the cylinder during vestibular inactivation may have promoted the cells to represent the environment as distinct from that of the baseline recordings. The repeated experience may have promoted "remapping" of place fields, a phenomenon in which some environmental change causes the place cell to cease firing or to adopt a firing field that is distinct from its original field (Bostock et al. 1991; Muller, 1996). Consistent with this interpretation, Shapiro and colleagues have shown that repeatedly subjecting rats to conflicting information from distal and local visual cues induces hippocampal place cells to remap (Shapiro et al., 1997; also see chapter 8 by Knierim). Together, these data demonstrate the importance of vestibular input for hippocampal representations of space. It will be of interest to test whether the nonspatial correlates of hippocampal neuronal activity (i.e., odor cues, cue approach, or behavioral choice in discrimination tasks as described by Wood et al. (1999) are also sensitive to vestibular lesion.

An interesting question is whether location-specific firing of hippocampal neurons would eventually recover in rats with a permanent lesion of the vestibular system. Bilkey and colleagues (2003) addressed this issue recently. Complex spike cells were recorded from hippocampal electrodes of Sprague Dawley rats 60 days after sham or mechanical labyrinthectomy surgery. Recordings revealed weak place-related firing by hippocampal neurons of lesioned rats, which was unstable across 10-min recording sessions as well as within a 30-min session (Russell et al., 2003). Similar instability of place fields in vestibular-lesioned rats was observed between recording sessions conducted with the room lights illuminated and those conducted in the dark. These data indicate that a lesion of the vestibular apparatus produces severe and lasting instability of hippocampal spatial representations.

Spatial Navigation   In the absence of visual cues, rodents' ability to return directly to a home locale after a circuitous outward journey is dependent upon self-motion cues (Mittelstaedt and Mittelstaedt, 1980; Etienne et al., 1985). A number of studies have attempted to determine which self-motion cues are most relevant for navigation. Repeated disorientation of rats, by rotation inside an opaque box before each trial, disrupts acquisition of spatial memory in an appetitive radial-arm maze task (Dudchenko et al., 1997; Martin et al., 1997). Lesions of the vestibular system (1) impair rats' ability to return to a goal location following passive transport (Miller et al., 1983); (2) disrupt spontaneous alternation performance (Potegal et al., 1977); and (3) impair spatial learning in a radial-arm maze task (Ossenkopp and Hargreaves, 1993). These findings suggest that vestibular input is an important self-motion cue for spatial behavior.

Although vestibular signals can influence navigation and the learning of spatial tasks, it is not clear in which situations this is required. One hypothesis is that vestibular signals improve spatial learning, by enabling associations between head position cues and external landmark cues (McNaughton et al., 1991; McNaughton et al., 1995; Samsonovich and McNaughton, 1997). To test this, we examined the effects of sodium arsanilate-induced vestibular lesion on spatial learning and memory in rats. Rats were trained to find water reward in one corner of a high-walled, black square enclosure (90 cm by 90 cm by 60 cm high). A large white cue card was present throughout training in a fixed position on one wall. Floor-to-ceiling curtains surrounded the enclosure to prevent the rats' use of cues outside of the enclosure. The goal location was fixed with respect to the cue card orientation. Each trial began by releasing the rat at the center of the enclosure, oriented toward a randomly selected wall. Hence the task *could not* be solved by a simple fixed motor response (i.e., always turn right). No attempt was made to disorient the rats prior to placing them in the enclosure at the start of each trial. Rats were placed in a holding box outside of the enclosure between each trial. There was no overall effect of the lesion on acquisition of this simple spatial task (Stackman and Herbert, 2002), which suggests that learning the predictive relationship between the orientation of a landmark and a goal location does not require vestibular input. However, in a probe test where the cue card was removed, the spatial behavior of the lesioned rats was impaired. In contrast, sham-lesioned control rats continued to choose accurately in the absence of the cue card. In a previous study using the same task (Golob et al., 2001), performance by intact rats in the probe test was significantly disrupted by slow (90° in 60 s) rotation of the rat inside the holding box 1 min before the probe test. Performance was not affected by fast (90° in 2–3 s) rotation before the probe test, suggesting that the rats remained oriented after the fast rotation, but were disoriented, or "misoriented," by the slow rotation. The impaired behavior of the vestibular-lesioned rats during probe tests (with no cue card) suggests that their accurate performance on standard trials was guided by the cue card. Stable probe test responses by intact rats may have been supported by internal representations of the goal location and by self-motion cues, with path integration from when the animal was removed from, until it was replaced in, the apparatus. The impaired probe test responses by lesioned rats may be due to a lesion-induced impairment of such path integration. In summary, the vestibular lesion did not prevent rats from learning the spatial relationship between a polarizing cue and the goal location in this task. The lesion did, however, disrupt spatial responding under a test condition that favored path integration.

Sodium arsanilate lesions of the vestibular system also impair performance of rats on a hippocampal-dependent path integration task (Wallace et al., 2002). Female Long-Evans rats were trained on a modified circular Barnes maze (Barnes, 1979) to leave a home nest box, find a randomly placed large food pellet, then carry the pellet back to the home box. The homing path of intact rats was generally a direct, efficient route, which was guided by extra-maze visual cues. Vestibular-lesioned rats exhibited homing behavior that was as efficient as the intact rats when extra-maze cues were available. However, in the dark the homing path of vestibular-lesioned rats was markedly longer and less direct than that of the intact rats (Wallace et al., 2002). These data showing that navigation by vestibular lesioned rats is dependent upon visual cues are consistent with several previous studies (Potegal et al., 1977; Miller et al., 1983; Stackman and Herbert, 2002). In summary, lesion of the vestibular apparatus abolishes the spatial firing properties of head direction cells and place cells, and impairs path integration. Of course, it remains to be determined whether the impaired spatial performance of the lesioned rats was due to the loss of normal head direction and place cell activity or can be attributed to some other consequence of the vestibular lesion.

Motor Efference

Several sources of information signal body displacement or self-movement. When a motor command signal is initiated along the corticospinal motor pathway, several other brain regions receive matching signals, referred to as motor efference copy. Motor efference copy is thought to provide sensory systems with information regarding the intended movement and is considered necessary for assuring accuracy of motor output and facilitating fine motor control (Von Holst, 1954; Miles and Evarts, 1979). Motor efference copy operates as an accurate anticipatory signal of body displacement, which allows the animal to determine whether a perceived change in orientation of some object results from the object having moved or from the viewer's movement. Thus, including motor commands, cues from receptors of muscle, tendon and joint, vestibular, and proprioceptive (limb position) cues, there are numerous sources of displacement information that will have an impact on navigation. The challenge, then, in understanding the role each of these motor signals in spatial behavior and the spatial firing correlates of limbic neurons, is to study the motor signal in isolation.

The first large-scale analyses of the relationships between hippocampal neuronal activity and behavior conducted in rats identified the close correspondence between certain automatic behaviors, such as walking or sniffing, and theta rhythm (Ranck, 1973)—a 4 to 12 Hz band within the hippocampal EEG. Hippocampal theta rhythm is also elicited by passive displacement and passive rotation of the animal (Gavrilov et al., 1995, 1996). Thus, movement, or cues associated with body displacement, triggers hippocampal theta, and in synchronizing the hippocampal circuitry, theta may represent a mechanism for the acquisition of information during exploration, such as that needed to update spatial maps.

The influence of motor cues on head direction cell and place cell activity has been studied, using several approaches. One has been to record these spatial units before, during, and after gentle but firm restraint. The discharge properties of most, but not all, post-subiculum and anterodorsal thalamic head direction cells are significantly reduced when rats are restrained in a towel and passively rotated through the cell's preferred firing direction (Taube et al., 1990; Knierim et al., 1995; Taube, 1995). In contrast, lateral dorsal thalamic head direction cells are not affected by restraint (Mizumori and Williams, 1993), suggesting regional differences in the sensitivity of head direction cells to motor cues. Place cell discharge is also disrupted during restraint (Foster et al., 1989). This restraint protocol arguably removes the possible influence of most volitional movements on neuronal firing. However, as conducted, the restraint manipulation has several potential confounds including stress, body pressure, the absence of postural tone, and the absence of paw contact with the floor. It is difficult to dissociate the changes in firing due to a lack of movement from those due to these other factors.

Despite these concerns, the findings outlined here have been interpreted as evidence that an animal's movement about space is a necessary requirement for the activation of place and head direction cells (Sharp et al., 1995; Wiener et al., 1995; McNaughton et al., 1996; Taube, 1998). Given the fact that active movement of the animal triggers theta, it is difficult to determine whether the decrease in spatial firing is due to the inability of the animal to move or to the lack of theta activity. In an intriguing "space clamping" experiment, hippocampal neurons were recorded from rats in a cage that included a running wheel. Place cells that had fields in the running wheel were recorded in order to address the issue of motor influences on place cell responses. The running wheel (29.5 cm dia, 10 cm wide) confined the running animal to a constant location in space and eliminated or reduced the contribution of linear and angular movement, optic flow, and other sensory stimuli on the firing of hippocampal neurons. Hippocampal place cells were identified while the rats ran in the wheel and moved about other areas of the cage. A subset of neurons exhibited place fields inside the running wheel that were comparable to those found outside the wheel. The firing rates of these "wheel" place cells were modulated by the running speed of the animals and, interestingly, the place cells ceased to fire when the rats stopped running in the wheel (Czurkó et al., 1999). Wheel running was associated with theta activity, and therefore these data suggest that theta activity, rather than active movement through space, is essential for place-related firing of hippocampal neurons.

Observations of place and head direction cell activity suggest that spatial firing is not particularly affected when the unrestrained animal is appropriately oriented or positioned, but motionless. Zugaro et al. (2001) have addressed this issue empirically by passively rotating unrestrained but immobile rats as they consumed water from a reservoir at the center of a circular platform. During passive rotations through the cells' preferred firing directions, the peak firing rate of anterodorsal thalamic head direction cells was significantly depressed by about 27% on average, compared to that observed during active movement on the platform (Zugaro et al., 2001). There was no change in preferred firing direction or the width of the directional response curves, despite the decreased firing rate. These data suggest an important contribution of motor initiation commands on the firing properties of thalamic head direction cells. The absence of such initiation of movement commands during passive rotations may then dampen head direction cell activity. These data are consistent with the notion that spatial navigation networks are more likely to be modulated by self-initiated movement commands than to those cues that follow passive rotation (i.e., rotational forces, postural corrections, etc.). Motor initiation and motor efference copy signals may act to set the gain of the response of thalamic directional discharge during active movement sequences. However, visual and vestibular information, which were maintained in these manipulations, are sufficient to establish head direction signals.

As these findings attest, motor (efference copy, motor command, and proprioceptive) cues influence the firing properties of head direction cells under standard cue conditions, such as in the presence of familiar cues. Recent studies have been conducted to determine how passive displacement might affect the location-specific responses of place cells under conditions that favor path integration. Gavrilov et al. (1998) recorded hippocampal neurons from male Long-Evans rats that were head-fixed with the body in a harness (permitting legs to dangle freely), as it was passively transported aboard a computer-controlled robot in an enclosed room. The robot accelerated and decelerated in 1 sec and otherwise moved at a constant velocity of 50 or 100 cm. The rat received a water reward when the robot moved it into a predetermined reward corner. Although firing rates were modulated during passive translation, the location-specific firing of hippocampal neurons was maintained in the absence of visual cues. These data suggest that, spatial information processing by the hippocampus remains stable under conditions that disrupt the animal's use of motor efference, proprioceptive, optic flow, and external visual cues (Gavrilov et al., 1998). The authors suggested that, with as many potential external cue sources controlled for in this study, the maintained place cell discharge (albeit with larger fields than found in unrestrained moving rats) was likely dependent upon vestibular and somatosensory cues. These findings indicate that the activity of limbic spatial neurons is modulated by motor signals under conditions that might favor path integration. In an interesting contrast, Nishijo and colleagues (1997) recorded hippocampal place-related activity from three macaque monkeys seated in a motorized cab inside an experimental room containing visual cues. The monkeys directed the movements of the cab by operating a joystick. Place fields were identified that were consistent from session to session and tightly coupled with landmark cues around the room. When the same neurons were recorded during passive translation of the cab, place-related firing was significantly diminished (Nishijo et al., 1997), suggesting that movement-related cues are necessary for location-specific firing of hippocampal neurons in this species. These data indicate that active movement or the self-motion cues resulting from it modulates the firing properties of hippocampal neurons. Taken together, these data suggest that other cues are sufficient to establish spatial signals, and the magnitude of these signals is correlated with motor state.

As previously reviewed, Taube and Burton (1995) found that preferred firing directions of head direction cells were stable (i.e., they shifted by no more than 18°) when rats walked from a familiar environment into a novel environment (Taube and Burton, 1995). Since familiar landmarks were not available to the rats as they left the cylinder and walked through a passageway into the novel rectangle, the relative stability of preferred firing directions was attributed to self-motion cues. To examine the degree to which motor efference copy and optic flow contribute to the preferred direction stability, we repeated the study of Taube and Burton (1995), using the same apparatus. This time, conditions were added to affect the rats' use of motor/proprioceptive and optic flow cues as they moved from the familiar cylinder to the novel rectangular arena (Stackman et al., 2003).

Rats could either walk or be passively transported inside a clear, Plexiglas container on a wheeled cart from the cylinder into the novel rectangular arena. A cue card was present in the cylinder in the "standard" (3 o'clock) position, and the rectangular arena contained a cue card positioned at 12 o'clock. The container on the cart limited but did not restrain the rats from moving during the passive transport of the cart. The rationale for using the passive transport manipulation was to disrupt the reliability of the match between the animals' motor efference/proprioception and vestibular cues with the animals' true orientation during movement into a novel environment, conditions thought to require path integration. That is, volitional linear and angular movements of animals on the cart during passive transport did not provide them with an accurate representation of their true orientation in the experimental apparatus. This passive transport manipulation was conducted with the room lights on for one group of rats, and in the dark for another group of rats. The light versus dark condition was designed to disrupt the rats' use of optic flow cues during the movement through the passageway into the novel rectangular arena. Together the experiment comprised three experimental conditions: *passive transport–lights on, passive transport–lights off, active movement–lights off*, and the control condition, *Active Movement/Lights On*. First, baseline activity was recorded in anterodorsal thalamic or postsubicular head direction cells in an 8 min "familiar cylinder" session. Next, one of the above manipulations was imposed. A "novel rectangle" recording session began upon arrival, or upon release of the rat in this arena. Figure 7.3 depicts the magnitude of shift in preferred firing direction between the original cylinder session and the novel rectangle session for each condition. Preferred firing directions shifted in the novel environment by an average of approximately 30° after locomotion from the familiar environment with the room lights off; by an average of about 70 after passive transport from the familiar environment with the room lights on; and by an average of approximately 67° after passive transport with the room lights off (Stackman et al., 2003). Further, the preferred firing direction shifts of passively transported rats were randomly distributed. The lighting condition had no significant additional influence on the shift in preferred firing direction over that of the passive transport.

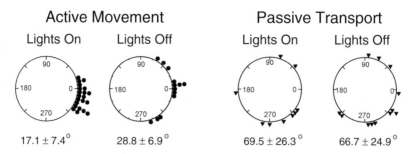

Figure 7.3
Polar plots depicting the distribution of head direction cell angular shifts in preferred firing direction between the familiar cylinder session and the novel rectangle session for the four experimental conditions. Head direction cells were recorded in the cylinder and then rats walked, or were passively transported, into the novel rectangle with the room lights on or off. The respective mean ± S.D. absolute shift in preferred firing direction is stated below each plot. (Redrawn with permission from Stackman et al., 2003.)

   All rats of the passive transport conditions had had previous experience being placed into the cart and wheeled around the cylinder. Therefore, it is unlikely that the stress of being on the cart can account for the magnitude of shift in preferred direction. Head direction cells that were monitored briefly during passive transport in the familiar cylinder did not exhibit a shift in preferred direction. It is more likely that the active movement of the rats in the cart during passive transport, together with the passive movement of the cart, provided the rats with complex stimuli confounding vestibular-based path integration. That is, the shift in preferred directions in the head direction cells observed in the novel environment was likely a consequence of disrupting the reliability of the match between the animals' motor efference and proprioceptive cues and the actual spatial orientation of the animals during the displacement into the novel environment. However, it is important to note that the passive transport manipulation did not allow the rats to have tactile contact with the novel passageway and rectangle while aboard the cart. (See also chapter 16 by Israël and Warren for discussion of podokinetic influences.) Thus, it is unclear to what degree tactile cue availability might have influenced the shift in the head direction cells' preferred firing direction under these conditions. It is interesting that the remaining self-motion cues that were available to the passively transported rats were not sufficient to permit stable preferred firing direction. Such cues are sufficient to support accurate navigation in passively transported rodents (Etienne 1980; Miller et al. 1983). If the rats had directed the cart from the familiar to the novel environment, perhaps they would have better tracked their orientation and head direction cells would have not exhibited such a large shift. Here, passive transport markedly affected directional firing in rats. It is also possible that further experience with passive transport might reduce the instability of head direction cells under these conditions.

Optic Flow

When an animal spontaneously turns its head, the visual field on its retinae rotates in the opposite direction. Conversely, visual field rotations can thus yield information about head motion in space. Indeed, perception of self-motion can be triggered by visual field rotation. This is what one experiences, for instance, in the famous illusion of self-motion provoked by the movement of an adjacent train while one is seated on a stopped train; such a perception is known as *vection*. One might suppose that the head direction signal could be updated by visual field motion. This hypothesis can be tested by inducing vection in immobile animals: the preferred directions are then expected to shift relative to absolute spatial coordinates by the same angle as did the visual field stimuli. However, this has not yet been proved in rats: no experiments have yet attempted to verify that the stimuli employed have actually provoked vection. In the train illusion, the sensation of movement disappears when the illusory movement arrives at the vestibular threshold, and the latter succeeds in dominating the resulting cue conflict. In general, the optimal visual stimuli for inducing such optokinetic effects have homogeneous contrasting patterns throughout the peripheral visual field. One typical experimental stimulus is a rotating cylinder with numerous alternating black and white stripes of the same widths and parallel to the axis of rotation, with the subject's head placed at the center of the axis of rotation. Note that this is to be distinguished from the stimuli used for landmark-based orientation, which have a reduced number of localized distinctive contrasts.

Distinct and complementary pathways process these two types of visual stimuli, which are likely to enter into the head direction circuit at two different loci. The brainstem vestibular nuclei receive peripheral optic field flow (as well as vestibular end organ and neck proprioceptive) signals and then transmit them to nucleus prepositus hypoglossi and the dorsal tegmental nucleus of Gudden. In contrast, the foveal processing pathway is presumed to pass through geniculocortical pathways to enter the head direction system through the postsubiculum and retrosplenial cortex. This is consistent with the finding that after postsubicular lesions, anterodorsal thalamic head direction cells have a reduced sensitivity to prominent visual landmark cues (Goodridge and Taube, 1997).

In order to study the potential influence of optic field flow on place cells and head direction cells, Blair and Sharp (1995, 1996) placed rats in a cylindrical apparatus decorated with four pairs of alternating black and white stripes (each subtending 45°). The wall of the apparatus was rotated by 90° (while the floor remained immobile), creating optic field flow that could trigger vection and thus alter the preferred directions of the head direction cells. Because of the symmetrical layout of the stripes, rotations by 90° resulted in permutation of the stripes, leaving the visual environment unchanged after the rotation. This was intended to ensure that any shift in preferred directions would be due to vection rather than to reorientation of visual landmarks. In most cases (8 place cells out of 14, and 6 head direction cells out of 8), the spatial selectivity of the neurons remained unchanged after rotations, indicating that optic flow may not contribute significantly to spatial responses. It may also be that this protocol did not provide optimal optic field flow; a more efficient stimulus could consist of smaller contrasts rotated for longer periods of time (Hess et al., 1985). Again, it may be that, although the contrasted stripes were indeed ambiguous spatial cues (e.g., all white stripes were similar as they were all the same size and each had a black stripe on its left and right), they did nonetheless provide a certain degree of polarization to the visual environment (the left and right edges of each stripe could be distinguished because they had different contrast successions, e.g., black, then white versus white, then black) which may have been used to correct potential shifts of preferred directions after the rotations.

Recently, Arleo et al. (2004) placed rats at the center of a darkened area surrounded by a cylindrical black curtain. They projected an irregular array of luminous points onto the curtain with a planetarium-like projector, then rotated this at 4.5 deg/s for a 90 s period (405°). In 28 sessions, rotation of the dot array provoked the directional responses of 14 anterodorsal thalamic neurons to drift in a direction coherent with circular vection. However, the drifts averaged only 204° (±54°), suggesting conflicts with other cues. This provides evidence that optic field flow does update head direction responses.

In the "space clamping" experiment of Czurkó et al. (1999) previously described, hippocampal place cells were recorded while a rat ran in a wheel. While running in the wheel the rat's head position remained stable, and therefore optic flow was essentially eliminated as an influence on the running animal. Place cell activity remained stable under this condition, which suggests that, in actively moving rats, optic flow is not necessary for hippocampal neurons to fire appropriate spatial responses.

Summary—Self-Motion Cues

The main findings of the respective self-motion manipulations are outlined in table 7.1. Vestibular manipulations seem to have the strongest effect on spatial firing. Lesions of the vestibular end organs abolish place and directional firing, even in the presence of external visual cues, suggesting that this self-motion signal is essential for spatial firing. Manipulations of motor efference copy and proprioceptive cues appear to differentially modulate head direction and place cell activity. Restricting volitional movements by tight restraint tended to suppress directional firing, but studies of immobile rats suggest that directional firing is preserved, even though peak firing rates are decreased. Passive transport of rats into a novel environment caused a significant shift in head direction cell preferred firing direction. These findings suggest that motor cues, such as efference copy, may exert a modulatory influence on direction- and location-specific firing. Finally, manipulation of optic flow cues seems to have the least significant consequence of the three. Exposing rats to apparent visual motion usually didn't affect place and head direction cell activity. Further, denying the rats' access to optic flow cues during path integration caused a mild but significant shift in head direction cell preferred firing direction.

Table 7.1
Summary of experimental evidence for self-motion cue influences on the head direction cell and place cell activity

Cue Source	Condition Type	Manipulation	Effect	Reference
Vestibular	Stimulation	Brief rotations above threshold in dark	ADN HD cell PFD stable	Blair & Sharp 1996; Knierim et al., 1998
			Striatal HD cell PFD shift	Wiener et al., 1993
			RSG/RSA HD cells PFD shift or lose directional firing	Chen et al., 1994
		Constant above threshold in dark	ADN HD cell PFD shift	Knierim et al., 1998
		Brief below threshold in dark	ADN HD cell PFD shift	Blair & Sharp 1996; Sharp et al., 1995;
			HPC place fields shift	Jeffrey et al., 1997
	Peripheral lesion	Sodium arsanilate lesion of vestibular apparatus	ADN HD cells permanently lose directional firing	Stackman & Taube, 1997
		Tetrodotoxin inactivation of vestibular apparatus	PoS HD cells lose directional firing	Stackman et al., 2002
		Mechanical destruction of vestibular apparatus	HPC place cells lose location-specific firing	Stackman et al., 2002
			Place fields of HPC neurons are unstable	Russell et al., 2003
Motor efference copy	Restraint	Wrapped tightly in a towel, passively rotated or moved	PoS & ADN HD cells PFR ↓	Taube et al., 1990; Taube 1995; Knierim et al., 1995
			LDN HD cells no effect	Mizumori and Williams 1993
			HPC place cells lose location-specific firing	Foster et al., 1989
	Immobile	Passively rotated while consuming water unrestrained	ADN HD cells remain directional, but PFR ↓	Zugaro et al., 2001

Table 7.1
(continued)

Cue Source	Condition Type	Manipulation	Effect	Reference
	Clamped to stationary position	While running in a stationary wheel	HPC place cell activity stable	Czurko et al., 1999
	Passive transport in a familiar environment	Rotations aboard a mobile robotic cart in the dark	HPC place fields stable, but FR ↓/↑	Gavrilov et al., 1998
		Aboard a wheeled cart	ADN + PoS HD cells stable	Stackman et al., 2003
		While seated in a cab actively guiding movements	HPC place-related activity impaired	Nishijo et al., 1997
	Passive transport into a novel environment	Wheeled from a familiar environment into a novel one aboard a cart	ADN + PoS HD cells shift PFD by ~70°	Stackman et al., 2003
Optic flow	Stimulation	Rapid rotation of cylinder wall with alternating B + W stripes	Most ADN HD cells PFD remain stable	Blair and Sharp, 1996
			Most place fields of HPC neurons remain stable	Sharp et al., 1995
	Obscured	Walked from a familiar environment into a novel one in the dark	ADN + PoS HD cells shift PFD by ~30°	Stackman et al., 2003
	Clamped to appear static	While running in a stationary wheel	HPC place cell activity stable	Czurko et al., 1999

Key: ADN, anterodorsal thalamic nuclei; B + W, black and white; FR, firing rate; HD, head direction; HPC, hippocampus; LDN, laterodorsal thalamic nuclei; PFD, preferred firing direction; PoS, postsubiculum; RSA, retrosplenial agranular cortex; RSG, retrosplenial granular cortex.

Cue Conflicts

As was discussed earlier, single sensory or motor cues can suffice to convey accurate spatial information. For instance, head rotations activate the vestibular semicircular canals, which trigger increased firing in type I vestibular neurons; conversely, this increased firing rate indicates that the head is turning in space. Another example would be that head rotations are accompanied by rotations of the visual scene in the opposite direction. Moreover, more information can be obtained by combining these vestibular and visual cues, for example, to disambiguate different possible causes for each individual signal. But consider the hypothetical case where the images on the retinas rotate, but type I vestibular neurons do not increase their firing rate. How should this be interpreted? Is the head turning, as the rotating retinal images seem to indicate, or is it immobile, which would be more compatible with the stable vestibular responses? This situation corresponds to a cue conflict, because vestibular and visual signals do not provide coherent information. More generally, a cue conflict occurs when two or more cues convey mutually contradictory information—in this instance, about the ongoing head direction.

Cue conflicts can occur in a number of natural situations. In the freely moving animal on a flat, solid substrate, motor signals to change the head direction lead to proportional vestibular signals in the same direction, and optic field flow in the opposite direction. But in darkness, when visual cues are diminished or invisible, coherent optic field flow is absent. Passive movements are another category: they occur, for example, in pups being carried by the dam, as well as in (currents in) aquatic and (winds in) arboreal environments. These situations also provide different somatosensory stimuli from the freely moving condition. The vestibular stimuli would be comparable to those arising during spontaneous active movements, but the accompanying motor command and feedback signals would be lacking (and in light conditions, the corresponding shifts of the visual field). Cue conflicts are a valuable experimental tool for studying multisensory and motor integration in the head direction system.

Goodridge and Taube (1995) compared the influence of self-motion cues (proprioceptive, vestibular, and motor efference copy) with visual information concerning familiar, visible landmarks. Head direction neurons in the postsubiculum and anterodorsal thalamic nucleus were recorded in female Long-Evans rats as they foraged in a gray cylinder with a white card subtending 100° along the inner wall. The rats were removed and disoriented, then replaced in the cylinder from which the card had been removed and the floor paper changed. Then, if the preferred direction had deviated by more than 30°, the cue card was installed in the original position. However, if the preferred direction had remained stable, the cue card was reinstalled at an angle rotated plus or minus 90° relative to the initial position. Further control sessions then followed according to the shift. In the 11 (of 20) sessions where the preferred direction shifted in the absence of the cue card, the return of the card to the original position provoked a shift of the preferred direction back to the initial value (Goodridge and Taube, 1995). In two other sessions, the preferred direction remained unchanged, and in the last case the preferred direction shifted to a position intermediate between the initial and new values. In the nine sessions in which the preferred direction did not shift when the disoriented rat was placed in the cylinder where the cue card was absent, the re-installation of the card at a deviation of 90° consistently induced a significant shift in the preferred direction, although the shift was less than 90° in all cases (mean 52.0° ± 9.5°; range: 6° to 84°). In the sessions in which the cue card, was absent the authors conclude that secondary sensory cues were employed, since shifts in preferred directions were not random and remained clustered near the original position (Goodridge and Taube, 1995). They note "dead-reckoning inputs also probably contributed to the maintenance of the cell's preferred direction during the course of the session." Since the reintroduction of the card frequently induced a return to the original values, they suggested, ". . . familiar cue-landmark information can override both internally driven directional information from idiothetic cues and other secondary landmark cues within the room".

Knierim et al. (1998) recorded anterodorsal thalamic head direction cells in male Fischer-344 rats. In one experiment, the rats foraged for food pellets in a gray cylinder with a white cue card subtending 100° along the inner wall. Then, the cylinder and its floor were rotated clockwise by either 45° or 180°, at about 90°/s to 180°/s. This created a conflict because the vestibular cues indicated that the animal had rotated in space, while the visual and substratal cues (cues on the floor surface, such as urine or feces, which were rotated together with the rats) appeared stable and thus contradicted vestibular cues. In general, the preferred directions followed the visual cues for the 45° rotations, but the 180° rotations were much less effective. However, in the latter cases, the preferred directions gradually migrated to follow the visual cues over the course of 5 to 8 minutes. The authors suggest: ". . . idiothetic cues are the primary sources of information that update head direction cells, with a secondary, corrective influence of static, external sensory cues, such as visual landmarks." It should, however, be recalled that the visual system of this albino strain of rats has visual deficits relative to pigmented rats, and this could account, in part, for the weaker influence of visual signals.

In a study by Zugaro et al. (2000) inspired by two previous studies (Sharp et al., 1995; Blair and Sharp, 1996), male Long-Evans rats were placed in a 76 cm diameter, 60 cm high, black-walled cylinder with a white card attached to the wall (covering 75°). As the rats foraged for food pellets, the wall (and card) was rapidly rotated by 90° while the floor remained fixed. The preferred directions of anterodorsal thalamic and postsubicular head direction cells shifted with these peripheral visual cues, but the angles of these shifts were consistently 10% smaller than the actual angle that the visual cue had moved (Zugaro et al., 2000). The same result was obtained when the wall and floor of the apparatus were rotated together by the same angle. This was interpreted to indicate that the visual cues have a dominant influence over the directional responses, but that the conflicting inertial (vestibular, somatosensory, and other force detectors) signals were responsible for the slight reduction in the shifts. This was confirmed by the fact that, in experiments where only the floor was rotated (and thus both the visual and inertial cues coherently indicated self-rotation), the preferred directions remained unchanged, i.e., they were fully controlled by visual and inertial cues.

However, the opposite result was found in a study by Chen and colleagues (1994a), who recorded posterior cortical head direction cells in rats that were confined in a small box. The lights were turned off, then the room cues were rotated. After the lights were turned on, the majority of the neurons remained unchanged or changed their firing properties unpredictably (Chen et al., 1994b). Thus, in this experiment the visual cues were ignored, and in the case of unchanged responses, the substratal and vestibular cues dominated. However, as stated earlier, albino rats have poorer vision than pigmented rats, which may account for the weaker influence of visual cues observed in this study.

Another contradictory result was obtained by Wiener (1993), who recorded head direction cells in the anteromedial part of the caudate nucleus (dorsal striatum) of male Long-Evans rats. The animals were required to make alternating visits between the respective corners and the center of a cubic-canopied enclosure with 60 cm sides. The task requirements were similar to a radial-arm maze task requiring working memory, where in each trial rewards were provided only once at each of the corners. Each trial (of four rewarded visits) began with a visit to the southeast corner and, periodically, all lights were extinguished and the arena was rotated by a multiple of 90° at velocities exceeding the vestibular system threshold. In all three neurons, the preferred direction generally rotated with the box, despite the fact that a contrasted card in the southeast corner was regularly lit with a small spotlight after the animal had correctly visited this corner at the beginning of each trial (Wiener, 1993). This indicates that in this paradigm, tactile and olfactory cues in the box exerted a greater influence than visual and vestibular cues. It is also possible that the completely enclosed apparatus may be responsible for the differences in head direction cell responses between this and other studies. It is noteworthy that in rare cases, the preferred direction shifted randomly: This occurred when the animal had left the center before the end of the arena rotation. In these cases, the summation of the vestibular signals from these simultaneous active and passive movements would have provided a complex and disorienting signal (similar to walking radially on a rotating carousel).

Another reason for the differences found in these studies may be the familiarity of the animals with the diverse cue manipulations. Indeed, Jeffery and O'Keefe (1999) showed that this could affect the relative influence of visual and inertial cues on place cells. In their study, rats were placed on a square box surrounded by circular curtains. A cue card served as the principal orienting cue. Place fields were compared before and after confining the rats on a rotating platter underneath an opaque container, then rotating the platter and the card by various amounts, to see whether the place fields would rotate with the card or with the rats. The rats belonged to one of three groups, depending on their behavioral training in preliminary sessions. For "uncovered" rats, the card had been visibly moved from trial to trial. "Covered" rats had not been exposed to visible card rotations: they either had no prior training at all, or had been covered for 3 min under an opaque container during card rotations. "Briefly covered" rats were also covered during card rotations, but for only 30 s. Place fields were always controlled by the cue card in covered rats. However, place fields of uncovered rats also rotated with the card at first, but by the last recording session the place fields usually rotated with the rat. For the briefly covered group, in half of the rats the place fields followed the card, while in the other half they behaved like those of the uncovered rats, which suggests the effect of covering the rats was time-dependent. In summary, the influence of the card was strongest in rats that had never seen it move and presumably perceived it as stable. In rats that had "learned" that the card was unreliable, idiothetic cues became dominant as the animals became more familiar with the card manipulations.

Summary—Cue Conflicts

From these data it remains unclear whether self-motion cues or familiar visual cues are the dominant signals that influence spatially tuned neurons under cue-conflict situations. Several issues may contribute to the differences in results among the above-mentioned studies, for example, rat strain differences in visual acuity, differences in brain region from which the cells were recorded, differences in apparatus and cue-conditions, or differences in training history and the animals' previous cue experience. With respect to this last point, it is possible that additional experience with cue-conflict situations may change the experimental outcome, meaning that head direction cells of an experienced animal may be predominantly influenced by self-motion cues, whereas visual cues may be the dominant influence in a less experienced animal. Further experimentation will be needed to more completely appreciate the influences on head direction cell firing under conflicting cue conditions and, importantly, whether such activity represents the status of an animal's spatial orientation.

Conclusions

We have reviewed the empirical findings regarding the influence of self-motion cues on head direction cell responses. These data can be summarized in the following manner: first, vestibular inputs play a fundamental role in the generation of the head direction cell signal, as vestibular lesions abolish directional firing responses altogether; second, although motor signals are not essential to the head direction cell system (directionality is preserved in passively rotated rats), motor signals do appear to help enhance the head direction cell signals when the ongoing behavior can benefit from it; third, in unfamiliar environments or in the absence of salient orienting cues (e.g., in darkness), path integration is the main mechanism for spatial orientation, and experimental evidence does show that under these conditions the head direction cells are influenced primarily by self-motion cues. However, in familiar environments, the influence of self-motion signals is superseded by that of environmental cues (e.g., visual landmarks), which indicates that there is some sort of selection of the best available source of spatial information that is modified with the animal's experience. Our chapter also reviewed data from similar studies of self-motion cue influences on hippocampal place cells. These studies reveal quite similar findings: the dependence of location-specific firing responses on vestibular input, and the modulatory influence of motor cues on place cell responses.

It has been theorized that self-motion cues support spatial orientation and spatial navigation under conditions where familiar landmarks are unavailable, such as in darkness or in unfamiliar environments (Gallistel, 1990; McNaughton et al., 1995). Inherent in this view is the idea that self-motion cues play a backup role to visual landmarks in controlling spatial navigation and its neural substrates. This interpretation does not appear to be supported by the findings reviewed here. As we have discussed, the degree to which self-motion cues influence neurophysiological correlates of spatial navigation depends on a number of factors. Ultimately, it appears that both landmark cues and self-motion cues are necessary for maintaining one's spatial orientation and for successful navigation. In order to orient by using landmarks, the animal must recall a learned association between landmarks and self-orientation (a landmark doesn't provide any orienting information, per se). In order to establish this relation, the animal must already be oriented when it perceives the landmarks for the first time; hence, path integration may be the initial enabling mechanism, rather than just a backup system.

Several studies have tested head direction cell responses under conditions in which different sensory cues provide conflicting spatial information to the animal. These cue conflict studies are essential for understanding how the brain resolves conflicts of incoming information. The latter may be fundamental to understanding the neural basis for motion sickness and spatial disorientation. In many cases, information from visual landmarks appears to exert a predominant influence on head direction cells over that of self-motion cues. In other cases, self-motion cues have been found to override influences of visual landmarks, such as when those landmarks are unstable. Further studies are needed to resolve the precise conditions under which self-motion cues prevail, and those under which visual landmarks control the response of head direction cells.

Acknowledgments

The authors would like to thank Drs. Jeffrey Taube and Sidney Wiener for their generous advice and support during our respective tenures in their labs. Much of our work summarized here was supported by grants from the NIH: DC00236 (RWS), MH48924 and

MH01286 (Taube), Ministère de la Recherche and Fondation pour la Recherche Médicale (MZ) and the Oregon Health Sciences Foundation and the Alzheimer's Research Alliance of Oregon (RWS).

References

Arleo A, Déjean C, Boucheny C, Khamassi M, Zugaro MB, Wiener SI (2004) Optic field flow signals update the activity of head direction cells in the rat anterodorsal thalamus. Us Society for Neuroscience Abstracts, 209.2.

Barlow JS (1964) Inertial navigation as a basis for animal navigation. J Theor Biol 6: 76–117.

Barnes CA (1979) Memory deficits associated with senescence: a neurophysiological and behavioral study in the rat. J Comp Physiol Psychol 93: 74–104.

Blair HT, Sharp PE (1995) Anticipatory head direction signals in anterior thalamus: Evidence for a thalamocortical circuit that integrates angular head motion to compute head direction. J Neurosci 15: 6260–6270.

Blair HT, Sharp PE (1996) Visual and vestibular influences on head-direction cells in the anterior thalamus of the rat. Behav Neurosci 110: 643–660.

Blair HT, Lipscomb BW, Sharp PE (1997) Anticipatory time intervals of head-direction cells in the anterior thalamus of the rat: Implications for path integration in the head-direction circuit. J Neurophysiol 78: 145–159.

Bostock E, Muller RU, Kubie JL (1991) Experience-dependent modifications of hippocampal place cell firing. Hippocampus 1: 193–205.

Chen LL, Lin LH, Barnes CA, McNaughton BL (1994a) Head-direction cells in the rat posterior cortex. II. Contributions of visual and ideothetic information to the directional firing. Exp Brain Res 101: 24–34.

Chen LL, Lin LH, Green EJ, Barnes CA, McNaughton BL (1994b) Head-direction cells in the rat posterior cortex. I. Anatomical distribution and behavioral modulation. Exp Brain Research 101: 8–23.

Chen YC, Pellis SM, Sirkin DW, Potegal M, Teitelbaum P (1986) Bandage backfall: Labyrinthine and non-labyrinthine components. Physiol Behav 37: 805–814.

Czurkó A, Hirase H, Csicsvari J, Buzsáki G (1999) Sustained activation of hippocampal pyramidal cells by "space clamping" in a running wheel. Eur J Neurosci 11: 344–352.

Darwin C (1873) Origin of certain instincts. Nature 9: 417–418.

Dudchenko PA, Goodridge JG, Seiterle DA, Taube JS (1997) Effects of repeated disorientation on the acquisition of two spatial reference memory tasks in rats: Dissociation between the radial arm maze and the Morris water maze. J Exp Psychol Anim Behav Process 23: 194–210.

Etienne AS (1980) The orientation of the golden hamster to its nest-site after the elimination of various sensory cues. Experientia 36: 1048–1050.

Etienne AS, Maurer R, Séguinot V (1996) Path integration in mammals and its interaction with visual landmarks. J Exp Biol 199: 201–209.

Etienne AS, Teroni E, Maurer R, Portenier V, Saucy F (1985) Short-distance homing in a small mammal: the role of exteroceptive cues and path integration. Experientia 41: 122–125.

Foster TC, Castro CA, McNaughton BL (1989) Spatial selectivity of rat hippocampal neurons: dependence on preparedness for movement. Science 244: 1580–1582.

Gallistel CR (1990) The Organization of Learning. Cambridge, MA: MIT Press.

Gavrilov VV, Wiener SI, Berthoz A (1995) Enhanced hippocampal theta EEG during whole body rotations in awake restrained rats. Neurosci Lett 197: 239–241.

Gavrilov VV, Wiener SI, Berthoz A (1996) Whole body rotations enhance hippocampal theta rhythmic slow activity in awake rats passively transported on a mobile robot. Ann NY Acad Sci 781: 385–398.

Gavrilov VV, Wiener SI, Berthoz A (1998) Discharge correlates of hippocampal complex spike neurons in behaving rats passively displaced on a mobile robot. Hippocampus 8: 475–490.

Golob EJ, Stackman RW, Wong AC, Taube JS (2001) On the behavioral significance of head direction cells: neural and behavioral dynamics during spatial memory tasks. Behav Neurosci 115: 285–304.

Goodridge JP, Taube JS (1995) Preferential use of the landmark navigational system by head direction cells in rats. Behav Neurosci 109: 49–61.

Goodridge JP, Taube JS (1997) Interaction between the postsubiculum and anterior thalamus in the generation of head direction cell activity. J Neurosci 17: 9315–9330.

Goodridge JP, Dudchenko PA, Worboys KA, Golob EJ, Taube JS (1998) Cue control and head direction cells. Behav Neurosci 112: 749–761.

Hess BJ, Precht W, Reber A, Cazin L (1985) Horizontal optokinetic ocular nystagmus in the pigmented rat. Neurosci 15: 97–107.

Hill AJ, Best PJ (1981) Effects of deafness and blindness on the spatial correlates of hippocampal unit activity in the rat. Exp Neurol 74: 204–217.

Jeffery KJ, O'Keefe JM (1999) Learned interaction of visual and idiothetic cues in the control of place field orientation. Exp Brain Res 127: 151–161.

Kaufman GD, Anderson JH, Beitz AJ (1992) Brainstem Fos expression following acute unilateral labyrinthectomy in the rat. Neuroreport 3: 829–832.

Knierim JJ, Kudrimoti HS, McNaughton BL (1995) Place cells, head direction cells, and the learning of landmark stability. J Neurosci 15: 1648–1659.

Knierim JJ, Kudrimoti HS, McNaughton BL (1998) Interactions between idiothetic cues and external landmarks in the control of place cells and head direction cells. J Neurophysiol 80: 425–446.

Martin GM, Harley CW, Smith AR, Hoyles ES, Hynes CA (1997) Spatial disorientation blocks reliable goal location on a plus maze but does not prevent goal location in the Morris maze. J Exp Psychol Anim Behav Process 23: 183–193.

Matthews BL, Campbell KA, Deadwyler SA (1988) Rotational stimulation disrupts spatial learning in fornix-lesioned rats. Behav Neurosci 102: 35–42.

McNaughton BL, Chen LL, Markus EJ (1991) "Dead reckoning", landmark learning, and the sense of direction: A neurophysiological and computational hypothesis. J Cogn Neurosci:190–202.

McNaughton BL, Knierim JJ, Wilson MA (1995) Vector encoding and the vestibular foundations of spatial cognition: Neurophysiological and computational mechanisms. In M Gazzaniga, ed., The Cognitive Neurosciences Cambridge, MA: MIT Press, pp. 585–595.

McNaughton BL, Barnes CA, Gerrard JL, Gothard K, Jung M, Knierim JJ, Kudrimoti HS, Qin Y, Skaggs WE, Suster M, Weaver KL (1996) Deciphering the hippocampal polyglot: the hippocampus as a path integration system. J Exp Biol 199: 173–185.

Miles FA, Evarts EV (1979) Concepts of motor organization. Annu Rev Psychol 30: 327–362.

Miller S, Potegal M, Abraham L (1983) Vestibular involvement in a passive transport and return task. Physiol Psychol 11: 1–10.

Mittelstaedt ML, Mittelstaedt H (1980) Homing by path integration in the mammal. Naturwissenschaften 67: 566–567.

Mizumori SJY, Williams JD (1993) Directionally selective mnemonic properties of neurons in the lateral dorsal nucleus of the thalamus of rats. J Neurosci 13: 4015–4028.

Muller RU (1996) A quarter of a century of place cells. Neuron 17: 813–822.

Nishijo H, Ono T, Eifuku S, Tamura R (1997) The relationship between monkey hippocampus place-related neural activity and action in space. Neurosci Lett 226: 57–60.

Olton DS, Becker JT, Handelmann GE (1979) Hippocampus, space, and memory. Behav Brain Sci 2: 313–365.

Ossenkopp KP, Hargreaves EL (1993) Spatial learning in an enclosed eight-arm radial maze in rats with sodium arsanilate-induced labyrinthectomies. Behav Neural Biol 59: 253–257.

Potegal M, Day MJ, Abraham L (1977) Maze orientation, visual and vestibular cues in two-maze spontaneous alternation of rats. Physiol Psychol 5: 414–420.

Quirk GJ, Muller RU, Kubie JL (1990) The firing of hippocampal place cells in the dark depends on the rat's recent experience. J Neurosci 10: 2008–2017.

Ranck JB, Jr. (1973) Studies on single neurons in dorsal hippocampal formation and septum in unrestrained rats. I. Behavioral correlates and firing repertoires. Exp Neurol 41: 461–531.

Russell NA, Horii A, Smith PF, Darlington CL, Bilkey DK (2003) Long-term effects of permanent vestibular lesions on hippocampal spatial firing. J Neurosci 23: 6490–6498.

Samsonovich A, McNaughton BL (1997) Path integration and cognitive mapping in a continuous attractor neural network model. J Neurosci 17: 5900–5920.

Save E, Cressant A, Thinus-Blanc C, Poucet B (1998) Spatial firing of hippocampal place cells in blind rats. J Neurosci 18: 1818–1826.

Saxon DW, Anderson JH, Beitz AJ (2001) Transtympanic tetrodotoxin alters the VOR and Fos labeling in the vestibular complex. Neuroreport 12: 3051–3055.

Shapiro ML, Tanila H, Eichenbaum H (1997) Cues that hippocampal place cells encode: dynamic and hierarchical representation of local and distal stimuli. Hippocampus 7: 624–642.

Sharp PE, Blair HT, Tzanetos DB (1995) Influences of vestibular and visual motion information on the spatial firing patterns of hippocampal place cells. J Neurosci 15: 173–189.

Stackman RW, Taube JS (1997) Firing properties of head direction cells in the rat anterior thalamic neurons: Dependence on vestibular input. J Neurosci 17: 4349–4358.

Stackman RW, Herbert AM (2002) Rats with lesions of the vestibular system require a visual landmark for spatial navigation. Behav Brain Res 128: 27–40.

Stackman RW, Clark AS, Taube JS (2002) Hippocampal spatial representations require vestibular input. Hippocampus 12: 291–303.

Stackman RW, Golob EJ, Bassett JP, Taube JS (2003) Passive transport disrupts directional path integration by rat head direction cells. J Neurophysiol 90: 2862–2874.

Stackman RW, Tullman ML, Taube JS (2000) Maintenance of rat head direction cell firing during locomotion in the vertical plane. J Neurophysiol 83: 393–405.

Taube JS (1995) Head direction cells recorded in the anterior thalamic nuclei of freely moving rats. J Neurosci 15: 70–86.

Taube JS (1998) Head direction cells and the neurophysiological basis for a sense of direction. Prog Neurobiol 55: 225–256.

Taube JS, Burton HL (1995) Head direction cell activity monitored in a novel environment and during a cue conflict situation. J Neurophysiol 74: 1953–1971.

Taube JS, Muller RU (1998) Comparisons of head direction cell activity in the postsubiculum and anterior thalamus of freely moving rats. Hippocampus 8: 87–108.

Taube JS, Muller RU, Ranck JB, Jr. (1990) Head-direction cells recorded from the postsubiculum in freely moving rats. II. Effects of environmental manipulations. J Neurosci 10: 436–447.

Von Holst E (1954) Relations between the central nervous system and the peripheral organs. Br J Animal Behav 2: 89–94.

Wallace DG, Hines DJ, Pellis SM, Whishaw IQ (2002) Vestibular information is required for dead reckoning in the rat. J Neurosci 22: 10009–10017.

Wiener SI (1993) Spatial and behavioral correlates of striatal neurons in rats performing a self-initiated navigational task. J Neurosci 13: 3802–3817.

Wiener SI, Korshunov VA, Garcia R, Berthoz A (1995) Inertial, substratal and landmark cue control of hippocampal CA1 place cell activity. Eur J Neurosci 7: 2206–2219.

Wood ER, Dudchenko PA, Eichenbaum H (1999) The global record of memory in hippocampal neuronal activity. Nature 397: 613–616.

Zugaro MB, Tabuchi E, Wiener SI (2000) Influence of conflicting visual, inertial and substratal cues on head direction cell activity. Exp Brain Res 133: 198–208.

Zugaro MB, Tabuchi E, Fouquier C, Berthoz A, Wiener SI (2001) Active locomotion increases peak firing rates of anterodorsal thalamic head direction cells. J Neurophysiol 86: 692–702.

Zugaro MB, Berthoz A, Wiener SI (2002) Peak firing rates of rat anterodorsal thalamic head direction cells are higher during faster passive rotations. Hippocampus 12: 481–486.

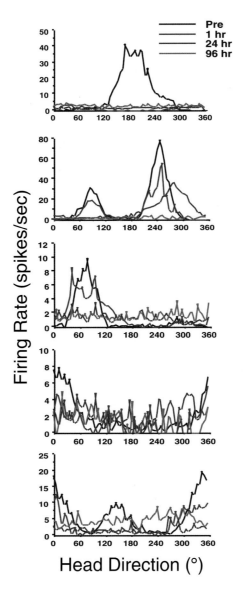

Plate 1 Lesion of the vestibular apparatus abolishes directional firing of anterior thalamic neurons. Five head direction cells were recorded before (Pre) and after (1–96 hr) transtympanic injection of the toxin sodium arsanilate. Rats displayed behaviors consistent with a loss of vestibular function within 24 hr of receiving sodium arsanilate, yet continued to move freely about the cylindrical arena during unit recording sessions. The isolation of each cell was maintained, and each cell's waveform was consistent over the entire course of each experiment. (Reproduced with permission from Stackman and Taube, 1997. Copyright by the Society for Neuroscience.) See chapter 7.

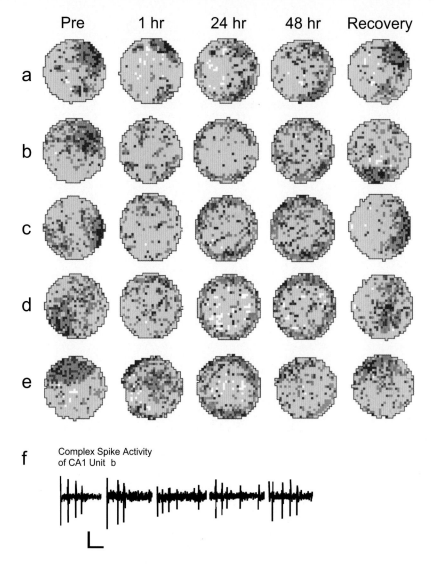

	Pre	1 hr	24 hr	48 hr	Recovery
a					
b					
c					
d					
e					

f   Complex Spike Activity
of CA1 Unit b

Plate 2 Temporary inactivation of the vestibular system disrupts location-specific firing of hippocampal neurons. Plot illustrates firing rate vs. location maps for five (a–e) representative hippocampal place cells recorded before (Pre), during (1–48 hr), and after (Recovery) tetrodotoxin-induced inactivation of the vestibular apparatus. For each map, increasing firing rates are coded from yellow, orange, red, green, blue, and purple, with yellow pixels depicting locations where no spikes were fired. Within 1 hr after vestibular inactivation the location-specific firing was substantially attenuated or abolished. The recovery of place fields occurred concomitant with the recovery of vestibular function, which took between 48 and 96 hr post injection. These plots also provide examples of the types of changes in place field location evident after recovery from vestibular inactivation (b and d). Despite the loss of location-specific firing, hippocampal neurons continued to exhibit a complex-spike pattern of discharge (f). The isolation of each cell was maintained, and each cell's waveform was consistent over the entire course of each experiment. Scale bars: 50 μV/10 ms (Reproduced with permission from Stackman et al., 2002. Copyright by Wiley Press.) See chapter 7.

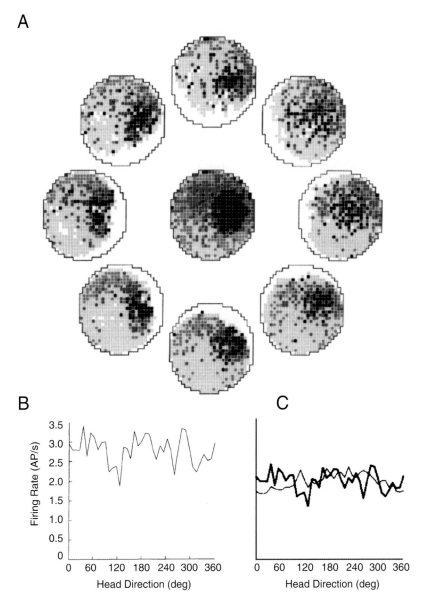

Plate 3 Direction-independent (center) and direction-specific firing rate maps for a place cell whose field is away from the cylinder wall. (A) Although there is some encroachment of the unsampled (white crescent) region on the area of the field, it is clear from the color code that firing was very similar in all 45° head direction sectors. This is therefore an example of a field whose omni-directional independence seems evident from the raw data. Median action potentials per second (AR/sec) by color categories: yellow, 0.0; orange, 0.40; red, 0.93; green, 1.7; blue, 3.2; purple, 6.5. (B) Firing rate as a function of head direction at higher (9°) resolution. (C) Comparison of observed values of firing rate as a function of head direction from (B) (thick line) with expected values. The rate variations are small and show no obvious systematic pattern, as expected from the maps in (A). The expected firing rate (thin line) is obtained from equation 9.1. See chapter 9.

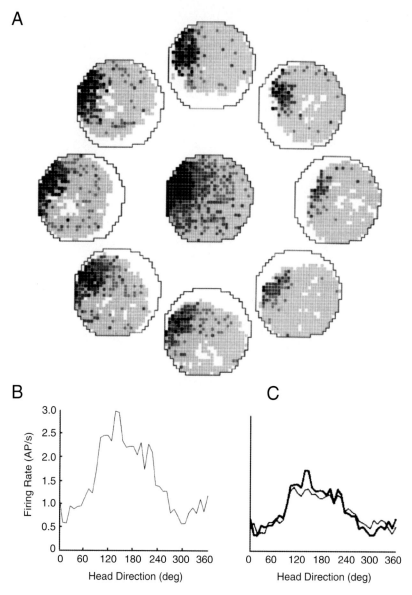

Plate 4 Direction-independent (center) and direction-specific rate maps for a place cell whose field is near the cylinder wall. In this case, the kinematically excluded region rotates so that it superimposes on the main area of the field. The result is the reduced firing for the direction-specific maps centered on 315° and 0°. Median action potentials per second (AP/sec) by color categories: yellow, 0.0; orange, 0.21; red, 0.55; green, 1.4; blue, 5.3; purple, 12.5. (B) Firing rate as a function of head direction at higher (9°) resolution. (C) Comparison of observed values of firing rate as a function of head direction from (B) (thick line) with expected values. The reduced firing at head directions between 300° and 60° is seen clearly when firing rate is plotted against head direction. The expected values (thin line) are obtained from equation 9.1. The key point is that the expected values conform closely to the observed values. See chapter 9.

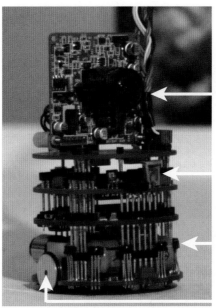

Vision system

Light detector

Infrared sensors

Odometer

Plate 5   The mobile Khepera miniature robot, a commercial platform produced and distributed by K-Team S.A. The Khepera has a cylindrical body with a diameter of 55 mm, and in the configuration used for the experiments is about 90 mm tall. Two DC motors drive two wheels independently, providing the robot with nonholonomic motion capabilities. The robot's sensory system consists of a vision system, which includes a CCD black and white camera with an image resolution of 768×576 pixels and a view field covering about 90° in the horizontal plane and 60° in the vertical plane; eight infrared sensors that can detect obstacles within a distance of about 40 mm (six infrared sensors span the frontal 180° of the robot and two sensors cover approximately 100° of the posterior side); a light detector placed in the front of the robot; and wheel rotation encoders (odometers) to estimate both linear and angular displacements. (From Arleo, 2000.) See chapter 19.

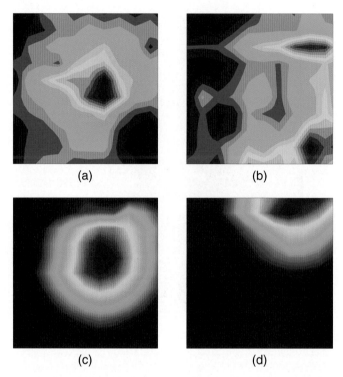

Plate 6 (a, b) Two samples of receptive fields obtained by recording from the vision-based place cell (ViPC) layer of the model. The squares represent overhead views of the environment. For each position visited by the robot, the corresponding mean firing rate of the recorded cell is plotted. Red regions indicate high activity whereas dark blue regions denote low firing rates. The receptive field in (a) codes for a localized spatial location. The cell in (b) is maximally active at two different locations (multipeak receptive field) because these purely vision-based representations are affected by the sensory aliasing problem. (c, d) Two typical place fields of cells in the CA3-CA1 layer of the model. Combining visual information and path integration yields stable place cell responses (single-peak receptive fields) solving the visual aliasing problem. (From Arleo, 2000.) See chapter 19.

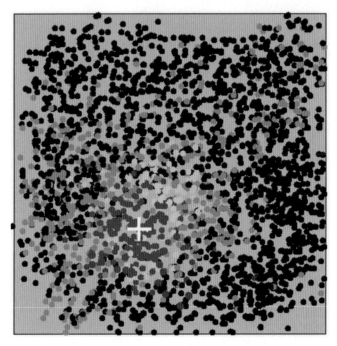

Plate 7 Sample of CA3-CA1 ensemble firing in the model. Each dot denotes the center of a place field. Red dots indicate highly active HP cells and dark blue dots denote silent neurons. The center of mass of the population activity (white cross) is used to reconstruct the robot's position. (From Arleo, 2000.) See chapter 19.

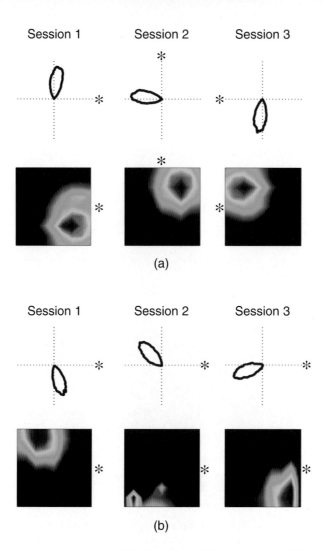

Plate 8 Intersession responses of one HD cell in the PoSC and one CA3-CA1 place cell of the model. At the beginning of each session the robot is disoriented. (a) During training the visual cue configuration (whose centroid is indicated by the asterisk) remains stable. Between probe sessions the constellation of visual cues undergoes a +90° rotation. Both the HD and the HP cell are controlled by the visual scene and reorient their receptive fields following the +90° intersession rotations. (b) The visual configuration is not stable during spatial learning. The data show that the disoriented robot fails to reactivate coherent representations across probe sessions, and remapping occurs. The directional and place selectivity does not maintain a fixed orientation relative to visual cues. See chapter 19.

8 Coupling between Head Direction Cells and Place Cells: Influences of Landmarks, Self-Motion, and Intrinsic Circuitry

James J. Knierim

A former New Yorker gets off a train at Grand Central Station. Remembering that the station is on 42nd Street, he knows that he must travel north to reach his final destination on 84th Street. With the skyscrapers blocking the sun and the street signs mysteriously removed, he has no way of ascertaining which direction to travel. Choosing one direction at random, he starts to walk, and twelve blocks later comes upon the Empire State Building. From his mental map of New York City, he knows that the Empire State Building is south of Grand Central Station, and that he must now reverse direction to head north.

This example illustrates the ability to navigate solely with a combination of known landmarks (Grand Central Station and the Empire State Building) and a map to localize the landmarks (a mental map of the grid of New York City streets). It would have been much easier on the traveler's feet, however, if he had a compass to give him his direction as he left the station. Such a compass would not only tell him whether he was facing north, south, east, or west as he walked, but would also allow him to align his mental map of the city with the visual landmarks he witnessed, thereby keeping him oriented with respect to their location.

O'Keefe and Nadel's (1978) cognitive map theory hypothesized that the place cell system of the hippocampus formed the animal's mental representation of the spatial layout of an environment. This theory was strengthened by Ranck's subsequent discovery of head direction cells in the dorsal presubiculum (or postsubiculum; see chapter 2 by Hopkins), an area that has extensive connections with the hippocampal formation (Ranck, 1985; Taube et al., 1990b). Head direction cells have subsequently been identified in numerous brain structures (Mizumori and Williams, 1993; Wiener and Berthoz, 1993; Chen et al., 1994; Taube, 1995), and they may serve as an "internal compass" used in tandem with the hippocampal place representation. Although anatomical and physiological data suggest that the place and head direction systems are closely related (Leutgeb et al., 2000), the precise nature of their interactions is still under investigation.

Under most conditions, the place cell system and the head direction cell system appear to be tightly coupled to each other, at least at the level of neural population activity. This coupling was suggested by early investigations, in which distal landmarks were rotated around the experimental apparatus. Both place cells (O'Keefe and Conway, 1978) and head direction cells (Taube et al., 1990a) were shown to be controlled in most cases by the rotation of the landmarks. Although these studies suggested a coupling of these systems, it was conceivable that the systems were independently controlled by the visual landmarks, with no direct connection between them. Knierim et al. (1995) addressed this issue by recording from CA1 place cells and anterior thalamic head direction cells simultaneously, under conditions in which the rat was disoriented prior to recording in a gray-walled cylinder with a single, white cue card covering 90° of the eastern wall. Under these conditions, the firing fields of place cells and the preferred directions of head direction cells sometimes adopted new, apparently arbitrary, orientations relative to the cue card (figure 8.1). In each case, the place fields and head direction cell tuning curves remained tightly coupled to each other, rotating by the same amount relative to the cue card (although partial remapping of the place cell representation sometimes complicated this conclusion; see following pages). Thus, in situations in which the cells' firing properties became decoupled from the external landmarks, they remained tightly coupled to each other.

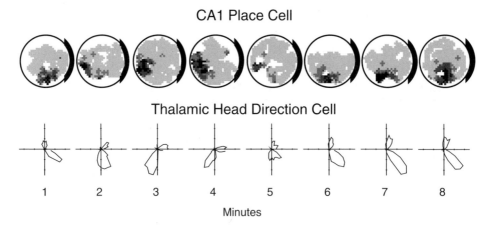

CA1 Place Cell

Thalamic Head Direction Cell

1   2   3   4   5   6   7   8

Minutes

Figure 8.1
Simultaneous recording of a place cell from CA1 and a head direction cell from the anterior dorsal nucleus of the thalamus. The rat foraged for food in a gray-walled cylinder, with a white cue card covering 90° of the east wall. The rat was disoriented before being placed in the cylinder, a procedure that tends to weaken the control of landmarks over place cells and head direction cells. The first 8 minutes of the recording session are broken down into 1-minute segments. During minute 2, both the place field and the head direction cell tuning curve began to rotate spontaneously approximately 90° counterclockwise (minutes 3–4). In minute 5, the cells' tuning properties rotated back to their original firing preferences. (Modified from Knierim et al., 1995. Copyright 1995 by the Society for Neuroscience; reproduced with permission.)

Because of the close relationship between the use of directional information and place information in navigation, and the close coupling between the two brain systems thought to represent this information, it is likely that a full understanding of one system will require an understanding of how it interacts with the other. This chapter reviews a number of studies of this interaction, focusing on how self-motion cues and visual landmarks interact to control place cells and head direction cells. Although other sources of information are also important (e.g., behavioral contingencies), most studies of the interactions between these systems have focused on these two classes of cues.

Visual Landmark Control over Place Cells and Head Direction Cells Depends on Experience

In their study on the effects of disorientation on the responses of place cells and head direction cells, Knierim et al. (1995) demonstrated that the strength of control by visual landmarks over these cells depended on the prior experience of the animal; that is, the relationship between the preferred locations/directions of these cells and their controlling external cues was learned. One group of rats was trained under conditions of disorientation: the rats were placed in a box and transported around the hallways and around the recording chamber while being gently rotated before being placed in the chamber. This procedure was intended to interfere with the animal's ability to use path integration mechanisms in order to accurately maintain its bearing between its holding platform and the recording room. Every time these animals entered the recording room for a training session, their internal sense of direction was presumably set at an arbitrary bearing. The other group of rats did not undergo this disorientation procedure, but instead was brought into the recording chamber directly from the holding platform. For this group, the internal sense of direction was presumably the same on each entry into the recording chamber. After many training sessions, recordings of place cells and head direction cells began; both groups of animals underwent the disorientation procedure before recording sessions. Thus, the recording conditions were identical for both groups, the only difference being the prior training history of the animals. The white cue card had much stronger control over the place cells and head direction cells in the group that had not been disoriented during training than the group that had been disoriented (figure 8.2). Knierim et al. (1995) interpreted these results as evidence that the animals had to learn that the cue card was a stable landmark in order for the card to exert control over the cells. They hypothesized that in a novel environment, place cells and head direction cells are controlled initially by idiothetic (self-motion) cues (McNaughton et al., 1991). As the rat explores the environment, visual landmarks perceived at different locations and heading directions begin to be associated with the place cells and head direction cells that encode these locations. Eventually, the synaptic connections between cells that represent the visual landmarks and the place/head direction cells become strong enough for the landmarks to control the cells directly. The

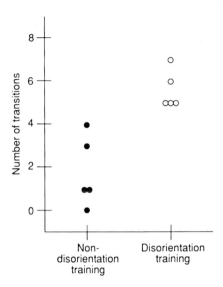

Figure 8.2
Cue-card control over place cells and head direction cells depends on the prior experience of the rat. In this experiment, 16 recording sessions were performed (4 sessions per day). A transition was defined as a change between sessions in the bearing of the head direction cell tuning curve or the place cell firing field relative to the white cue card. Rats that had been disoriented during training displayed many more transitions than rats that had been trained without disorientation. (From Knierim et al., 1995. Copyright 1995 by the Society for Neuroscience; reproduced with permission.)

function of this learned landmark control is to allow the animal to correct for cumulative error in its inertial navigation system (path integration) by taking "visual fixes" of the environment (Barlow, 1964; Gallistel, 1990).

   Why does the disorientation procedure disrupt this control? Knierim et al. (1995) reasoned that when the animal is disoriented, its head direction system is set at an arbitrary bearing each time it enters the environment. Thus, even though the cue card is stable relative to the world, on every session the rat's own internal sense of direction rotates relative to the cue card. Because there is no stable relationship between the orientation of the cue card and the bearing of the head direction cells and place cells, no strong learning occurs, and the cue card never develops strong control over the cells. Subsequent studies by Goodridge et al. (1998) demonstrated that it takes a few minutes of experience in an environment before landmarks begin to gain strong control over head direction cells (see chapter 3 by Taube). Another relevant set of studies by Jeffery and colleagues (Jeffery et al., 1997; Jeffery, 1998; Jeffery and O'Keefe, 1999) explicitly gained control over the animal's sense of direction by placing it in a covered bucket and slowly rotating the bucket 90°, below the vestibular threshold, between recording sessions. When the animal was returned to the recording environment after the rotation procedure, it experienced a conflict between its internal direction sense and the salient visual landmark in the environment. Under these conditions, hippocampal place fields tended to stay aligned with the animal's presumed sense of direction if the animal had explicitly witnessed the cue card being moved on prior occasions (i.e., the animal learned that the cue card was unstable). However, the ability of the cue card to control the place fields was enhanced the longer the animal stayed in the covered bucket between recording sessions. It was as if the strength of the internal direction signal (or the animal's "confidence" in it) decreased over time in the absence of visual feedback. In behavioral experiments, Dudchenko et al. (1997) and Martin et al. (1997) have demonstrated that disorientation can prevent the animal's ability to use a stable landmark to solve an appetitive spatial task on a normal substrate, but the procedure has no effect on the ability of the animal to solve an aversive task in water (such as the Morris water maze). The factors that account for this intriguing difference in behavioral task performance as a result of the disorientation procedure are not understood.

Head Direction Cells and Hippocampal Remapping

Although Knierim et al. (1995) showed directly that place cells and head direction cells were strongly coupled to each other, this relationship is complicated by the phenomenon known as "remapping" in the hippocampus. That is, changes to the environment or to some internal state variable can cause the hippocampus to form a new representation of an environment (Muller, 1996; Knierim, 2003). For example, changing the color or shape of a recording chamber (Muller and Kubie, 1987; Bostock et al., 1991), or changing the rules of the animal's task (Markus et al., 1995), can cause a complex reorganization of place fields in the environment. Some place cells become silent, other place cells that were previously silent develop a strong field, and other place cells shift their firing fields to unpredictable locations. Knierim et al. (1995) demonstrated that a shift in the orientation of the head direction cell system relative to the external landmarks is one of the internal variables that can occur in conjunction with remapping in the hippocampus (figure 8.3). Thus, the hippocampal representation becomes, in one sense, decoupled from the head direction cell system. Individual place fields change their relationship to each other, as well as to the preferred directions of head direction cells. However, no laboratory has reported that the hippocampal place cell representation can rotate in a direction different from that of the head direction cell network and maintain its own internal coherence (i.e., not remap). Thus, at a network level, the two systems are strongly coupled. Under most conditions, they rotate in register. Under some conditions, however, when a conflict is introduced between the head direction cell system and external environment, the hippocampus will react in one of two ways: its representation will rotate along with the head direction cells, independent of the external cues, or it will respond to the conflict by remapping.

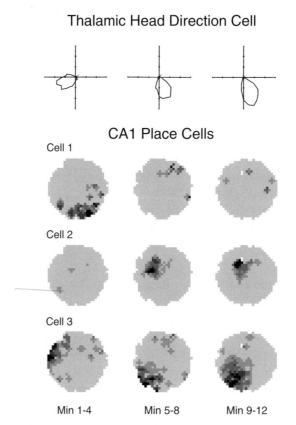

Figure 8.3
Misorientation of the head direction cells correlates with hippocampal remapping. A 12-minute recording session is broken down into three 4-minute segments. Between the first and second segments, the head direction cell tuning curve spontaneously rotated approximately 90° counterclockwise. Simultaneously recorded place cells displayed a partial remapping. Cell 1 lost its place field, cell 2 gained a place field, and the place field of cell 3 rotated 90° along with the head direction cell's tuning curve. No changes occurred in the head direction cell or the place cells in the third segment. (Modified from Knierim et al., 1995. Copyright 1995 by the Society for Neuroscience; reproduced with permission.)

Drift in Place Cells and Head Direction Cells

The preferred firing locations/directions of place cells and head direction cells are not always stable within a recording session. Rather, these tuning curves can rotate over time relative to the external environment, either spontaneously or as the result of an experimental manipulation (e.g., figures 8.1 and 8.3). Knierim et al. (1995) reported in their disorientation study that head direction cell tuning curves rotated by 30° to 130° in 30% of the recording sessions, usually in the first few minutes. When it was possible to look at both place cells and head direction cells recorded simultaneously, the preferred firing location/direction of both sets of cells rotated in synchrony. The prevalence of drift in these experiments is most likely the result of the disorientation procedure, as most other studies do not report such firing instability relative to the environmental landmarks. Nonetheless, these results reinforce the ease with which the systems can become decoupled from the external environment, while maintaining their internal coherence with each other.

Another type of intrasession drift occurred when the floors and wall of a cylindrical chamber with a white cue card were abruptly rotated while the rat foraged for food inside the chamber (Knierim et al., 1998). In separate groups of rats, head direction cells or CA1 place cells were recorded. In some of the 180° rotation sessions, the tuning curves of place cells and head direction cells rotated to follow the cylinder. In the other sessions, the place cells remapped the cylinder, and the head direction cell tuning curves either stayed in the same location relative to the external laboratory environment or adopted a new, arbitrary orientation. When the head direction cells that were controlled by the intracylinder cues were examined with high temporal resolution, an interesting phenomenon was unveiled. In all cases, the cells initially maintained the same preferred firing direction relative to the external laboratory. Over the course of 1 minute or so, the cells' preferred directions drifted smoothly 180° until they were realigned to the intracylinder cues (e.g., the cue card).

A particularly interesting example is shown in figure 8.4. In this case, the cell initially responded to the abrupt cylinder rotation by a reduction in firing rate (minute 3), but the preferred direction remained stable relative to the external laboratory environment. After 3 minutes, the cylinder was rotated slowly clockwise, below the vestibular threshold of the rat (minute 6). Interestingly, the cell's preferred direction began to shift counterclockwise, rotating relative to both the external laboratory environment and the local, intracylinder environment, until the cell's preferred direction was realigned to its original bearing relative to the cylinder (minute 8). From this point, the preferred direction began to rotate clockwise with the slow rotation of the cylinder, as the cell's tuning curve became locked into the standard configuration with the cylinder cues.

These results argue strongly that after the fast rotation, the original sensory stimulus used to update the preferred direction of the head direction cells in this experiment was an idiothetic signal, such as vestibular activation or optic flow from potential cues outside the cylinder (McNaughton et al., 1991; McNaughton et al., 1995; Stackman and Taube, 1997). The rat sensed the rotation of the cylinder and itself, and its head direction system was updated according to its new bearing relative to the laboratory. The preferred directions stayed at the new bearing relative to the cylinder cues in some sessions, whereas in other sessions the preferred directions eventually rotated to realign with the initial orientation relative to the cylinder. This result provides evidence for the notion that head direction cells are updated dynamically by idiothetic information, with a powerful, correcting influence of visual landmarks (McNaughton et al., 1996).

Limitations on the Ability of Landmarks to Correct for Error in the Head Direction Cell Bearing

In many studies of visual landmark control over place cells and head direction cells, distal cues are rotated relative to the behavioral apparatus to test whether the firing fields/ preferred directions rotate along with the cues (O'Keefe and Conway, 1978; Taube et al., 1990a). These types of studies provided the original evidence for a strong influence of distal visual landmarks over both place cells and head direction cells. A number of subsequent studies have demonstrated that the strength of this control can depend on the angle by which the cues were rotated from their original position. It appears that there is a threshold around 45° to 90°, below which the landmarks (if they are considered stable) almost always have strong control over the cells. Rotations above this threshold can give variable results. Rotenberg and Muller (1997) rotated a white cue card in the presence of the rat in 45° or 180° increments, and showed that place fields always rotated with the card after the 45° rotations but never after the 180° rotations. Knierim et al. (1998) rotated the entire apparatus and rat abruptly, and showed a similar result. That is, when the apparatus was quickly rotated 45°, the tuning curves of place cells and head direction cells almost always rotated by 45°. When the apparatus was rotated 180°, the tuning curves rotated with the apparatus in only about half the sessions; in the other half, head direction cell tuning curves stayed in the same frame relative to inertial cues (or laboratory cues), and place cells remapped the environment (as described above). Although place cells and head direction cells were not recorded simultaneously in this experiment, the similar pattern of results for the two cell types supports the coupling between these systems.

In another set of studies, Knierim et al. (1998) recorded head direction cells while a rat either foraged for food on an open platform or was passively rotated on a raised platform. In this experiment, there were a number of salient landmarks on the walls of the laboratory. After recording the preferred firing directions of head direction cells, the lights were extinguished. The firing directions of the cells were monitored until they drifted a certain amount from the original direction, and the lights were turned back on to see if the tuning curves would return to their original direction relative to the room cues. When the drift was greater than 45°, in most cases the preferred directions stayed at their new settings when the lights came on, as if the distal landmarks had no control over the cells. When the drift was 45° or less, however, the tuning curves rotated to realign with the landmarks in about half of the cases. In this experiment, a number of light-dark-light sessions were recorded in succession. The 45° drifts were subsequently analyzed to see whether the preferred direction started in the initial (and presumably most common) direction in the room, or whether it started from a different direction to which it had rotated in a previous test. When the cell drifted 45° from the original direction, it reset back to that direction when the lights were turned on in 10 of 13 cases; when it drifted 45° from a different direction, it reset back to that direction in only 4 of 17 cases. Thus, there appeared to be a single

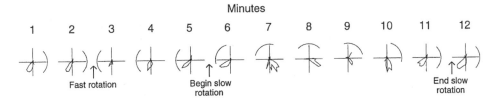

Figure 8.4
Delayed cue control over head direction cells. A head direction cell from the anterior dorsal thalamic nucleus fired at the southwest direction for the first 2 minutes of recording in a gray-walled cylinder with a white cue card at the east. After the second minute, the entire cylinder (with the rat near the center) was abruptly and quickly rotated 180°. The cell initially reduced its firing rate, but maintained its firing in the southwest direction, independent of the new orientation of the cue card. After minute 5, the cylinder was rotated slowly clockwise. The head direction tuning curve rotated counterclockwise until it realigned with its initial orientation relative to the cue card (minute 8). From this point on, it was controlled by the cue card and rotated clockwise. (From Knierim et al., 1998. Copyright 1998 by the American Physiological Society; reproduced with permission.)

preferred direction to which the cell's tuning curve would usually reset when it drifted to a new direction in the dark; this corrective reset when the lights were turned back on typically occurred only when the drift was relatively small.

This phenomenon helps explain the data of the drifting tuning curve of figure 8.4. After the fast rotation of the cylinder, the cell was controlled by the rat's idiothetic cues and stayed in the same firing direction, 180° out of register with the cue card's new position. With the system out of its learned alignment with the landmarks, it behaved as if it were in the dark: the preferred direction began to drift, as the system accumulated error in a counterclockwise-biased manner (the reason for the counterclockwise bias is not known). When the system's drift took it within the 45° window of control of the landmarks, the system "snapped" back into place with the visual cues, and it was controlled by the slowly rotating landmark from that point forward (see also chapter 7 by Stackman and Zugaro).

Double-cue Rotations: Local Versus Distal Landmarks

Early investigations into place cells concluded that the cells were controlled predominantly by distal landmarks (O'Keefe and Conway, 1978; Muller and Kubie, 1987). In these experiments, rotation of the landmarks typically caused the place fields to rotate by the same amount, whereas rotation of the behavioral apparatus (e.g., radial maze) or the floor of a recording chamber caused the place fields to maintain their locations relative to the distal landmarks. In these experiments, the cues on the apparatus or on the floor were typically not very salient. More recent experiments have shown that salient local cues can control the location of place fields (Young et al., 1994; Shapiro et al., 1997; Knierim and McNaughton, 2001; Knierim, 2002). These salient cues can be textured floors, odors, or changes in the three-dimensional orientation of the maze. Thus, when salient local cues and salient distal cues are rotated relative to each other, there is a competition in the place cell network to determine whether the representation will follow the local cues or the distal landmarks. Shapiro et al. (1997) suggested that within an individual data set, some place fields could rotate with the local cues, whereas other fields could rotate with the distal landmarks. These results were important for theories that proposed the existence of attractor networks in the hippocampus (see chapters 14 by Rolls, 18 by Touretzky, and 19 by Arleo and Gerstner) as a strong attractor might prevent the hippocampal representation from splitting in the way suggested by the Shapiro et al. (1997) data.

We investigated this issue further by recording ensembles of place cells as a rat ran a circular track with four distinct, textured inserts on the track (Knierim, 2002). Along the walls of the room were salient visual landmarks. After extensive training in a standard configuration of landmarks and the track, we performed manipulations in which the track was rotated counterclockwise by varying amounts (22.5°, 45°, 67.5°, and 90°), while the distal landmarks were rotated clockwise by an equal amount. In these experiments, we replicated the results of Shapiro et al. (1997), in that simultaneously recorded cells could follow either set of cues. Some cells split their place fields, firing in two locations on the track in the double-rotation sessions (see also O'Keefe and Burgess, 1996). Although these results were not predicted by models of attractor networks, they were not necessarily inconsistent with them either. Many attractor network models of place cells proposed a role for external landmarks in calibrating the orientation of the representation relative to the external landmarks (Skaggs et al., 1995; Touretzky and Redish, 1996; Zhang, 1996; Samsonovich and McNaughton, 1997). Thus, if the influence of the external landmarks was strong enough, it could override the attractor network and cause the splitting. Interestingly, the place cells responded differently to a 45° mismatch of the local and distal cues compared to larger mismatches (figure 8.5). With the small mismatch, the representation appeared to maintain some degree of coherence, as the distribution of place field rotation angles was unimodal and centered around 0°; the place fields split into two distinct representations only with the larger mismatch amounts. This is yet another example of the 45° threshold; somewhere between a mismatch amount of 45° and 90°, the system switched from maintaining a degree of coherence to splitting its representation.

The splitting of the place field representation may indicate a situation in which the place field representation and the head direction representation can become uncoupled. If one assumes that head direction cell tuning curves rotated with either the local or distal landmarks, then the place fields that rotated with the other set of cues may have maintained their relative coherence with each other, but they became decoupled from the head direction cell system. Alternatively, it is possible that the head direction cells also split their representations, and some place fields were coupled to local-cue-dominated head direction cells and other place fields were coupled to distal-cue-dominated place fields. We have recently begun to address whether the head direction cell representation can also be split in the double rotation paradigm, or whether these cells always maintain a unitary repre-

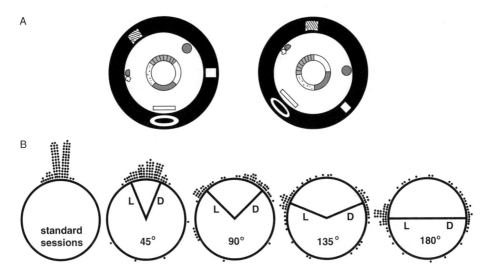

Figure 8.5
(A) Place cells were recorded on a circular, textured track in a standard environment (left) and in a mismatch environment in which the track was rotated counterclockwise (in this case 45°) and the distal landmarks were rotated clockwise (in this case 45°), for a total mismatch of 90°. The inner ring represents the circular track with the four textures. The outer, black ring represents the curtains at the perimeter of the recording room. (B) Rotation angles of place fields recorded from eight rats. L indicates the rotation angle of the local cues and D indicates the rotation angle of the distal landmarks. When the local and distal cues were counterrotated 45° relative to each other, the distribution of place field rotation angles centered around 0°, but the dispersion of the distribution was greater than between two standard session. For larger cue mismatches (90–180°), the representations split, with some place fields following the distal landmarks and other place fields following the local cues. (Modified from Knierim, 2002. Copyright 2002 by the Society for Neuroscience; reproduced with permission.)

sentation of a single direction. Although the data are still preliminary, to date we have demonstrated that (1) preferred directions in ADN cells can rotate clockwise or counterclockwise in this experiment, but (2) to date we have seen no examples of the head direction representation splitting (D. Yoganarasimha, unpublished data). This result remains tentative until more conclusive data are obtained, however.

Cue Rotations Versus Translations

Most studies of the impact of visual landmarks on place cells and head direction cells have rotated the distal landmarks relative to the behavioral apparatus being used (an eight-arm maze, a Y-maze, a cylindrical chamber, etc.). Under these conditions, in which there are typically few salient local cues, the place cells are dominated by the distal landmarks. These results led to the idea that place cells represented the configurations of distal landmarks; that is, a given place cell fired at its place field because it was sensitive to the exact configuration of sensory input that reached the animal at that location. A place field located a few cm away would be sensitive to the slightly different configuration of inputs that reached the animal at that location. Although subsequent studies that emphasized the role of path integration mechanisms and local surface cues modified these views, it is still commonly held that place cells are responsive to configurations of distal landmarks. Moreover, it is often commonly held that animals use these configurations to solve such tasks as the Morris water maze. O'Keefe and Nadel (1978) proposed a different role for distal landmarks in their cognitive map theory. They argued that distal landmarks were not good sources of information to define precise locations, because the relationships between these landmarks did not change much as the animal moved from one location to an adjacent location. They argued that local cues and self-motion cues are more appropriate for defining precise locations. Distal landmarks, in their view, are important for providing directional information to the cognitive map, to allow the internal representation of the environment to be aligned with the external world.

If place fields are defined primarily by the configurations of distal landmarks that occur at a given location, then place fields should change dramatically if a behavioral apparatus is shifted relative to the distal landmarks. O'Keefe (1979) reported anecdotally that some place fields remained bound to the distal landmarks when a small platform was moved in the room, whereas other fields remained bound to the platform. Few details were given about this finding, however. O'Keefe and Burgess (1996; Lever et al., 2002) reported that when a high-walled, square chamber was moved relative to the room, a minority of place fields remained at the same location in room coordinates. Again, few details were given, and it is unclear whether there were any salient, distal landmarks in the room that were visible within the high-walled chamber. We investigated this issue while the rat ran on a rectangular or circular track in a room with salient visual landmarks (Knierim and Rao, 2003). Between recording sessions, the track was shifted to different locations in three dimensions in the room. In some cases, the tracks occupied completely nonoverlapping regions of the room in different sessions, separated by distances greater than the average size of a place field. Nevertheless, in most cases the place fields remained bound to the track when it was shifted across the room. In some instances, some place fields remapped, but typically the remapped field now became bound to the track when it was again shifted to a new location. There was limited evidence of place fields that were bound to a location defined by configurations of distal landmarks. Rather, in most cases, the place fields appeared to be bound to the track itself.

When the experiment was run on a circular track, the landmarks were rotated around the track in 45° increments, and the place fields tended to follow the rotation of the landmarks. This result showed that the cells were sensitive to the distal landmarks in this experiment, arguing against the possibility that the cues were not salient or were invisible to the rat. We have recently repeated this experiment with simultaneous recordings of CA1 place cells and ADN head direction cells. As predicted in the literature (Ranck, 1985; Taube, 1998), the head direction cells had the same preferred direction regardless of the location of the track in the room, although the preferred directions were controlled by the distal landmarks when the landmarks were rotated (Yoganarasimha and Knierim, 2005). These data provide support for O'Keefe and Nadel's ideas on the relative importance of distal and proximal landmarks (O'Keefe and Nadel, 1978). Landmarks at the periphery, far removed from the rat, are more useful to control the overall orientation of the place cell representation of the environment rather than to define precise locations. Local cues, such as geometry, or path integration mechanisms are more suitable for providing precise location information to the place fields. Thus, when the rat is placed on the track, the distal landmarks orient the head direction system; this orientation, in combination with local cues, allows the rat to localize where it is on the track (e.g., the northeast or northwest corner). When the track is translated, the head direction cells are not affected, and therefore the place cells still fire at the same location on the track. When the landmarks are rotated, however, the head direction cells are reoriented, which causes a corresponding rotation of the hippocampal representation (see also Burgess et al., 2000; Hartley et al., 2000; Save and Poucet, 2000; Zugaro et al., 2001; Cressant et al., 2002) (see chapter 4 by Zugaro and Wiener).

Place Cell Firing in Three-Dimensional Space

Place Fields on an Inclined Track

Head direction cells are known to fire as a function of direction in the horizontal (azimuth) plane only (Taube et al., 1990a, 1990b) (see chapter 3 by Taube). If the animal is facing in the preferred direction of a cell, the cell will continue to fire if the animal's head direction changes in the pitch or roll axes ($\pm90°$). It will change firing only if the head direction changes in the yaw axis. Taube (1998) graphically illustrated the three-dimensional tuning curve of a head direction cell as a hemi-torus. Because of the close coupling between head direction cells and place cells, it is natural to question whether place fields are two-dimensional or three-dimensional entities. That is, if an animal moves along a path, will the cell fire differently if the path is flat as opposed to inclined? Head direction cells apparently do not distinguish the two situations (at least in terms of their preferred orientations; they may distinguish the two, based on firing rate; Stackman et al., 2000). Few experiments have asked similar questions of place fields.

Knierim and McNaughton (2001) recorded the activity of place cells as the rat ran on a rectangular track, which could be either flat or tilted 40° to 45°, such that the rat had to climb up an incline on the long side of the rectangle, traverse a flat short side, run down the other long side, and traverse the final, flat, short side. When the track was tilted from flat incline to a 45° incline, the place cell representation underwent a partial remapping. Some cells maintained the same place field on the tilted track, even in locations in which the track occupied a different location in three-dimensional space; other cells shut off or, if they were previously silent, gained a place field anew. The partial remapping demonstrated that the hippocampal representation was sensitive to the altered environment when the track was tilted; it is not clear whether the important changes were the altered geometry of the track, the altered behavioral patterns necessary to negotiate a flat track versus a steeply tilted incline, or the changes in visual input that arise from the different three-dimensional locations traversed. Because head direction cells are presumably not affected by this manipulation (this was not directly tested in this experiment, but see Stackman et al., 2000; Taube, 1998), these results may indicate another situation where individual place cells and head direction cells can decouple because of the systemic remapping induced in the hippocampus.

In further experiments, the flat and tilted tracks were rotated 180° or 90° in the yaw axis between sessions, while the animal was out of the recording room. When the flat track was rotated 180°, place fields stayed at the same locations relative to the distal landmarks on the walls. When the tilted track was rotated 180°, however, the place cell ensemble representation underwent partial remapping. Some place fields maintained the same firing location relative to the azimuthal orientation of the distal landmarks. That is, the cells fired in the same x,y coordinates of the room, regardless of the z-axis. For example, one cell fired at the southeast corner of the track in one session, when the south side of the track was in the down position and the north side of the track was in the raised position. When the track was rotated 180°, the south side was now in the raised position and the north side was in the down position. Nonetheless, even though the southeast corner now occupied a different location in three-dimensional space (its location differed in the z-axis), the cell continued to fire on the southeast corner. In contrast, other cells responded to the manipulation by remapping the track, either gaining a new place field or becoming silent after the rotation. Thus, the three-dimensional geometry of the track had a major influence on the responses of the cells to a 180° rotation of the track. When the track was flat, the rotation had no effect on how the cells fired relative to the distal room cues (even though there were polarizing cues on the apparatus, such as the lift mechanism that raised it to the tilted position, which the rats attended and explored). This result is consistent with many results in the literature. When the tilted track was rotated, however, the cells responded with a partial remapping, as cells either maintained their fields relative to the x-y coordinates of the room or remapped. No more cells than would be expected by chance retained their fields relative to the track.

The 90° rotation of the *flat* rectangular track differed from the 180° rotation of the flat track in that it provoked a partial remapping. In this case, the cells that did not remap maintained their firing fields in the same location relative to the room. That is, a cell that fired on the southeast corner of the standard track remained firing on the southeast corner of the rotated track, even though these were two geometrically distinct corners of the rectangle. Note that, because the track was rotated along the axis in the center of the rectangle, the southeast corner in each case occupied somewhat different locations relative to the distal landmarks in the room (see also Rettenmaier et al., 1999; Cressant et al., 2002).

Thus, it appears that the cell was sensitive to the local geometry of the track (i.e., a corner) and fired at whichever corner of the track occupied the southeast location, relative to the distal landmarks. No more cells than would be expected by chance retained their place fields in the reference frame of the rotated track. When the tilted track was rotated 90°, a more complete remapping was obtained. No cells retained their fields relative to the x,y coordinates of the room than would be expected by chance.

Lost in Space

The coupling between place cells and head direction cells, and the insensitivity of head direction cells to turns in the pitch axis (Stackman et al., 2000; Taube, 1998), formed the basis of an experiment on place cells performed on the Space Shuttle Columbia in April 1998 (Knierim et al., 2000, 2003). In this experiment, rats ran on a three-dimensional track that interspersed three 90° turns in the yaw axis with three 90° turns in the pitch axis. As a result, when the rat completed one complete circuit of this track and returned to its starting location, it had completed only 270° of turns in the yaw axis. It was predicted that in this unfamiliar environment, with little chance for the external landmarks to gain control over the cells, a place cell that fired at the start would not fire again until the animal completed the fourth 90° yaw turn (for a total of 360° yaw); thus, the whole place field representation would shift by one-third of the track on each lap. This predicted result was not obtained, however. Rather, on the first day of recordings in space (four days into the mission), place cells fired apparently normally in one animal (i.e., firing selectively at a single location on the track) and abnormally in the remaining two animals (Knierim et al., 2003). In one of the latter animals, about one-third of the cells fired on the track with little spatial specificity; the other cells were inactive. In the other animal, some cells fired with well-defined place fields, but only when the rat's head was off the track, investigating the walls of the recording chamber and the objects on them. Cells that fired on the track itself had place fields that were unable to distinguish the symmetrical locations on the track. Two cells fired at all three locations where the animal made a pitch turn, and another cell fired in all three locations where the animal made a yaw turn. On the second day of recording (nine days into the mission), the place cells of these two animals were normal, firing selectively on a single location on the track. This difference between the two days of recording suggests some adaptive process that allowed the hippocampus to create a stable representation of the three-dimensional track over time (Knierim et al., 2000). It is not known whether the animals created separate, two-dimensional representations of each plane of the track, or whether the representation was truly three-dimensional. Nor is it known why the abnormal firing on the first day of recordings occurred. Knierim et al. speculated that, even though the recording environment was novel, the animals still had a few minutes of experience in the chamber before starting to run on the track. Because Goodridge et al. (1998) showed that landmarks begin to gain control over the firing of head direction cells in only a few minutes, Knierim et al. (2003) speculated that the three-dimensional trajectories caused the head direction cell system and place cell systems to receive conflicts between their idiothetic sources of input and the landmarks on each lap. In the face of this conflict, the place cells of one rat lost all spatial tuning. The place cells of the other rat displayed normal spatial tuning when the rat was actively investigating the walls, which had distinguishing local landmarks. When the rat was on the track, however, the cells could not distinguish identical locations on the track (e.g., the 90° yaw and pitch locations). Knierim et al. (2003) speculated that these place cells received local-cue information about the track itself (e.g., yaw corners), but with a head direction system functioning improperly because of the cue conflicts, the place cell firing fields were unable to disambiguate each of the three identical corners (see also Taube et al., 1999; Burgess et al., 2000; Hartley et al., 2000; Save and Poucet, 2000; Cressant et al., 2002).

External Landmarks and Intrinsic Circuitry: A Conceptual Model

Figure 8.6 shows a conceptual model of the interaction between idiothetic input onto head direction cells and the learned input from external landmarks in the environment, drawing on the work of numerous investigators (Skaggs et al., 1995; McNaughton et al., 1996; Zhang, 1996; Redish et al., 1996; Sharp et al., 2001). In the absence of strong external cues, such as in the dark (figure 8.6A1), the system is driven purely by the intrinsic connectivity and idiothetic inputs, as hypothesized attractor dynamics form a "bump" of activity at a single location (in the figure, firing rate is signified by the size of the circle, and the strength of connections is signified by the thickness of the arrows). Under such conditions, the system integrates angular velocity signals (not shown in the figure), which can arise from vestibular input, optic flow input, or motor efference copy, to move the bump around to signal new head directions. The bump can also drift relative to the external world, as the system accumulates error over time (figure 8.6A2).

In a new environment, the system is hypothesized to be controlled exclusively by such attractor circuits and idiothetic input (McNaughton et al., 1991, 1996). After a short period of exploration, Hebbian mechanisms increase the strength of the connections between neural ensembles that represent the landmarks at each location and the currently active head direction cells (figure 8.6A3). As a result, the external landmarks quickly begin to exercise some control over the head direction cell network. This control can help to prevent the bump from drifting relative to external world whenever the animal takes a visual fix of its environment. Note that this initial period of learning is required, for it is impossible for the system to know in advance what landmarks will be present in each new environment, and it must thus learn this relationship for each new place the animal visits and each head direction. With repeated exposure to a stable environment, the connections between the landmark representation and the head direction cells become stronger (figure 8.6A4).

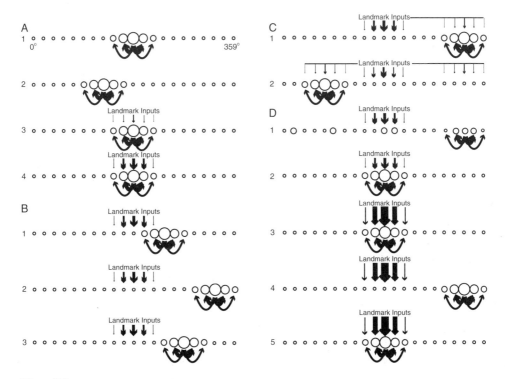

Figure 8.6
Hypothetical interaction between intrinsic, attractor circuitry and modifiable inputs from external cues on the firing of head direction cells (Skaggs et al., 1995; McNaughton et al., 1996; Zhang, 1996; Redish et al., 1996; Sharp et al., 2001). The circles represent an array of head direction cells, with the cell that represents 0° on the left and the cell that represents 359° on the right. The firing rate of the cell is signified by the size of the circle, and the strength of connections is signified by the thickness of the arrows. (A) Hypothesized attractor networks and experience-dependent strengthening of visual landmark inputs onto head direction cells. For clarity of illustration, inhibitory connections that are necessary to form a stable attractor are omitted. (B) Ability of visual landmarks to correct for small drifts of the head direction cell activity bump. (C) Formation of multiple, learned bearings of the attractor bump relative to visual landmarks in an unstable environment. (D) Ability of visual landmarks to correct for large drifts of the head direction cell activity bump.

When the visual landmark connections become strong enough, they are able to correct for errors that can be introduced between the head direction cells and the landmarks. Thus, when the system drifts out of calibration by a small amount (in momentary darkness, for example) (figure 8.6B1), or if the visual landmarks are rotated by a small amount, the combination of the visual input and the attractor circuitry can cause the bump to realign itself with the landmarks (i.e., the system returns to figure 8.6A4). If the error is too large, however, the bump can move outside of the range of control by the landmarks; if the attractor circuitry is stronger than the visual inputs, the system will remain in the new location (figure 8.6B2) or may even drift around as if the system were in the dark (figure 8.6B3).

If the system continues to drift, it may eventually realign itself by chance with the visual landmarks, at which time the landmarks will resume control over the bump. Such a situation appears to be demonstrated in figure 8.4 and may also explain the delayed cue control seen in all sessions when the cylinder was rotated abruptly with the rat inside (Knierim et al., 1998).

In other cases, however, the system may maintain its new orientation relative to the external world. In this case, the landmark representations that once were coactive with the initial bump of activity are now coactive with the new bump. As a result, the connections between the landmark inputs and the active head direction cells increase (as in figure 8.6A3-A4), while the previous connections can weaken by a long-term depression (LTD) mechanism (figure 8.6C1–C2). In a particularly unstable environment (due to repeated cue manipulations in an experiment, or due to repeated disorientation of the animal), a number of stable states may appear in the network, each corresponding to a different bearing of the head direction cell network relative to the visual landmarks (figure 8.6C2) (see Taube and Burton, 1995). Depending on the initial starting point, the system will lock into the nearest stable configuration, but may be easily decoupled from that configuration (e.g., figure 8.1 and 8.3).

A number of investigators (e.g., Taube and Burton, 1995; Zugaro et al., 2003) have demonstrated that even large discrepancies between the visual landmarks and the head direction cells can be corrected in a very short time (unlike the situation reported by Knierim et al. (1998), in which correction of large errors was always delayed). There are a number of possible mechanisms to produce such immediate corrections. One possibility is that an error signal or some contextual signal (i.e., entry into a new environment, turning on the lights) can cause a brief decrease in the inhibition in the attractor network. This decrease may cause a momentary breakdown in the attractor (figure 8.6D1); when the inhibition returns, the system will recoalesce into a stable attractor state that is aligned with the landmarks, as the input from the landmarks biases the location where the attractor bump forms (figure 8.6D2) (Zhang, 1996). Relevant to this hypothesis, Knierim et al. (1998) showed that when the head direction cell signal became erratic in the dark (perhaps as the result of a breakdown in the attractor), the visual landmarks regained good control of the cells when the lights were turned back on; in contrast, when the head direction cells retained a well-formed tuning curve in the dark, the landmarks in general had poor control over the cells when the lights were turned on. Another possibility is that the inputs from the landmarks become much more powerful than the internal attractor circuitry (figure 8.6D3). This can occur in a very stable, very familiar environment, or in an environment in which the landmarks are particularly salient and powerful in controlling the animal's sense of direction (Etienne et al., 1995a, 1995b; Song and Wang, 2005). When there is a mismatch (figure 8.6D4), the powerful inputs from the visual landmarks immediately override the attractor bump, and the bump returns to the original bearing relative to the landmarks (figure 8.6D5).

This model shows how attractor dynamics in the head direction cell network, combined with learned input from visual cues, work together to control the orientation of the head direction cells relative to the external environment. The dynamic nature of the influence of the landmarks can explain discrepant results that have been reported in the literature. In some cases, the landmarks have strong control over the head direction cells, and in other cases the control is strong only for small errors. Studies strongly support the idea that the control over place cells and head direction cells by external landmarks is learned (Knierim et al., 1995; Jeffery et al., 1997; Jeffery, 1998; Goodridge et al., 1998; Jeffery and O'Keefe, 1999); idiothetic inputs presumably control the system exclusively upon initial exploration of an environment, before the landmarks rapidly begin to exert influence as well.

What is the relationship between the bearing of head direction cells and the orientation of the place cell representation in the hippocampus? Knierim et al. (1995, 1998) have shown that when the head direction cells change their orientations relative to the external landmarks, the place cell ensemble representation sometimes changes its orientation by the same amount, thus maintaining internal coherence between place cells and head direction cells while decoupling from the external world. In other cases, the place cell representation remaps (completely or partially) when the head direction cell tuning curves drift relative to the external environment. The reason for the differing responses of hippocampal cells is not known. Knierim et al. (1998) suggested that place cells and head direction cells each receive independent, modifiable inputs from external landmarks. For both systems, the function of these inputs is to calibrate the idiothetic updating of the systems and keep them aligned with the external world. In cue-conflict situations, the head direction cells may be controlled by the landmarks, in which case the place cells will also be controlled by the landmarks. In other cases, when the landmark input to the head direction cells is weak, the head direction cells may decouple from the landmarks, and the hippocampal response will depend on the strength of landmark inputs to place cells. If these inputs are also weak, the place cells will be controlled by the head direction cells, and the representation will rotate with the head direction cells. If the inputs are strong, however, the hippocampus will experience a conflict between the directional information provided by head direction cells and by the external landmarks. The hippocampus may respond to this conflict by creating a new representation of the environment, either completely or partially independent. Remapping was also proposed by Redish and Touretzky (1997) to result from a mismatch between local view and path integration systems (see also Mittelstaedt, 2000).

The foregoing discussion assumes that the orientation of the head direction cell system determines the orientation or remapping of the place cells. It is also possible, and perhaps likely, that the coupling goes the other way as well. That is, the place information in the hippocampus, by way of feedback projections from the subiculum, may be involved in resetting the orientation of the head direction cells. McNaughton et al. (1991) proposed this very role for place cells in an early model, in which they viewed place cells as local view detectors. Such an influence would be of clear use in a situation in which there is only one polarizing landmark in an extended environment. Our hypothetical traveler in New York, for example, would be able to orient himself directionally by viewing the Empire State Building only if he already knew his location relative to the building. To use the visual fix of this landmark to set his internal compass, the viewer must know whether he is seeing the building from a southern location (in which case he is facing north) or from a northern location (in which case he is facing south). Without this place information, the use of single landmarks (perhaps represented in visual association cortex) to calibrate the internal compass is impossible (McNaughton et al., 1995). Thus, place information can be used to disambiguate directions, and direction information can be used to disambiguate places. The interaction between place cells, head direction cells, and external landmarks is likely to be a complex process that involves many brain areas and is modulated by behavioral contingencies, variability in external landmarks, and experience-dependent changes in synaptic strengths.

Acknowledgments

Many of the experiments reported here were performed in the laboratories of Bruce McNaughton and Carol Barnes. The work from the author's laboratory is supported by PHS grants RO1 NS39456 and K02 MH63297. I thank Geeta Rao, Inah Lee, and D. Yoganarasimha for comments on the manuscript.

References

Barlow JS (1964) Inertial navigation as a basis for animal navigation. J Theor Biol 6: 76–117.

Bostock E, Muller RU, Kubie JL (1991) Experience-dependent modifications of hippocampal place cell firing. Hippocampus 1: 193–205.

Burgess N, Jackson A, Hartley T, O'Keefe J (2000) Predictions derived from modelling the hippocampal role in navigation. Biol Cybern 83: 301–312.

Chen LL, Lin LH, Green EJ, Barnes CA, McNaughton BL (1994) Head-direction cells in the rat posterior cortex. I. Anatomical distribution and behavioral modulation. Exp Brain Res 101: 8–23.

Cressant A, Muller RU, Poucet B (2002) Remapping of place cell firing patterns after maze rotations. Exp Brain Res 143: 470–479.

Dudchenko PA, Goodridge JP, Seiterle DA, Taube JS (1997) Effects of repeated disorientation on the acquisition of spatial tasks in rats: dissociation between the appetitive radial arm maze and aversive water maze. J Exp Psychol Anim Behav Process 23: 194–210.

Etienne AS, Joris-Lambert S, Dahn-Hurni C, Reverdin B (1995a) Optimizing visual landmarks: two- and three-dimensional minimal landscapes. Anim Behav 49: 165–179.

Etienne AS, Joris-Lambert S, Maurer R, Reverdin B, Sitbon S (1995b) Optimizing distal landmarks: horizontal versus vertical structures and relation to background. Behav Brain Res 68: 103–116.

Gallistel, CR (1990) The organization of learning. Cambridge, MA: MIT Press.

Goodridge JP, Dudchenko PA, Worboys KA, Golob EJ, Taube JS (1998) Cue control and head direction cells. Behav Neurosci 112: 749–761.

Hartley T, Burgess N, Lever C, Cacucci F, O'Keefe J (2000) Modeling place fields in terms of the cortical inputs to the hippocampus. Hippocampus 10: 369–379.

Jeffery KJ (1998) Learning of landmark stability and instability by hippocampal place cells. Neuropharm 37: 677–687.

Jeffery KJ, Donnett JG, Burgess N, O'Keefe JM (1997) Directional control of hippocampal place fields. Exp Brain Res 117: 131–142.

Jeffery KJ, O'Keefe JM (1999) Learned interaction of visual and idiothetic cues in the control of place field orientation. Exp Brain Res 127: 151–161.

Knierim JJ (2002) Dynamic interactions between local surface cues, distal landmarks, and intrinsic circuitry in hippocampal place cells. J Neurosci 22: 6254–6264.

Knierim JJ (2003) Hippocampal remapping: Implications for spatial learning and navigation. In KJ Jeffery, ed., The Neurobiology of Spatial Behaviour Oxford: Oxford University Press, pp. 226–239.

Knierim JJ, Kudrimoti HS, McNaughton BL (1995) Place cells, head direction cells, and the learning of landmark stability. J Neurosci 15: 1648–1659.

Knierim JJ, Kudrimoti HS, McNaughton BL (1998) Interactions between idiothetic cues and external landmarks in the control of place cells and head direction cells. J Neurophysiol 80: 425–446.

Knierim JJ, McNaughton BL (2001) Hippocampal place-cell firing during movement in three-dimensional space. J Neurophysiol 85: 105–116.

Knierim JJ, McNaughton BL, Poe GR (2000) Three-dimensional spatial selectivity of hippocampal neurons during space flight. Nat Neurosci 3: 209–210.

Knierim JJ, McNaughton BL, Poe GR (2003) Ensemble neural coding of place in Zero-G. In: JC Buckey and JL Homick, eds., The Neurolab Spacelab Mission: Neuroscience Research in Space Houston: National Aeronautics and Space Administration, pp. 63–68.

Knierim JJ, Rao G (2003) Distal landmarks and hippocampal place cells: Effects of relative translation versus rotation. Hippocampus 13: 604–617.

Leutgeb S, Ragozzino KE, Mizumori SJ (2000) Convergence of head direction and place information in the CA1 region of hippocampus. Neuroscience 100: 11–19.

Lever C, Wills T, Cacucci F, Burgess N, O'Keefe J (2002) Long-term plasticity in hippocampal place-cell representation of environmental geometry. Nature 416: 90–94.

Markus EJ, Qin YL, Leonard B, Skaggs WE, McNaughton BL, Barnes CA (1995) Interactions between location and task affect the spatial and directional firing of hippocampal neurons. J Neurosci 15: 7079–7094.

Martin GM, Harley CW, Smith AR, Hoyles ES, Hynes CA (1997) Spatial disorientation blocks reliable goal location on a plus maze but does not prevent goal location in the Morris maze. J Exp Psychol Anim Behav Process 23: 183–193.

McNaughton BL, Barnes CA, Gerrard JL, Gothard K, Jung MW, Knierim JJ, Kudrimoti H, Qin Y, Skaggs WE, Suster M, Weaver KL (1996) Deciphering the hippocampal polyglot: the hippocampus as a path integration system. J Exp Biol 199: 173–185.

McNaughton BL, Chen LL, Markus EJ (1991) "Dead reckoning", landmark learning, and the sense of direction: A neurophysiological and computational hypothesis. J Cognit Neurosci 3: 190–202.

McNaughton BL, Knierim JJ, Wilson MA (1995) Vector encoding and the vestibular foundations of spatial cognition: neurophysiological and computational mechanisms. In: MS Gazzaniga, ed., The Cognitive Neurosciences Cambridge, MA: MIT Press, pp. 585–595.

Mittelstaedt H (2000) Triple-loop model of path control by head direction and place cells. Biol Cybern 83: 261–270.

Mizumori SJ, Williams JD (1993) Directionally selective mnemonic properties of neurons in the lateral dorsal nucleus of the thalamus of rats. J Neurosci 13: 4015–4028.

Muller R (1996) A quarter of a century of place cells. Neuron 17: 813–822.

Muller RU, Kubie JL (1987) The effects of changes in the environment on the spatial firing of hippocampal complex-spike cells. J Neurosci 7: 1951–1968.

O'Keefe J (1979) A review of the hippocampal place cells. Prog Neurobiol 13: 419–439.

O'Keefe J, Burgess N (1996) Geometric determinants of the place fields of hippocampal neurons. Nature 381: 425–428.

O'Keefe J, Conway DH (1978) Hippocampal place units in the freely moving rat: why they fire where they fire. Exp Brain Res 31: 573–590.

O'Keefe J, Nadel L (1978) The hippocampus as a cognitive map. Oxford: Clarendon Press.

Ranck JB, Jr (1985) Head direction cells in the deep cell layer of dorsal presubiculum in freely moving rats. In G Buzsàki and CH Vanderwolf, eds., Electrical Activity of Archicortex Budapest: Akademiai Kiado, pp. 217–220.

Redish AD, Elga AN, Touretzky DS (1996) A coupled attractor model of the rodent head direction system. Network Comput Neural Sys 7: 671–685.

Redish AD, Touretzky DS (1997) Cognitive maps beyond the hippocampus. Hippocampus 7: 15–35.

Rettenmaier BB, White AM, Doboli S, Minai AA, Best PJ (1999) Place fields of hippocampal pyramidal cells in rats show hysteresis. Soc Neurosci Abstr 25: 1380–1380.

Rotenberg A, Muller RU (1997) Variable place-cell coupling to a continuously viewed stimulus: evidence that the hippocampus acts as a perceptual system. Philos Trans R Soc Lond B Biol Sci 352: 1505–1513.

Samsonovich A, McNaughton BL (1997) Path integration and cognitive mapping in a continuous attractor neural network model. J Neurosci 17: 5900–5920.

Save E, Poucet B (2000) Involvement of the hippocampus and associative parietal cortex in the use of proximal and distal landmarks for navigation. Behav Brain Res 109: 195–206.

Shapiro ML, Tanila H, Eichenbaum H (1997) Cues that hippocampal place cells encode: dynamic and hierarchical representation of local and distal stimuli. Hippocampus 7: 624–642.

Sharp PE, Blair HT, Cho J (2001) The anatomical and computational basis of the rat head-direction cell signal. Trends Neurosci 24: 289–294.

Skaggs WE, Knierim JJ, Kudrimoti HS, McNaughton BL (1995) A model of the neural basis of the rat's sense of direction. Adv Neural Inf Process Syst 7: 173–180.

Song P, Wang X (2005) Angular path integration by moving "hill of activity": a spiking neuron model without recurrent excitation of the head-direction system. J Neurosci 25: 1002–1014.

Stackman RW, Taube JS (1997) Firing properties of head direction cells in the rat anterior thalamic nucleus: dependence on vestibular input. J Neurosci 17: 4349–4358.

Stackman RW, Tullman ML, Taube JS (2000) Maintenance of rat head direction cell firing during locomotion in the vertical plane. J Neurophysiol 83: 393–405.

Taube JS (1995) Head direction cells recorded in the anterior thalamic nuclei of freely moving rats. J Neurosci 15: 70–86.

Taube JS (1998) Head direction cells and the neurophysiological basis for a sense of direction. Prog Neurobiol 55: 225–256.

Taube JS, Burton HL (1995) Head direction cell activity monitored in a novel environment and during a cue conflict situation. J Neurophysiol 74: 1953–1971.

Taube JS, Muller RU, Ranck JB, Jr. (1990a) Head-direction cells recorded from the postsubiculum in freely moving rats. II. Effects of environmental manipulations. J Neurosci. 10: 436–447.

Taube JS, Muller RU, Ranck JB, Jr. (1990b) Head-direction cells recorded from the postsubiculum in freely moving rats. I. Description and quantitative analysis. J Neurosci 10: 420–435.

Taube JS, Stackman RW, Oman CM (1999) Rat head direction cell responses in 0-G. Soc Neurosci Abstr 25: 1383.

Touretzky DS, Redish AD (1996) Theory of rodent navigation based on interacting representations of space. Hippocampus 6: 247–270.

Wiener SI, Berthoz A (1993) Forebrain structures mediating the vestibular contribution during navigation. In A Berthoz, ed., Multisensory Control of Movement Oxford: Oxford University Press, pp. 427–456.

Yoganarasimha D, Knierim JJ (2005) Coupling between place cells and head direction cells during relative translations and rotations of distal landmarks. Exp Brain Res 160: 344–359.

Young BJ, Fox GD, Eichenbaum H (1994) Correlates of hippocampal complex-spike cell activity in rats performing a nonspatial radial maze task. J Neurosci 14: 6553–6563.

Zhang K (1996) Representation of spatial orientation by the intrinsic dynamics of the head-direction cell ensemble: a theory. J Neurosci 16: 2112–2126.

Zugaro MB, Arleo A, Berthoz A, Wiener SI (2003) Rapid spatial reorientation and head direction cells. J Neurosci 23: 3478–3482.

Zugaro MB, Berthoz A, Wiener SI (2001) Background, but not foreground, spatial cues are taken as references for head direction responses by rat anterodorsal thalamus neurons. J Neurosci 21: RC154(1–5).

9 Directional Responses in Place Cells

Nicolas Brunel and Robert U. Muller

A great many of the pyramidal cells of hippocampal areas CA3 and CA1 are called "place cells" because their activity is strongly correlated with the animal's location in its surroundings (O'Keefe and Dostrovsky, 1971). Each place cell discharges when the rat's head is in an environment-specific, simply shaped, stable region called the "place field" or "firing field" and is nearly silent when the head is elsewhere. The strength of the place cell signal, its localization to a brain structure characterized by synaptic plasticity, the notion that "location-specific firing" underlies navigation by rats, and the possibility that navigation is analogous to more complex memory and cognitive processes conspire to ensure great and growing interest in place cells.

Although firing fields are categorized primarily by location, they also differ from each other according to shape, size, and intensity (peak firing rate), although the significance of this variance is unknown. This chapter is devoted to yet another fundamental property of place cells: remarkably, place cells show directional selectivity in some circumstances, but are unselective under others. In brief, most if not all place cells are omnidirectional when the rat is in an open, unobstructed space. In contrast, many and perhaps all place cells discharge preferentially while the rat runs on a linear track in one direction but not in the other.

We proceed in the following way: First, we outline the empirical evidence concerning the directional firing properties of place cells; next, we review several models that account for the ability of place cells to be directional on tracks but omnidirectional in open space. These models focus on how directionality can shift depending on the structure of the available space, but do not address the significance of variable directional selectivity. We then briefly touch on relationships among directionality, phase precession, and the backwards shift of activity as a rat runs repetitive cycles on a topologically circular track. Finally, we speculate on the significance of the variable directionality of place cells.

Directional Properties of Place Cells: Experimental Evidence

In one of the first place cell papers, O'Keefe (1976) stated that some of these neurons discharge, regardless of which way the rat faces. This report of omnidirectional firing gave the first strong evidence that place cells are not just very sophisticated sensory units but rather may signal something as abstract as the animal's location in space (O'Keefe, personal communication). In contrast to the initial, anecdotal description of place cells as omnidirectional, the first work to use automatic video/computer tracking of a rat's head found that most cells showed strong directional selectivity as rats ran in or out on the arms of an eight-arm maze (McNaughton et al., 1983). In a later paper using one-spot tracking to detect the rat's head position, but not head direction, in open apparatuses, direct observation of firing during retrieval of pellets that were dropped from above indicated that discharge did not depend on head direction (Muller et al., 1987).

The discovery of head direction cells (Ranck, 1984; Taube et al., 1990a,b) motivated construction of a two-spot tracker to detect head direction as well as position. After work on head direction cells, this device was used by Muller et al. (1994) to determine the directional properties of place cells in two conditions: (1) as rats chased food pellets in a 76 cm diameter, 50 cm high cylinder; (2) on an eight-arm maze in which each arm was 61 cm by 10 cm with a regular octagonal center 14 cm on a side.

Firing rate for head direction cells (not shown here) and place cells was illustrated in two ways. First, firing rate was plotted as a function of head direction at high resolution, as shown in figures 9.1B and 9.2B (see plates 3, 4). Second, the discharge pattern was summarized with nine rate maps, a direction-independent map surrounded by eight direction-specific rate maps on the vertices of a regular octagon. Each of the direction-specific maps showed activity for the 45° range of head angles centered on the direction from the center of the octagon to the map. Examples of this display are shown in figures 9.1A and 9.2A.

Three key observations on place cell directionality were made in the cylinder. First, the modulation of firing by head direction varied greatly; some cells showed minor variations in firing rate with head direction (figure 9.1) whereas others showed strong variations (figure 9.2). Second, the degree of firing rate modulation by head direction was systematic: modulation was low for centrally located fields and high for fields that encroached on the cylinder wall. Third, rate variations as a function of head direction were closely associated with the location of the firing field near the edge of the cylinder: rates were lowest for head directions facing away from the wall at the location of the field.

Why do directional firing variations have these specific properties? A numerical analysis shows that differences in depth of modulation with field eccentricity, the predictability of the direction of minimum rate and, most important, the precise form of the rate versus head direction function can all be explained with two assumptions: (1) in the cylinder, firing is *independent* of head direction; at any point in the environment, firing rate is

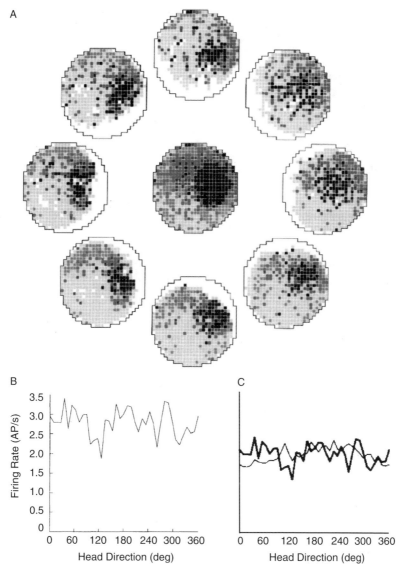

Figure 9.1
Direction-independent (center) and direction-specific firing rate maps for a place cell whose field is away from the cylinder wall. (A) Although there is some encroachment of the unsampled (white crescent) region on the area of the field, it is clear from the color code that firing was very similar in all 45° head direction sectors. This is therefore an example of a field whose omnidirectional independence seems evident from the raw data. By color category, median action potentials per second (AP/sec) are as follows: yellow, 0.0; orange, 0.40; red, 0.93; green, 1.7; blue, 3.2; purple, 6.5. (B) Firing rate as a function of head direction at higher (9°) resolution. (C) Comparison of observed values of firing rate as a function of head direction from B (thick line) with expected values. The rate variations are small and show no obvious systematic pattern, as expected from the maps in A. The expected firing rate (thin line) is obtained from equation 9.1. See plate 3 for color version.

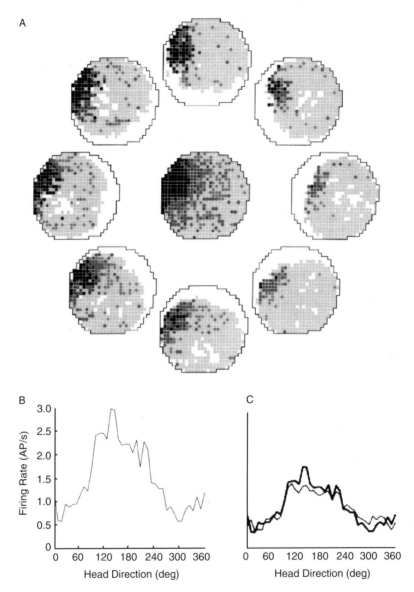

Figure 9.2
Direction-independent (center) and direction-specific rate maps for a place cell whose field is near the cylinder wall. In this case, the kinematically excluded region rotates so that it superimposes on the main area of the field. The result is the reduced firing for the direction-specific maps centered on 315° and 0°. By color categories, median action potentials per second (AP/sec) are as follows: yellow, 0.0; orange, 0.21; red, 0.55; green, 1.4; blue, 5.3; purple, 12.5. (B) Firing rate as a function of head direction at higher (9°) resolution. (C) Comparison of observed values of firing rate as a function of head direction from B (thick line) with expected values. The reduced firing at head directions between 300° and 60° is seen clearly when firing rate is plotted against head direction. The expected values (thin line) are obtained from equation 9.1. The key point is that the expected values conform closely to the observed values. See plate 4 for color version.

the same regardless of which way the head points, and (2) the rat does not spend equal amounts of time with its head pointing in all directions everywhere in the cylinder, certainly because the cylinder wall precludes certain postures and possibly because the rat may prefer certain head directions at certain places.

The origins of directional firing variations near the wall despite ideal direction-independence can be seen in the rate maps of figure 9.2A. The central map shows a firing field centered near ten o'clock at the cylinder wall. The direction-specific maps show evidence of the firing field at all head directions, but the field is strongly attenuated at three o'clock and to a lesser extent in both directions away from three o'clock toward the maps at ten-thirty and nine o'clock, where it is most intense. The reason for this pattern of attenuation is the excluded (white-coded) region in each map between the cylinder wall and the rest of the apparatus. The excluded region rotates systematically with head direction because the rat cannot be at the wall pointing inwards toward the cylinder center since its body cannot penetrate the wall; the excluded region is purely a result of the fact that the rat is not a point but an extended body.

The origin of the directional firing rate modulation shown in figure 9.2A may now be evident: the low rates in the angular range $300°$ to $60°$ (centered on three o'clock) occur because the rat cannot sample the entire firing field at such head directions, and especially the intense region near the wall. It is important to note that the excluded region is also visible in figure 9.1A, but that it induces hardly any directional rate modulation for this centrally located firing field, as seen in figure 9.1B.

To ascertain whether the apparent variations in directional selectivity have mechanical rather than neural origins, we used a quantitative method, as follows: assuming that place cell discharge is truly direction-independent so long as the head direction occurs at any given position, the number of action potentials N_p expected at any place p with the head pointing in the direction θ is:

$$N_p(\theta) = R_p T_p(\theta),$$

where R_p is the direction-independent rate at location p and $T_p(\theta)$ is the time spent at p as a function of head direction. For any extended region, including a firing field, the expected number of action potentials as a function of head direction is:

$$N(\theta) = \sum_p (R_p T_p(\theta)),$$

where the sum is over all locations p in the firing field. The total time as a function of head direction in the extended region is $T(\theta) = \Sigma_p(T_p(\theta))$, so the average firing rate in the extended region as a function of head direction is:

$$R(\theta) = N(\theta)/T(\theta) = \sum_p (R_p T_p(\theta)) / \sum_p (T_p(\theta)). \tag{9.1}$$

Note that in general, R depends on θ even though the R_p are independent of θ, because space is sampled differently at different head orientations, due to the physical constraints of the environment and behavioral tendency of the rat to avoid certain head directions at certain places. Equation 9.1 therefore predicts firing rate as a function of head direction using only rate as a function of position and the distribution of dwell time as a function of position and head direction. The results of this calculation are shown as thin lines in figures 9.1C and 9.2C, where it is evident that the matches between the predicted and observed results are extremely close. The conclusion that place cells are omnidirectional in an open environment is supported by an analysis in which observed firing rates are accurately predicted by equation 9.1 for most firing fields in a cylinder with one or three cue cards on the wall (Muller et al., 1994).

In the same study, recordings using the two-spot tracker for rats running on a conventional eight-arm maze tell a somewhat different story. Cells on the central platform were omnidirectional, whereas cells on the arms were often but not always directionally selective. Interestingly, an individual cell could be non-directional in the open field but directionally selective on the eight-arm maze.

The study of place cell directionality was enhanced by the work of (Markus et al., 1995) who used single-spot tracking methods. Markus et al. (1995) found that only a small fraction of place cells (approx. 15%) show directional selectivity in a cylinder. They saw that a marginally larger fraction (approx. 20%) were directional on a 1.22 m diameter disk, but also that most of the cells (approx. 65%) were selective on an eight-arm maze. Thus, although the method of determining direction was very different from that used by Muller et al. (1994), the basic results were in agreement. Note that some cells with fields on the central platform showed directional selectivity, as did most cells at the ends of the arms. A later study reported that fields at the ends of arms tend to be non-directional (Redish et al., 2000).

Markus et al. (1995) also reported a fascinating finding: that the nature of the task performed by the rat influences place cell directionality. Thus, when rats learned to follow a square-shaped trail on the open disk, the fraction of directional fields increased, mainly due to the addition of new fields. Recordings on a plus-maze with two wide arms perpendicular to two narrow arms revealed no differences in directional selectivity on arms of different width, reinforcing the idea that the unidirectional running behavior and not the physical constraints imposed by the apparatus was the major determinant of directional selectivity. Finally, although beyond the scope of this paper, changing the behavioral requirements of the task caused a significant fraction of the cells to undergo changes in their firing locations, an interesting example of partial remapping (Muller et al., 1991). Changes in directionality and field location take place rapidly, on a scale of minutes (Markus et al., 1995).

More recently, two studies asked how directionality is affected by various lesions. Brun et al. (2002) removed almost all input from CA3 to CA1, leaving the direct pathway from entorhinal cortex as the predominant spatial input to CA1. Lesioned and control animals learned to collect food scattered in an open field and to run on linear tracks where they received reward at the ends. In both environments, pyramidal cells in CA1 of the lesioned rats had sharp, stable firing fields whose directional properties were similar to place cells in normal rats; they were nondirectional in the open field but directional on the linear track. The implication is that CA3 is not necessary for generation of normal place fields and that directional properties are generated outside CA3. In a second study, Calton et al. (2003) lesioned two areas that contain head direction cells, namely, anterodorsal thalamic nuclei (ADN) and postsubiculum (PoS), in separate groups of animals. Although place cells from lesioned animals did not differ from controls in many regards, such as field size and in-field firing rate, the signal was significantly degraded with respect to measures of out-of-field (background) firing rate, spatial coherence, and information content. Surprisingly, place cells from lesioned animals were more likely modulated by the rat's head direction. This work implies that the hippocampal representation of the environment is surprisingly independent of the head direction cell system. It leaves open the question of whether there are spatial tasks that are refractory to damage of the head direction system, and how such tasks might be accomplished using only the remaining positional system.

Directional Place Fields in Hippocampal Models

Despite the abundance of computational models of the hippocampus (see reviews by Trullier et al. 1997, Tsodyks 1999, Redish 2001), few models explicitly address the problem of the directionality of place cells. Our focus here is on models that tackle place cell directionality.

Feedforward Models with Plastic Synapses

Sharp (1991) proposed a three-layer feedforward network with binary units and competitive learning in the second and third layers. The input to the network (the first layer) consisted of "sensory neurons" tuned to individual landmarks along the periphery of a simulated cylindrical environment. Half of these sensory neurons were also tuned to the orientation of the animal with respect to the landmarks. She found that the simulated place cells tended to be nondirectional in open environments but directional in an eight-arm maze, in agreement with the data. In this model, competitive learning tends to associate "clusters" of similar local views into a single category that will be represented by one place cell. When the rat makes random movements, it can occupy a given place while assuming many different orientations. This forms a group of related local views that are each sufficient to trigger the firing of the same single place cell, even though local views of opposite orientations at the same place are rather different. In contrast, on the arms of a maze, by far the most common orientations are outward and inward. Since the corresponding local views are too different from each other, each view will activate a different place cell.

Although this model predicts directional selectivity in constrained environments and omnidirectional firing in open fields, such a purely feedforward model is not adequate to describe many place cell properties since they can continue firing after cue removal or in the dark. We therefore turn to networks with attractor dynamics that can explain the persistence of activity after removal of all salient cues (for a tutorial on attractor networks, see chapter 18 by Touretzky).

Models with Prewired Synaptic Connectivity That Support "Charts"

Another class of models assumes that the synaptic connectivity of area CA3 of the hippocampus endows the network dynamics with two-dimensional attractors called "charts" (McNaughton et al., 1996; Samsonovich and McNaughton, 1997; Redish and Touretzky, 1998; Battaglia and Treves, 1998). For the network dynamics to implement attractors, the strength of connection (or the probability of connection) of two neurons must be a decreasing function of the distance between their fields (Muller et al., 1991). In this class of models, the connectivity is assumed to be prewired. Upon first entrance into a novel environment, the network dynamics select one of the ready-made charts at random. The state of the network can be represented as a hill of activity on the chart that represents the current environment. The cell set that currently supports the activity hill is updated by self-motion information, visual and other sensory cues, or a combination of these. In a given chart, cells are intrinsically nondirectional and since a single chart is used in an open field environment, place cells appear nondirectional. This class of models needs, however, an ad hoc mechanism to explain directional selectivity on a linear track. A proposed solution is to change the chart or "internal map" such that one group of place cells is active when the rat is moving in one direction, whereas a second group is active while the rat is moving in the other direction. The shift from one set of place cells to the other set has been proposed to be due to a "shift of attention" at established reward locations where the animal changes movement direction (McNaughton et al., 1994; Markus et al., 1995). Unfortunately, these models do not propose a mechanism that can easily be tested explicitly. Furthermore, the idea of abrupt switching between two charts seems difficult to reconcile with the finding that place fields are nondirectional at the end of linear tracks (Redish et al., 2001). Extensions of the model to networks storing attractors with different topologies (both one-dimensional and two-dimensional attractors) would be needed to bring them into line with the empirical observations.

Models with Plastic Synapses in Recurrent CA3 Circuitry

Brunel and Trullier (1998) and Kali and Dayan (2000) proposed a model with Hebbian plasticity in the recurrent CA3 circuitry, in which place cells are initially directional, due to local-view type inputs. In these models, directionality disappears in some cases as the result of the cooperative dynamics of interconnected place cells. The crucial element of the model is the presence of fast Hebbian synaptic dynamics, which modulate the efficacy of recurrent connections between cells as a function of the activity of pre- and postsynaptic cells. These modifications depend on both the position and orientation specificities of each pair of cells connected by these synapses. They, in turn, induce changes in the activity patterns of these cells, thereby changing their selective discharge properties. To explain the absence of directionality in new environments, as measured from recordings of about 20 minutes, the dynamics of synaptic modifications must be fast enough so that increases in synaptic efficacy are already present after a few passes of an animal through any given place field (typically a few minutes, assuming realistic exploration dynamics). The dynamics of such a network have been tested in simulated environments that resemble those often used in experimental studies: an open-field, an eight-arm maze, and a plus maze. In each case, sessions with random or directed movements have been compared. This class of models shows that the same place cells can appear directional or nondirectional, depending upon the locomotor activity of the simulated rat. In particular, (1) most cells appear omnidirectional in the case of random movements in the open field, whereas most cells appear directional on the plus or eight-arm maze; (2) cells can be either directional or nondirectional on the center of mazes; (3) when the simulated rat switches from random to directed motion in the open field, the average directionality of cells increases; and the same switch induces no significant changes in directionality on the plus maze; and (4) significant changes in directional properties occur after about 3 minutes of (simulated) exploration. Note that in these simulations, the generated representations usually consist of directional and omnidirectional cells because head directions at particular locations are not sampled uniformly by the animal.

The computational models of Brunel and Trullier (1998) and Kali and Dayan (2000) thus account for a large body of experimental data on the directionality of place cells. Furthermore, the dynamics of the model and the synaptic learning mechanisms also account for other properties of place cell activity, such as an increase in the place cell peak firing rates (Brunel and Trullier 1998), as observed by Mehta et al. (1997, 2000) and place field stretching in an enlarged environment (Kali and Dayan, 2000) as observed by Muller and Kubie (1987) and O'Keefe and Burgess (1996). These models predict that a blockade of plasticity in hippocampus would cause place fields in a novel open environment to be more directional than usually observed. In contrast, the place cells in a familiar open environment should stay omnidirectional. The idea that directionality properties depend on CA3 recurrent circuitry seems in contradiction with the recent study of Brun et al. (2002), which showed that directionality properties of CA1 neurons are unaffected by lesions of the CA3–CA1 pathway. However, the synaptic plasticity mechanisms described by Brunel and Trullier (1998) and Kali and Dayan (2000) could be implemented downstream, e.g., in entorhinal cortex. Alternatively, directional properties might be due to plasticity of feedforward connections such as the entorhinal cortex–CA1 direct pathway, as in the Sharp (1991) model. More experimental data in entorhinal cortex is needed to clarify these issues.

In summary, two classes of models have been proposed to explain the directional properties of place cells. In one class, a fixed synaptic structure implements a set of continuous attractors. In another class of models, the connectivity is initially random and the synaptic structure is learned during exploration of the environment (Muller et al., 1996), leading to plasticity of directionality properties as a function of the types of movements performed by the animal.

These considerations are only part of the story. An interesting but unexplored hypothesis is that the hippocampus could play a transitional role. In early stages in life, a rat might form a multiplicity of continuous attractors in a recurrent synaptic structure that reflect its experiences in open spaces or constrained trajectories along specific routes. These attractors might serve as the charts in the first class of models, although there would be both two-dimensional and one-dimensional charts, unlike those in the Samsonovich and McNaughton model. Upon entering a new environment, the animal would select one of the stored attractors that best corresponds to the current environment, two-dimensional in an open field, one-dimensional in a constrained environment. In this scenario, cells would be nondirectional immediately after entering a new environment, as opposed to the models of Brunel and Trullier (1998) and Kali and Dayan (2000). However, synaptic plasticity mechanisms might still be present in the adult brain and modulate the connectivity formed in the early stage. These plasticity mechanisms might lead, for example, to changes in directionality as the rat switches from random to directed moves in an open field, as in the Markus et al. (1995) experiment.

Consequences of Directionality in Hippocampal Models

One consequence of directionality is the appearance of asymmetry of place fields in models with spike-timing dependent synaptic plasticity: the firing rate is low as the rat enters the field but high as it exits (Mehta et al., 1997, 2000). Tsodyks et al. (1996) and Wallenstein and Hasselmo (1997) have shown that asymmetry in the synaptic structure of a CA3 model leads in turn to phase precession: the average phase of the spikes of a cell with respect to the theta EEG rhythm advances as the rat passes through its place field (O'Keefe and Recce 1993, Skaggs et al., 1996). However, an asymmetry in the synaptic structure is probably not the only mechanism responsible for phase precession, since this phenomenon is also present in the open field, where no such asymmetry is to be expected (Skaggs et al., 1996).

Discussion

Although additional information concerning the directionality of place cells will certainly be discovered, at the time of this writing the basic properties seem to be clear. Regardless of whether directionality is measured according to head angle in the environment (Muller et al., 1994) or the progression of the whole animal through the environment (McNaughton et al., 1983; Markus et al., 1995), it seems generally agreed that place cells are directionally unselective in open environments and directionally selective on linear tracks. Moreover, it appears that directional selectivity is enhanced if the rat walks along a narrow, closed path even if it does so on an open surface (Markus et al., 1995). Thus, to some degree, the fraction of directional cells depends not purely on whether the rat is mechanically constrained to walk along a narrow path, but rather whether it in fact does so, even if other, more complex paths are available.

We have already reviewed theoretical models that explain how the switch between the directional and nondirectional firing modes might occur. In this context, a key question is whether switching depends on NMDA receptor-based glutamatergic transmission, on transmission mediated by other glutamatergic receptors, on non-glutamatergic transmission, or whether the switching process does not require synaptic strength changes at all. On the current evidence that the expansion and backward motion of firing fields recorded during running on topologically circular tracks can be blocked by the NMDA receptor antagonist CPP [(6)-3-(2-carboxypiperazin-4-yl)propyl-1-phosphonic acid] (Ekstrom et al., 2001), a similar mechanism may account for directionality shifts. Nevertheless, why such shifts occur is an entirely different issue. We close with speculations about why hippocampal place cells switch their directional selectivity.

The viewpoint we adopt arises from the idea that the hippocampus is in a fundamentally different state when place cells are omnidirectional on the one hand, or directionally selective on the other. In the simplest case, the environment is uniformly represented by omnidirectional cells, as in a cylinder, or by directional cells as on a linear track. It is also possible for the representation to be a composite of omnidirectional and directional place cells, as on an eight-arm maze where cells are omnidirectional on the center but directional in its arms. The two kinds of place responses also exist simultaneously when a rat runs on a narrow path in an open area (Markus et al., 1995) where the original omnidirectional cells are supplemented by additional directional cells that develop as the number of laps run by the rat grows.

The first order picture is therefore quite simple: the directionality of the local set of place cells may reflect the effective connectivity of the space to which the rat has access. Thus, omnidirectional place cells may be used when it is possible to go from any place to any other place, as in a foraging area where the rat may find food scattered in various places. In contrast, directional cells may be used to represent the route from one foraging area to a second, or from a foraging area to home.

How are paths from one place to another represented? One possibility is that a path is, in fact, a sequence of place cells connected by synapses whose strength represents the distance from one firing field to another. The required relationship between synaptic strength and distance will form if the synapses that connect place cell pairs are Hebbian. In this case, synapses that connect cells with overlapping fields will strengthen since the cells will tend to fire together, whereas synapses that connect cells with widely separated fields will remain weak (Muller et al., 1991, 1996; Brunel and Trullier, 1998; Kali and Dayan, 2000).

Given this synaptic strength rule and a randomly connected network of omnidirectional place cell-like units in an open environment, an optimal path from any place to any other place can be found by searching the network for the cell sequence that minimizes the sum of the synaptic resistance along the path (Muller et al., 1996). The same rule about synaptic strength applied to firing fields along a linear track would produce a linear sequence in which, if followed by the rat, each step would take it from its current location to a neighboring position. The fact that the individual place cells are directionally selective ensures that selected paths representing oppositely directed motions will interact minimally. This is because cells that are tuned to discharge with the rat moving in opposite directions will not fire at the same time, preventing synapses between such cells from strengthening. A prediction of this model is that the rat will not recognize the same point along a linear track as the same place when it is moving in opposite directions. In particular, a rat trained to stop, or otherwise indicate arrival at a certain location going in one direction, would not in general stop at the same location going in the opposite direction.

In summary, our speculations on directional switching arise from a belief that one of the major functions of the rat hippocampus is the task of forming a map of the environment (O'Keefe and Nadel, 1987). It is our further belief that the features of this map correspond in surprisingly concrete ways to the surroundings; the hippocampal representation of the rat's environment is unexpectedly veridical. The fact of location-specific firing, the use of cells with linear or crescent shaped fields at boundaries, and the simple rules by which stimulus combinations control place cells all suggest that the across-cell representation is in many ways a copy of the surroundings. Further evidence in this direction comes from experiments in which a different class of pyramidal cells appear to discharge in association with a movable barrier, with the effect that the ensemble of cells can flexibly and realistically represent different configurations of an arena and the location of its contents (Muller et al., 2001; Lenck-Santini et al., 2003).

To these considerations we would like to add the idea that the directional properties of place cells reflect the local structure of space, the actions carried out by the rat, or both. One value of this arrangement is clear: it means that paths are suited to the surroundings. A second benefit comes from the reduced computational resources required to find optimal paths in kinematically constrained circumstances. But in the end, variable directionality is yet another reason to treat the rat hippocampus as both a spatial computational machine and a model for more complex cognitive processes.

Acknowledgments

This work was supported by NIH grant NS20686 and an MRC (UK) Overseas Initiative Grant to RUM.

References

Battaglia FP, Treves A (1998) Attractor neural networks storing multiple space representations: a model for hippocampal place fields. Phys Rev E 58: 7738–7753.

Brun VH, Otnass MK, Molden S, Steffenach HA, Witter MP, Moser MB, Moser EI (2002) Place cells and place recognition maintained by direct entorhinal-hippocampal circuitry. Science 296: 2243–2246.

Brunel N, Trullier O (1998) Plasticity of directional place fields in a model of rodent CA3. Hippocampus 8: 651–665.

Calton JL, Stackman RW, Goodridge JP, Archey WB, Dudchenko PA, Taube JS (2003) Hippocampal place cell instability after lesions of the head direction cell network. J Neurosci 23: 9719–9731.

Ekstrom AD, Meltzer J, McNaughton BL, Barnes CA (2001) NMDA receptor antagonism blocks experience-dependent expansion of hippocampal place fields. Neuron 31: 631–638.

Gothard, KM, Skaggs WE, McNaughton BL (1996) Dynamics of mismatch correction in the hippocampal ensemble code for space: interaction between path integration and environmental cues. J Neurosci 16: 8027–8040.

Hollup SA, Molden S, Donnett JG, Moser MB, Moser EI (2001) Place fields of rat hippocampal pyramidal cells and spatial learning in the water maze. Eur J Neurosci 13: 1197–1208.

Kali S, Dayan P (2000) The involvement of recurrent connections in area CA3 in establishing the properties of place fields: a model. J Neurosci 20: 7463–7477.

Knierim JJ, Kudrimoti HS, McNaughton BL (1998) Interactions between idiothetic cues and external landmarks in the control of place cells and head direction cells. J Neurophysiol 80: 425–446.

Lenck-Santini PP, Muller RU, Poucet B (2003) Place cell activity and exploratory behavior following spatial and non-spatial changes in the environment. Program Nr. 198.4 Abstract Viewer, Soc. for Neuroscience.

Markus EJ, Barnes CA, McNaughton BL, Gladden VL, Skaggs WE (1994) Spatial information content and reliability of hippocampal CA1 neurons: effects of visual input. Hippocampus 4: 410–421.

Markus, E. J., Y.-L. Qin, B. Leonard, W. E. Skaggs, B. L. McNaughton, and C. A. Barnes (1995) Interactions between location and task affect the spatial and directional firing of hippocampal neurons. J Neurosci 15: 7079–7094.

McNaughton, BL, Barnes CA, Gerrard JL, Gothard K, Jung MW, Knierim JJ, Kudrimoti H, Qin Y, Skaggs WE, Suster M, and Weaver KL (1996) Deciphering the hippocampal polyglot: the hippocampus as a path integration system. J Exp Biol 199: 173–186.

McNaughton BL, Barnes CA, O'Keefe J (1983) The contribution of position, direction, and velocity to single unit activity in the hippocampus of freely-moving rats. Exp Brain Res 52: 41–49.

Mehta MR, Barnes CA, McNaughton BL (1997) Experience-dependent, asymmetric expansion of hippocampal place fields. Proc Natl Acad Sci USA 94: 8918–8921.

Mehta MR, Quirk MC, Wilson MA (2000) Experience-dependent asymmetric shape of hippocampal receptive fields. Neuron 25: 707–715.

Muller RU, Bostock EM, Taube JS, Kubie JL (1994) On the directional firing properties of hippocampal place cells. J Neurosci 14: 7235–7251.

Muller RU, Kubie JL (1987) The effects of changes in the environment on the spatial firing of hippocampal complex-spike cells. J Neurosci 7: 1951–1968.

Muller RU, Kubie JL, Bostock EM, Taube JS, Quirk GJ (1991) Spatial firing correlates of neurons in the hippocampal formation of freely moving rats. In: J Paillard, ed., Brain and Space New York: Oxford University Press, pp. 296–333.

Muller RU, Kubie JL, Ranck JB Jr (1987) Spatial firing patterns of hippocampal complex-spike cells in a fixed environment. J Neurosci 7: 1935–1950.

Muller RU, Poucet B, Rivard B (2001) Sensory determinants of place cell firing fields. In: PE Sharp, ed., The Neural Basis of Navigation: evidence from Single Unit Recording. Boston: Kluwer Academic Publishers.

Muller RU, Stead M (1996) Hippocampal place cells connected by Hebbian synapses can solve spatial problems. Hippocampus 6: 709–719.

O'Keefe J (1976) Place units in the hippocampus of the freely moving rat. Exp Neurol 51: 78–109.

O'Keefe and Burgess (1996) Geometric determinants of the place fields of hippocampal neurons. Nature 381: 425–428.

O'Keefe J, Conway DH (1978) Hippocampal place units in the freely moving rat: why they fire where they fire. Exp Brain Res 31: 573–590.

O'Keefe J, Dostrovsky J (1971) The hippocampus as a spatial map. Preliminary evidence from unit activity in the freely moving rat. Exp Brain Res 34: 171–175.

O'Keefe J, Recce ML (1993) Phase relationship between hippocampal place units and the EEG theta rhythm. Hippocampus 3: 317–330.

Ranck JB Jr (1984) Head-direction cells in the deep cell layers of the dorsal presubiculum in freely moving rats. Soc Neurosci Abstr 10: 599.

Redish AD (2001) The hippocampal debate: are we asking the right questions? Behav Brain Res 127: 81–98.

Redish AD, McNaughton BL, Barnes CA (2000) Place cell firing shows an inertia-like process. Neurocomputing 32–33: 235–241.

Redish AD, Touretzky DS (1998) The role of the hippocampus in solving the Morris water maze. Neural Comput 10: 73–111.

Samsonovich A, McNaughton BL (1997) Path integration and cognitive mapping in a continuous attractor neural network model. J Neurosci 17: 5900–5920.

Sharp PE (1991) Computer simulation of hippocampal place cells. Psychobiology 19: 103–115.

Skaggs WE, McNaughton BL, Wilson MA, Barnes CA (1996) Theta phase precession in hippocampal neuronal populations and the compression of temporal sequences. Hippocampus 6: 149–172.

Taube JS, Muller RU, Ranck JB Jr (1990a) Head-direction cells recorded from the postsubiculum in freely moving rats. I. Description and quantitative analysis. J Neurosci 10: 420–435.

Taube JS, Muller RU, Ranck, JB Jr (1990b) Head-direction cells recorded from the postsubiculum in freely moving rats. II. Effects of environmental manipulations. J Neurosci 10: 436–447.

Trullier O, Wiener SI, Berthoz A, Meyer J-A (1997) Biologically-based artificial navigation systems: review and prospects. Prog Neurobiol 51: 483–544.

Tsodyks M (1999) Attractor neural network models of spatial maps in hippocampus, Hippocampus 9: 481–489.

Wallenstein GV, Hasselmo ME (1997) GABAergic modulation of hippocampal population activity: sequence learning, place field development, and the phase precession effect. J Neurophysiol 78: 393–408.

Wan HS, Touretzky DS, Redish AD (1994) Towards a computational theory of rat navigation. In M Mozer, P Smolensky, DS Touretzky, JL Elman, and A. Weigend, eds., Proceedings of the 1993 Connectionist Models Summer School, New York: Lawrence Erlbaum Associates, pp. 11–19.

III RELATIONS BETWEEN THE HEAD DIRECTION SYSTEM, SPATIAL ORIENTATION, AND BEHAVIOR

10 Head Direction Codes in Hippocampal Afferent and Efferent Systems: What Functions Do They Serve?

Sheri J. Y. Mizumori, Corey B. Puryear, Kathryn M. Gill, and Alex Guazzelli

The discovery of head direction cells in many limbic and limbic-afferent structures could lead one to suggest that the limbic system is specialized for spatial analysis, and in particular the processing of directional orientation. Considering this hypothesis, it becomes important to know whether head direction codes are unique to the limbic system. Previous chapters provide convincing evidence that the mechanism for the generation of head direction signals involves sequential processing through the tegmentum, mammillary nucleus, anterior dorsal thalamus (ADN), and postsubiculum circuit. Precisely how ADN or postsubicular head direction codes impact hippocampal (or other downstream) directional processing is less clear. Here, we present the possibility that a neural code for directional heading in structures located outside of the tegmentum-to-postsubicular circuit represents a fundamental unit of spatial information that can enter into diverse neural computations. That is, perhaps a broad set of neural systems ultimately receives and uses a common directional signal. As such, the collective operation of these neural systems may contribute to the generation of a common spatial reference frame. One function of such a global spatial reference frame is that it allows the coordination of multiple processes, such as interpreting allocentric sensory information within an egocentric coordinate system, eventually transforming it back to an allocentric coordinate system during the execution of behaviors.

According to the above hypothesis, head direction representations within the tegmentum-to-postsubiculum circuit serve a fundamental function that is different from other brain areas that also contain head direction cells (figure 10.1). Evidence that the tegmentum-to-postsubiculum circuit is involved in the initial generation of a head direction signal includes the finding that cells early in the circuit appear to anticipate specific orientations by some 38 to 95 ms, while cells later in the circuit show little or no such anticipatory firing (Blair et al., 1998; Blair and Sharp, 1995, 2002; Stackman and Taube, 1998; Taube, 1998; Taube and Muller, 1998; chapter 1 by Sharp). Such an anticipatory

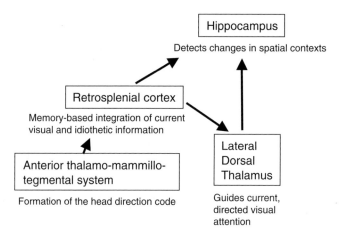

Figure 10.1
Schematic illustration of a model that distinguishes head direction cell functions in structures afferent to the hippocampal complex.

firing relationship between head direction signals and behavior might be expected if these signals were destined for subsequent use by efferent structures to direct ongoing sensory processing and behavioral output. If this were the case, head direction cells found within hippocampal afferent systems that do not include the tegmentum-to-subicular circuit may function to orient visual spatial attention, while head direction cells found within hippocampal efferent systems may help to define the orientation of appropriate behavioral responses. Head direction firing by cells that contribute to attentional processes may be expected to be sensitive to changes in spatial context, and therefore more directly related to ongoing choice accuracy. In contrast, head direction cells in hippocampal efferent systems might be uniquely related to ongoing egocentric movement (e.g., movement velocity) when compared to head direction cells in the tegmentum-to-postsubicular attention circuit. This property may make head direction codes in hippocampal efferent structures more directly related to ongoing behaviors.

This chapter evaluates the extent to which the properties of head direction cells recorded within the tegmentum-to-postsubicular circuit differ relative to properties of head direction cells in other hippocampal afferent and efferent structures. In particular, we will discuss whether head direction cells within the lateral dorsal thalamus (LDN; a structure afferent to hippocampus, yet outside of the tegmentum-to-postsubicular circuit) behave in a manner that is consistent with the view that they contribute to spatial attention processes (Mizumori and Williams, 1993). Then, we will describe head direction representations within hippocampal efferent systems such as the striatum and the PrCM (medial precentral cortex; also known as FR2, AGm cortex, or secondary motor cortex; Wiener, 1993; Mizumori et al., 1999a, 2000b; Ragozzino et al., 2001; Guazzelli et al., 2000) to determine whether their firing properties are consistent with the view that they function to orient appropriate behavioral responses.

General Method

The experiments described in the following pages involve recording single unit activity from rats as they perform various tasks on an open, elevated eight-arm radial maze. The version of the task most frequently used is the spatial working memory task in which rats must retrieve food reward located at the ends of the maze arms. For each trial, reward is provided only once at each arm. The first four choices vary for each trial, and are presented sequentially in a predetermined order. The remaining choices are made when rats have full access to all eight maze arms. After the rats obtain rewards from all eight maze arms, a trial ends and a 2-min intertrial interval begins. Rats perform between 10 and 20 trials per recording session, depending upon the specific experiment. Other variations on this basic training procedure will be described individually for separate experiments.

When possible, recordings involve the simultaneous recording of hippocampal units along with units from other brain regions (e.g., striatum or PrCM). Single unit records were obtained with either the stereotrode or tetrode methodologies. These electrodes were loaded onto moveable microdrives that allowed the recording of unit activity across multiple test sessions. A given cell's sensitivity to changes in the spatial context is tested by varying visual cue arrangements or cue accessibility.

Head Direction Cells of the Lateral Dorsal Nucleus of the Thalamus

The lateral dorsal nucleus of the thalamus (LDN) comprises a key component of the comparatively large tectocortical visual system of the rat (Linden and Perry, 1983; Sefton and Dreher, 1985; Sripanidkulchai and Wyss, 1986; van Groen and Wyss, 1992). LDN receives direct projections from the superior colliculus and projects to posterior cortical areas, such as the retrosplenial cortex, parietal cortex, the subicular complex, and visual association cortex area 18b (Vogt and Miller, 1983; Vogt et al., 1986; Thompson and Robertson, 1987a; van Groen and Wyss, 1990a,b, 1992). The connections between LDN and posterior cortex appear to be reciprocal, with retrosplenial cortex providing rather extensive feedback. Retrosplenial cortex is also a major efferent target of the ADN (van Groen and Wyss, 1995). Since LDN does not appear to receive the type of vestibular input that occurs within ADN (reviewed in Taube et al., 1996), the LDN is probably not directly involved in the initial creation of head direction signals as is ADN. Rather, ADN head direction signals may be passed onto retrosplenial cortex, and then to LDN (see chapter by Hopkins). The overall pattern of anatomical connections of the LDN is similar to those of the pulvinar nucleus in primates (Thompson and Robertson, 1987b). The pulvinar has been shown to play an important role in visual spatial attention (Ungerleider and Christensen, 1979; Petersen et al., 1987). In particular, Desimone et al. (1990) suggested that the pulvinar may functionally gate extrastriate responses to distracting stimuli, thereby focusing one's attention within the visual environment. Perhaps LDN directional signals perform a comparable attentional orientation function within the domain of adaptive navigation.

When rats perform in a familiar test environment, the directional tuning of LDN head direction cells appears similar to that reported for ADN and postsubicular head direction cells (Taube et al., 1990a,b; Mizumori and Williams, 1993; Blair and Sharp, 1995; Taube, 1995). However, features of LDN head direction firing can be shown to be different from ADN head direction firing when access to familiar cues is eliminated (either by imposed darkness or the removal of extramaze cues). In one test situation, if rats were not allowed to view the test room before or during maze trials that were performed in darkness, many LDN head direction cells showed little or no evidence of directional firing. When the room lights were turned on, directional firing appeared as it was during prior training with the lights on (Mizumori and Williams, 1993). This pattern was unexpected, considering that, theoretically, a directional code could be established exclusively with idiothetic information. Identified ADN and postsubicular head direction cells did not appear to lose the fundamental property of head direction firing when tested in rats that were blindfolded after a period of exposure to the familiar environment (Goodridge et al., 1998). It is not known whether head direction firing would have been observed had the rats not had the exposure to the environment prior to being blindfolded. Our hypothesis that head direction cells within the tegmentum-to-postsubicular circuit are closely tied to the generation of a directional heading neural code, while LDN head direction cells serve to direct attention within a visual context, predicts that ADN head direction firing would be observed if blindfolded rats were not allowed to view the environment before being blindfolded.

Another pattern of responses that distinguishes LDN cells from ATN/postsubicular cells is seen when rats are allowed to view the visual environment before the room lights are turned off. Under these testing conditions, directional firing by LDN neurons was initially maintained during the period of darkness. However, within a couple of minutes (or after the first maze trial performed in darkness), we almost always observed the directional preference of LDN head direction cells to systematically rotate either in the clockwise or counterclockwise direction by increments of about 45° per trial (Mizumori and Williams, 1993; figure 10.2). Control tests showed that the symmetry of the radial maze may have contributed to the rather rapid shift in directional preference. If rats were restricted to a single asymmetric (i.e., rectangular) maze arm in darkness, the original directional preferences were maintained throughout the 30 min test period. If rats were restricted to the round central platform in darkness, the directional preferences were maintained for only 2 to 3 min.

The finding that LDN head direction firing requires visual input to become established, but that once established, visual or nonvisual input can be used to align the directional

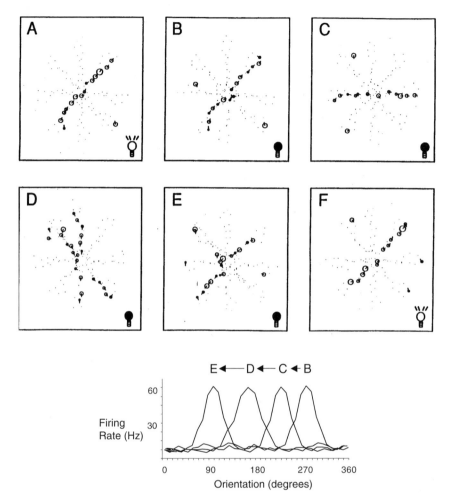

Figure 10.2
Example of an LDN head direction cell response to imposed dark trials after first viewing the test environment. (Top) A top down view of the radial maze apparatus reveal positions occupied by the rat (dots) and local firing rates (indicated by circles that are proportional in size to the firing rate). Vectors indicate the direction of movement on the maze. In panel A, it can be seen that when the lights are on, the preferred orientation of the cell was toward the northeast corner of the room. During the first dark trial, the preference remained unchanged (B). Panels C to E show the systematic clockwise rotation of the directional preference with continued training in darkness. The original preference of the cell was restored when the room lights were turned back on (F). (Bottom) Head direction preferences are illustrated when firing rates are plotted relative to orientation within the room. Such plots make more clear the unidirectional shift in directional preference of head direction cells when tested under the conditions described for the top portion of the figure.

firing, is consistent with the view that LDN directional codes may be related to memory-guided visual attention processes. In our usage of the term, this attention process is important not only for establishing directional preferences, but also for maintaining the representation in the face of partial sensory input. Accordingly, upon initial exposure to the spatial context visual input may be required to activate directional firing by LDN neurons. Once activated, directional firing could be maintained in darkness after the rat viewed the room, because it had retrieved a visual association-based spatial memory of the environment, perhaps via retrosplenial cortex (Cooper et al., 2001; Mizumori et al., 2000a). The retrosplenial cortex-activated association between previously experienced visual and idiothetic input could be used to maintain firing relative to head orientation, and to stabilize directional preferences in the face of partial sensory input (i.e., when rats were restricted to a maze arm in darkness). That is, a pattern completion-like process may have taken place. In the absence of both reliable and salient visual and somatosensory cues, the directional preferences of LDN head direction cells began to drift.

While the effects of retrosplenial cortex lesion or inactivation are not known for LDN cells, it is known that such retrosplenial cortex disturbances disrupt (presumably learned) visual cue control over ADN head direction cells (Bassett and Taube, 1999). Disruption of retrosplenial cortex function also results in drifting head direction preferences of ADN cells (Golob and Taube, 1999), induces the reorganization of hippocampal place fields (Cooper and Mizumori, 2001), and impairs spatial learning when tested in darkness, but not in light conditions (Cooper and Mizumori, 1999). Thus, retrosplenial cortex may confer a mnemonic property to ADN, LDN, and hippocampal spatially correlated neurons. However, this influence may differ for different efferent targets, resulting in distinct responses in times of restricted input. For example, when ADN and postsubicular head direction cells were recorded in blindfolded rats, only a slight shift was observed in the directional preference of cell firing (Goodridge et al., 1998). This response appears qualitatively different from that of LDN cells after cue removal by imposed darkness. Future studies utilizing the same behavioral tests and same environmental probes are necessary to determine whether these differences are due to the structure being recorded or to different experimental conditions. If LDN and ADN truly respond qualitatively differently in the absence of familiar cues, this would be consistent with the view that LDN head direction cells serve a different function than ADN/postsubicular head direction cells. There are no known direct connections between ADN and LDN head direction cells, and it has been shown that LDN lesions do not alter cue control over ADN head direction cells (Golob et al., 1998). Thus, LDN head direction signals are either downstream from ADN processing, or these structures operate in parallel. Both LDN and ADN head direction signals appear to contribute to the stability of hippocampal place fields (Mizumori et al., 1994; Calton et al., 2003).

Consistent with the view that head direction codes in LDN and ADN/postsubiculum serve different purposes, are the results of tests that examine the extent to which head direction firing by LDN and ADN cells are related to behavioral accuracy. However, it is important to note that tests of experience-related head direction firing have been conducted with very different behavioral paradigms (for a review, see Muir and Taube, 2002 and chapter 11 by Dudchenko, et al.). Consequently, additional work is needed to resolve this issue. The evidence initially provided by Mizumori and Williams (1993) for mnemonic-related head direction firing came in different forms. For example, a significant negative correlation was found between the number of errors made during acquisition of a spatial working memory task on a radial maze, and the directional specificity of LDN head direction cells. However, no relationship was found between ADN head direction cell firing and an animal's behavioral choices on relatively simple reference and working memory spatial tasks (Golob et al., 2001; cf. Dudchenko and Taube, 1997). Perhaps a relationship was not found because head direction cells within the tegmentum-to-postsubiculum circuit may contribute a more basic function that defines orientation within specific contexts and does not guide directed attention or precise behavioral orientation. Cells that contribute to attention or behavioral expression functions might be expected to be more directly related to details of an animal's behavior within a familiar environment.

Other evidence supporting the view that LDN head direction codes represent a learned association between visual and nonvisual input is the finding that the original directional preference was maintained in darkness if rats were given reliable nonvisual cues (previously described). It also was shown that rats needed to view the entire visual environment, rather than just the view associated with the directional preference of the cell being tested, for peak directional firing to be achieved. Consistent with these data, Goodridge et al. (1998) showed that ADN and postsubicular head direction cells quickly come to reflect an association between idiothetic information and landmark cues when a rat is placed in a novel environment (see chapter 3, Landmark Control).

It is important to note that the many differences in LDN and ADN head direction properties do not necessarily preclude the possibility that they operate within a common and broadly defined neural system. Indeed, there are also important similarities in the responses of LDN and ADN/postsubicular head direction cells when tested in a lighted, familiar environment. For example, for both populations, the directional preferences of the LDN and ADN head direction cells shift in accordance with a rotation of the prominent visual cues (e.g., Mizumori and Williams, 1993; Taube et al., 1990b). Also, when a rat is led to an adjacent environment (or room) from a familiar environment, the original directional preference is maintained (Taube and Burton, 1995; Mizumori, unpublished data). These similarities support the view that different head direction cell populations may function cooperatively within a single spatial reference frame.

We have suggested earlier that the LDN may serve to direct current attention to salient aspects of a spatial context. Indeed, LDN head direction codes were found to be more sensitive to changes in a familiar environment than head direction cells of the tegmentum-to-postsubicular circuit. Now, we evaluate the possibility that head

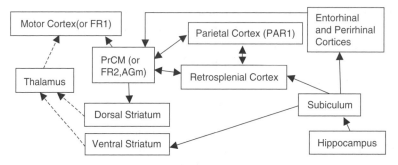

Figure 10.3
Hippocampal processing may impact ongoing behavior according to the two routes shown here. From the subiculum, output directly to ventral striatum may modulate behavioral output, especially during new learning. In addition, subicular output to neocortical systems may comprise an important behavioral control circuit. From posterior neocortex, relevant hippocampal information may be fed forward to frontal regions (e.g., PrCM), which in turn may impact motor cortex directly (solid lines) or indirectly (via dorsal striatum; dashed lines). Head direction codes are found in the retrosplenial cortex and PrCM, and these may contribute to the memory-guided mediation of ongoing behavior.

direction cells found in hippocampal efferent systems may serve to provide orientation guidance to ongoing behaviors. We will focus on the main routes by which hippocampal information may have an impact on ongoing behavior: the striatum and neocortex (figure 10.3).

Striatal Head Direction Cell Properties

The most widely studied hippocampal efferent system concerns the hippocampal projection to striatum, especially ventral striatum. For over two decades, it has been hypothesized that limbic information becomes interfaced with motivational and motor systems via the subicular output to ventral striatum (e.g., Mogenson, 1980). During this time, much anatomical, behavioral, and neurophysiological data has accumulated to support this view. For example, accumbens neurons were found to show not only egocentric movement responses, but also location and reward-related firing (Lavoie and Mizumori, 1994). In addition, we explored the possibility that dorsal striatum may contribute by recording dorsal striatal neural activity during the performance of hippocampal-dependent tasks, such as the spatial working memory task on a radial maze. We found evidence for behavioral correlates that appeared similar to those recorded from primates, such as reward and egocentric movement-related codes (Hikosaka et al., 1999; Schultz et al., 2003). In addition, in agreement with Wiener (1993), we found evidence for spatial codes that appear similar to what had been reported for limbic system structures: place cells and head direction cells (Mizumori et al., 1999a, 2000b; Ragozzino et al., 2001). Location-specific neurons were found throughout dorsal striatum, while head direction cells were found only in the dorsomedial sector. The fact that such cell correlates had not yet been described for primates may reflect the fact that rodents were tested while they moved about freely within a spatially extended test environment.

Many characteristics of striatal place fields were similar to those observed for hippocampal place fields. For example, peak in-field firing rates and the reliability of the fields were comparable. In our usage of the term, "reliability" refers to the proportion of trials in which the cell fired maximally when the rat traversed the field location. However, other characteristics were found to be different, such as the average size of the place field. Striatal fields tend to be larger than hippocampal fields. Another characteristic of hippocampal place fields is that they undergo a partial reorganization of the locations of the fields following cue manipulations (e.g., rearranging cues, removing cues, or turning lights off). That is, about half of the hippocampal place fields do not change locations following cue manipulations, while the remaining fields do change locations (Mizumori et al., 1999b). One interpretation of the partial reorganization phenomenon is that some hippocampal cells are driven more by a memory of the spatial context, while others are driven more by the currently available information. In this way, the hippocampus may compute the extent to which the expected and experienced spatial contexts differ. In contrast, striatal place fields almost always changed in response to alterations in the visual spatial context (Mizumori et al., 2000b), perhaps reflecting the fact that striatal place cells encode information relative to the current visual context more than to a memory of the spatial context. It may be that such a continual update of the current contextual situation is critical in order for the striatum to perform its more global function of evaluating the reinforcement consequences that are expected for the current context (e.g., Mizumori et al., 1999a; Schultz et al., 2003).

Dorsal striatal head direction cells appeared very similar to those described in limbic regions. This was the case in baseline firing properties (e.g., specificity and reliability of directional tuning), and in the cells' sensitivity to changes in the visual environment. For example, when access to visual cues is eliminated by imposed darkness, most striatal head direction cells showed only modest peak rate changes (figure 10.4). Only on occasion did we observe a significant shift in the directional preference of these cells. When visual cues were rotated, we most often observed a concurrent rotation of the directional preference of the cell (Mizumori et al., 2000b).

One prediction of the hypothesis that hippocampal efferent head direction signals may provide orientation information to guide context-relevant behavioral responses is that they may be uniquely related to specific aspects of egocentric movement. We tested this hypothesis by comparing, across structures known to contain head direction cells, the relationship between firing rate and movement velocity (or running speed) when rats were oriented within 40° of the preferred orientation of the cell being recorded. A majority of striatal head direction cells analyzed (about 73% or 11/15 cells evaluated thus far) showed significant linear correlations not only with head orientation but also movement velocity. Further, 87% of the cells showed significant correlations with acceleration. An illustration

A. Directional tuning during LD test

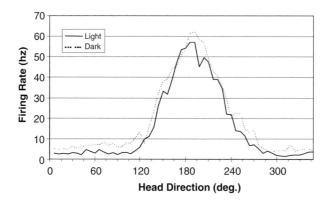

B. Velocity tuning during LD test

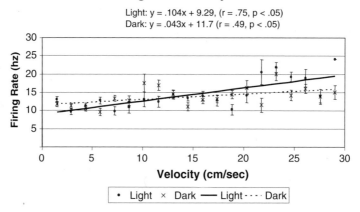

Figure 10.4
Dorsal striatal head direction cells respond very little to changes in a familiar context. (A) This was the case when assessing head direction tuning curves of one striatal cell before and after lights are turned off (Light and Dark, respectively). (B) A single cell example of the finding that a majority of striatal head direction cells show a significant correlation with movement velocity (i.e., running speed). This correlation (although reduced) remains significant when the lights are turned off.

of the velocity correlate of a striatal head direction cell is shown in figure 10.4B. Correlations between angular head velocity (i.e., velocity during head turns) had been described for head direction cells within the tegmentum-to-postsubiculum circuit (Blair and Sharp, 1996; Stackman and Taube, 1998; Knierim et al., 1998; Taube, 1995). Since our velocity measure included not only head turns, but also forward movement, and since rats performing our maze task spend much more time moving forward through space than making turns, we assume that our velocity measure is more directly related to linear velocity during forward locomotion. Past studies have not consistently reported the number of head direction cells that showed correlated firing with running (linear) velocity. However, a population average showed that head direction cells within the tegmentum-to-postsubiculum circuit are modestly correlated with linear velocity (Stackman and Taube, 1998). This conclusion needs to be tested more conclusively, however, by using similar tests and analyses when recording in the many brain areas that contain head direction cells.

If it is the case that, unlike head direction codes in hippocampal afferent systems, a common striatal neural code incorporates a combination of directional heading and movement velocity, this could indicate that striatal head direction cells convey information about a behavioral state (i.e., the velocity of locomotion when oriented in a particular direction) rather than contribute to directional attention functions or the generation of head direction signals. Such behavioral state information could become incorporated in intrastriatal computations that evaluate changes in reinforcement contingencies, relative to ongoing behaviors exhibited in a particular context. Interestingly, the velocity correlates of striatal head direction cells did not change as a function of visual context (17 cells tested so far), suggesting that other correlate types (e.g., striatal place cells) may provide such information to the striatal analysis.

PrCM Head Direction Cell Properties

The hippocampus may impact ongoing behavior not only via its striatal connections, but also via neocortical routes that ultimately reach motor cortex (Delatour and Witter, 2002). Recently, we have been focusing on what is arguably one of the more direct paths that extends from the subicular complex to retrosplenial cortex (Van Groen and Wyss, 1990b), and then to the medial precentral cortex (PrCM, or FR2, AGm; Vogt and Miller, 1983; Swanson and Kohler, 1986; Reep et al., 1990; Van Groen and Wyss, 1990a; Zilles and Wree, 1995). From PrCM, information can move directly to primary motor cortex (or FR1; Donoghue and Parham, 1983; Zilles and Wree, 1995; Reep et al., 1997). The PrCM also projects directly to dorsal striatum (Reep et al., 1984; Sesack et al., 1989; Reep and Corwin, 1999; Zheng and Wilson, 2002). Thus, PrCM may be strategically situated to allow for the integration of basal ganglia and frontal cortical movement control systems influenced by hippocampal output.

In order to facilitate direct comparisons across studies, rats were trained according to the same spatial working memory task as described earlier for LDN and striatal experiments. The firing of PrCM neurons was clearly correlated with a number of behaviors, including heading direction, egocentric movements such as turns and forward motion, and reward. The present discussion concerns only the head direction cells. When rats performed a known task in a familiar environment, the properties of the PrCM head direction cells very much resembled those described for other brain areas (including striatum), in terms of signal specificity and reliability. Also, the specific behavior in which the rat was engaged (e.g., grooming, eating, drinking, etc.) did not impact the head direction signal. As a test of the visual sensitivity of PrCM head direction cells, the salient visual cues were rotated by 180° to determine the extent to which cues determine the directional preference of the cell. Similar to what has been reported for head direction cells found in other brain areas, the preferred direction of the cells rotated on average about 174°. The uniqueness of PrCM head direction cells, however, became evident when the cells' responses to changes in the spatial context were tested. Unlike what had been found to be typical for head direction cells in the striatum (Mizumori et al., 2000b), hippocampus proper (Leutgeb et al., 2000), retrosplenial cortex (Chen et al., 1994b), and the tegmentum-to-postsubicular circuit (see earlier discussion), a large proportion (74%) of recorded PrCM head direction cells showed a significant response when the lights were turned off. These included changes in the ratio between peak and background firing rates, the half amplitude width of the Gaussian function in the directional tuning curve, and/or directional preference. Figure 10.5A provides an example of a PrCM head direction cell response during a single recording session in which trials were first performed with the lights on, then with the lights off.

In addition to testing the reliance of PrCM head direction cells on the available visual cues, we analyzed the relationship between cell firing and movement velocity and acceleration. Similar to what are found for striatal head direction cells, we found that 76% of the cells analyzed (22/29 cells) showed significant linear correlations with movement velocity, and 83% of the cells showed significant correlations with acceleration. Thus, similar to striatal head direction cells, PrCM head direction cells also encode rather complex idiothetic-based computations relative to an animal's behavior.

Unlike striatum, the velocity and acceleration aspects of the PrCM head direction neural codes appear dependent at least in part on spatial context (Nadel and Wilner, 1980; Mizumori et al., 1999b) information. Figure 10.5B also shows that the relationship between cell firing and velocity can change dramatically if the spatial environment changes. That is, for some units, a change in the visual environment resulted in the loss or appearance of velocity-correlated firing even though clear head directional discharge was observed before and after the environmental alteration. It appears, then, that the velocity and/or acceleration modulation of head direction cell discharge may be gated by information concerning the current context. In other words, an important function of the PrCM may be to provide orientation guidance to ongoing behavior in a context-dependent

A. Directional tuning during LD test

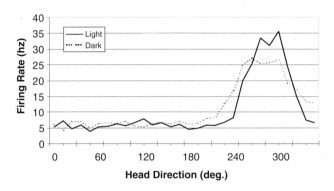

B. Velocity tuning during LD test

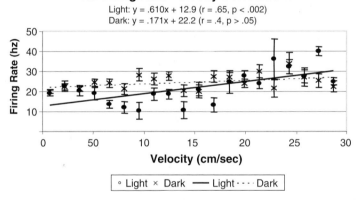

Figure 10.5
In contrast to striatal head direction cells, PrCM head direction cells appear sensitive to changes in visual spatial context. This is shown in (A) when a significant change in the Gaussian function is observed when the room lights are turned off. Also, in (B) the velocity correlation of PrCM head direction cells was observed to change after the lights were turned off. In this example, the velocity correlation essentially disappeared in darkness even though the animal continued to perform the task.

manner. In this way, PrCM may effectively contribute to the selection of the appropriate behavioral response.

Summary and Conclusions

Neuronal firing associated with heading direction has been identified in many brain structures located across diverse neural systems. A variety of results is consistent with the view that the tegmentum-to-postsubicular circuit is important for the initial formation of head direction signals in the brain. The functional significance of head direction cells found elsewhere in the brain remains enigmatic. Here, we suggest that the initial directional heading signal provided by the tegmentum-to-postsubicular circuit is one that other neural systems incorporate into local neurocomputational landscapes. We have provided two examples of the manner in which directional signals could be used to guide spatial attention (perhaps via the LDN), or to impact the selection of ongoing behaviors (via striatal and/or frontal cortical processing). The unusual sensitivity of LDN head direction cells to visual manipulations (relative to head direction cells within the tegmentum-to-postsubicular circuit) is consistent with an attention hypothesis of LDN function. Also, striatal and PrCM head direction discharge was significantly correlated with egocentric parameters such as velocity and acceleration of movement. That is, PrCM head direction cells either engage path integration operations, or their firing reflects path integration computations performed elsewhere in the brain. Functionally, striatal and PrCM head direction cells may contribute to the orientation of ongoing behaviors in a velocity/acceleration-dependent manner. Such a contribution appears to be spatial context-dependent for only PrCM cells.

Anatomical, behavioral, and physiological evidence suggest that the retrosplenial cortex may be critical for the memory-dependent gating of context information in LDN and PrCM. Interestingly, head direction cells are also found in retrosplenial cortex (Chen et al., 1994a,b; Cho and Sharp, 2001). Preliminary evidence from this laboratory shows that about 57% (4/7 cells analyzed thus far) of recorded retrosplenial cortex head direction cells are also correlated with linear velocity (Smith and Mizumori, unpublished data). This is a lower percentage than that found for head direction cells in the striatum or PrCM. Head direction cell firing in the tegmentum-to-postsubicular circuit is reported to be mildly correlated with velocity (Stackman and Taube, 1998). In order to make direct comparisons across brain structures, in the future it will be important to conduct a linear velocity analysis on cells within the tegmentum-to-postsubicular circuit when rats are performing a spatial memory task. If it is found that a larger proportion of head direction cells show linear movement velocity correlations as one moves closer to behavioral output systems, this would support the general hypothesis that head direction cells serve different purposes depending on the structure in which they are found. More specifically, it supports the view that head direction cells in hippocampal efferent structures use directional heading codes to help guide ongoing behaviors. It is important to keep in mind that findings of regional differences do not mean that each brain area operates independently. Rather, it may be that there is a common spatial metric or reference frame that is used to engage parallel and multiple neural systems during the performance of complex behaviors such as adaptive navigation (Mizumori et al., 2000a).

Acknowledgments

This work was supported by NIH grant 58755. We are grateful to many students who, over the years, made empirical and theoretical contributions to this work. Most recently, we thank Dr. David Smith and Chris Higginson in this regard.

References

Bassett JP, Taube JS (1999) Retrosplenial cortex lesions disrupt stability of head direction cell activity. Soc Neurosci Abstr 25: 1383.

Blair HT, Cho J, Sharp PE (1998) Role of the lateral mammillary nucleus in the rat head irection circuit: A combined single-unit recording and lesion study. Neuron 21: 1387–1397.

Blair HT, Sharp PE (1995) Anticipatory head-direction signals in anterior thalamus: Evidence for a thalamocortical circuit that integrates angular head motion to compute head direction. J Neurosci 15: 6260–6270.

Blair HT, Sharp PE (1996) Visual and vestibular influences on head-direction cells in the anterior thalamus of the rat. Behav Neurosci 110: 643–660

Blair HT, Sharp PE (2002) Functional organization of the rat head-direction circuit. In PE Sharp ed., The Neural Basis of Navigation. Evidence from Single Cell Recording. Boston: Kluwer, Academic Publishers, pp. 163–182.

Calton JL, Stackman RW, Goodridge JP, Archey WB, Dudchenko PA, Taube JS (2003) Hippocampal place cell instability after lesions of the head direction cell network. J Neurosci 23: 9719–9731.

Chen LL, Lin L-H, Green EJ, Barnes CA, McNaughton BL (1994a) Head-direction cells in the rat posterior cortex: I. Anatomical distribution and behavioral modulation. Exp Brain Res 101: 8–23.

Chen LL, Lin L-H, Barnes CA, McNaughton BL (1994b) Head-direction cells in the rat posterior cortex: II. Contributions of visual and idiothetic information to the directional firing. Exp Brain Res 101: 24–34.

Cho J, Sharp PE (2001) Head direction, place, and movement correlates for cells in the rat retrosplenial cortex. Behav Neurosci 115: 3–25.

Cooper BG, Mizumori SJY (1999) Retrosplenial cortex inactivation selectively impairs navigation in darkness. NeuroReport 10: 625–630.

Cooper BG, Mizumori SJY (2001) Temporary inactivation of retrosplenial cortex causes a transient reorganization of spatial coding in hippocampus. J Neurosci 21: 3986–4001.

Delatour B, Witter MP (2002) Projections from the parahippocampal region to the prefrontal cortex in the rat: evidence of multiple pathways. Eur J Neurosci 15: 1400–1407.

Desimone R, Wessinger M, Thomas L, Schneider W (1990) Attention control of visual perception: cortical and subcortical mechanisms. Cold Spring Harbor Symp Quant Biol 55: 963–971.

Donoghue JP, Parham C (1983) Afferent connections of the lateral agranular field of the rat motor cortex. J Comp Neurol 217: 390–404.

Dudchenko PA, Taube JS (1997) Correlation between head direction cell activity and spatial behavior on a radial arm maze. Behav Neurosci 111: 3–19.

Golob EJ, Taube JS (1999) Head direction cells in rats with hippocampal or overlying neocortical lesions: evidence for impaired angular path integration. J Neurosci 19: 7198–7211.

Golob EJ, Wolk DA, Taube JS (1998) Recordings of postsubicular head direction cells following lesions of the lateral dorsal thalamic nucleus. Brain Res 780: 9–19.

Golob EJ, Stackman RW, Wong AC, Taube JS (2001) On the behavioral significance of head direction cells: Neural and behavioral dynamics during spatial memory tasks. Behav Neurosci 115: 285–304.

Goodridge JP, Dudchenko PA, Worboys KA, Golob EJ, Taube JS (1998) Cue control and head direction cells. Beh Neurosci 112: 749–761.

Guazzelli A, Ragozzino K, Leutgeb S, Cooper BG, Kunz B, Mizumori SJY (2000) Firing correlates of anterior cingulate and medial precentral cortex neurons of the rat. Soc Neurosci Abstr 26: 473.

Hikosaka O, Nakahara H, Rand MK, Sakai K, Lu X, Nakamura K, Miyachi S, Doya K (1999) Parallel neural networks for learning sequential procedures. Trends Neurosci 22: 464–471.

Knierim JJ, Kudrimoti HS, McNaughton BL (1995) Place cells, head-direction cells, and the learning of landmark stability. J Neurosci 15: 1648–1659.

Lavoie AM, Mizumori SJY (1994) Spatial-, movement-, and reward-sensitive discharge by medial ventral striatum neurons of rats. Brain Res 638: 157–168.

Leutgeb S, Ragozzino KE, Mizumori SJY (2000) Convergence of head direction and place information in the CA1 region of hippocampus. Neurosci 100: 11–19.

Linden R, Perry VH (1983) Massive retinotectal projection in rats. Brain Res 272: 145–149.

Mizumori SJY, Cooper BG, Leutgeb S, Pratt WE (2000a) A neural systems analysis of adaptive navigation. Molec Neurobiol 21: 57–82.

Mizumori SJY, Miya DY, Ward KE (1994) Reversible inactivation of the lateral dorsal thalamus disrupts hippocampal place representation and impairs spatial learning. Brain Res 644: 168–174.

Mizumori SJY, Pratt WE, Ragozzino KE (1999a) Function of the nucleus accumbens within the context of the larger striatal system. Psychobiol 27: 214–224.

Mizumori SJY, Ragozzino KE, Cooper BG (2000b) Location and head direction representation in the dorsal striatum of rats. Psychobiol 28: 441–462.

Mizumori SJY, Ragozzino KE, Cooper BG, Leutgeb S (1999b) Hippocampal representational organization and spatial context. Hippocampus 9: 444–451.

Mizumori SJY, Williams JD (1993) Directionally-selective mnemonic properties of neurons in the lateral dorsal nucleus of the thalamus of rats. J Neurosci 13: 4015–4028.

Mogenson GJ, Jones DJ, Yim CY (1980) From motivation to action: functional interface between the limbic system and motor system. Prog Neurobiol 14: 69–97.

Muir GM, Taube JS (2002) The neural correlates of navigation: Do head direction and place cells guide spatial behavior? Behav Cog Neurosci Rev 1: 297–317.

Nadel, L, Wilner J (1980) Context and conditioning: a place for space. Physiol Psychol 8: 218–228.

Petersen SE, Robinson DL, Morris JD (1987) Contributions of the pulvinar to visual spatial attention. Neuropsychologia 25: 97–105.

Ragozzino KE, Leutgeb S, Mizumori SJY (2001) Dorsal striatal head direction and hippocampal place representations during spatial navigation. Exp Brain Res 139: 372–376.

Reep RL, Corwin JV (1999) Topographic organization of the striatal and thalamic connections of rat medial agranular cortex. Brain Res 841: 43–52.

Reep RL, Corwin JV, Hashimoto A, Watson RT (1984) Afferent connections of medial precentral cortex in the rat. Neurosci Lett 44: 247–252.

Reep RL, Corwin JV, Hashimoto A, Watson RT (1997) Efferent connections of the rostral portion of medial agranular cortex in rats. Brain Res Bull 19: 203–221.

Reep RL, Goodwin GS, Corwin JV (1990) Topographical organization in the corticocortical connections of medial agranular cortex in rats. J Comp Neurol 294: 262–280.

Schultz W, Tremblay L, Hollerman JR (2003) Changes in behavior-related neuronal activity in the striatum during learning. Trends Neurosci 26: 321–328.

Sefton AJ, Dreher B (1985) Visual system. In G Paxinos ed., The Rat Nervous System, vol 1, Forebrain and Midbrain. Sydney: Academic Press, pp. 169–221.

Sesack SR, Deutch AY, Roth RH, Bunney BS (1989) Topographical organization of the efferent projections of the medial prefrontal cortex in the rat: An anterograde tract-tracing study with *Phaseolus vulgaris* leucoagglutinin. J Comp Neurol 290: 213–242.

Sripanidkulchai K, Wyss JM (1986) Thalamic projections to retrosplenial cortex in the rat. J Comp Neurol 254: 143–165.

Stackman RW, Taube JS (1997) Firing properties of head-direction cells in the rat anterior thalamic nucleus: dependence on vestibular input. J Neurosci 17: 4349–4358.

Stackman RW, Taube JS (1998) Firing properties of rat lateral mammillary single units: head direction, head pitch, and angular head velocity. J Neurosci 18: 9020–9037.

Swanson LW, Kohler C (1986) Anatomical evidence for direct projections from the entorhinal area to the entire cortical mantle in the rat. J Neurosci 6: 3010–3023.

Taube JS (1995) Head direction cells recorded in the anterior thalamic nuclei of freely moving rats. J Neurosci 15: 70–86.

Taube JS (1995) Place cells recorded in the parasubiculum in freely-moving rats. Hippocampus 5: 569–593.

Taube JS (1998) Head direction cells and the neurophysiological basis for a sense of direction. Prog Neurobiol 55: 225–256.

Taube JS, Burton HL (1995) Head direction cell activity monitored in a novel environment during a cue conflict situation. J Neurophysiol 74: 1953–1971.

Taube JS, Goodridge JP, Golob EJ, Dudchenko PA, Stackman RW (1996) Processing the head direction cell signal: review and commentary. Brain Res Bull 40: 477–486.

Taube JS, Muller RU (1998) Comparisons of head direction cell activity in the postsubiculum and anterior thalamus of freely moving rats. Hippocampus 8: 87–108.

Taube JS, Muller RU, Ranck JB Jr (1990a) Head-direction cells recorded from the postsubiculum in freely moving rats: I. Description and quantitative analysis. J Neurosci 10: 420–435.

Taube JS, Muller RU, Ranck JB Jr (1990b) Head-direction cells recorded from the postsubiculum in freely moving rats: II. Effects of environmental manipulations. J Neurosci 10: 436–447.

Thompson SM, Robertson RT (1987a) Organization of subcortical pathways for sensory projections to the limbic cortex. I. Subcortical projections to the medial limbic cortex in the rat. J Comp Neurol 265: 175–188.

Thompson SM, Robertson RT (1987b) Organization of subcortical pathways for sensory projections to the limbic cortex. II. Afferent projections to the thalamic lateral dorsal nucleus in the rat. J Comp Neurol 265: 189–202.

Ungerleider LG, Christensen CA (1979) Pulvinar lesions in monkeys produce abnormal eye movements during visual discrimination training. Neuropsychologia 17: 493–501.

Van Groen T, Wyss JM (1990a) Connections of the retrosplenial granular a cortex in the rat. J Comp Neurol 300: 593–606.

Van Groen T, Wyss JM (1990b) The postsubicular cortex in the rat: Characterization of the fourth region of the subicular cortex and its connections. Brain Res 529: 165–177.

Van Groen T, Wyss JM (1992) Projections from the laterodorsal nucleus of the thalamus to the limbic and visual cortices in the rat. J Comp Neurol 324: 427–448.

Van Groen T, Wyss JM (1995) Projections from the anterodorsal and anteroventral nucleus of the thalamus to the limbic cortex in the rat. J Comp Neurol 358: 584–604.

Vogt BA, Miller MW (1983) Cortical connections between rat cingulate cortex and visual, motor, and postsubicular cortices. J Comp Neurol 216: 192–210.

Vogt BA, Sikes RW, Swadlow HA, Weyand TG (1986) Rabbit cingulate cortex: cytoarchitecture, physiological border with visual cortex, and afferent cortical connections of visual, motor, postsubicular, and intracingulate origin. J Comp Neurol 248: 74–94.

Wiener SI (1993) Spatial and behavioral correlates of striatal neurons in rats performing a self-initiated navigation task. J Neurosci 13: 3802–3817.

Zheng T, Wilson CJ (2002) Corticostriatal combinatorics: The implications of corticostriatal axonal arboriza-
tions. J Neurophysiol 87: 1007–1017.

Zilles K, Wree A (1995) Cortex: Areal and laminar structure. In G Paxinos ed., The Rat Nervous System, San
Diego, CA: Academic Press, pp. 649–685.

Zugaro MB, Berthoz A, Wiener SI (2002) Peak firing rates of rat anterodorsal thalamic head direction cells are
higher during faster passive rotations. Hippocampus 12: 481–486.

11 What Does the Head Direction Cell System Actually Do?

Paul A. Dudchenko, Gary M. Muir, Russell J. Frohardt, and Jeffrey S. Taube

The firing of head direction (HD) cells is one of the clearest, most robust, neural signals observed in the mammalian brain. As discussed in the preceding chapters, we know much about how the activity of these cells is controlled by cues in the animal's environment, and we are beginning to understand the critical circuitry underlying the processing of this signal. However, an obvious question with regard to this signal remains: what is its purpose? This chapter provides a review of the data on the relationship between head direction cells and behavior. (The interested reader may wish to consult Muir and Taube (2002) for a review that also addresses how place cells might guide behavior.) This chapter will be concerned primarily with electrophysiological studies. (A review of the behavioral effects of lesions to the HD cell system can be found in chapter 13 by Aggleton.) As the findings described in this chapter will show, although initial studies have demonstrated a clear relation between HD cells and behavior, recent work has shown that this link does not apply in all spatial tasks.

Before considering individual findings, we would like to note that the studies linking HD cells and behavior, and indeed hippocampal place cells and behavior, are correlational. That is, we, as experimenters, observe changes in the HD or place cell representation of an environment, and look for corresponding changes in the animal's behavior. The assumption underlying this approach is that such a correspondence is consistent with (but certainly does not prove) the notion that the HD cell system guides specific behaviors. On the other hand, a negative effect—a lack of correlation—provides strong evidence against the participation of this system in a given behavior. More direct means of testing the system by, for example, electrically stimulating individual neurons, may seem like an attractive alternative. However, given that HD cells are found in a variety of brain regions, a negative effect—a lack of change in behavior following stimulation of the HD cells in a particular brain region—would be quite difficult to interpret.

Of Rats and Mazes: Correlation between Head Direction Cells and Behavior

Since the first maze studies by Small (1901), many psychological studies have capitalized on the exceptional ability of rats to use spatial information to solve spatial tasks. Even in the early studies of Watson (1907) it was recognized that "the so-called 'sense of position' ('sense of direction') in this animal is extremely well marked" (p. 85). Lashley (1929) suggested that in learning to run a maze, rats developed "some central organization by which the sense of general direction can be maintained in spite of great variations of posture and of specific direction in running" (p. 138). Later work also provided evidence that rats use "spatial direction cues" when alternating on a T-maze (Douglas, 1966, p. 179). These behavioral observations, of course, were made well in advance of the discovery of head direction (HD) cells in the 1980s.

Does the HD cell system underlie a spatial direction sense? Surprisingly, only a few studies have addressed this question. The purpose of this chapter is to examine these data, first considering supporting evidence, then considering refuting evidence, and then attempting to reconcile the two. We will conclude with a brief discussion of related findings from experiments using disorientation.

An initial attempt to relate HD cells and spatial behavior is found in the study by Mizumori and Williams (1993), which describes HD cells in the lateral dorsal thalamus. In two animals, they observed an increase in the directionality of HD cells that correlated with a decrease in the number of mistakes made in learning a radial arm maze task.

In a more explicit study of the relationship between HD cells and behavior, Dudchenko and Taube (1997) trained rats to select a single reinforced maze arm on a plus- or radial-arm maze (comparable to the 1987 study by O'Keefe and Speakman of hippocampal place cells). The maze was curtained off from the remainder of the recording environment, and a white curtain occupying 48° of the black-curtained enclosure served as a salient visual landmark in the environment. The question these authors asked was, can a rat's behavior on the maze be predicted by the behavior of its HD cells?

To test this, once rats had learned to select readily the maze arm that contained reinforcement, the white "cue" curtain was rotated by 90° or 180° (in the absence of the rat). If this cue anchored the head direction cell system, then the preferred firing direction of individual HD cells would be expected to rotate by 90° or 180°. If the cue curtain also exerted stimulus control over the rats' spatial behavior, then the rats would be expected to choose an arm with a 90° or 180° orientation relative to the maze arm chosen prior to curtain rotation.

An example of the results from these manipulations can be seen in figure 11.1. Following training, the rat in this example reliably selected maze arm 1 on six consecutive trials, and then chose the opposite (180°) arm following the 180° rotation of the cue curtain (figure 11.1A). (On two trials the rats first entered the arm that they faced when placed on the center of the maze, before entering arm 5 on their second choice.) The firing of a HD

A   Behavior

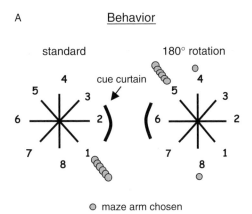

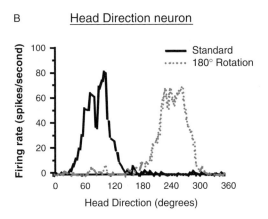

Figure 11.1

Correlation between head direction cell activity and behavior on the radial arm maze. (A) Maze arm choices (shown as dots) of a rat trained to select arm 1. Following a 180° rotation of the cue curtain, this rat selected maze arm 5, the arm with the same spatial relationship to the cue curtain as the trained arm; (B) The firing direction of an HD cell recorded during these trial also shifted by 180° during the curtain rotation trials. (From Dudchenko and Taube, 1997 with permission. Copyright American Psychological Association.)

cell during these maze choices is shown in figure 11.1B. As is evident in this figure, 180°
rotation of the cue curtain resulted in a corresponding rotation of the direction in which
this cell fired. Thus, the shift in the HD cell preferred direction correlated with the shift
in the rat's spatial behavior. Over both 90° and 180° rotations this correlation was robust
(r = .816; p < .01; cells were recorded in either the anterior dorsal thalamus or the postsubiculum of eight rats).

Although it is possible that these changes in HD cell preferred direction and spatial
behavior were independent, the observed correlation between the two is consistent with
the view that HD cells provide a directional framework that can be used to guide the rats'
spatial behavior. Subsequent studies, however, have suggested that this conclusion may
not apply to all spatial tasks.

A Lack of Correlation between Head Direction Cells and Spatial Behavior

An important study by Golob et al. (2001) has suggested that the link between HD cells
and spatial behavior is *not* universal. The authors used a spatial reference memory
task where they first trained water-deprived rats to run to one corner of a square, gray
box to receive a water reward. The rats were placed in the box at different entry points
for each trial. Different rats were trained to run to different corners, but for each rat the
correct (reinforced) corner of the box maintained a constant spatial relationship with a
white cue card mounted on one wall of the box. After the rats had learned to readily run
to the reinforced corner of the box (77% correct responses), they were given a probe
session in a rectangular box (see figure 11.2). This novel rectangular box was similar to
the square, gray box in that it also contained a white cue card, and the rat was also reinforced for choosing the corner that possessed the same spatial relationship with the cue
card.

The idea behind the experiment was as follows: previous work had shown that moving
a rat from a square to a rectangular apparatus causes HD cells to adopt a different pre-

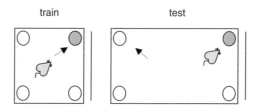

Figure 11.2
Schematic of the spatial task used by Golob et al. (2001). Rats were trained to find a reward in one corner of a
square box with a cue card (train, left figure). Upon being placed in a rectangle with a similar cue card (test,
right figure), the rats selected the corner of the apparatus with the same spatial relationship to the cue card, even
though their HD cells shifted to a different firing direction (arrows). Vertical bars in both figures indicate position of cue card from an overhead view. The shaded circle indicates the corner in which reward was available.

ferred direction (Taube et al., 1990). The question posed by Golob et al. was the following: If the preferred firing direction of HD cells shifts in the rectangle, will the corner that the rat chooses also shift a similar amount?

The surprising answer was "no." In 12 of 13 (92%) of the rectangle sessions, the HD cell's preferred firing direction shifted relative to the square. Most of these shifts were of at least 90°. The behavior of the rats, however, did not change. Rats selected the correct corner as accurately in the rectangle (78%) as they had in the square (77%). Moreover, the rats began choosing the correct corner in their first trials in the rectangle, suggesting that their spatial learning had generalized from the square.

A second experiment using a spatial working memory task produced a similar result. Golob et al. trained water-restricted rats on a delayed matching-to-position task in a rectangular apparatus. As before, the rectangle contained a white cue card and the animal's task on a given trial was to remember which corner was rewarded. Previous work with this task had shown that disoriented rats tend to use the shape of the environment, as opposed to visual landmarks, to guide their responses (Cheng, 1986; Margules and Gallistel, 1988). Thus, rats (and young children; Hermer and Spelke, 1994) tend not to distinguish between the correct corner of the rectangle and the corner located symmetrically opposite to this. That is to say, if a rat has been trained to go to a specific corner of a rectangular apparatus, it will use the shape of the apparatus, as opposed to a cue card, to guide its behavior.

In the Golob et al. study, after the sample phase of a trial, the rat was removed from the rectangle for a short delay. The rat was then replaced in the rectangle for the choice phase of the trial, in which its task was to remember which corner of the rectangle had provided a water reward. This task differed from the square → rectangle task previously described in that different corners were rewarded in different trial blocks. The authors found that the spatial relationship between the corner chosen by the rat and the firing direction of its HD cells was maintained on the choice phase in only 23 of 70 (33%) of the trials in which an HD cell was recorded. Thus, the rat's choice could not be predicted on the basis of its HD cells.

Interim Summary
The experiments of Golob et al. suggest that knowing the direction or change in preferred direction of individual HD cells does not allow one to predict a rat's spatial behavior in the square or rectangular chamber. Similar results have also been reported with hippocampal place cells (Jeffery et al., 2003). How can these results be reconciled with the strong correlation between HD cell-firing direction changes and maze arm choices observed by Dudchenko and Taube (1997)?

A necessary conclusion is that rats do not always make their choices using the same information that HD cells use to establish their firing directions. In the Dudchenko and Taube study, the radial maze did not possess a polarizing geometry. That is, there was nothing about the shape of the maze that provided information about which direction the rat was facing. Thus, the rats in this study may have been more inclined to use the only polarizing cue available, the white cue curtain, to anchor the HD cell system and to guide spatial responses. In contrast, in the square and rectangular apparatuses used by Golob et al., the geometry of the apparatus provided polarizing information in addition to the cue card. Thus, the HD cell system could at times anchor itself to one of the corners of the square or rectangle, instead of the cue card, even though the animal's behavior was guided by the other polarizing cue. Support for this view comes from the observations of Golob et al. that in the square apparatus (1) the preferred firing directions of HD cells occasionally rotated on baseline sessions even though the cue card was not moved, (2) the preferred firing direction appeared to rotate less reliably with rotation of the cue card, compared to similar experiments they conducted in a cylindrical chamber, and (3) shifts of the preferred firing directions were usually in multiples of 90°. Similarly, in the rectangle, HD cells maintained the same preferred direction across sample and choice trials only 56% of the time, even though the cue card was in the same place. These observations suggest that the cue card exerted much less stimulus control over the HD cell system in the square and rectangle than is typically observed in nongeometrically polarized environments such as the cylinder.[1]

The results of Golob et al. demonstrate that the HD cell system and the rats' spatial behavior are not tightly linked in all instances. The outstanding question then is, under what conditions, if any, is the HD cell system used? More recent work has attempted to address this issue, using different types of spatial tasks.

Do HD Cells Underlie Different Types of Spatial Behavior?

The Dudchenko and Taube (1997) and Golob et al. (2001) experiments used landmark navigation tasks that required associative learning, and found that HD cell orientation and behavior are not always coupled. However, in the absence of visual landmarks, rodents can make a spontaneous, direct return to a homesite following an excursion from that site (Etienne et al., 1988; Whishaw et al., 2001). It is thought that this ability is based on *path integration*—the integration of self-motion information provided by vestibular, kinesthetic, motor efference, and visual flow senses. There is also evidence that rats can maintain a sense of direction when they cross between different environments to solve a spatial task (Douglas, 1966; Dudchenko and Davidson, 2002). Finally, rats may be able to construct a cognitive map of an environment to take a "shortcut" to a goal location (Tolman et al., 1946). If such tasks depend on a stable direction sense then we might expect to find a tighter coupling between HD cell orientation and behavior. Next, we describe three experiments designed to test the relationship between the HD cell system and these types of spatial cognition.

Path Integration in the Circular Maze

One spatial task that appears to rely on path integration is the "food-carrying task" designed by Whishaw and Tomie (1997). The task is a modification of the original circular holeboard maze task of Barnes (1979) that required animals to escape into a "safe" escape hole on a circular platform that contained about 18 other blocked holes spaced evenly around its periphery. The task as originally designed by Barnes involved aversive avoidance, where rats tried to avoid bright lights by escaping down into the hole. Whishaw and colleagues modified this task by using appetitive reinforcement (comparable to experimental designs of Etienne et al., 1988). Their apparatus was similar to the circle-holeboard maze, but the rat started from a nesting box beneath one of the holes. It climbed through the hole onto the platform and explored until it located a large-sized food pellet placed in one of 10 to 15 small cups positioned randomly over the platform. The pellet was too large to be consumed quickly; the rats preferred to carry it back to the nest and consume it there. The task was frequently run in the dark or with a blindfold on the rats so that path integration was the only strategy the animals could use to keep track of their orientation and return to the nest directly. Thus, it is a good task for assessing whether HD cells underlie non-landmark-based navigation. Indeed, a recent study showed that animals with lesions of the anterior dorsal thalamic nucleus (ADN) had poor heading angles on their return to the nest in the blindfold version of this task, but not in the visual version when landmarks were available, suggesting that the ADN is critically involved in path integration (Frohardt et al., 2001).

In a preliminary study, Frohardt et al. (2002) modified the food-carrying task to make it compatible with single-unit recording. The 6-foot diameter platform was positioned in the center of an 8-foot diameter, floor-to-ceiling black curtain. A white curtain that subtended approximately 30° was attached to the inside of the black curtain along one side and served as the most prominent polarizing visual cue during light conditions. Instead of holes located around the periphery, there were eight evenly spaced doorways, with each doorway covered by a black curtain (figure 11.3A). Only one doorway led to the nesting box, while the other seven doorways were blocked with pieces of wood. Once the rats were proficient at the food-carrying task in the light, they were habituated to wearing blindfolds and further trained to perform the task without visual cues. Following training, proficiency was evaluated over the course of several days in both the visual and blindfolded versions of the task. Each rat then received an electrode implantation aimed at the ADN. Once the rats recovered from surgery, they were screened daily for HD cells in a standard cylinder that rested on top of the food-carrying apparatus in the same room. After an HD cell was identified, it was recorded first in the cylinder, then during four trials in the food-carrying task, and again back in the cylinder. Four types of sessions were conducted for the food-carrying task: (1) *standard*—four trials with the refuge in the original training position; (2) *blindfold*—identical to the standard session except the rat wore a blindfold, and an additional cylinder baseline session was recorded before the food-carrying session;

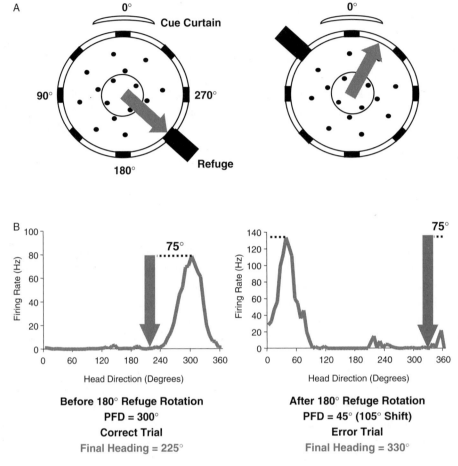

Figure 11.3
Consistency between the preferred firing direction of a head direction cell and the rat's behavioral choice after refuge rotation (A) Schematic of the food-carrying apparatus and the cue curtain located at 0°. Left: The refuge is initially located at 225° during the original training sessions. Right: The refuge and rat are rotated 180° prior to the start of the rotation session. The arrows indicate the rat's final heading during a correct trial (left) and an incorrect trial (right). (B) Corresponding firing rate vs. head direction plots from a head direction cell recorded during the sessions shown in *A*. Left graph: Correct trial. The final path heading of the rat (arrow) and the HD cell's preferred firing direction are 75° apart. Right graph: Error trial following 180° rotation of the refuge. The preferred firing direction of the HD cell shifted 105° CCW instead of 180°. Note, however, that the final path heading of the rat (arrow) and the HD cell's preferred firing direction remained 75° apart. PFD, preferred direction.

(3) *dark*—identical to the blindfold session except darkness (room lights out) was substituted for the blindfold, and (4) *rotation*—identical to standard, except the refuge was moved to a position either 90° or 180° from the original training position, relative to the room and curtain. The purpose of the blindfold and dark sessions was to determine the rat's performance and how HD cells respond in a task that must be solved using only path integration. In contrast, the purpose of the rotation sessions was to determine under lit conditions which cues were controlling the cell's preferred firing direction and guiding the animal's behavior—allothetic cues (i.e., the cue curtain) or idiothetic/other intramaze cues. Rotations were conducted with the rat outside the apparatus, between the baseline cylinder session and the first trial of the food-carrying task session. For each rotation session there were four trials in which we monitored the cell(s) as the rat searched for and retrieved a food pellet. There was no attempt to disorient the rat or prevent it from observing the refuge rotation in most cases; however, in cases when the rotations occurred with the rat in another room, there was no difference in the amount the preferred firing direction shifted compared to sessions when the rat was present during the rotation. Returning to the wrong doorway was counted as an error, and the angular displacement from the correct doorway was recorded. Errors were scored and the firing properties of HD cells were monitored during each session.

HD cell recordings in the food-carrying task provided interesting insights into how rats use HD cells for navigation. First, HD cells did not shift their preferred firing direction between the baseline cylinder sessions and the food-carrying sessions for the standard, blindfold, or dark conditions, but did shift during the Rotation condition. The amount of shift in the preferred firing direction in the rotation session usually corresponded to the amount the refuge position was moved from the training position (e.g., 90° or 180°), suggesting that under light conditions the HD cells were using the refuge as a landmark for orientation. Second, the rats rarely made errors during the food-carrying task while an HD cell was being recorded. On trials when the rat returned to the correct doorway, the cell's preferred firing direction usually did not shift, and was therefore consistent with the choice behavior of the rat (standard: 89%, blindfold: 100%, dark: 100%, rotation: 90%). However, during trials in which the rat made an error the cell's preferred firing direction usually did *not* shift to correspond to the behavioral choice; for example, if the animal returned to a doorway that was located 90° clockwise (CW) from the correct doorway, the preferred firing direction of the recorded HD cell did *not* shift 90° CW. Thus, the rat made a behavioral error, even though HD cell discharge remained constant compared to previous trials. The percentage of error trials in which the HD cell's preferred firing direction shifted a similar amount as the behavioral choice were as follows: standard: 14%, blindfold: 0%, dark: 0%, rotation: 17%. These results again demonstrate that the animal's behavioral response is not always coupled with the spatial information encoded by the HD cell network.

Some evidence of a relationship between the HD cell system and path integration was found, however, in the initial errors made following rotation of the refuge. As previously mentioned, the preferred firing direction of an HD cell would often rotate 180° if the refuge (and hence the starting point) was moved 180° opposite from the original training position, and in these cases the rat's choice behavior was similar to the other conditions (i.e., errors were rare). However, in a number of sessions the preferred firing direction did not shift completely with the amount of rotation of the refuge (i.e., underrotation). In these sessions, the rat made an error on the first one or two trials of the four-trial session, and in each case it made the behavioral error in a direction consistent with the amount of underrotation of the HD cell's preferred firing direction. Figure 11.3B shows one such example. In this case, the cell had an initial preferred firing direction of 300° and the rat's directional heading upon selecting a doorway was 225°, which was 75° CW from the cell's preferred firing direction. Following a 180° rotation of the refuge, the cell's preferred firing direction shifted by only 105°. However, the final directional heading of the rat as it approached the periphery to make a door choice *also* shifted by 105°. Thus, the final directional heading of the rat could be predicted by the shift in the cell's preferred firing direction.

This subset of results is consistent with the view that shifts in the preferred firing direction of the HD cell signal may initially guide a rat's choice behavior when it perceives a change in the surrounding environment, and if the preferred firing direction of the HD cell is misdirected, then the choice behavior is misdirected as well (figure 11.4). However, it was also found that, once the rat began making rotationally correct choices (i.e., choices oriented 180° relative to the initial doorway), the cell's preferred firing direction did not shift, and remained relatively stable throughout the four-trial session. One possibility is that, after the rat has selected the incorrect (and closed) doors, it started choosing other doors on subsequent trials, without a shift in its HD cell orientation.

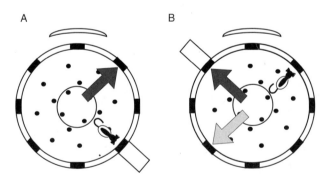

Figure 11.4
Relationship between the preferred firing direction and errant choice in a rotation session. The white cue curtain remained fixed between the initial standard session (A) and the subsequent rotation session (B), while the refuge was rotated 180° from the standard position. (A) During the standard session the preferred firing direction of the HD cell (dark gray arrow) was anchored ~90° relative to the behavioral choice of the rat (doorway to the refuge). (B) During the first trial of the 180° refuge rotation the preferred firing direction of the HD cell shifted by only 90° (dark gray arrow) instead of the full 180° (light gray arrow). The rat's behavior (as shown) appeared to correlate with the shift in the firing direction of its HD cells, and not the shift in the refuge location.

It is worth considering the behavioral steps involved between the rat's perception of the cue on a rotation trial and the moment the rat makes a navigational choice. During rotation trials shortly after the rat emerged from the refuge, the preferred firing direction of the HD cell shifted some amount. If the amount of shift nearly matched the amount of refuge rotation (i.e., 180° for both), the rat did not make a behavioral error. If, however, the preferred firing direction underrotated (e.g., 90° cell rotation for a 180° refuge rotation), then the rat made one, or two, behavioral mistakes in the direction indicated by the information encoded by the HD cell, that is, to the place where the refuge should have been, as indicated by the underrotated HD cell, two doors away from the real refuge (figure 11.4). After the error(s) were made, there appeared to be a sudden realization that something was amiss, and on subsequent trials the rat made the correct choice. Nonetheless, this change in behavioral response did not affect the preferred firing direction of the recorded HD cell, which remained stable across all the rotation trials. It appears that the problem during the error trials was a combination of two processes: (1) the HD cell's preferred firing direction was not correctly anchored to the extra-maze cue curtain once the rat left the refuge (i.e., the HD cell was registering the cue as west instead of south), and (2) the HD cell's preferred firing direction had shifted from its original orientation in the refuge, therefore, the rat followed the errant HD cell system signal on its return trip. It is unlikely that the error was the result of the HD cell network incorrectly guiding the rat's behavior because the information provided by the HD cell network appeared to initially guide the navigational choice on the first couple of trials.

The Maintenance of a Sense of Direction across Environments by the HD Cell System

A second experiment was designed to test whether the HD cells system might allow the rat to use spatial information across two environments. This experiment (Dudchenko and Zinyuk, 2002) was based on the ability of rats to alternate directions on a T-maze. In this maze, a rat is typically given two consecutive runs from the base of the T, and there is a strong tendency for the animal to select different arms of the T on each run. Rats will do this even without training; this behavior is known as spontaneous alternation.

In an intriguing set of experiments, Douglas (1966) attempted to find out what cues the rats used to remember which arm of the T they had entered on their first run. To preclude the use of any olfactory or local cues, he gave rats their second run on a separate T-maze located in a different room. In doing this, Douglas made a striking observation: rats would alternate reliably when the two T-mazes were oriented in the same direction, but alternated at chance levels when the mazes were oriented in different directions relative to each other. This suggests that the rats were not simply making alternate egocentric responses (e.g., left on one maze, then right on the other), because this would be successful regardless of the second maze's orientation. Rather, Douglas concluded that the rats must be alternating arms based on a sense of direction that was carried across environments. This strategy would allow the rats to alternate when the mazes were parallel to one another, but would be insufficient when the mazes were in a different orientation.

To test whether the HD cell system could be the basis for this directional sense, Dudchenko and Zinyuk (2002) recorded from HD cells on T-mazes located in adjacent environments. The data shown in figure 11.5 are examples from one rat, and the results were consistent across subjects.

As is evident in figure 11.5A, when the rat was carried from a T-maze in one environment to a parallel T-maze in a second environment, the preferred direction of an HD cell was maintained. In figure 11.5B, however, it is clear the when the T-maze in the second room was rotated by 90°, the direction of the cell shifted by 90°. Thus, the HD cell was anchored to the maze and was not maintaining a sense of direction across environments. This result would be inconsistent with the hypothesis that the HD cell system underlies alternation across environments. However, alternation performance levels were low in both the parallel and perpendicular maze recording trials, so it is difficult to draw a firm conclusion about the relationship between HD cells and alternation across mazes.

The apparent anchoring of the HD cell system to the T-mazes raises an additional question: Why did the HD cells not carry their preferred directions across environments? In this study, no attempt was made to disorient the animals as they were carried from one T-maze to the other. Indeed, they were carried between these mazes in a shallow, clear plastic container. One possibility is that the reliable shifts in the cell's preferred direction to agree with the orientation of the second T-maze is an indication that familiar landmarks exert much more stimulus control over the HD cell system than does self-motion information (Dudchenko and Zinyuk, 2003).

HD Cells and the Tolman Sunburst Maze

In a recent experiment, Muir and Taube (2004) tested whether the information provided by the HD system was used to guide behavior in a navigational task requiring a cognitive mapping strategy. The firing properties of ADN and postsubicular (PoS) HD cells were recorded as rats performed a navigational task based on the classic "sunburst" maze study of Tolman et al. (1946). By training animals on a fixed maze configuration, then altering the maze by blocking the old route to the reward and introducing a new route, Tolman was able to demonstrate that rats could use a previously unavailable shortcut to reach a goal. This was seen as critical evidence to support the notion that animals possess an internal representation of space, or "cognitive map," that can be used by the animal while navigating. Muir and Taube adapted Tolman's maze by reducing the number of novel maze arms available from 18 to 8 to increase the angular difference between arms, and by removing the light from above the goal location which may have acted as a beacon in the original study.

Once trained on a maze configuration (e.g., figure 11.6A), animals ran three additional training trials along the elevated maze route in the same configuration to locate a water

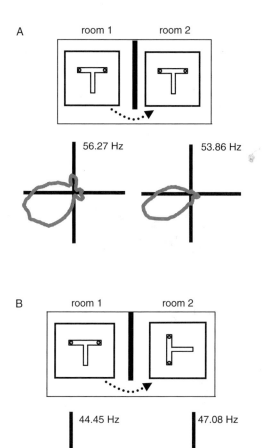

Figure 11.5
An anterior thalamic HD cell recorded across T-mazes in adjacent environments. This HD cell maintained a constant firing direction across environments when the T-mazes were parallel (A), but not when the mazes were perpendicular to one another (B) (Dudchenko and Zinyuk, 2002). The polar plots are in the absolute reference frame of the room.

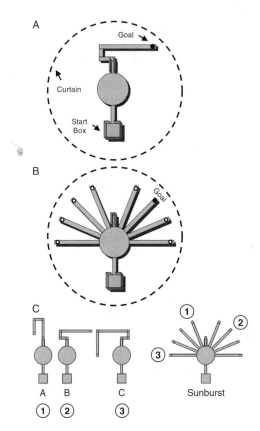

Figure 11.6
(A) An example of a maze configuration used during training trials. (B) The sunburst maze configuration. Note that the goal is in the same spatial location in the room as in A. (C) Each training maze used has a differ- ent path that is associated with a different correct shortcut arm (shortest path) on the sunburst trial, as shown on the numbered arms of the sunburst configuration on the right. (Reproduced from Muir and Taube, 2004, with permission.)

reward in a fixed location. The maze was enclosed within a black circular curtain through- out training and testing. Training trials began with an initial period during which animals were confined to the start box, followed by a period when the animal had access to the maze. Upon reaching the goal, the animal was returned to the start box and a lid placed over it for a delay. These three training trials were followed by a sunburst trial in which the normal route to the reward was blocked and eight novel routes introduced; one being a direct path (shortcut) to the reward's previous location (figure 11.6B). Animals that can utilize an accurate cognitive map of the environment should have been able to use the novel shortcut route to reach the reward. Once a sunburst trial was completed, the animal began training on a new maze configuration (figure 11.6C) with a different arm as the "correct" shortcut. For each configuration, data from the three training trials were combined and compared to data from the sunburst trial to determine the amount of shift in the cell's preferred firing direction.

The results showed that throughout the sunburst trial, the preferred direction of both ADN and PoS HD cells remained stable relative to the training trials and was not related to the accuracy of the behavioral choice(s) made by the animal. For example, when one animal was exposed to the sunburst maze for the first time and correctly selected the novel shortcut to the rewarded arm, the preferred firing direction of its HD cell did not shift, compared to the training trials on the first maze (figure 11.7A). Similarly, another animal that made seven errors before selecting the correct arm showed stable HD cell activity across trials on the maze, both compared to the training trials and to the sunburst trial (figure 11.7B). Overall, the preferred firing direction of HD cells on the sunburst maze was shifted, on average, by less than 1° (figure 11.7C) from that seen during the training trials, while animals averaged 5.5 errors (range: 0–25) per sunburst trial.

Additional probe trials conducted on cells by rotating the maze 180° relative to the room showed that the firing of the HD cells was related to the orientation of the maze and not the room, suggesting that the animals were using the maze as an orienting cue. If animals were indeed using the maze as a cue to orient by, and given that the central platform of the maze and the start box, in particular, remained constant from the training trials to the sunburst trials, it is not surprising that the HD cell activity also remained unaltered from training to sunburst trials. Although the animals may have lacked sufficient experience with the novel "sunburst" component of the task to perform well, one animal that experienced the sunburst maze nine times consistently showed HD cell activity unrelated to its behavioral choice across all nine sunburst trials. The results clearly show that HD cell activity, at least in the PoS and ADN, remained robust throughout all phases of the task, independently of whether the animal performed well or poorly. This finding stands in contrast to the results reported by Mizumori and Williams (1993), who suggested that HD cells in the LDN developed a more robust directional signal as an animal learned the task. However, these data are consistent with those of Golob et al. (2001): the animal may have reliably encoded directional information about its orientation upon entry into the environment, but this information may not necessarily have been used to guide the animal's navigation to a goal.

A Digression: the Head Direction Cell System and Disorientation

HD Cells and Landmark Learning
We have seen that in a nonpolarized apparatus such as the radial arm maze, the same extramaze cue—a white curtain—can exert stimulus control over the rats' spatial behavior and the preferred firing direction of their HD cells. In this type of situation, how do landmarks in the environment come to anchor the preferred firing direction of HD cells? One hypothesis is that this stimulus control is the result of a learned association between visual

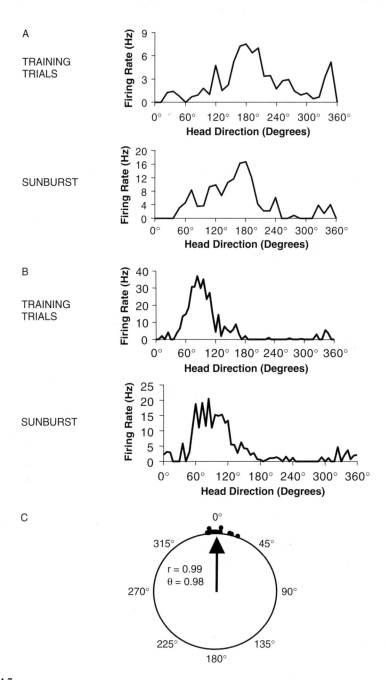

Figure 11.7
(A) On this sunburst trial, the animal chose the correct shortcut arm on the first choice, and the preferred firing direction (although less clear due to the low firing rate and short sampling times for this cell) remains stable from the training trials to the sunburst trial. (B) The preferred firing direction of this ADN HD cell was unaltered from the training trials to the sunburst trial, during which the animal made seven errors before choosing the correct shortcut arm. This HD cell stability was consistent for the duration the animal was on the maze. (C) Distribution of shifts in the preferred firing direction of HD cells from training trials (=0°) to the sunburst trial. The shift for each given cell is shown as a filled circle on the outside of the unit circle with degrees marked. As is apparent, the average amount of shift was negligible (~1°), with very little angular deviation observed. r, mean vector length; θ, mean phase angle. (Reproduced from Muir and Taube, 2004, with permission.)

landmarks, and a sense of orientation derived from self-motion cues (McNaughton et al., 1991, 1996).

Empirical support for this view came from an experiment conducted by Knierim et al. (1995; also see chapter 8 by Knierim). They sought to break the link between the rat's sense of orientation and a cue card in a cylinder by repeatedly disorienting the rat before it was placed in the cylinder and after it was removed. Disorientation took the form of gentle rotation of the rat in an opaque container as the experimenter approached the cylinder. The authors observed that HD cells and hippocampal place cells in rats that had been repeatedly disoriented were less likely to be anchored to the cue card in the cylinder. This weakening of the cue control appeared to persist even when the disoriented rats were subsequently trained under nondisorientation conditions.

As Knierim et al. suggest, this result is slightly counterintuitive: one might expect that a disoriented rat would be more, not less, likely to derive its orientation from a stable visual landmark. Indeed, in other studies (using a different strain of rats), disorientation prior to recording appeared to have less effect on the stimulus control of a visual landmark over the preferred firing direction of HD cells and the place fields of hippocampal place cells (Taube, 1995; Dudchenko et al., 1997b; Golob and Taube, 1997). However, the results of Knierim et al. would imply that disoriented rats would have difficulty learning to use extra-maze landmarks to guide their spatial behavior.

To test this, Dudchenko et al. (1997a) trained disoriented and nondisoriented rats on a landmark-based, eight-arm radial maze task. The maze was curtained off from the remainder of the environment, and a white curtain served as the sole extra-maze landmark available to the rats. A single maze arm contained a water reward, and the rat's task was to reliably select this arm when placed on the center of the maze. Although seven out of eight animals in one of the nondisoriented groups learned the task, none of the eight disoriented animals learned it.

This behavioral result supports the view that landmarks are learned by their association with a stable internal sense of orientation. One would predict, then, that rats should be impaired on any type of landmark-based task when they are first disoriented prior to the task. However, this prediction appears not to be the case. Both in the Dudchenko et al. study, and a study done at the same time by Martin et al. (1997), disoriented rats readily learned to use a landmark to solve a Morris water-maze task. This interaction between disorientation and type of spatial task—aversive versus appetitive—has also been replicated in landmark navigation tasks in a circular arena (Gibson et al., 2001) and a rectangular pool (Golob and Taube, 2002). In addition, disoriented rats can learn to solve an aversive plus maze task (Hynes et al., 2000).

Interim Summary

The stimulus control of visual landmarks over HD cell preferred firing appears to be learned, and learned relatively quickly, within a minute or two (see chapter 3 by Taube).

Disruption of this association by disorientation weakens this stimulus control in some situations, and results in a clear impairment in the use of landmarks to guide spatial behavior in appetitive spatial tasks. Why landmarks can be learned by disoriented animals when they are placed in aversively motivated tasks, remains an open question. However, one implication of this dissociation is that, in the disoriented rat, neural systems in addition to the HD cell and place cell systems can be used to guide spatial behavior when escape from an aversive condition is required. In support of this notion, recent work in *Drosophila* shows that there are two independent neurotransmitter systems for learning appetitive (octopamine) and aversive (dopamine) olfactory tasks (Schwaerzel et al., 2003).

Disorientation and HD Cell Activity   The issue of behavioral disorientation raises the question: What are the neural correlates for disorientation? How do HD cells respond when an animal is behaviorally (or perceptually) disoriented? Do HD cells lose their direction-specific firing? If so, do the cells become completely quiescent (i.e., total absence of discharge) or is there a tonic rate of firing that is elevated above background firing levels? Understanding the neural correlates of disorientation is also important in the context of the three-dimensional locomotion experiments described in chapter 3 by Taube. These experiments showed that when the rat locomoted on the ceiling in 1 g, or on the wall or ceiling in 0 g, there was a loss of direction-specific firing (Calton et al., 2000; Taube et al., 2004). Were these animals "perceptually" disoriented at the same time? A better understanding of the neural correlates underlying spatial disorientation would help to resolve this issue.

Three forms of spatial disorientation have been identified in humans (Gillingham and Previc, 1996). Type I spatial disorientation involves a misperception of one's orientation and is unrecognized by the observer. Assuming the activity of HD cells reflects the sense of direction of the animal, direction-specific firing of HD cells would presumably be maintained in this situation, albeit at an incorrect orientation with respect to the environment. Type II spatial disorientation entails a conscious recognition by the subject that he or she is disoriented and attempts are then made to become oriented by using any available information. Type III spatial disorientation occurs when the subject becomes so disoriented that he or she is incapacitated. This type of spatial disorientation can occur when the subject is experiencing rapid and continual rotations that lead to confusion, or when the subject experiences severe motion sickness or oscillopsia that makes it difficult to override these compelling conditions. In contrast to type I spatial disorientation, types II and III spatial disorientation would be expected to lead to a disruption of normal HD cell discharge. Indeed, type I spatial disorientation would more appropriately be labelled a "misorientation" rather than disorientation. The type of disorientation that is relevant to the questions posed here is most closely associated with types II or III.

Knierim et al. (1998) reported that HD cell firing occasionally (2 out of 10 cases) became "erratic, firing with no directional specificity" when rats were spun continuously in one direction (unidirectional) on a rotating pedestal in the dark. While continuing to spin the rats, cell firing was also described as erratic in 6 out of 10 cases when the lights were turned back on and the animal could view a prominent landmark within the room. Erratic cell firing was also occasionally observed (5 out of 16 cases) after some time when rats were spun irregularly back-and-forth (bidirectional) for several minutes. The erratic discharge observed in these cells could best be described as cell firing that occurred in many different directions, although detailed analyses over small time intervals was not conducted. It should be noted that these experiments were conducted on Fischer-344 rats, animals that are thought to have poor vision (Munn, 1950). This fact may have contributed to the poor control the landmark exerted over cell firing once the lights were turned back on.

To address this issue more extensively, Steven and Taube (2002) spun Long-Evans rats back and forth on a turntable while recording HD cell responses. Long-Evans rats have better visual capacities than Fischer-344 rats (Munn, 1950). In addition, cell firing was analyzed with a greater temporal resolution than in the Knierim et al. study. The animals were either blindfolded and spun in the dark, or were spun without blindfolds in the light with a prominent visual cue that has been shown to exert control over HD cell preferred firing directions. Spinning speeds were either slow (approx. 90°/s) or fast (approx. 240°s). The results were quite clear. When rats were spun under blindfold conditions at either slow or fast speeds, HD cells quickly lost their direction-specific firing within one to two revolutions and cell activity varied between states of increased tonic firing at all head directions to total quiescence (figure 11.8). In contrast, when rats were spun without blindfolds in the light, direction-specific firing was maintained and the cells' preferred directions remained in alignment with the prominent visual cue.

These results raise the interesting chicken and egg question: Which comes first? Do the HD cells lose their direction-specific firing and therefore the animal perceives that it is disoriented? Or, does the animal become disoriented as a result of the rotary stimulation, and therefore HD cells lose their direction-specific firing? Of course, the answer to this question is not clear from these experiments, but one would like to think that the neural circuitry responsible for detecting angular velocity was not capable of following the constant irregular rotary stimulation. This incapacity then led to erroneous signals being passed on to the HD cell network, which in turn resulted in the loss of direction-specific discharge. The readout from the HD cell network thus did not provide accurate information concerning directional heading, and the animal would subsequently perceive itself to be disoriented. Alternatively, it is also possible that circuitry outside the HD cell network might have been disrupted by the rotary stimulation, and this disruption in turn would have led to erroneous signals being passed onto the HD cell network. To distinguish these possibilities, future experiments might test whether it is possible to dissociate HD cell discharge from the perception of disorientation. For example, can conditions be created where either (1) HD cell activity is disrupted without the animal perceiving that it is disoriented?

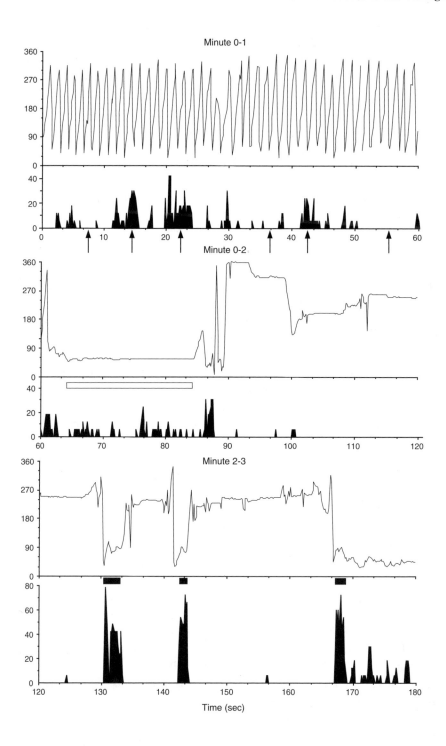

or (2) where the animal perceives itself to be disoriented despite normal HD cell discharge? If it proves impossible to create either of these conditions, then this result would support the notion that the loss of direction-specific firing is the neural correlate of perceived disorientation.

Secondary Correlates of HD Cells on the Radial-Arm Maze

A number of previous studies have shown that hippocampal place cells contain additional, nonspatial neuronal correlates when tested under the right conditions (e.g., West et al., 1981; Berger et al., 1983; Breese et al., 1989; Wiener et al., 1989; Young et al., 1994; Wood et al., 2000). For example, Wiener et al. (1989) demonstrated that place cell firing can be correlated to more than one behavioral or spatial event, depending on the type of behavioral task the animal is performing. Consequently, one might ask whether HD cells show nonspatial correlates when also tested under the right conditions. The limited work that has addressed this issue has not shown any evidence for such activity, at least in ADN HD cells. Dudchenko and Taube (1997) recorded eight HD cells on the radial-arm maze task and explicitly looked for activity that was modulated by the rat's behavior other than directional heading. Specifically, they looked for evidence of goal-approach or reward-consumption correlates in HD cell activity as the rat travelled down a reinforced arm and consumed a water reward at the end of the arm. The activity that was observed was always related to the rat's head direction, and this activity did not appear to be modulated by the approach to or consummation of the reward. Thus, in contrast to place cells, there was no evidence that ADN HD cell firing was modulated by the rat's behavior other than directional heading in this spatial reference memory task.

What Does the Head Direction Cell System Do?

The clear, robust activity of HD cells would appear to make this neural system an ideal substrate for spatial cognition. However, attempts to link the behavior of HD cells to the

Figure 11.8
Firing rate and head direction by time plot of a HD cell for a 3-minute session. During the first minute (top graph), a blindfolded rat was spun clockwise continuously on a turntable at approximately 270°/s. Direction-specific firing was lost, and cell firing could be characterized as either silent (black-filled arrows) or increased tonic, background firing (open arrows). After 1 minute the platform rotation was stopped and the rat was free to move around for 2 minutes to retrieve small pellets that were randomly dropped onto the floor of the platform (middle and bottom graphs). Direction-specific firing returned quickly with a preferred firing direction at 78°. Note that when the rat's head was pointing in the preferred firing direction, firing rate peaked at about 80 spikes/s (black-filled bars, bottom graph). When the rat maintained a head direction for about 16 sec that pointed about 20° clockwise of the cell's preferred firing direction (open bar, middle graph), the cell fired constantly at a rate below the peak firing rate. Firing rates during the first minute when the rat was spun never approached the level of peak firing during nonrotation conditions, although the cell occasionally fired at a relatively high rate for several seconds before going through subsequent silent periods.

rat's spatial behavior have been only partially successful. Although a correlation between HD cells and behavior was observed by Dudchenko and Taube (1997), and to an extent by Frohardt et al. (2002), studies by Golob et al. (2001), and Muir and Taube (2004) show a clear lack of correlation. Importantly, a similar lack of correlation has also been seen in hippocampal place cells (Jeffery et al., 2003).

What, then, does the head direction system do? It seems likely that the HD cell system, like the place cell system, can use different types of cues to orient relative to an environment. In environments that do not possess a polarizing layout, such as the cylinder or radial maze, a polarizing cue (such as a cue card) will control the direction in which HD cells fire. If such a cue is not available or is ambiguous, as in the blindfold and dark trials on the circular maze of Frohardt et al., HD cells may anchor themselves to the point from which the rat enters the environment. However, in environments such as a square, rectangle, T-maze, or sunburst maze, the shape of the environment itself is a strong cue that can "anchor" the HD cell system. Thus, the likelihood that the HD cell system and the animal's spatial behavior are related depends on the aspect of the environment to which the spatial behavior is oriented. If, for example, a rat is trained to find a goal location that is defined by a spatial association with a cue card, the likelihood that this cue card will also anchor the rat's HD cell system depends on the shape of the environment. HD cells may automatically orient to particular aspects of the environment, such as a corner; rats, on the other hand, may be trained to make spatial associations with other cues in an environment.

A stronger test of the capacity of the HD cell system to guide behavior would require that the rat make a spatial response based on this system. As has been done with hippocampal place cells (O'Keefe and Speakman, 1987), this may be tested by assessing rats in an environment that lacks directional landmarks, and observing that the behavior can be predicted by the direction in which a given HD cell fires. The circular maze of Frohardt et al. is an attempt to do this, although the rats' HD cell systems appeared to anchor themselves to the start locations. Tests in which the HD cell system shifts from trial to trial, and in which a corresponding shift in the animal's spatial behavior is observed, would provide support for a role of this system in guiding spatial behavior.

Note

1. The relative influence of landmarks versus the geometry of the environment in controlling spatial behavior may present a challenge to traditional learning theory. Recent results by Pearce et al. (2001) and Hayward et al. (2003) suggest that the shape of the environment is not overshadowed or blocked by landmarks.

References

Barnes CA (1979) Memory deficits associated with senescence: A neurophysiological and behavioral study in the rat. J Comp Physiol Psychol 93: 74–104.

Berger TW, Rinaldi PC, Weisz DJ, Thompson RF (1983) Single-unit analysis of different hippocampal cell types during classical conditioning of rabbit nictitating membrane response. J Neurophys 50: 1197–1219.

Breese CR, Hampson RE, Deadwyler SA (1989) Hippocampal place cells: Stereotypy and plasticity. J Neurosci 9: 1097–1111.

Calton JL, Tullman ML, Taube JS (2000) Head direction cell activity in the anterodorsal thalamus during upside-down locomotion. Soc Neurosci Abstr 26: 983.

Cheng K (1986) A purely geometric module in the rat's spatial representation. Cogn 23: 149–178.

Douglas RJ (1966) Cues for spontaneous alternation. J Comp Phys Psychol 62: 171–183.

Dudchenko PA, Davidson M (2002) Rats use a sense of direction to alternate on T-mazes located in adjacent rooms. Animal Cogn 5: 115–118.

Dudchenko PA, Goodridge JP, Seiterle DA, Taube JS (1997a) Effects of repeated disorientation on the acquisition of spatial tasks in rats: dissociation between the appetitive radial arm maze and aversive water maze. J Exp Psychol: Anim Behav Proc 23: 194–210.

Dudchenko PA, Goodridge JP, Taube JS (1997b) The effects of disorientation on visual landmark control of head direction cell orientation. Exp Brain Res 115: 375–380.

Dudchenko P, Taube JS (1997) Correlation between head-direction single unit activity and spatial behavior on a radial arm maze. Behav Neurosci 111: 3–19.

Dudchenko PA, Zinyuk LE (2002) Head direction cell orientation after cue card separation, and after transport between two mazes. Soc Neurosci Abstr 28: 584.5.

Dudchenko PA, Zinyuk LE (2003) Do head direction cells rely more on landmarks than path integration when a rat walks between environments? Soc Neurosci Abstr 29: 91.2.

Etienne AS, Maurer R, Saucy F (1988) Limitations in the assessment of path dependent information. Behaviour 106: 81–111.

Frohardt RJ, Marcroft JL, Taube JS (2001) Lesions of the anterior thalamus impair path integration performance on a food-carrying task. Soc Neurosci Abstr 27: 315.11.

Frohardt RJ, Marcroft JL, Taube JS (2002) Do head direction cells guide spatial navigation in rats? An electrophysiological investigation in a path integration task. Soc Neurosci Abstr 28: 584.1.

Gibson BM, Shettleworth SJ, McDonald RJ (2001) Finding a goal on dry land and in the water: differential effects of disorientation on spatial learning. Behav Brain Res 123: 103–111.

Gillingham KK, Previc FH (1996) Spatial orientation in flight. In R Dehard ed., Fundamentals of Aerospace Medicine. 2nd ed. Baltimore: Williams and Wilkins, pp. 309–397.

Golob EJ, Taube JS (1997) Head direction cells and episodic spatial information in rats without a hippocampus. Proc Nat Acad Sci USA 94: 7645–7650.

Golob EJ, Taube JS (2002) Differences between appetitive and aversive reinforcement on reorientation in a spatial working memory task. Behav Brain Res 136: 309–316.

Golob EJ, Stackman RW, Wong AC, Taube JS (2001) On the behavioral significance of head direction cells: neural and behavioral dynamics during spatial memory task. Behav Neurosci 115: 285–304.

Hayward A, McGregor A, Good MA, Pearce JM (2003) Absence of overshadowing and blocking between landmarks and the geometric cues provided by the shape of the test arena. Quart J Exp Psychol 56B: 114–126.

Hermer L, Spelke ES (1994) A geometric process for spatial reorientation in young children. Nature 370: 57–59.

Hynes CA, Martin GW, Harley CW, Huxter JR, Evans JH (2000) Multiple points of entry into a circular enclosure prevent place learning despite normal vestibular orientation and cue arrays: evidence for map resetting. J Exp Psychol: Anim Behav Proc 26: 64–73.

Jeffery KJ, Gilbert A, Burton S, Studwick A (2003) Preserved performance in a hippocampal-dependent spatial task despite complete place cell remapping. Hippocampus 13: 175–189.

Knierim JJ, Kudrimoti HS, McNaughton BL (1995) Place cells, head direction cells, and the learning of landmark stability. J Neurosci 15: 1648–1659.

Knierim JJ, Kudrimoti HS, McNaughton BL (1998) Interactions between idiothetic cues and external landmarks in the control of place cells and head direction cells. J Neurophys 80: 425–446.

Lashley KS (1929) Brain mechanisms and intelligence. Chicago: University of Chicago Press.

Margules J, Gallistel CR (1988) Heading in the rat: Determination by environmental shape. Anim Learn Behav 16(4): 404–410.

Martin GW, Harley CW, Smith AR, Hoyles SE, Hynes CA (1997) Spatial disorientation blocks reliable goal location on a plus maze but does not prevent goal location in the Morris maze. J Exp Psychol: Anim Behav Proc 23: 183–193.

McNaughton BL, Chen LL, Markus EJ (1991) "Dead Reckoning," landmark learning, and the sense of direction; a neurophysiological and computational hypothesis. J Cogn Neurosci 3: 190–201.

McNaughton BL, Barnes CA, Gerrard JL, Gothard K, Jung MW, Knierim JJ, Kudrimoti H, Qin Y, Skaggs WE, Suster M, Weaver KL (1996) Deciphering the hippocampal polyglot: the hippocampus as a path integration system. J Exp Biol 199: 173–185.

Mizumori SJY, Williams JD (1993) Directionally selective mnemonic properties of neurons in the lateral dorsal nucleus of the thalamus of rats. J Neurosci 13: 4015–4028.

Muir GM, Taube JS (2004) Head direction cell activity and behavior in a navigation task requiring a cognitive mapping strategy. Behav Brain Research, in press.

Muir GM, Taube JS (2002) The neural correlates of navigation: do head direction and place cells guide spatial behavior? Behav Cogn Neurosci Rev 1: 297–317.

Munn NL (1950) Handbook of Psychological Research on the Rat. Boston, MA: Houghton Mifflin, pp. 155–156.

O'Keefe JA, Speakman A (1987) Single unit activity in the rat hippocampus during a spatial memory task. Exp Brain Res 68: 1–27.

Pearce JM, Ward-Robinson L, Good M, Fussell C, Aydin A (2001) Influence of a beacon on spatial learning based on the shape of the test environment. J Exp Psychol: Anim Behav Procs 27: 329–344.

Small WS (1901) Experimental study of the mental processes of the rat. II. Am J Psychol 12: 206–239.

Schwaerzel M, Monastirioti M, Scholz H, Friggi-Grelin F, Birman S, Heisenberg M (2003) Dopamine and octopamine differentiate between aversive and appetitive olfactory memories in *Drosophila*. J Neurosci 23: 10495–10502.

Steven MS, Taube JS (2002) Head direction cell discharge during periods of disorientation. Soc Neurosci Abstr 28: 584.3.

Taube JS (1995) Head direction cells recorded in the anterior thalamic nuclei of freely moving rats. J Neurosci 15: 70–78.

Taube JS, Muller RU, Ranck, JB Jr. (1990) Head direction cells recorded from the postsubiculum in freely moving rats. II. Effects of environmental manipulations. J Neurosci 10: 436–447.

Taube JS, Stackman RW, Calton JL, Oman CM (2004) Rat head direction cell responses in 0-G parabolic flight. J Neurophys, in press.

Tolman EC, Ritchie BF, Kalish D (1946) Studies in spatial learning. I. Orientation and the short-cut. J Exp Psychol 36: 13–24.

Watson JB (1907) Kinaesthetic and organic sensations: their role in the reactions of the white rat to the maze. Psych Rev (Monog Supp) Vol. 8, no. 2

West MO, Christian E, Robinson JH, Deadwyler SA (1981) Dentate granule discharge during conditioning. Exp Brain Res 44: 287–294.

Whishaw IQ, Tomie JA (1997) Piloting and dead reckoning dissociated by fimbria-fornix lesions in a rat food-carrying task. Behav Brain Res 89: 87–97.

Whishaw IQ, Hines DJ, Wallace DG (2001) Dead reckoning (path integration) requires the hippocampal formation: evidence from spontaneous exploration and spatial learning tasks in light (allothetic) and dark (idiothetic) tests. Behav Brain Res 17: 49–69.

Wiener SI, Paul CA, Eichenbaum H (1989) Spatial and behavioral correlates of hippocampal neuronal activity. J Neurosci 9: 2737–2763.

Wood ER, Dudchenko PA, Robitsek RJ, Eichenbaum H (2000) Hippocampal neurons encode information about different types of memory episodes occurring in the same location. Neuron 27: 623–633.

Young BJ, Fox GD, Eichenbaum H (1994) Correlates of hippocampal complex-spike cell activity in rats performing a nonspatial radial maze task. J Neurosci 14: 6553–6563.

12 Behavioral Studies of Directional Orientation in Developing and Adult Animals

Sidney I. Wiener and Françoise Schenk

Signals concerning directional orientation of the head and body in space are essential in order to elaborate efficient navigation behaviors, in particular, orienting displacements to reach a given goal. In addition to directional information, most real-life and maze navigation tasks also require distance estimations. Orientation and distance information are treated at several levels of signal processing before they actually are applied to displace the body in the appropriate direction toward the desired place. The principal focus here is on the ontogenesis of capacities for processing and applying head orientation information. This is difficult, since orienting is rarely measured in isolation. Furthermore, developmental studies to date have differed substantially both in their theoretical bases and their experimental designs. This has given rise to widely varying results, for example, in estimates of the age at which water maze learning occurs. To resolve these discrepancies, it will be helpful for us to first make a brief critical overview of what the brain actually must do in processing spatial information on the basis of head orientation, as well as linear translation information, in light of the fact that these two are often combined in everyday experience (although they are disambiguated in distinct types of neural processing). This will help clarify how the interpretations of some previous results have been confounded by discrepancies between non-specificity of experimental measures and the richness and complexity of the underlying processes. For reviews of related topics see O'Keefe and Nadel (1979), Gallistel (1990), Thinus-Blanc (1996), Trullier et al., (1997), Poucet and Cressant (1998), Sharp (2002), Jacobs and Schenk (2003), and Jeffery (2003).

Overall, the current state of knowledge concerning the ontogenesis of directional orientation is incomplete and fragmentary. The results from various approaches, such as neuroanatomy, physiology, and behavior appear in many cases to be inconsistent. These various results will be briefly reviewed, followed by suggestions that could help future studies to be more easy to reconcile.

From Directional Representations to Navigation Skills: A Modular View

The Bottom-Up View: Hierarchical Embedding of Direction Processing Modules

In order to analyze the ontogenesis of directional representations and orientation behaviors, it is useful to take a "module"-oriented approach wherein particular brain structures as well as integrated groups of these structures are assumed to make distinct contributions to signal processing and elaboration of behaviors. Such functional units can also be grouped together sequentially and hierarchically as "hypermodules" and systems that mediate specific processes so that, for example, head direction representations could be engaged for path integration or even spatial mapping. Characterizing and determining the mechanisms of these contributions is a goal of modern neuroscience, and the formulations below are provisional, intended to provide a useful framework for future modification. Such a modular view helps to reduce the complexity of the problem, because these elements can be recombined in various ways to elaborate the diverse strategies for the many types of spatial orientation. Furthermore, as the brain matures, these mechanisms are likely to come into play at different ages, permitting an understanding of the step-by-step progression in the animal's behavioral and cognitive capacities.

The Top-Down View: Navigation Performance Is Limited by the Weakest Link

In the present context, navigation will be considered as the process of getting from one point to a goal that is not immediately detectable from the origin. Path direction will thus be defined as a maintained orientation relative to the goal, or to an intermediate milestone, during the journey. A sense of directional orientation is required to determine an initial angle of departure from a starting point, and to guide subsequent reorienting along the way. This can be implemented via several different means, drawing upon individual or combinations of modular functions. In the adult, the criteria for selection among these mechanisms may depend upon the available sensory and memorized information about the layout of the environment, as well as the individual's position within it. Other decisive factors include the capacities and limitations of the locomotor apparatus relative to environmental affordances (such as obstacles and existing paths), as well as the animal's intrinsic and previously learned signal processing faculties. Because of these multiple factors, behavioral measures of the precision of directional orientation can yield values of resolution that are lower than those of the underlying internal representations, thus underestimating capacities for processing of head direction. In the interest of disambiguating these factors, it is essential to design experimental protocols that best permit the identification of the cues being employed as well as the types of brain computations and strategies being employed.

A Framework for Hierarchical Embedding of Modular Systems for Navigation

When adult subjects patrol environments containing spatially fixed sources of reinforcement, they learn the spatial relations between different places, which enables them to later choose optimal paths for reaching specific targets. This can be analyzed in terms of strategies carried out with the following modules (adapted from Trullier et al., 1997).

1. One elemental strategy involves the continuous estimation of one's distance and heading angle relative to a point of origin exclusively on the basis of self-movement information. Examples of this include measuring number of paces or swimstrokes, angles turned, and duration of movements at constant velocity, as in *path integration*. Note that no information concerning the environment is required, except frictional resistance of the substrate to forces applied against it during locomotion.

2. *Guidance* involves displacements toward perceptible targets, also referred to as "beacons," which can signal the position of the goal or, in complex routes, intermediate milestones on the way to the goal.

3. *Place-triggered reorientation* occurs in a familiar environment, where a single asymmetric cue or the relations between several different cues can be used to situate one's position and orientation relative to the goal location. Memory of the relation between the cues and the direction to go, coupled with other high-level spatial signal processing, would trigger reorientation and displacement toward the appropriate direction. These could be chained together as sequences of several cue/direction associations.

4. Finally, these various strategies must be able to be summoned successively as required and interlaced, allowing for the emergence of a hypothetical fourth "hyperstrategy". Such an integrated module (presumably involving prefrontal cortex and associated areas) would permit planning, and help increase performance accuracy, flexibility, and robustness by permitting learning. This would also provide a benefit by reducing computational requirements. As an example of this interlacing, in the preceding strategy the progress of a displacement command could be taken in charge by the first (self-movement tracking) module. Then, after a number of paces and the inevitable drift-related path deviations, this could trigger a new assessment of position and appropriate reorientation by the third strategy. Once near the goal, the second strategic system could then instruct the process of homing in on the target. *Late development of any of these processes could hence be responsible for inefficient navigation in young animals, and it is essential that experimental designs permit distinguishing among them.*

Roles for Learning and Memory Processes

Multiple learning and recall capacities are implicit to each of these respective processes, and these may involve distinct or overlapping neural mechanisms. Furthermore, episodic memory traces can concern particular paths, while procedural memory would increase efficiency and accuracy in strategies for acquiring experience with new paths and reproducing them. Certain other intrinsic and learned memorization processes are also called upon, for example, incidental learning about the spatial relations within an environment during exploration, or while performing other nonspatial tasks. Note that such latent learning occurs automatically in the absence of rewards or punishing contingencies. This can occur quite rapidly in an enclosed area where the relative distances of the various borders are perceptible. One means by which places can be identified, stored, and re-recognized is on the basis of visual patterns of light-dark profiles (or *contrast panoramas*), as has been proposed in honeybees (Cartwright and Collett, 1983; Collett, 1992). Another possible substrate involves specific modules, such as those identified in human parahippocampal cortex, that are selectively active during landmark recognition (Aguirre et al., 1996; Takahashi and Kawamura, 2002). Anatomical homologs of these zones exist in the rodent and other mammals.

Head Direction Processing with Perceived and Remembered Environmental Signals

As alluded to earlier, orientation information can come from polarization of the environment (surface slopes, celestial markers such as atmospheric light polarization, moss on the north side of trees, or even laboratory computer hum), asymmetries of landmarks (the front of a statue on a public square, or natural topographic elements), or configurations of cues. The latter are particularly informative since they vary from different viewpoints, especially when the immediately previous history of views and movements are taken into account. The accuracy of orientation estimates could be constrained by the sensory information available because of limited sensory capacities and the poverty of environmental cues, as well as the quality of the signal processing. All of these factors can confound estimates of directional capacities on the basis of maze performance.

This is complemented by recall of relevant information. This can include (1) recognition of position and orientation from individual or combinations of viewpoint data, (2) recall of memories concerning spatial relations of goals and landmarks relative to this position, (3) recall or computation of relative coordinates (e.g., by triangulation or panorama matching) in order to compute the optimal orientation for the angle of departure from the current position, and (4) the organization of the interlacing of these components. It is likely that signals from the head direction system could have an impact on these processes at several different levels. Furthermore, these systems may mature successively over time, and interexperiment variations in behavioral measures, as well as in experimental protocols, could be responsible for biasing performance measures towards different subsets of the above processes.

Cognitive Processing

Another critical form of high-level processing that can be associated with many of these processes is generalization. This can occur in identifying a single landmark or a place characterized by multiple cues. It is rare, or even impossible, to experience the precisely identical sensory signals, to occupy the same precise location or viewpoint, or to perform the identical reorientation or displacement movement. Generalization processes would permit matching of actual input signal patterns with stored traces, despite differences due to scaling and perspective shifts (due to deviations between the actual position and the point where the trace was first acquired). Examples of such generalization of responses are found in perspective and size-independent object-selective neurons of inferotemporal cortex in monkeys, and also in hippocampal neurons that respond when the rat occupies the same place with different bearings, thus experiencing varying local views. This matching could also occur despite differences due to changes in the scene since it was initially viewed (objects missing, added, shifted, or altered in appearance). Thus, it is vital that stimuli and behaviors be generalizable, particularly under conditions when inputs from certain sensory modalities are occluded, or when new constraints or liberties for locomotion are imposed. It is expected that generalization will occur and continue to improve throughout later phases of maturity. This is yet another confounding factor that must be disambiguated in behavioral studies of the ontogenesis of directional orienting mechanisms.

The Ongoing Challenge of Developing Behavioral Assays for Spatial Navigation Processing Modules

Place-learning tasks in open field environments (rather than mazes with alleys) permit assessments whether and how accurately subjects can orient when permitted continuous selection and modification of angular orientations during displacements. However, the unstructured nature of these tasks can also lead to progressive improvements in performance when strategies are employed that do not require directional accuracy. The resulting learning curves thus do not necessarily provide evidence for the particular spatial skill for which the task was designed. For this reason, final performance levels and behavioral patterns must also be taken into account.

In the water-maze navigation task developed by Richard Morris (Morris, 1981, 1984; Schenk, 1998), there are two popular measures of the level of spatial cognitive capacities. First, a progressive reduction in *escape latency* (the time elapsed from the point where the animal was placed in the water to when it climbs onto the hidden, submerged escape platform) during training is taken as an indication of some kind of spatial learning. Second, during probe trials where the expected reinforcement (the escape platform) has been removed, the duration of time and the spatial accuracy with which the rats *persist at the former target location* is considered as an indicator of *place memory*, as elaborated by

O'Keefe and Nadel (1979). Other parameters can be measured and compared with the optimal direct path, including *escape path length, overall path direction*, and *starting orientation*. These measures can be particularly revealing when a novel departure point is introduced, and also while a new goal location is learned (assuming that it is not clearly marked, even by line-of-sight background cues; cf. Tolman, 1948).

Spatial Cues in the Water Maze

The exact nature and disposition of the available cues are critical to performance quality, and variations in these may be responsible for some apparent inconsistencies among results of different studies of young animals. Figure 12.1 (top) illustrates the diversity of visual panoramas offered in different experiments on immature subjects. In order to distinguish the emergence of guidance versus place-recognition–triggered reorientation processes during ontogenesis, Schenk and colleagues compared the tendencies of rats of different ages to rely on particular cues, either inside the arena or around it, to learn a reinforced position. Placing a salient cue in the test arena allows the experimenter to assess whether it could serve as a *beacon* (in direct proximity to goal) or rather as a distinct *guidepost* or *milestone* serving as an intermediate goal and reference point along the route.

The working hypothesis for precocious development of guidance strategies, which are then followed by place-triggered reorientation, is based upon the observation that even very young rats have a strong tendency to approach salient objects, particularly if they are novel. If the position of this object remains fixed relative to the target goal, then a fixed route from it to the goal can be learned. While the animal first follows this sequence, it can then learn to orient relative to such milestones without actually visiting them. Distant, distinct cues can thus be employed to compute the orientation of a less visible goal. This could mark the beginning of the use of distinctive place-specific panoramic views (sometimes referred to as "snapshots") as well as the relations between landmark cues to identify intermediate stations along the route to a goal. Such a strategy can be demonstrated by analyses of the frequency of paths oriented toward this object (which would be considered as a simple taxislike guidance behavior) and from there to the goal, versus that of direct paths. After an intra-maze object is removed, changes in orientation behavior can reveal how critical the object's presence was for goal location. Thus, it can be useful to assess whether such a cue facilitates spatial memory, or whether it induces *overshadowing* in reducing acquisition of information from distant cues.

Multiple Confounding Strategies in the Water Maze

Several different strategies permit performance improvements in various measures in the Morris water maze (see also Lalonde, 1997; Lindner, 1997; Dalm et al., 2000; D'Hooge and DeDeyn, 2001; Gerlai et al., 2001, 2002; Baldi et al., 2003). Surprisingly, animals can learn over time to adopt more effective search strategies to locate the escape platform, even while ignoring spatial navigation cues. This can be tested in control trials by continually varying the location of the platform, and testing for improvements in search strategies (Baldi et al., 2003). These strategies can exploit the facts that the border of the pool provides information about both direction (since the escape platform is typically at one of only four fixed angles from departure point) and distance of the escape platform (since it is always the same distance from the wall). Furthermore, numerous training trials could facilitate automatization of stimulus-response strategies along specific paths with very limited generalizability to novel maze configurations. Since there are typically only four departure points and the escape platform location is fixed, the animal could learn to first orient itself toward the center (by a motor strategy or using border cues), take a visual fix of the environment, and depart in a direction toward cues learned to be in the line of sight of the submerged platform. The rodent would be required to learn only four such place-triggered reorientation movements. Alternatively, the animal could learn four independent sets of line-of-sight cues to orient directly to the platform from the departure points. (While efficient, this is not the type of spatial memory that most investigators intend to study with this task.) Another possibility is that if the animal has learned the distance of the platform from the wall (see Dalm et al., 2000), it need only swim to that distance, then circle the pool at this distance to reach the platform. It is also possible that the animal employs the relation between a single external cue and the border of the pool, or the panorama of contrasts, or the combination of configural cues, to determine a general direction to head to. This could be followed by a continuous or stepwise series of scanning and reorientation steps (since pointing errors have fewer grave consequences over shorter trajectories). While this is interesting, it does not require a cognitive map of space. Alternatively, the rat could swim at random until near the platform site (such random search behavior also improves over time; Baldi et al., 2003). The place-recognition processing near and at the goal site would elicit continuous swimming in this region, the size of which indicates the degree of recognition of the place, and the quality of the recalled memory of it. Note that while such recognition is a vital module for navigation, its presence does not presuppose the active function of any of the other processes discussed above.

These considerations underline the need for a modular approach in developing experimental design to determine how subjects of different ages orient in the test arenas, based on the available spatial information (uncontrolled and controlled extra- and intra-maze landmarks). Cue guidance, route and place learning can then be assessed, respectively, with greater precision. Furthermore, it is necessary to compare these different spatial abilities with observations in mature adult subjects in order to meaningfully interpret measures of performance during the ontogenesis of orientation capacities.

Directional Orientation in Adult Animals

This section will review experimental methodologies and the results of several studies. Our goal is to demonstrate the types of approaches already employed to test directional capacities. Some of these could potentially be adapted to test the ontogenesis of certain of the directional processing modules previously described.

Comparison of Two of the Principal Experimental Paradigms

The Morris water-navigation task remains a popular tool for assessing spatial learning. Questions remain concerning the generalization of these results to tasks requiring walking rather than swimming. Since vestibular and kinesthetic information, as well as substratal resistance, may provide less reliable information during swimming, optic flow might play a more critical role in this paradigm. Motivation and stress levels are likely to be different, favoring alternate neural mechansims (see, e.g., Golob and Taube, 2002). Two other terrestrial spatial learning tasks have been designed in which the reinforcement is an escape hole leading to a refuge from an open platform that contains other identically appearing, but blocked, holes (figure 12.1). In the holeboard task developed by Carol Barnes (1979), rats are released from the center of the table, and their accuracy in reaching the reinforced hole can be measured from their heading direction. In the homing board described later (Schenk, 1989), the escape hole is placed at a certain distance from the circular wall and the animal can be released at several different points.

Several studies have determined the capacities for directional discrimination in adult experimental animals. Under light conditions, this would be expected to depend upon the availability of orienting cues, and the animal's capacity to detect, represent, and apply this directional information in a given paradigm. Many studies in radial mazes have shown that freely moving rats are able to discriminate between arms separated by 45° (Olton et al., 1978) or even only 10° (Tolman, 1948, although the latter evidence appears to be inconclusive, since a prominent cue was positioned behind the goal arm).

Klement and Bures (2000) placed rats on a rotating platform (at 9°/s), where they were restricted to a 60° sector by transparent barriers mounted on the platform. This operant conditioning chamber contained a bar which, if pressed when the chamber was oriented in a particular 60°-wide "reward sector", triggered delivery of a food reward. Bar pressing increased when the chamber arrived at 60° before the reward sector boundary, regardless of the direction of rotation. During extinction, there was more bar pressing in the central 30° of the reward sector (this greater precision was probably due to the absence of delays imposed in the reward condition). This demonstrates a capacity to discriminate directions even in the absence of active navigation. Matthews et al. (1989) tested rats in a six-arm radial maze where only one arm was rewarded. The rats were enclosed in the center in the absence of visual cues and rotated by varying angles (thus this maze can evaluate orientation capacities with precision to 60°). Performance was above chance levels,

Water maze setups

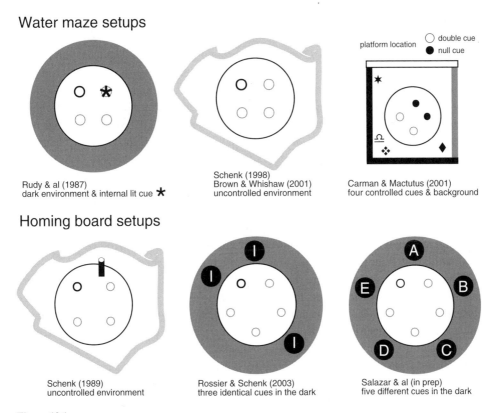

Homing board setups

Figure 12.1
(Top) Comparison of three different environmental setups for water mazes to test juvenile rats' spatial abilities. The setup used by Rudy et al. (1987) provided few distant cues because only the pool was illuminated and a cup was hanging in the center of the quadrant adjacent to the target platform. The apparatus used by Brown and Whishaw (2001) was placed in an open environment with uncontrolled room cues perceptible from the water surface. The small pool (diameter 40 cm) used by Carman and Mactutus (2001) was surrounded by contrasting curtains and four salient objects that were either nearest to the platform (double cue) or distant from it (null cue). (Bottom) Schemas of the homing board setups discussed here with external and internal cues available, or with only a configuration of three identical or five different triplets of LEDs placed on panels regularly placed around the table. Four or five different start areas are used. Parameters measured include the occupation time, number of reorientations, and start orientation.

and it increased over training. Vestibular lesions markedly impaired performance in this task.

Studies in open (rather than structured) environments permit observations of angular discrimination at finer levels of resolution. Mittelstaedt and Mittelstaedt (1980), in one of their classic papers on path integration, showed that a female desert mouse, after following a circuitous path to find one of its pups that had been displaced by 130 cm, is able to direct a return trajectory to the nest with home components of 0.94 to 0.98 (calculated as the mean vector length multiplied by the cosine of the direction of the mean vector). Standard deviations ranged from 10° to 20°. Mather and Baker (1980) studied the orientation of captured wood mice relative to the capture point (considered as home) after they were displaced in a specially designed cage. The animals maintained a mean orientation of 21° relative to home. These corresponded to mean deviation angles of 28° relative to the direction in which the animals escaped after release.

Etienne and colleagues (Seguinot et al., 1993) trained female golden hamsters to follow a dimly lit, baited rod along a linear trajectory to a cache of nuts at distances of 1.41 or 2.42 m from the nest. In the unguided return trajectories under (invisible) infrared lighting, the magnitude of the deviations from a beeline, direct course averaged 13.6° ± 7.4° (SEM, these figures have been calculated from data presented in the manuscript). Although there is some variability among trials, adult rats are capable of almost perfect trajectories in the holeboard and water maze tasks (e.g. figure 12.3; Morris, 1981; Schenk, 1987; Schenk, 1989). Whishaw and colleagues have developed a related task that is a hybrid of the Etienne and Barnes paradigms, where the animal's nest is connected to one of the holes. It forages on the table for a large food morsel, which the rats tend to consume in the security of the nest. The animals were observed to run more rapidly along a direct route to return to the escape hole. The angular deviation of the trajectories is negligible in light or dark (infra-red) conditions (Wallace et al., 2002).

Ontogeny of Spatial Orientation Behaviors in the Rat

Complexities of Ontogenetic Studies

One reason to study the ontogenesis of spatial orienting skills is to provide fundamental understanding of the underlying neurobiological processes. This is accomplished by comparing behavioral observations indicating keynote signal processing and cognition-related mechanisms with the maturation of brain regions that elaborate them. Ironically, a potential pitfall in such investigations is that most types of behavioral measures provide experiences likely to facilitate training, which in turn can stimulate maturation of the neural substrates under study. This confounds interpretation of repeated measures on the same individual. There is also a risk that a direct causal relationship may be inferred when particular anatomical, physiological, or behavioral milestones occur at the same time, especially when there are so many other possibly confounding crucial parameters. Comparisons among studies can also be confounded by differences in strain (albino strains have visual anomalies, for example), weaning date, cage size, environmental richness, nutrition, and stress (in particular prenatal stress in the rat dam). These many sources of variability underline the interest in focusing on specific modular capacities, rather than complex behaviors, which may be influenced in multiple ways by these factors. We have not included many other behavioral ontogeny studies in our review since they do not directly concern the issue of directional capacities.

Studies in Rats

The experimental model of the laboratory rat has the advantage of being an already popular subject for numerous studies at behavioral, anatomical and physiological levels. The timescale of development to adulthood over only a few months is advantageous for organizing experimental studies. The present review will sketch the state of the art while also pointing out important, but as yet missing, elements of the directional ontogeny story. Inbred strains provide a low degree of genetic diversity, but there remain other sources of variability, for example, among the 8 to 12 littermates. This is due to differential placement (and hence nourishment levels) within the rat uterus, and during nursing, when preferential placements are at more nourishing nipples. Thus, animals of the same age can have different weights and levels of development.

First, the development of the fundamental sensory and motor capacities will be presented. The rat pups are born weighing only a few grams and are transported by the dam, which generally holds a pup's loose skin at the back of the neck in her teeth. This provides the pup with its initial postpartum locomotor experiences. Young rats aged only 10 days can be trained to approach their dam (which is anesthetized for the experiment) along an alley 32 cm long and 8 cm wide (Amsel et al., 1976), presumably using olfactory cues. Even newborns of several species are able to make local displacements in order to attach to the nipple. Rats aged 5 days that are forced to alternate between the dam's 12 nipples perform better at the Olton radial-arm maze (Olton et al., 1978) at the age of 42 days than those that only alternated among four (Cramer et al., 1988). Thus experience at early ages can have long-term effects. Young rat pups are only capable of crawling with the ventral body contacting the floor. On the eleventh day, quadruped walking begins, and this is mastered by the seventeenth day. In the first two weeks the primary sensory inputs are tactile, thermic, olfactory, and gustatory. The principal behaviors are suckling, attaching, rolling, sleeping, etc. On the fifth day, the animals are already sensitive to differences in brightness and to tones of different frequencies. The eyes open sometime between the fifteenth and seventeenth days. Only two days after the eyes have opened, on P17, rats are able to orient and approach nearby visible targets (Rudy et al., 1987).

After rats are weaned and have begun exploring the environment, they express spatial abilities like spontaneous alternation earliest at ages of 27 to 28 days (Douglas et al., 1973; Egger, 1973; Blozovski and Hess, 1989). The radial-arm maze (requiring nonrepeated visits to each of the arms; Olton et al., 1978) presents a particular problem for ontogeny studies, since even in normal adults it can take 10 days to learn this. Thus, while it can be employed with rats as young as 20 days (Rauch and Raskin, 1984) it is difficult to pin-point ages of transitions in performance, and there are difficulties in interpretation due to the effects of cumulative training. The Morris water-escape task is better adapted because it can be learned in 8 to 10 trials (in adults). Another advantage is that young rats are able to rapidly orient to a unique goal such as the submerged platform in the Morris naviga-tion task (Schenk, 1985, 1987; Rudy et al., 1987).

Brown and Whishaw (2000) compared young rats aged 18, 19, and 20 days in cued versus place-learning versions of the Morris water task. In the cued-place task, the plat-form is visible, and it is not moved from trial to trial. This permits both place and cue strategies, in contrast to the classic place-learning task which leaves the imperceptible platform at the same location with the intention of requiring only place strategies (pre-sumably employing configuration cues in the environment) for optimal escape. Previous studies had suggested that the optimal strategies for these two tasks depend upon distinct neural circuits, which mature at different ages. Training methodologies were adapted, with many trials in the same day, but assuring that body temperatures returned to normal between trials. In both tasks, 18-day-old rats performed significantly worse than 19- and 20-day olds on the second two blocks of four trials. Comparisons of performance between first and last blocks showed significant learning only in the two groups of older animals. While escape latencies understandably were more rapid in the (easier) cued task than in the hidden platform task, the learning rates were comparable for the two tasks in the two groups that learned the tasks. Thus, this result does not provide support for distinct neural substrates with different ontogenetic timings (although different mechanisms could exist that have similar timings, or there could be a common limiting process) during this age window. The young ages of rats that showed improvements in the Morris water task here may be credited to the favorable timing of the training protocol (note, also, that the timing of training to avoid hypothermia may have favored learning; cf. Kraemer and Randall, 1995; Commins et al., 2003). The authors quantified performance in terms of a special measure that expresses a bias toward a quadrant (although comparison values of these measures in mature subjects are not presented). It is noteworthy that these animals did not demonstrate direct swim paths from the release point to the goal in cued or hidden plat-form conditions, and further study is required to determine exactly what spatial capacities these very young animals have. All groups demonstrated a tendency to swim at a fixed distance from the pool border, which, as noted above, could facilitate alternative water maze strategies.

Carman and Mactutus (2001) described spatial abilities of 19-day-old rats in a small pool (diameter 40 cm), with a salient complex visual panorama composed of four distinct curtains, four salient objects placed around the pool wall, and a paper cutout of a point-ing hand suspended 6 cm above water level at the center of the tank. In this experiment these rats were capable of distinguishing and selecting the target quadrant from the opposite quadrant if the platform was close to the salient objects (their "distal-double-cue" condition), but not when it was in the other half of the pool (the "distal-null-cue" condition). This indicates that the visual panorama around the pool plays an important role and that the ease with which the young rats can learn the escape platform position depends on how well it can be associated with surrounding cues.

This short overview tends to suggest that juvenile rats' poor long-term memory (Brown and Kraemer, 1997), limited ability to thermoregulate, and maturing visual capacities also contribute to discrepancies in the identification of clear-cut steps in the development of adultlike spatial discrimination and orientation capacities. Furthermore, even rats with hippocampal lesions can express spatial capacities provided they are trained in special conditions (see for example Morris et al., 1990; Whishaw et al., 1995), suggesting alternate mechanisms that may be employed by the several subsystems involved in spatial memory.

Perhaps the successive maturation of skills supported by these subsystems has led authors to observe discrete steps toward the development of adult levels of performance. The expression of these different skills might depend on the richness of visual cues in the arena or immediately around it, as well as early training and experience of the animal. A related hypothesis is that there is a critical period during development during which spatial experience is crucial to the full development of potential capacities in the adult. In a manner analogous to critical periods in the visual system, depriving rats of spatial experience during these periods would lead to irrecuperable performance deficits in adulthood. An extension of this hypothesis is that rats raised in hypogravity environments (not polarized along a vertical yaw axis) will possess head direction cells selective in the pitch and roll planes, as well as the yaw plane that governs responses in terrestrially reared animals.

Further Studies of the Ontogeny of Orientation Processing Modules in Juvenile Rats in Two Place-Learning Tasks

Schenk and colleagues have conducted behavioral studies in which two place navigation tasks were compared (e.g., Schenk, 1987, 1998; Schenk et al., 1995; Chevalley, 1999). Young hooded (pigmented) rats of the PVG strain were either trained to swim to a submerged, non-visible platform in a cylindrical pool, that is the classical Morris navigation task, or they were allowed to walk on a circular platform to find the escape hole (among many sealed holes) that would permit them to return to their home cage, as shown in figure 12.1 (the "homing task," Schenk, 1989). Both arenas were of the same size (diameter 160 cm) and were surrounded by a circular wall (extending 40 cm above the water or table surface). This permitted elevated cues within the room to be viewed and engaged for orientation.

The homing task may be the more relevant of the two for studies of young subjects because it seems better adapted to the response and motivation repertoire of an immature animal, and also because it presents considerably less risk of hypothermia (see Iivonen et al., 2003 or Satinoff, 1991), since it has been reported that young rats do not thermoregulate well (Spear and Riccio, 1994). Moreover, stress-related variability in the results can be reduced, since the rats are gently deposited on the table where they can take some time for reorientation and are not abruptly forced to swim in order to breathe. (And, since responses to stress may also change with age, it is important to disambiguate this factor as much as possible.) As shown by Chevalley and Schenk (1987), this task also permits measures of the orientation of the subjects in the start area and the heading direction of their initial trajectory towards the goal.

Results obtained from the two different experimental approaches will be summarized. First, the spatial abilities of different age groups are compared in the aquatic and terrestrial environments, in the presence or absence of a salient intra-arena cue, in a room that also contained multiple uncontrolled cues. Second, a visually controlled environment was employed to assess the age when young rats become capable of relying on an elemental configuration of visual cues for place learning.

Place Learning in the Homing Board Task and in the Water Maze with Three Types of Available Cues

Experimental Conditions   Four (or five) age groups were trained during four days in the respective tasks, and no individuals were tested in both tasks. Performance differences were assessed in groups presented with three different combinations of intra- and extramaze cues. In all cases, the room visible from the homing board or pool contained a variety of uncontrolled multimodal cues. The intramaze controlled cue was a metal cylinder (20 cm high and 6 cm diameter), either suspended above the water or placed on the table. Note that since the cylinder is symmetric, it provides no directional information in a direct way. However, such information can be derived from its position relative to the arena walls (except when placed in the exact center) and uncontrolled room cues. In the first condition, the cylinder was *proximal* to the target (submerged platform or escape hole). In the second condition, the cylinder was placed at a fixed horizontal distance and angle (*distant*) from it (Chevalley and Schenk, 1988; Chevalley, 1999). A third *extra-arena cues only* condition allowed assessments of spatial behavior in the absence of the cylinder cue. In all three conditions, the table was rotated between trials to render olfactory cues irrelevant.

Stress Factors   As previously mentioned, aversive components were limited as much as possible, although the task is based on the principle that entering the home cage through the connected hole is reinforcing, since it reduces the stress of being in an open field. Along the course of training, when spatial memory and skills improve escape performance, and there is more familiarity with the environment, the animals are likely to be less anxious, as would also be the case in the water maze. Since stress responses and related effects on spatial performance and learning may vary with age, this could remain an inevitable confounding factor in these experiments.

Capacities of Different Age Groups in Different Conditions

Figure 12.2 (left) shows escape path length after four days of training in the three conditions for both of the tasks. In both tasks, the youngest subjects followed circuitous escape paths several times longer than the direct path from start to the goal. They did not develop systematically direct escape paths until the beginning of the second month of life. However, as evident in figure 12.2 (right), during probe trials (with no hidden platform or no escape hole connected), even the youngest rats, aged 21 days, showed a significant bias toward the training sector (ANOVAs of the time spent in the training sector as compared to the other three irrelevant ones). This indicates that the youngest subjects expressed a spatially differentiated behavior oriented toward the previously reinforced position, in the water or on solid ground, on the basis of distal room cues only. This bias was significantly stronger in the older groups.

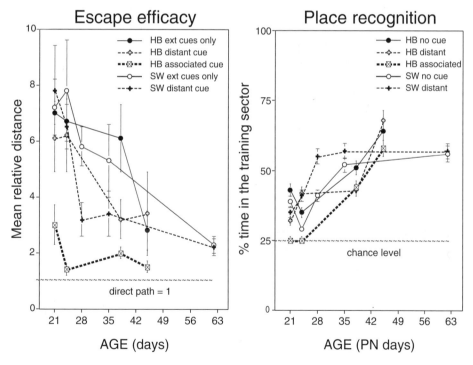

Figure 12.2
(Left) Escape performance in the two tasks as a function of age (mean relative distance during the session on the fourth training day); HB, homing board; SW, water maze. Exact age (PND) at the time of testing is indicated whereas training started when the rats were three days younger. (Right) Bias toward the training sector during probe trials as a function of age (time in the training area related to the total time spent in four symmetrically dispersed positions). (Data from Chevalley, 1999.)

As with a visible platform, training in the condition where there was a *cue proximal* to the goal helped all the rats to reach the escape hole along shorter paths, resembling those of the oldest rats in the *extra-arena cue only condition* (figure 12.2, left). This facilitation was particularly evident in the 24-day-old group. However, removal of this cue during the probe trial prevented the expression of a spatial bias toward the training position in the two youngest groups (figure 12.2, right), possibly as a consequence of an overshadowing effect during training (as discussed by Schenk, 1998), or poor reliance on distant cues at this age. However, this overshadowing by a cue placed at the goal is not observed in the more mature subjects (see also Schenk, 1985, 1989). It is again evident in senescent (24-month-old hooded) rats in the homing task (Schenk et al., 1990).

When the *cue was distant from the goal position*, in the pool or on the homing board, it also facilitated escape by reducing path length. This effect was particularly evident in 28-day-old rats in the swimming task (figure 12.2, left). In contrast to the cued goal condition, however, this placement of the intra-arena landmark did not overshadow spatial discrimination based on extra-arena cues, as its removal did not reduce the expression of a spatial bias toward the training sector. In fact, figure 12.2 (right) shows that the spatial bias was stronger in these rats than in the matched subjects trained with no intra-maze cue (*extra-arena cue only condition*). More generally, an object placed in a fixed position in the arena (hole board or pool) facilitates escape performance and improves the residual spatial bias in the probe trial in 28-day-old rats, even if situated in the exact center of the pool (Chevalley, 1999). This suggests that the single cue was used in conjunction with its different backgrounds when approached from various angles. In contrast, an asymmetric configuration of three *identical* suspended cues had no facilitatory effect.

In these experiments, only the oldest age groups (i.e., more than 40 days PN) showed no measurable improvement in performance in the presence of the intra-arena cue, and expressed no overshadowing when the goal cue was removed.

Detailed Analyses of Start Orientation

Detailed analyses of the rats' behavior in the three training conditions on the homing board revealed that the subjects remained in the start area for some time before walking toward the goal (figure 12.3). For each trial, the rat was placed 30 cm away from the wall, in one of four possible starting positions (figure 12.3A), facing the center of the arena to prevent circling along the wall ("thigmotaxis"). They often spent a few seconds in the start area, reorienting their head or body axes in different directions before starting to aim for the escape hole (figure 12.3B). Figure 12.3C shows that the youngest subjects spent more time in the start area, changing their orientation 2 to 3 times. However, the time spent facing the exact direction of the cued escape hole was lower in the youngest subjects (Chevalley and Schenk, 1988). As might be expected from the circuitous nature of the paths, figure 12.3B confirms that the 21-day-old rats showed little consistency or accuracy in their starting orientation in any of the three training conditions. However, their final approach to the

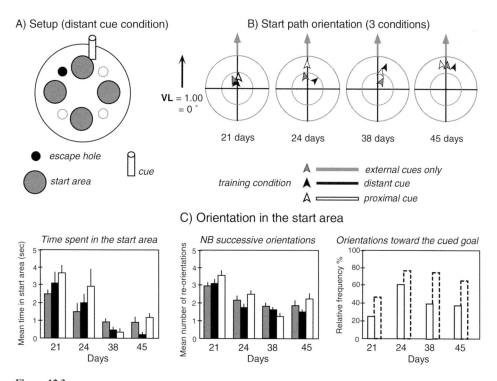

Figure 12.3
(A) Schematic of homing apparatus used by Chevalley and Schenk (1987). (B) Start orientations (averaged vector sums and net directions) as a function of age in the homing task in three different experimental conditions: intra-maze cues proximal or distant to the goal, or with cues external to the maze only. The arrow to the left calibrates maximum possible vector length (VL) and optimal angle of 0°. This direction is also indicated by the gray arrows above the individual polar plots. (C) Quantitative measures in the start area prior to displacement. (Left) Time spent in the start area of the homing board during the fourth training session as a function of age in the three conditions. (Middle) Number (NB) of different head orientations as defined in Chevalley and Schenk (1987). The key for the left and middle histograms is in the middle row to the right. (Right) In the proximal goal experiment only, head orientations relative to the cued goal in the start area as a function of age. The solid-edged bars correspond to a high accuracy criterion (training hole center ±10 cm) and the dashed bars are for a less precise criterion (±30 cm).

cued goal was frequently a direct one. This was observed (but not quantified) as a sudden acceleration and a straight approach from diverse positions on the table, as if they had just faced the cue and were attracted to it.

If trained in the *proximal cue* condition, the 24-day-old rats, but not the 21-day-old rats, were very systematic about facing the cued hole. During this short phase of reorientation before leaving the area, the 24-day-old rats faced the cued hole most of the time, as shown on figure 12.3C. Rats of this age were also highly systematic in following direct approach paths (see figures 12.2, left and 12.3B) from the release area when the target hole was cued, but not in the other two conditions. Moreover, these rats were frequently observed to run to, and to rear up against, the cue before entering into the escape hole, suggesting that their primary aim was the cue itself. However, this was not observed when the cue was placed at a distance from the escape hole (*distal cue* condition) although there was a high probability of "visits" to the cue. When the cue was distant from the target hole, the 24-day-old rats systematically passed near the object before approaching the escape hole ($69 \pm 6\%$ of their trials), which might have contributed to the longer escape paths. In contrast the 38-day-old rats appeared very accurate in initial orientation in both intra-arena cue conditions. This is particularly interesting in the distal cue condition since the animals were apparently capable of computing the geometric relations between their start position, the cue and the remembered position of the goal, often after a transitory phase in which they were observed to start in the direction of the cue and to correct their heading direction "en route" to reach the goal more directly. It is worth mentioning that the three oldest groups tended to start in a direction that was slightly biased toward the position of the cue, which was offset relative to the direct path to target hole (*distal cue* condition). In the *extra-arena cues only* condition (in the absence of maze landmarks), only the young adults (aged 38 days) were significantly oriented toward the escape hole when they left the start area.

Orienting with a Controlled Cue Configuration

In the experiments we have reported, we made no attempt to control the extra-arena room cues, but it was clear that salient contrasts in the room environment (dark versus light walls, uncontrolled asymmetrical illumination) were available to facilitate more direct escape paths. Here, we used rats of the PVG strain, whereas most studies use the Long Evans hooded rats as subjects. In a second phase, we used Long Evans rats in the homing task with controlled cue conditions in order to study more precisely the development of orientation capacities during the second month of life (Rossier, 2002).

In most laboratory environments, it is difficult to determine which of the variety of salient room cues in the panoramic view perceptible from the release point are actually being associated with the target. To clarify this, in a second series of experiments with the homing task, we worked in an environment in which the visual and olfactory cues could be controlled (Rossier, 2002). In brief, experiments were conducted in the dark, under infrared illumination (invisible to rats but permitting tracking measurements), and only three distant small light cues (LEDs) were made available as landmark cues (see figure 12.1, bottom). First, we found that in comparison with 4-month-old adult rats, subjects aged around 50 days were still unable to learn to go to a goal position on the table using only a configuration of three LEDs, distributed asymmetrically at a distance from the table (Rossier and Schenk, 2003). However, the same visual cues were sufficient to orient these rats if they had been coupled with distributed olfactory cues deposited at regular intervals on the table during the first three training sessions. This strongly suggests that the difficulty was not due to a perceptual problem, but to a deficit in relying on a pure configuration of visual cues.

In another series of experiments (Salazar et al., in preparation) we used five different visual cues to provide a comparison with the experiments by Rossier and Schenk (2003), in which five regularly placed olfactory cues allowed to efficient orientation in this age group. We found that rats aged around 48 days did not show a significant bias toward the escape hole position during the probe trials after training with a configuration of five different triplets of LEDs placed around the tables, as in figure 12.1B. However, the rats were capable of detecting the distant visual cues because they were observed to systematically start in the exact direction of a specific cue nearest to the goal position. Indeed, following removal of the two cues most tightly linked with the target hole (as in the null cue situation of Carman and Mactutus, 2001; see also figure 12.1C) there was no longer a preferential starting direction. This was measured as an abrupt decrease in mean vector length during this probe trial (Salazar et al., in preparation).

This series of experiments confirmed that rats aged around 50 days are not yet capable of relying on spatially distributed visual cues in the form of small LEDs, although they appear to express excellent spatial abilities when provided with a cue-rich room environment. Moreover, they indicate that visible cues in close association with the escape hole are attractive and might support an oriented approach strategy.

An Integrated Perspective of the Ontogenesis of Spatial Capacities

This first series of observations confirmed that the youngest rats, aged between 18 and 21 days, and trained in a visually rich environment, could develop a bias toward a particular region of the table or of the pool with help of distant uncontrolled room cues. However, they did not systematically orient toward the cued hole from the start, perhaps because of table and cue size (160 cm in diameter, 14 cm high object).

Around the age of 24 days, possibly starting from 22 days, as in the Rudy et al. (1987) study, rats are clearly attracted by salient objects or contrasts in the test arena. When closely associated with the target (*proximal cue* condition), the cue improves escape accuracy from the age of 24 days (see also Carman and Mactutus, 2001). This is accompanied by a high frequency of head orientations toward the goal in the release area and by highly directional escape paths. The critical role played by this object in attracting the young rat is highlighted by the lack of spatial bias toward the reinforced sector during the probe trial after it has been removed (see also Brown and Whishaw, 2000). When the object is at some distance to the hole (*distant cue* condition), however, its presence does not significantly improve escape efficiency in rats aged 24 days, confirming that it acts as a simple attractor for guidance strategies, which might help organizing invariant approach paths for which the surrounding landscape becomes relevant. The results obtained by Rudy et al. (1987) suggest that when the room cues are minimized due to direct illumination of the pool only, such cues may already facilitate the development of a significant spatial bias.

An abrupt change occurs between 24 and 28 days of age, where the distant object improves orientation in a very significant manner, as if the rats were able to benefit from following a route to the goal, and meanwhile learn about the position of the escape hole or platform in relation to external cues. Schenk et al. (1995) interpreted this by postulating that in this phase, juvenile rats might be guided by salient cues to develop organized invariant trajectories from the cue to the goal, during which they have a high rate of successful approaches. It is thus possible that even constrained approach paths, such as training with a single start point, are better at promoting memory of the target position than are disorganized and highly variable ones. Interestingly, this type of spatial learning strategy permits behavioral orientation capacities very similar to those of mature animals relying on external cues only. This suggests that during ontogeny, a tendency to systematically orient toward salient objects might play an organizational role in facilitating the selection of relevant spatial information.

Brandner (1999) proposed that accurate spatial orientation and memory requires that all possible cues be integrated to optimize spatial processing. This implies that the most "intense cues" (large ones, with high contrast and high reinforcing value, such as the target cue) be somewhat attenuated in order to allow for the integration of less salient but possibly relevant ones together with more salient ones. Immature and senescent rats, as well as those with lesions of the medial septum, behave as if they had been impressed by the most salient cues and tend to ignore the others; this could be responsible for the marked overshadowing effect (Schenk, 1998; Brandner, 1999).

Adult rats are known to develop highly organized exploratory movements with identifiable home bases when allowed free movement on a large surface (Eilam and Golani, 1989). Their selection of successive directions on a partially open tunnel maze appears also to be highly constrained (Schenk et al., 1990; Schenk and Grobéty, 1992), and the guidance phase observed in juvenile subjects might represent a first step in this organization.

Finally, as in Schenk (1985), more recent results (figure 12.3B) indicate that accurate orientation relative to a configuration of distant room cues is not common in juvenile rats. Moreover, since young adult subjects aged around 50 days cannot rely on an elemental visual configuration to discriminate the escape position (Rossier and Schenk, 2003), but can nevertheless start in the direction of the goal by relying on specific visual cues, we can suggest that orientation mechanisms underlying spatial memory in young rats are still undergoing a functional maturation involving calibration and learning processes. However, in environments in which a salient cue may be associated with the target, when the subject is at this precise location—resting on the escape platform or sitting near the goal hole— immature subjects might appear to be as accurate as adults. Their difficulty in relying on a configuration of discrete cues (Rossier and Schenk, 2003)—and the facilitation induced by transitory coupling with olfactory cues—indicates that a diversity of redundant strategies can be used for spatial orientation in rich environments. Moreover, this delayed maturation of sophisticated orientation mechanisms suggests a late maturation of the brain systems involved in orientation, possibly related to adjustments between complementary memory systems (White and McDonald, 2002) or between intrahippocampal parallel mapping systems, as proposed by Jacobs and Schenk (2003).

Anatomy and Function of Sensory and Motor Systems in Rats

Data concerning the ontogenesis in rats of brain systems related to directional representations are summarized below. No experimental studies examine the relation between these specific events and the ontogenesis of directional processing capacities.

Sensory Systems
In the somatosensory system the peripheral receptors are present at birth, while thalamocortical projections mature by the fifth day. In the olfactory system, the vomeronasal division matures first, while the principal olfactory system is more complex. By 30 days, lamination is present in the primary olfactory cortex. Normal function is found in the primary vestibular nuclei by 22 days while the auditory system anatomy appears mature at 10 to 15 days postnatal.

Motor Systems
A review of the ontogenesis of locomotor function can be found in Westerga and Gramsbergen (1990). On P5, the first corticospinal tract fibers arrive at lumbar segments (Gribnau et al., 1986; Joosten et al., 1987; Schreyer and Jones, 1988). The major increase in sensorimotor cortex connectivity occurs between 12 and 20 days (Eayrs and Goodhead, 1959; Hicks and D'Amato, 1975). The cerebellar Purkinje cell firing characteristics and histochemical appearance arrive at mature levels during the same period that free walking appears (Woodward et al., 1969; Altman, 1982). This is of interest for motor as well as spatial orientation function, since the cerebellum is implicated in the mathematical integration of velocity to head angle signals as well as in the elaboration of certain spatial cognitive strategies (Rondi-Reig et al., 2002). Gomez-Pinilla et al. (1994) found that basic fibroblast growth factor (bFGF; important for establishing neuronal connections) immunoreactivity does not reach adult levels until P20.

Head Direction System

Using the tritiated thymidine methods, Altman and Bayer (Bayer and Altman, 1995) determined that the anterodorsal thalamic nucleus neurons are generated on E15 through E17 (in their system E1 is the morning after mating and E22 the final day before birth, rather than E0 used by some authors). Lateral mammillary neurons appear on days E12 through E15 while the dorsal tegmental nucleus of Gudden develops on E13 through E16. Postsubiculum (called superficial presubiculum) neurons appear on E17 through 19, as do fields CA1 and CA3 of hippocampus, while most dentate granule cells are generated on days P0–15. Neurogenesis gradually diminishes with the dentate gyrus taking on a mature appearance by P21, which corresponds to the time of weaning. Dentate gyrus neurons continue to be generated into adulthood.

Hippocampal Pathways

In the albino rat, myelination in the anterior thalamus and fornix starts on P14. Cingulum bundle myelinization matures between days 21 and 25 (Jacobson, 1963). Hippocampal connections develop during the first weeks of life (Crain et al., 1973; Pokorny and Yamamoto, 1981) and synaptogenesis continues there over several months. Hippocampal metabolic levels arrive at adult levels by P30 (Meibach et al., 1981) but changes continue until 40–60 days.

Ontogeny of Head Direction and Place Responses in Rats

Martin and Berthoz (2002) recorded head direction unit activity in the cingulum bundle of a young rat on postnatal days 28, 30 and 31. Since the head is growing so rapidly at these ages, it was not possible to record more than a few days from the same animal. On the basis of the relations between the responses on the individual tetrode wires, the authors speculate that the first recording was near a cingulate cortex neuronal soma while the others were axonal fibers, perhaps from (anterodorsal) thalamic afferents to cortex. Figure 12.4 indicates that the ranges of the directional responses were 90°, 71°, and 123°, respectively, consistent with observations in adult rats. The peak firing rates of the neurons were 8.9 Hz, 7.1 Hz, and 141 Hz, while baseline firing rates (that is, for angles outside of the range of the preferred direction) were 2.2 Hz, 1.5 Hz, and 51 Hz. The third neuron is among the highest of the peak directional rates ever observed in recordings in adult rats, while the other two are at the low end of the range observed in adults. The baseline firing rates are higher than those typically reported in adults, and in the case of the neuron recorded on day P31 are extraordinary, exceeding the peak firing rates of many directional neurons in adult rats. Martin and Berthoz (2002) posit that head direction information may be present in even younger rats, permitting them to perform simple proximal cue navigation tasks. The earliest age at which HD cell responses appear is not yet known. Perhaps future studies could succeed at more recordings by focusing on other species that are born precociously (such as ferrets).

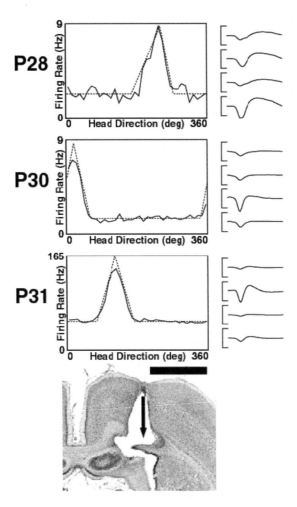

Figure 12.4
Head direction responses in cingulum recordings in a 1-month-old rat (age at recording shown at left). Tetrode waveforms are shown to right (vertical scale bars 222 μV, 50 μV, and 121 μV respectively); histology is below (bar: 2 mm). (From Martin and Berthoz, 2000. Copyright © Wiley-Liss, Inc. Reproduced by permission of Wiley-Liss, Inc., a subsidiary of John Wiley & Sons, Inc.)

In contrast, adultlike place responses in hippocampal neurons were not observed until after the rats were 45 days old. Intriguingly, this corresponds to the observations of Bronzino et al. (1987) that hippocampal theta EEG (4–11 Hz) shows a significant increase in peak power from 14 to 45 days of age. Martin and Berthoz also found that position-selective activity was also less stable in young rats. This is consistent with Golob and Taube's (1997) conclusions, about adult rats with lesions of the hippocampus that head direction signals in the anterodorsal thalamic nucleus and the postsubiculum are independent of hippocampal position responses. However, it was suggested that the low selectivity and poor stability of the hippocampal responses impaired performance in tasks requiring integration of distal cue configurations.

Closing Remarks

This brief overview demonstrates that there remains much work to be done in this area. It is difficult to draw conclusions on the basis of the fragmentary and contradictory data. The results for the various approaches suggest certain ages as key transition points, but they are not consistent, perhaps because data was sampled from different age groups, or because variations in housing conditions and experience produced variations in the rate of development among the rat populations. Furthermore, the variation in results from behavioral studies can be resolved only by efforts to make housing and animal care conditions more uniform among laboratories, and continue to refine theory and methodology to provoke studies that focus upon the specific skills associated with identifiable anatomical and physiological milestones during the animals' development.

Overall, certain tendencies have emerged. Maturation of directional accuracy is precocious in certain conditions, and this may promote heading for salient features in the environment. Such a strategy reduces variability in approach routes and helps learning about the relation between features of the environment. Moreover, as proposed by Jacobs and Schenk (2003), the accuracy of information provided by head directional units might be a condition for the development of sketch maps, that is, local maps in which the subjects process the spatial relation between salient cues, based on an accurate reference/calibration signal from head orientation. The late maturation of navigation based exclusively on learning the relation between particular features of the environment (in the dark) provides further evidence of a modular development in which a critical step is the processing of accurate directional orientation in the environment which then allows for more topological assessment of local maps or sketch maps (Jacobs and Schenk, 2003).

The studies reviewed here have highlighted certain crucial periods in the first months of life of the rat for development of spatial orientation and navigation capacities. However, it is clear that future studies need to focus more specifically upon the timing of the beginning of active functioning of specific modular functions. Further work also is required to identify the anatomical and physiological substrates of these systems, and eventually to experimentally link their maturation with that of their associated functions.

Acknowledgments

Thanks to the French Centre National d'Etudes Spatiales for grant support. This research was supported by a grant from the Fonds National Suisse de la Recherche Scientifique No 3100-061938.00 to FS.

References

Aguirre GK, Detre JA, Alsop DC, D'Esposito M (1996) The parahippocampus subserves topographical learning in man. Cereb Cortex 6: 823–829.

Altman J (1982) Morphological development of the rat cerebellum and some of its mechanisms. In SJ Palay and V Palay, eds., The Cerebellum—New Vistas, Berlin: Springer-verlag, pp. 8–49.

Amsel A, Burdette DR, Letz R (1976) Appetitive learning, patterned alternation, and extinction in 10-day-old rats with non-lactating suckling as a reward. Nature 262: 816–818.

Baldi E, Lorenzini CA, Bucherelli C (2003) Task solving by procedural strategies in the Morris water maze. Physiol Behav 78: 785–793.

Bayer SA, Altman J (1995) Neurogenesis and neuronal migration. In G Paxinos, ed., The Rat Nervous System, New York: Academic Press, pp. 1041–1078.

Blozovski D, Hess C (1989) Hippocampal nicotinic cholinergic mechanisms mediate spontaneous alternation and fear during ontogenesis but not later in the rat. Behav Brain Res 35: 209–220.

Brandner C (1999) Effets promnésiant de traitements stimulant le développement et le maintien du système cholinergique chez le rat. Doctoral thesis, Faculty of SSP, University of Lausanne.

Barnes CA (1979) Memory deficits associated with senescence: a neurophysiological and behavioral study in the rat. J Comp Physiol Psych 93: 74–104.

Bronzino JD, Siok CJ, Austin K, Austin-Lafrance RJ, Morgane PJ (1987) Spectral analysis of the encephalogram in the developing rat. Dev Brain Res 35: 257–267.

Brown RW, Kraemer PJ (1997) Ontogenetic differences in retention of spatial learning tested with the Morris water maze. Dev Psychobiol 30: 329–341.

Brown RW, Whishaw IQ (2000) Similarities in the development of place and cue navigation by rats in a swimming pool. Dev Psychobiol 37: 238–245.

Carman HM, Mactutus CF (2001) Ontogeny of spatial navigation in rats: a role for response requirements? Behav Neurosci 115: 870–879.

Cartwright BA, Collett TS (1983) Landmark learning in bees. Experiments and models. J Compar Physiol A 151: 521–543.

Chevalley AF (1999) Les capacités d'orientation spatiale chez le rat en cours de développement: utilisation de différents types de repères. pp. 1–221. Ph.D. Thesis, Faculty of Science, University of Lausanne.

Chevalley AF, Schenk F (1987) Immature processes of spatial learning in hooded rats. Soc Neurosci Abstr 17: 184.5.

Chevalley AF, Schenk F (1988) Ontogénèse du comportement d'orientation spatiale chez le rat. Sci Tech Anim Lab 13: 49–52.

Collett TS (1992) Landmark learning and guidance in insects. Phil Trans R Soc Lond B 337: 295–303.

Commins S, Cunningham L, Harvey D, Walsh D (2003) Massed but not spaced training impairs spatial memory. Behav Brain Res 139: 215–223.

Crain B, Cotman C, Taylor D, Lynch G (1973) A quantitative electron microscopic study of synaptogenesis in the dentate gyrus of the rat. Brain Research 63: 195–204.

Cramer CP, Pfister JP, Haig KA (1988) Experience during suckling alters later spatial learning. Dev Psychobiol 21: 1–24.

Dalm S, Grootendorst J, deKloet ER, Oitzl MS (2000) Quantification of swim patterns in the Morris water maze. Beh Res Meth, Instr & Cptrs 32: 134–139.

D'Hooge R, DeDeyn PP (2001) Applications of the Morris water maze in the study of learning and memory. Brain Res Rev 36: 60–90.

Douglas RJ, Peterson JJ, Douglas DP (1973) The ontogeny of a hippocampus-dependent response in two rodent species. Behav Biol 8: 27–37.

Eayrs JT, Goodhead B (1959) Postnatal development of the cerebral cortex in the rat. J Anat 93: 385–402.

Egger GJ (1973) Novelty induced changes in spontaneous alternation by infant and adult rats. Dev Psychobiol 6: 431–435.

Eilam D, Golani I (1989) Home base behavior of rats (Rattus norvegicus) exploring a novel environment. Behav Brain Res 14: 199–211.

Gallistel CR The Organization of Learning. 1990. Cambridge, MA: MIT Press/Bradford Books.

Gerlai R (2001) Behavioral tests of hippocampal function: simple paradigms complex problems. Behav Brain Res 125: 269–277.

Gerlai RT, McNamara A, Williams S, Phillips HS (2002) Hippocampal dysfunction and behavioral deficit in the water maze in mice: an unresolved issue? Brain Res Bull 57: 3–9.

Golob EJ, Taube JS (1997) Head direction cells and episodic spatial information in rats without a hippocampus. Proc Nat Acad Sci (USA) 94: 7645–7650.

Golob EJ, Taube JS (2002) Differences between appetitive and aversive reinforcement on reorientation in a spatial working memory task. Behav Brain Res 136: 309–316.

Gomez-Pinilla F, Lee JW, Cotman CW (1994) Distribution of basic fibroblast growth factor in the developing rat brain. Neurosci 61: 923.

Gribnau AAM, DeKort EJM, Dederen PJWC, Nieuwenhuys R (1986) On the development of the pyramidal tract in the rat. II. An anterograde tracer study of the outgrowth of the corticospinal fibers. Anat Embryol 175: 101–110.

Hicks SP, D'Amato CJ (1975) Motor-sensory cortex-cortico-spinal system and developing locomotion and placing in rats. Am J Anat 143: 1–42.

Iivonen H, Nurminen L, Harri M, Tanila H, Puolivali J (2003) Hypothermia in mice tested in Morris water maze. Behav Brain Res 141: 207–213.

Jacobs LF, Schenk F (2003) Unpacking the cognitive map: the parallel map theory of hippocampal function. Psych Rev 110: 285–315.

Jacobson S (1963) Sequence of myelinization in the brain of the albino rat: cerebral cortex, thalamus and related structures. J Comp Neurol 121: 5–29.

Jeffery, KJ The Neurobiology of Spatial Behaviour. 2003. New York: Oxford University Press.

Joosten EAJ, Gribnau AAM, Dederen PJWC (1987) An anterograde tracer study of the developing corticospinal tract in the rat: three components. Dev Brain Res 36: 121–130.

Klement D, Bures J (2000) Place recognition monitored by location-driven operant responding during passive transport of the rat over a circular trajectory. Proc Nat Acad Sci (USA) 97: 2946–2951.

Kraemer PJ, Randall CK (1995). Spatial learning in preweanling rats trained in a Morris water maze. Psychobiology 23: 144–152.

Lalonde R (1997) Visuospatial abilities. Int Rev Neurobiol 41: 191–215.

Lindner MD (1997) Reliability, distribution, and validity of age-related cognitive deficits in the Morris water maze. Neurobiol Learn Mem 68: 203–220.

Martin PD, Berthoz A (2002) Development of spatial firing in the hippocampus of young rats. Hippocampus 12: 465–480.

Mather JG, Baker RR (1980) A demonstration of navigation by small rodents using an orientation cage. Nature 284: 259–262.

Matthews BL, Ryu JH, Bockaneck C (1989) Vestibular contribution to spatial orientation. Acta Otolaryngol 468: 149–154.

Meibach RC, Ross DA, Cox RD, Glick SD (1981) The ontogeny of hippocampal metabolism. Brain Research 204: 431–435.

Mittelstaedt M, Mittelstaedt H (1980) Homing by path integration in a mammal. Naturwiss 67: 566–567.

Morris RG (1981) Spatial localization does not require the presence of local cues. Learn Motiv 12: 239–260.

Morris RG, Schenk F, Tweedie F, Jarrard LE (1990) Ibotenate lesions of hippocampus and/or subiculum: Dissociating components of allocentric spatial learning. European Journal of Neuroscience 2: 1016–1028.

Morris RGM (1984) Development of a water-maze procedure for studying spatial learning in the rat. J Neurosci Meth 11: 47–60.

O'Keefe J, Nadel L (1979) The hippocampus as a cognitive map, Behav Brain Sci 2: 487–533.

Olton DS, Branch M, Best PJ (1978) Spatial correlates of hippocampal unit activity. Exp Neurol 58: 387–409.

Pokorny J, Yamamoto T (1981) Postnatal ontogenesis of hippocampal CA1 area in rats: I Development of dendritic arborization in pyramidal neurons. II Development of ultrastructure in stratum lacunosum and moleculare. Brain Res Bull 7: 113–130.

Poucet B, Cressant A (1998) On the spatial information used by the neural substrates of navigation. Curr Psych Cogn 17: 901–919.

Rauch SL, Raskin LA (1984) Cholinergic mediation of spatial memory in the preweanling rat: Application of the radial arm maze paradigm. Behav Neurosci 98: 35–43.

Rondi-Reig L, Le Marec N, Caston J, Mariani J (2002) The role of climbing and parallel fibers inputs to cerebellar cortex in navigation. Behav Brain Res 132: 11–18.

Rossier J. Représentation et mémoire de l'espace chez le rat: une analyse multimodale et développementale. 2002. University of Lausanne, Faculté des Sciences Sociales et Politiques.

Rossier J, Schenk F (2003) Olfactory and/or visual cues for spatial navigation through ontogeny: olfactory cues enable the use of visual cues. Behav Neurosci 117: 412–425.

Rudy JW, Stadler-Morris S, Albert P (1987) Ontogeny of spatial navigation behaviors in the rat: Dissociation of "proximal"- and "distal"-cue-based behaviors. Behav Neurosci 101: 62–73.

Satinoff E (1991) Developmental aspects of behavioral and reflexive thermoregulation. In: Developmental psychobiology: new methods and changing concepts (Shair HN, Barr GA, Hofer MA, eds.), pp. 169–188. New York: Oxford Univ. Press.

Schenk F (1985) Development of place navigation in rats from weaning to puberty. Behav Neur Biol 43: 69–85.

Schenk F (1987) Dissociation between components of spatial memory in the rat during ontogeny. In P Ellen and C Thinus-Blanc, eds., Cognitive Processes and Spatial Orientation in Animal and Man, Dordrecht: M. Nijhoff, pp. 160–167.

Schenk F (1989) A homing procedure for studying spatial memory in immature and adult rodents. J Neurosci Meth 26: 249–258.

Schenk F (1998) The Morris water maze (is not a maze). In M Foreman and N Gillett, eds., Interacting with the Environment: a Handbook of Spatial Research Paradigms and Methodologies, Hove, UK: Psychology Press.

Schenk F, Contant B, Grobéty M-C (1990) Angle and directionality affect rat's organization of visit sequences in a modular maze. Learn Motiv 21: 164–189.

Schenk F, Grobéty M-C (1992) Interactions between directional and visual environmental cues in a radial maze task and in spontaneous alternation tests. Learn Motiv 23: 80–98.

Schenk F, Grobéty M-C, Lavenex P, Lipp H-P (1995) Dissociation between basic components of spatial memory in rats. In E Alleva, A Fasolo, H-P Lipp, L Nadel and L Ricceri, eds., Dissociation between Basic Components of Spatial Memory in Rats. Boston: Kluwer Press.

Schreyer DJ, Jones EHG (1988) Topographic sequence of outgrowth of corticospinal axons in the rat: a study using retrograde axonal labeling with Fast blue. Dev Brain Res 38: 89–101.

Seguinot V, Maurer R, Etienne AS (1993) Dead reckonong in a small mammal: the evaluation of distance. J Comp Physiol A 173: 103–113.

Sharp P (ed.) The Neural Basis of Navigation: Evidence from Single Cell Recording. 2002. Boston: Kluwer Press.

Spear NE, Riccio DC. Memory: Phenomena and Principles. 1994. Needham Heights, MA: Allyn and Bacon.

Takahashi N, Kawamura M (2002) Pure topographical disorientation—the anatomical basis of landmark agnosia. Cortex 38: 717–725.

Thinus-Blanc C. Animal Spatial Cognition: Behavioral and Neural Approaches. 1996. Singapore: World Scientific Publishing.

Tolman EC (1948) Cognitive maps in rats and men. Psych Rev 55: 190–208.

Trullier O, Wiener SI, Berthoz A, Meyer J-A (1997) Biologically based artificial navigation systems: Review and prospects. Prog Neurobiol 51: 483–544.

Wallace DG, Hines DJ, Whishaw IQ (2002) Quantification of a single exploratory trip reveals hippocampal formation mediated dead reckoning. J Neurosci Methods 113: 131–145.

Westerga J, Gramsbergen A (1990) The development of locomotion in the rat. Dev Brain Res 57: 163–174.

Whishaw IQ, Cassel JC, Jarrard LE (1995) Rats with fimbria-fornix lesions display a place response in a swimming pool: a dissociation between getting there and knowing where. J Neurosci 15: 5779–5788.

White NM, McDonald RJ (2002) Multiple parallel memory systems in the brain of the rat. Neurobiol Learn Mem 77: 125–184.

Woodward DJ, Hoffer BJ, Lapham LW (1969) Correlative study of electrophysiological, neuropharmacological, and histochemical aspects of cerebellar maturation in rat. In RR Llinas, ed., Neurobiology of Cerebellar Evolution and Development, Chicago: AMA. pp. 725–742.

13 Cognitive Deficits Induced by Lesions of Structures Containing Head Direction Cells

John P. Aggleton

Although the head direction signal is generated prior to reaching the hippocampal formation, it is within the hippocampus that this signal is often thought to primarily affect spatial processing and, hence, behavior. This specific aspect of hippocampal function can be placed within the broader context of the central role of the hippocampus in memory and, in particular, in "episodic memory." The term episodic memory refers to our remembrance of autobiographical events that have a specific spatial and temporal context, the loss of which is the hallmark feature of anterograde amnesia. The importance of the hippocampus for memory raises the question of the extent to which head direction signals, and the regions that generate them, might also have a broader role in cognition. While head direction and memory may seem an unlikely pairing, there is an apparent overlap between brain sites containing head direction cells (mammillary bodies, anterior thalamic nuclei, posterior cingulate/retrosplenial cortex, hippocampal formation) and sites that, when damaged, can cause amnesia. This relationship is the focus of this chapter.

This review considers both human and animal studies that describe the consequences of lesions in structures that contain head direction cells. Of these structures, the postsubiculum will receive little attention as it is embedded within the hippocampal formation, and so it is inevitably more difficult to distinguish its separate contribution from that of the structure within which it is contained. Nevertheless, there is evidence that neurotoxic lesions of the rat postsubiculum are sufficient to produce mild impairments on tests of spatial reference memory (water maze) and spatial working memory (radial-arm maze) (Taube et al., 1992). It should also be noted that the large majority of the lesion studies in other areas containing head direction cells will involve damage to nuclei in addition to those containing head direction cells. For this reason the cognitive deficits need not reflect a loss of head direction cells per se. A further problem specific to studies with rodents is that standard tests of memory rely very heavily on spatial processes, so distinguishing a mnemonic deficit from a navigational deficit can be remarkably difficult. This is a two-way problem, given that spatial/navigational tests will invariably have mnemonic demands.

Figure 13.1 shows sites that contain head direction cells and their anatomical relationships. This indicates not only the structures but also the tracts that, when damaged, may disrupt the head direction signal. In the case of several structures (e.g., the anterior thalamic nuclei and the mammillary bodies), head direction cells are confined to a specific subregion or nucleus within the structure. Wherever possible, the lesion evidence will focus on this subregion, but in many instances this information is lacking and so it is necessary to consider the effects of damage to the structure as a whole. For this reason, it can sometimes be more informative when a null result is obtained because this can help to rule out the critical importance of the head direction signal for that task. A further issue is that research on head direction cells, and the regions containing them, is heavily biased towards the rodent brain. Comparable research on the primate brain is usually lacking (but see chapter 14 by Rolls). A final point is that this analysis will examine one structure at a time, and it is quite possible that the broader impact of a loss of head direction signals is

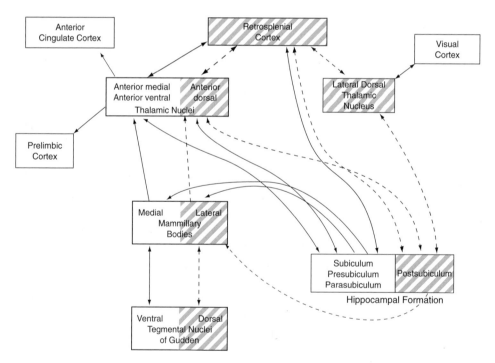

Figure 13.1
Diagrammatic representation of the major connections interlinking structures containing head direction cells in the rat brain. Those subregions that contain head direction cells are shown with diagonal lines, and their interconnections are distinguished by dashed lines. The arrows reflect the direction of the connections.

only fully evident when several sites afferent to the hippocampus are simultaneously removed. Such studies have rarely been conducted (but see Wilton et al., 2001; Van Groen et al., 2002b).

Mammillary Bodies

The mammillary bodies are composed of two major nuclei, and head direction cells are restricted to only one, the lateral mammillary nucleus (Blair et al., 1998; Stackman and Taube, 1998). While lesion studies in rats have shown that destruction of the lateral mammillary nucleus results in a loss of the head direction signal in the anterior thalamic nuclei (Blair et al., 1999), to which the lateral mammillary nucleus projects via the mammillothalamic tract (MTT), very little else is known about the selective effects of damage in this nucleus. Thus, to gain an insight into the potential contributions to cognition of head direction cells in this nucleus, it is necessary to consider the outcome of lesions that involve the entire mammillary bodies, or lesions of the mammillothalamic tract. A problem is that the medial mammillary nuclei may themselves contribute to cognitive processes given that they receive very dense inputs from the hippocampal formation. This underlines the need to distinguish the contributions from the two subregions.

Clinical Evidence

Evidence that the mammillary bodies are important for cognitive processes dates back to studies of the neuropathology of Korsakoff's syndrome (Gudden, 1896; Gamper, 1928). The most striking, cognitive feature of this syndrome is a severe amnesic state that typically involves both anterograde and retrograde amnesia (Delay and Brion, 1969; Kopelman, 1995). The pathology associated with this persistent amnesia can be variable, but one invariant feature is the shrinkage and necrosis found in the mammillary bodies (Delay and Brion, 1969; Victor et al., 1971; Mair et al., 1979; Mayes et al., 1988; Rigges and Boles, 1944). There has been much debate whether this pathology is sufficient to account for some or all of the memory loss in Korsakoff's syndrome. Some claim that it is possible that there are cases with mammillary body pathology in which there is not a persistent amnesia (Victor et al., 1971; Davila et al., 1994; Harding et al., 2000). This suggests that mammillary body damage is not sufficient to produce the memory loss. This carries the assumption that the memory loss is either the consequence of damage elsewhere (Victor et al., 1971; Victor, 1988) or is the result of the combination of mammillary body damage with pathology in some other site. A third claim is that some alcoholic Korsakoff cases have only mammillary body damage (Rémy, 1942; case A6 of Delay and Brion, 1969; Torvik, 1987) and that this therefore must be sufficient for the memory loss.

Even though many studies have been carried out on patients with Korsakoff's syndrome, it has proved very difficult to resolve these varying views. Difficulties are posed both by the likelihood of diffuse, additional pathology, e.g., in the frontal lobes, and the lack of cases with detailed histopathology combined with comprehensive, qualitative analyses of memory loss (but see Mair et al., 1979; Mayes et al., 1988). A solution to these short-comings is to consider other forms of mammillary body damage. Although such cases are rare, evidence from this source supports the view that mammillary body damage does con-tribute to the memory loss, but that additional damage is necessary to produce the per-sistent, catastrophic memory loss seen in Korsakoff's syndrome.

Perhaps the most dramatic support comes from patient BJ who, in a fight, had a snooker cue pushed up his left nostril and into the mammillary body region (Dusoir et al., 1990). BJ suffered bilateral damage to the mammillary bodies, with some sparing on the right. There was also some additional damage to the pituitary and adjacent posterior hypothal-amic nuclei (Dusoir et al., 1990). While it is not specified whether the lateral mammillary nuclei were involved, there was possible involvement of the mammillothalamic tract (MTT). BJ showed clear deficits when recalling new information but did not suffer from retrograde amnesia, except for the period immediately surrounding the accident. He also showed a relative sparing of recognition memory (Dusoir et al., 1990). His memory loss affected the recall of both verbal and nonverbal material, though this was most noticeable for verbal material. This is consistent with the laterality of his pathology. A strikingly similar pattern of cognitive deficits, including the relative sparing of nonverbal memory, was observed in patient NA, who had a miniature fencing foil pushed up his nose (Squire et al., 1989). Once again, there was bilateral damage to mammillary bodies, but unlike the case of BJ, there was additional left thalamic pathology (Squire et al., 1989).

Other relevant evidence comes from people with tumors in the region of the mammil-lary bodies (Kahn and Crosby, 1972; Tanaka et al., 1997; Kapur et al., 1998; Hildenbrandt et al., 2001). Once again, these cases have appreciable memory problems but they are not as severe as those in alcoholic Korsakoff's syndrome. Examples of this difference from Korsakoff's syndrome include a relative sparing of recognition memory (Aggleton and Shaw, 1996; Kapur et al., 1998; Hildebrandt et al., 2001), a lack of retrograde amnesia (Kapur et al., 1996, 1998; Tanaka et al., 1997; Hildebrandt et al., 2001), and less severe recall deficits (Dusoir et al., 1990; Kapur et al., 1998). This memory profile strongly sug-gests that pathology in addition to that found in the mammillary bodies is responsible for the additional memory problems typically found in Korsakoff's syndrome. Candidate regions include the anterior thalamic nuclei (Harding et al., 2000), the medial dorsal thal-amic nucleus (Victor et al., 1971; but see Kapur et al., 1996), the parataenial thalamic nucleus (Mair et al., 1979; Mayes et al., 1988), and the intralaminar thalamic nuclei (Mair, 1994). In addition, imaging studies have revealed widespread patterns of cortical abnor-mality (Paller et al., 1997). It should be noted that these candidate regions are not mutu-ally exclusive, and given the range of memory impairments in Korsakoff's syndrome it seems more likely that multiple sites are compromised.

It is pertinent to consider whether pathology in the region of the mammillary bodies disrupts spatial as well as nonspatial memory. Tests on the subject BJ have indicated a greater impairment for delayed matching-to-place than delayed matching-to-sample (Holdstock et al., 1995), as well as an impairment on a visual location task that required the participants to identify those items in a picture that had changed location (Kapur et al., 1994). Clearly, it would be of considerable benefit to know more about the nature of any spatial deficits following mammillary body damage.

Of special relevance to the question at the center of this review, namely, the contribution from head direction cells to memory, is the location of the pathology in Korsakoff's syndrome within the mammillary bodies. In their classic monograph, Victor, Adams and Collins (1971) examined 47 brains of Korsakoff cases. Histological assessment revealed lesions in the medial mammillary nucleus in all 47 cases. In contrast, the lateral mammillary bodies were affected in only one of the 47 cases. The knowledge that the lateral mammillary nuclei are typically preserved in this syndrome might at first appear to preclude their contribution to memory functions. In fact, this finding simply means that Korsakoff's syndrome is unlikely to depend on a loss of the mammillary head direction cells, and it cannot determine whether lateral mammillary nucleus pathology can contribute to the memory disorder.

In conclusion, the human clinical data do support a role for the mammillary bodies in the new learning of both spatial and nonspatial material. While this leaves open the possibility that damage to the lateral mammillary nuclei contributes to these memory problems, there is no direct support for this view. The only direct test would be to examine the outcome of selective lateral mammillary pathology and, as yet, no such cases have been reported. While there is much evidence about the nature of Korsakoff's syndrome, this is relevant for the medial and not the lateral mammillary nuclei.

Animal Lesion Studies
The effects of mammillary body lesions have been examined in a range of species. The most consistent finding is that the surgery results in mild, but appreciable, deficits on tests of spatial memory (Vann and Aggleton, 2004a). These deficits on tests of spatial memory are found (in monkeys: Holmes et al., 1983a,b; rats: Rosenstock et al., 1977; Aggleton et al., 1990, 1995; Saravis et al., 1990; Sziklas and Petrides, 1998; and mice: Beracochea and Jaffard, 1995). In addition, lesions of the mammillary bodies and fornix were found to produce comparable deficits on an automated object-in-place task (Parker and Gaffan, 1997a), which involves monkeys learning object discriminations displayed on a computer screen. This task may capture elements of episodic memory as the objects are set in distinctive "scenes" designed to aid the acquisition of the individual discriminations. Because this task has no navigational component, it might be expected to make little or no demand on head direction information.

A number of attempts have been made to define the nature of the mammillary spatial memory deficits more precisely, with the largest body of data coming from studies with rats. Research from various groups has helped to confirm the importance of the mammillary body region in rats for tests that can be solved using allocentric spatial information (Sutherland and Rodriguez, 1989; Neave et al., 1997; Sziklas and Petrides, 1998). While spatial tests of reference memory typically yield deficits that can be partially overcome (Sutherland and Rodriguez, 1989; Santin et al., 1999; Vann and Aggleton, 2003), more persistent deficits are observed on tests of working memory that tax allocentric spatial processes (Santin et al., 1999; Vann and Aggleton, 2003). Such results have led to the notion that mammillary body damage results in less efficient encoding of distal spatial cues that could, in turn, lead to increased proactive interference (as contextual cues that distinguish episodes are poorly encoded). In this way, it can be seen that mammillary body damage could have quite broad, indirect effects on memory processes.

Once again, a problem with many experimental studies of mammillary body damage is the likelihood of damage to other, adjacent regions. Of special concern is the supramammillary nucleus, which lies immediately dorsal to the mammilllary bodies and is often involved in mammillary body lesions (e.g., Saravis et al., 1990; Aggleton et al., 1991; Sziklas and Petrides, 1998). As this nucleus regulates hippocampal theta rhythm (Kirk, 1998), it is all the more important to spare this area. To avoid this problem and to more precisely focus on the projections from the mammillary bodies to the anterior thalamic nuclei, a recent study (Vann and Aggleton, 2003) measured the behavioral effects of MTT section in rats. Bilateral lesions of the MTT led to deficits on allocentric spatial tasks just as severe as those seen after combined lateral and medial mammillary body lesions. These deficits were characterized as a delayed or inefficient use of allocentric spatial cues (Vann and Aggleton, 2003).

Nonspatial deficits have been observed in a series of studies that also examined the effects of MTT lesions. These tract lesions impaired the retention and learning of active avoidance responses in cats (Kriekhaus, 1964; Kriekhaus and Chi, 1966), rats (Kriekhaus et al., 1968), and rabbits (Gabriel et al., 1995). Deficits have been found both for runway avoidance and lever-press avoidance by cats (Kriekhaus and Chi, 1966; Kriekhaus and Lorenz, 1968). Related studies have shown that these deficits are not due to excessive freezing or to a lack of emotional responsivity as measured by conditioned emotional suppression (Kriekhaus and Chi, 1966; Kriekhaus and Lorenz, 1968). Several points are worthy of note. The avoidance deficits do not mirror those sometimes observed after hippocampal or fornix pathology, which are principally for one-way active avoidance (Gray and McNaughton, 1983). Furthermore, in the case of lever-press avoidance there appears to be little or no spatial element, i.e., the deficits are unlikely to reflect a loss of head direction information. Intriguingly, Kriekhaus (1964) notes that avoidance deficits were observed after unilateral MTT lesions, and suggests that this may reflect the importance of the lateral mammillary nucleus, given its crossed projection to the thalamus (figure 13.1). However, evidence of avoidance deficits after selective lesions in the anterior ventral thalamic nucleus, which does not receive inputs from the lateral mammillary nucleus, would argue against this view (Gabriel et al., 1995).

Additional information comes from the finding that mammillary body lesions spare a variety of learning tasks. For such null results to be informative, it is vital that the lateral mammillary nuclei are included in the lesions, and in some cases (e.g., Aggleton and Mishkin, 1985, Zola-Morgan et al., 1989) there is at least partial sparing. Examples of tests seemingly unaffected by mammillary body lesions include visual discrimination learning (in monkeys, Zola-Morgan et al., 1989; in rats, Saravis et al., 1990), concurrent object discrimination learning (in monkeys, Zola-Morgan et al., 1989), visual discrimination reversal (in monkeys, Holmes et al., 1983b; in rats, Saravis et al., 1990), delayed response (in monkeys, Zola-Morgan et al., 1989); conditioned taste aversion (in rats, Sziklas and Petrides, 1993), conditional learning tasks in which object A is associated with either turning in a constant direction (in rats, Sziklas and Petrides, 1998) or to a constant location (in rats, Sziklas and Petrides, 2000), and delayed matching-to-position (in rats, Harper et al., 1994), and delayed nonmatching-to-position (in rats, Aggleton et al., 1991) for levers in an automated apparatus. For object recognition, mammillary body damage sometimes has little or no effect (in monkeys, Aggleton and Mishkin, 1985; in rats, Aggleton et al., 1990), although other studies of mammillary body lesions or MTT section in monkeys do suggest a mild recognition impairment (Aggleton and Mishkin, 1983a; Zola-Morgan et al., 1989). In addition, MTT lesions do not appear to affect passive avoidance (in rats, Kriekhaus et al., 1968); lever pressing for an appetitive reward (in cats, Kriekhaus and Lorenz, 1968); or the retention of a preoperatively acquired brightness discrimination (in rats, Kriekhaus et al., 1968). The logical conclusion is that mammillary body head direction cells are not necessary for the learning or performance of these tasks.

Anterior Thalamic Nuclei

The anterior thalamic nuclei are composed of the anterior medial (AM), anterior ventral (AV), and anterior dorsal (AD) nuclei (see chapter 2 by Hopkins). The adjacent lateral dorsal thalamic nucleus (LD), which shares many anatomical features with the anterior thalamic nuclei, is sometimes regarded as a fourth member of the group (Van Groen and Wyss, 1992). Head direction cells are confined to the region of the anterior dorsal nucleus (Taube, 1995; Blair et al., 1997) and the lateral dorsal nucleus (Mizumori and Williams, 1993). For the purposes of this chapter, AD and LD will be treated separately. This is because AD, but not LD, appears to be necessary for the postsubicular head direction signal (Taube et al., 1996; Goodridge and Taube, 1997; Golob et al., 1998). Furthermore, direct projections from the lateral mammillary nuclei go to AD rather than LD (Cruce, 1975; Seki and Zyo, 1984; Shibata, 1992). These findings suggest that there may be functional differences between the respective head direction cell areas.

Clinical Evidence

Although the effects of selective pathology to the anterior thalamic nuclei in humans remain largely unknown (Aggleton and Saghal, 1993; Aggleton and Brown, 1999), there are good grounds to believe that damage to these nuclei can result in anterograde amnesia. It is known that rostral thalamic pathology caused by vascular accidents can sometimes produce a marked, anterograde amnesia. Attempts to localize the thalamic region most consistently associated with amnesia have revealed the importance of the MTT (Von Cramon et al., 1985; Gentilini et al., 1987; Van der Werf et al., 2000, 2003). It should be added that the anterior thalamic nuclei themselves are often spared in these vascular accidents because they have multiple arterial sources and so are less vulnerable to strokes. When, however, the pathology is more localized to the anterior thalamic nuclei, then anterograde amnesia is reported (Clarke et al., 1994; Schnider et al., 1996). At present, however, nothing is known about the specific nature of any spatial deficits associated with those rare instances when the pathology is most closely associated with the anterior thalamic nuclei.

Evidence that the anterior thalamic nuclei are crucial for memory also accords with a recent, highly detailed study of Korsakoff's syndrome (Harding et al., 2000). Pathology in the anterior thalamic nuclei was found to be the best predictor of memory loss. The conclusion, that the anterior thalamic nuclei are more crucial than the mammillary bodies, may well relate to the connections of these two structures with the hippocampal formation (figure 13.1). Both regions receive dense inputs from the subicular cortices of the hippocampal formation, but while the anterior thalamic nuclei also project directly back upon the hippocampal formation, the mammillary bodies do not do so, their main efferents being to the anterior thalamic nuclei. This pattern of connections means that anterior thalamic pathology is very likely to be the more disruptive, since the mammillary bodies are almost entirely dependent on the anterior thalamic nuclei, while the converse is not true.

Animal Lesion Studies

Studies with monkeys have shown that lesions centered in the anterior thalamic nuclei can impair object recognition tests and exacerbate the effects of other thalamic damage (Aggleton and Mishkin, 1983a,b). These lesions were, however, produced by aspiration, so there is inevitable tract damage, along with damage to adjacent midline nuclei. Studies using cytotoxins are needed to confirm these effects. More discrete anterior thalamic lesions in monkeys were found to impair an automated object-in-place task (Parker and Gaffan, 1997b) in which the deficit was comparable to that found after mammillary body lesions (Parker and Gaffan, 1997a).

It has been shown repeatedly that anterior thalamic nucleus lesions in rats produce severe deficits on standard tests of spatial memory (Sutherland and Rodriguez, 1989; Aggleton et al., 1995; Aggleton et al., 1996; Warburton et al., 1997). Deficits are found on spatial tasks whether training occurred before or after surgery (Warburton and Aggleton, 1999). A common feature of these tasks is that they can be solved using allocentric spatial information, that is, using the relative positions of distal stimuli to identify current position. Furthermore, these deficits do not extend to egocentric spatial information. For example, Sziklas and Petrides (1999) trained rats on a conditional task in which they were required to learn that particular objects contain reward when they are in certain locations within an arena, but do not contain food when they are presented in other locations in the arena. Electrolytic lesions of the anterior thalamic nuclei impaired the ability of rats to learn this spatial conditional discrimination, but not their ability to learn another conditional task involving the use of egocentric spatial information.

Unlike what is true for the mammillary bodies, research has been done into the behavioral effects of more selective lesions within the anterior thalamic nuclei. So far, five studies, all using rats, have compared different subregions within the anterior thalamic nuclei on tests of spatial learning. This information is vital if one is to contrast the effects of damage in those regions that do or do not contain head direction cells. In two of these studies, lesions centered within either AV or AM nuclei were directly compared (Aggleton et al., 1996; Byatt and Dalrymple-Alford, 1996). In both studies the AV-centered lesions consistently included AD, i.e., they included the head direction area. These studies demonstrated that lesions of the AM region (sparing head direction cells) are sufficient to induce deficits on working memory tasks in the T-maze and radial-arm maze (Aggleton et al., 1996; Byatt and Dalrymple-Alford, 1996). They also showed that lesions of AV/AD also impair these same tasks, and typically give somewhat greater deficits (Aggleton et al., 1996; Byatt and Dalrymple-Alford, 1996). The greatest impairments were, however, associated with combined damage to all three nuclei (Aggleton et al., 1996). This pattern of results is supported by a third study showing that the ability to find a platform in a water maze is mildly impaired by AV/AD lesions, but that a more complete deficit is found after the addition of AM damage (van Groen et al., 2002a). These findings clearly show that performance on these tests of spatial memory does not solely reflect a contribution from head direction information. Rather, there is a separate contribution from the other anterior thalamic nuclei.

In a fourth study (Wilton et al., 2001), lesions were placed in AD but included the rostral portions of LD. Thus, the surgery more selectively removed those thalamic nuclei containing head direction cells. In addition to establishing that these AD/LD lesions disrupted performance in a conventional T-maze alternation task, the rats were also tested in a novel water-maze task that assesses the ability to learn a specific heading vector and distance (Pearce et al., 1998). Rats with AD/LD lesions were impaired on this second task (Wilton et al., 2001), which does not rely on allocentric memory as it can be solved effectively by rats with extensive hippocampal (dentate gyrus, CA1–3) lesions (Pearce et al., 1998). These results suggest that the head direction cells in AD and LD are required for accurate spatial navigation and that this involvement in spatial performance may be quite general (see also, Mizumori et al., 1994; Dudchenko and Taube, 1997). Further support for this view comes from the finding that, while the AD/LD lesions did not affect object recognition, they did impair the ability to distinguish an object moved to a novel location (Wilton et al., 2001). This deficit is informative as the task involves minimal navigational demands. Finally, there is evidence that lesions confined to AD are sufficient to impair a path integration task (Frohardt et al., 2001). As noted previously, these findings do not, however, show that removal of the AD and LD nuclei is sufficient to induce the full anterior thalamic lesion deficit. This is because selective lesion studies have shown that AM also contributes to the spatial memory deficit (Aggleton et al., 1996; Byatt and Dalrymple-Alford, 1996). Further support comes from a recent c-fos imaging study showing that all three anterior thalamic nuclei (AV, AM and AD) have increased levels of gene activation during performance of a spatial task in the radial-arm maze (Vann et al., 2000). These findings again point to the combined role of these nuclei in spatial tests of learning and memory.

The conclusion, that damage to the head direction regions contributes to the spatial memory deficits, but does not produce the full spatial deficit, receives support from another class of evidence. Because of the anatomical relationship between the anterior thalamic nuclei and mammillary bodies, it is possible to make the following assumption: When the disruptive effects of anterior thalamic lesions are greater than those of mammillary body lesions, they are likely to reflect a contribution from that part of the anterior thalamic nuclei not involved in processing head direction information. This can be concluded because anterior thalamic head direction cells are dependent on the lateral mammillary nucleus for their inputs, and so a task that solely taxes head direction information will produce equivalent deficits after mammillary body and anterior thalamic lesions. Thus, the finding that anterior thalamic nuclei lesions can produce significantly greater deficits on T-maze alternation (Aggleton et al., 1995; Aggleton and Brown, 1999) and delayed nonmatching-to-position in an operant chamber (Aggleton et al., 1991), reveals a contribution from the rest of the anterior thalamic nuclei (i.e., not from the head direction area).

Finally, other information about the contribution of head direction nuclei comes from tasks spared after anterior thalamic damage. In these cases the presence of additional damage should not be a confounding factor. Examples of sparing include the learning of egocentric discriminations (in rats, Aggleton et al., 1996 and Warburton et al., 1997) and egocentric conditional tasks (in rats, Sziklas and Petrides, 1999 and Chudasama et al., 2001), as well as visual discriminations (in monkeys, Aggleton and Mishkin, 1983b and Ridley et al., 2002) and their reversals (in rats, Chudasama et al., 2001); concurrent object discriminations (in monkeys, Ridley et al., 2002); visual-visual conditional learning tasks (in monkeys, Ridley et al., 2002), tests of attention (in rats, Chudasama and Muir, 2001), and sensory preconditioning (in rats, Ward-Robinson et al., 2002). The last task is of potential interest as it can be classified as "relational" (Eichenbaum et al., 1994), a category of learning tasks that may depend on hippocampal activity (Eichenbaum et al., 1994).

Lateral Dorsal Thalamic Nucleus

At present, very little is known about the effects of LD lesions, and our current knowledge is limited to studies of rats and spatial learning. An important discovery was that inactivation of LD resulted in increased errors in the radial-arm maze and a disruption of hippocampal place cells (Mizumori et al., 1994), although postsubicular head direction cells are not dependent on the integrity of LD (Golob et al., 1998). In addition, it has been found that ibotenic acid lesions of LD induce relatively mild deficits on a water-maze task (van Groen et al., 2002b). The severity of these water-maze deficits is appreciably greater if the lesions extend into AD, indicating that both nuclei contribute in a nonredundant manner to spatial learning (van Groen et al., 2002b). This pattern of results accords with that reported by Wilton et al. (2001), who found that the effects of combined AD plus LD lesions on T-maze alternation are more severe than those observed after AD/AV lesions (Aggleton et al., 1996; Wilton et al., 2001). Likewise, it was found that the addition of LD damage to complete anterior thalamic lesions led to increased deficits on T-maze alternation (Warburton et al., 1997), although this increase was not significant, possibly due to floor effects. This additivity is consistent with evidence that the LD and AD head direction systems have different connectivities (figure 13.1), and are differentially sensitive to visual and vestibular cues (Mizumori et al., 2000; see chapter 10).

One obvious difficulty in interpreting these results is that, unlike the case of mammillary bodies or the anterior thalamic nuclei, no distinctive subregion within LD contains head direction cells. Head direction cells are concentrated in the dorsal aspect of the caudal two-thirds of LD in the rat (Mizumori and Wiliams, 1993), which means that all attempts to lesion LD have included other regions of the nucleus. This potential problem of added pathology can be discounted only when there is no lesion effect, e.g., for delayed matching-to-sample with retractable levers (Burk and Mair, 1999). For these reasons, it is difficult to make any firm conclusions apart from the likelihood that LD damage summates with AD damage to disrupt spatial learning tasks; that is, they are not redundant.

Retrosplenial Cortex

The retrosplenial cortex is densely connected to the anterodorsal and laterodorsal thalamic nuclei (van Groen et al., 1993), and like those thalamic nuclei it contains head direction cells (Chen et al., 1994; Cho and Sharp, 2001). In order to interpret lesion data it is important to appreciate the distribution of head direction cells within the retrosplenial cortex. At present, a precise answer is lacking. In the study by Cho and Sharp (2001) the position of the electrodes from bregma (−5.7 mm) suggests that the recordings were taken from the caudal retrosplenial cortex in the rat (although this does not preclude other areas from containing head direction cells). Additional information comes from the report that head direction cells and direction-dependent place cells are found in both granular and dysgranular parts of area 29 (Chen et al., 1994; Cho and Sharp, 2001). These head direction cells make up only a small proportion (9%) of the rodent retrosplenial cortex (Chen et al., 1994), which is thought to have multiple functions (Vogt et al., 1992). Unlike primates, the rat does not contain a distinct posterior cingulate region (area 23). Rather, the entire area is regarded as area 29 (Vogt and Peters, 1981). Finally, it should be noted that damage to the retrosplenial cortex often extends to the adjacent cingulum bundle, and this may add to the cognitive disturbances that are observed.

Clinical Evidence

Like the anterior thalamic nuclei and the mammillary bodies, damage to the region of the retrosplenial cortex can impair human memory. The first reported case (Valenstein et al., 1987) involved a man who developed both anterograde and retrograde amnesia following a hemorrhage in the region containing the left retrosplenial cortex and cingulum bundle. While the duration of the retrograde amnesia diminished to a period of about one year before the injury, his anterograde amnesia persisted (Valenstein et al., 1987). In addition, he showed a marked deficit in learning the temporal order of events (Bowers et al., 1988). Other cases also indicate that retrosplenial pathology, typically bilateral, can lead to anterograde amnesia (Rudge and Warrington, 1991; Von Cramon and Schuri, 1992). There is, however, at least one case where right retrosplenial pathology is associated with both verbal and nonverbal memory deficits (Yasuda et al., 1997). A different profile was observed in the patient described by Gainotti et al., (1998) who had bilateral retrosplenial pathology, but whose memory deficits were principally a retrograde amnesia combined with a failure to learn new nonverbal information. A problem in many of these cases is that there is associated fornix damage, making it very difficult to define precisely the retrosplenial contribution. For this reason it is important to note that increased retrosplenial cortex activity is often observed in neuroimaging studies of memory (Maguire 2001b), including studies of autobiographical event recall (Maguire 2001a).

Perhaps of more direct relevance to the issue of head direction information are reports that damage to the retrosplenial area can lead to topographic amnesia. An example is provided by Takahashi et al. (1997), who described three patients with focal hemorrhages extending from the right retrosplenial area to the medial parietal lobe. While they did not appear to have perceptual or mnemonic problems for buildings or landscapes, they had great difficulty remembering the directions from one location to another. In contrast, they could determine and remember the locations of objects when standing in one place (e.g., furniture inside a room). These and other cases have been reviewed by Maguire (2001b), who notes a number of common features in ten cases of topographic amnesia associated with retrosplenial damage. In eight of these cases, the pathology was in the right hemisphere. The patients were all able to recognize landmarks in their neighborhoods, that retained a sense of familiarity. Nevertheless, none of the patients were able to find their way around this familiar environment. There was good evidence that the condition improved over a number of weeks after initial onset, indicating that another region could support this function. None of these cases was amnesic, i.e., general memory performance was intact (Maguire 2001b). Additional support for a role in navigation has come from functional imaging (Maguire 2001b; Burgess 2002). This support includes studies looking at large-scale navigation e.g., using film footage or virtual reality. Of 14 such studies identified by Maguire (2001b), retrosplenial activation was observed in 12. Thus, unlike the regions previously considered (mammillary bodies and anterior thalamic nuclei), there is direct clinical evidence that the retrosplenial cortex may have a specific role in spatial processes, in addition to a more general role in memory function.

Animal Lesion Studies

As might be predicted, the rodent retrosplenial cortex (area 29) is important for spatial learning and memory. Evidence comes from the lesion-induced deficits found for both reference and working memory tests in the water maze (Sutherland et al., 1988; Sutherland and Hoesing, 1993; Whishaw et al., 2001; Harker and Whishaw, 2002; Vann and Aggleton, 2002; Vann et al., 2003), and for tests of spatial working memory in the radial-arm maze (Vann and Aggleton, 2002, 2004b; Vann et al., 2003). Retrosplenial lesion deficits are also found for tests of path integration that tax idiothetic spatial behavior (Cooper and Mizumori, 1999, 2001; Whishaw et al., 2001) and for tests in recognizing the location of objects (Vann and Aggleton 2002). These findings indicate a broader role in spatial processing.

A potentially important point is that the consequences of retrosplenial lesions on tests of spatial memory depend critically on the extent of area 29 that has been removed. Complete lesions reveal deficits that may not be seen with more selective lesions (Vann and Aggleton 2002, 2004b), and it appears that inclusion of the most caudal part of area 29 can be crucial (Vann et al., 2003). Linked to this is evidence that damage to the cingulum bundle can influence the outcome of retrosplenial lesions (Aggleton et al., 1995; Warburton et al., 1998).

General Conclusions

A number of key facts emerge from this review. Perhaps the most important is confirmation that bilateral damage to regions containing head direction cells can produce memory impairments in humans. The resulting anterograde amnesia affects both spatial and nonspatial forms of memory. While this association is found repeatedly for anterograde amnesia, there are enough cases to show that the same pathology need not produce retrograde amnesia. At the same time, it is vital to appreciate that there is no clinical evidence that selective pathology in a specific subregion containing head direction information (e.g., lateral mammillary nucleus or anterior dorsal thalamic nucleus) is sufficient to induce amnesia. Nevertheless, the link that the mammillary bodies, anterior thalamic nuclei, and retrosplenial cortex all have with amnesia is striking.

In the case of the anterior thalamic nuclei, there is good evidence that those nuclei not containing head direction cells (AV, AM) contribute to learning and memory. This has been shown most directly in lesion studies in rats. These studies have revealed how selective damage to these nuclei impair tests of spatial learning and memory. Other support comes from brain activity imaging in monkeys (Friedman et al., 1990) and rats (Vann et al., 2000), as well as electrophysiological studies in rabbits (Gabriel, 1993). Thus, not only are these anterior thalamic nuclei physically adjacent to the head direction cells in AD but they can also influence similar (e.g., spatial) learning tasks, albeit in different ways. As a consequence, the effects of combined lesions of these nuclei are additive. In view of the anatomical connections between the mammillary bodies and the anterior thalamic nuclei, it is most likely that the same arrangement applies to the mammillary bodies, i.e., that both medial and lateral mammillary nuclei contribute to learning and memory but in different ways.

From this summary two main questions emerge: (1) Can a spatial/navigation deficit lead to more widespread cognitive problems and thus explain the apparent importance of head direction cells for more general aspects of memory? and (2) Does the repeated arrangement of head direction cells next to a nucleus (nuclei) in the same structure that is also engaged in the same overall process, confer any particular advantage?

The first question is how a loss of head direction information might have a broader impact on memory processes. The resolution of this question depends crucially on the way in which head direction information interacts with, and is necessary for, other forms of spatial information (see chapters 10, 11, and 12). If it is the case that head direction information and place information are closely coupled (Knierim et al., 1995), and that accurate place information depends on the integrity of the head direction system (Mizumori et al., 1994; but see Golob et al., 2001), then it is relatively easy to envisage a link between head direction signals and episodic memory. A characteristic of episodic information is that event information is set within a distinctive context or scene, which is defined both spatially and temporally. If setting a scene depends on these interactive spatial processes, then damage to head direction nuclei could disrupt the acquisition of distinctive episodes (Gaffan, 1992; Aggleton and Pearce, 2001).

A more specific hypothesis has been advanced by Burgess (2002). He argues that the retrieval of spatial information, and hence spatial episodes, requires the setting of a particular viewpoint. This, in turn, depends on the representation of head direction and, hence, the input from the head direction system. The parietal cortex and retrosplenial cortices are given special prominence in this model as they represent regions where there is an integration of different spatial systems (allocentric, egocentric, body orientation). As a consequence, information about current head direction makes it possible to translate allocentric representations into egocentric ones and vice versa (Burgess, 2002). This, in turn, helps to create distinctive episodes of information.

Such models can also explain the relative sparing of recognition that is associated with mammillary body damage both in animals and humans. It has been argued that recognition relies on two processes, one dependent on familiarity detection the other on the recollection of the recognized event (Mandler, 1980; Yonelinas, 2002). From this, a relative sparing of recognition memory after mammillary body damage is to be predicted (Aggleton and Brown, 1999) if damage to this region affects only the recollective component, that is, there is a sparing of familiarity. This accords with the idea that the recollective component is scene based (Perfect et al., 1996), while the feeling of familiarity is not (Brown and Aggleton, 2001). Consistent with this account are rat studies showing that combined removal of AD and LD does not affect object recognition but does impair the ability to distinguish an object moved to a novel location, thus creating a new scene (Wilton et al., 2001). Complete retrosplenial lesions produce the same pattern of results (Vann and Aggleton, 2002).

A strong version of the model proposed by Burgess (2002) is that the effects of mammillary body and anterior thalamic damage upon memory are solely the consequences of a loss of frame of reference. As has repeatedly been observed, evidence from a variety of sources shows that the non-head direction nuclei (medial mammillary nucleus, AV, AM) also contribute to learning (e.g., Gabriel, 1993; Gabriel et al., 1995). This indicates that the model of Burgess (2002) can only partially explain the effects of lesions in the mammillary bodies and anterior thalamic nuclei. This brings me to the second question: Why are head direction cells found next to nuclei in the mammillary bodies and anterior thalamic nuclei that are also engaged in the same overall process but in different ways?

The physical proximity of these functional regions is unlikely to be coincidental since it is repeated in both structures. A more likely account is that it derives from common connections that serve the different subregions within these structures. Uppermost among these connections are those with the hippocampus. The hippocampal formation (via the subiculum complex) projects to all nuclei within the anterior thalamic region as well as the mammillary bodies. This interaction is reciprocal, as the anterior thalamic nuclei project directly to the hippocampal formation, although the return connections from the mammillary bodies are indirect, as they are principally via the anterior thalamic nuclei.

While the "lateral" system (lateral mammillary bodies and AD) is now known to be important for head direction, evidence about the functions of the "medial" system (medial mammillary bodies, AM, AV) remains scarce (Vann and Aggleton, 2004a). Electrophysiological studies suggest that the medial mammillary nuclei may be important for relaying theta (Kocsis and Vertes, 1994; Kirk et al., 1996) to the anterior thalamic nuclei and, indirectly, beyond. There is increasing agreement that theta rhythm within the hippocampus is important for memory, and that this may be linked to theta activity in a number of circuits, including that via the medial mammillary nuclei (Kirk and Mackay, 2003). One suggested function is that this theta signal may reduce interference by separating episodes (Hasselmo et al., 2002). Recent studies have shown that there are theta-sensitive cells in all three anterior thalamic nuclei, most of which increase their firing rates during theta (Albo et al., 2003). Although AV appears to contain the highest numbers of theta-related cells (Albo et al., 2003), the presence of both head direction cells and theta responsive cells in AD points to a potential interaction between these signals.

Another source of relevant data comes from electrophysiological and lesion studies of signaled avoidance behavior (foot step) by rabbits (Gabriel, 1993). From this it has been proposed that the connections from the mammillary bodies to the anterior thalamic nuclei and, thence, to the posterior cingulate cortex form part of a mnemonic "primacy" system. This system helps to retain the primary or original encoding of a learning event, but is inflexible to subsequent changes in that event. It has, for example, been shown that neurons in both AV and the superficial layers of the posterior cingulate cortex show discriminative activity in the later stages of behavioral learning (Gabriel et al., 1980). The fact that this function is not associated with a spatial task suggests that these are properties of the medial system. Consistent with this, lesions of not only the MTT but also AV stop the training induced neural activity in the posterior cingulate cortex and impair acquisition of the avoidance task (Gabriel, 1993; Gabriel et al., 1995).

The conclusion that there are two parallel mammillary body–anterior thalamic systems (medial and lateral) that contribute to learning raises questions as to how and where these two systems interact. Studies by Gabriel (1993) suggest that this interaction does not occur within the posterior cingulate cortex since the primacy system is still distinct. While it is possible that there is interaction within the anterior thalamic nuclei themselves (Albo et al., 2003), the most likely convergence point is within the hippocampal formation as AV, AD and LD all project to the presubiculum. Finally, the effects of damage to the anterior thalamic nuclei on memory are sometimes most dramatic when they are in combination with damage to another site, for example, with the medial dorsal thalamic nucleus (Aggleton and Mishkin, 1983a,b; Ridley et al., 2002). This highlights the ways in which selective lesion evidence might sometimes underestimate the importance of a specific structure to cognition, and this may include regions providing head direction signals.

References

Aggleton JP, Brown MW (1999) Episodic memory amnesia and the hippocampal anterior thalamic axis. Behav Brain Sci 22: 425–466.

Aggleton JP, Hunt PR, Nagle S, Neave N (1996) The effects of selective lesions within the anterior thalamic nuclei on spatial memory in the rat. Behav Brain Res 81: 189–198.

Aggleton JP, Hunt PR, Shaw C (1990) The effects of mammillary body and combined amygdalar-fornix lesions on tests of delayed non-matching-to-sample in the rat. Behav Brain Res 40: 145–157.

Aggleton JP, Keith AP, Saghal A (1991) Both fornix and anterior thalamic but not mammillary lesions disrupt delayed non-matching-to-position memory in rats. Behav Brain Res 44: 151–161.

Aggleton JP, Mishkin M (1983a) Memory impairments following restricted medial thalamic lesions in monkeys. Exp Brain Res 52: 199–209.

Aggleton JP, Mishkin M (1983b) Visual recognition impairment following medial thalamic lesions in monkeys. Neuropsychologia 21: 189–197.

Aggleton JP, Mishkin M (1985) Mamillary-body lesions and visual recognition in monkeys. Exp Brain Res 58: 190–197.

Aggleton JP, Neave N, Nagle S, Hunt PR (1995) A comparison of the effects of anterior thalamic mammillary body and fornix lesions on reinforced spatial alternation. Behav Brain Res 68: 91–101.

Aggleton JP, Neave N, Nagle S, Sahgal A (1995) A comparison of the effects of medial prefrontal cingulate cortex and cingulum bundle lesions on tests of spatial memory: evidence of a double dissociation between frontal and cingulum bundle contributions. J Neurosci 15: 7270–7281.

Aggleton JP, Pearce JM (2001) Neural systems underlying episodic memory: Insights from animal research. Phil Trans Roy Soc 356: 1467–1482.

Aggleton JP, Sahgal A (1993) The contribution of the anterior thalamic nuclei to anterograde memory. Neuro-psychologia 31: 1001–1019.

Aggleton JP, Shaw C (1996) Amnesia and recognition memory: a re-analysis of psychometric data. Neuropsy-chologia 34: 51–62.

Albo Z Di Prisco GV, Vertes RP (2003) Anterior thalamic unit discharge profiles and coherence with hippocampal theta rhythm. Thal Rel Sys 2: 133–144.

Beracochea DJ, Jaffard R (1995) The effects of mammillary body lesions on delayed matching and delayed non-matching to place tasks in the mice. Behav Brain Res 68: 45–52.

Blair HT, Cho J, Sharp PE (1998) Role of the lateral mammillary nucleus in the rat head direction circuit: a com-bined single unit recording and lesions study. Neuron 21: 1387–1397.

Blair HT, Cho J, Sharp PE (1999) The anterior thalamic head-direction signal is abolished by bilateral but not unilateral lesions of the lateral mammillary nucleus. J Neurosci 19: 6673–6683.

Blair HT, Lipscomb BW, Sharp PE (1997) Anticipatory time intervals of head-direction cells in the anterior thal-amus of the rat: implications for path integration in the head direction circuit. J Neurophys 19: 495–502.

Blair HT, Sharp PE (1995) Anticipatory head direction signals in anterior thalamus: Evidence for a thalamocor-tical circuit that integrates angular head motion to compute head direction. J Neurosc 15: 6260–6270.

Bowers D, Verfaellie M, Valenstein E, Heilman KM (1988) Impaired acquisition of temporal information in retrosplenial amnesia. Brain Cogn 8: 47–66.

Brown MW, Aggleton JP (2001) Recognition memory: what are the roles of the perirhinal cortex and hippocampus? Nature Rev Neurosci 2: 51–61.

Burgess N (2002) The hippocampus space and viewpoints in episodic memory. Quart J Exp Psychol 55A: 1057–1080.

Burk JA, Mair RG (1999) Delayed matching-to-sample trained with retractable levers is impaired by lesions of the intralaminar or ventomedial but not laterodorsal thalamic nuclei. Psychobiol 27: 351–363.

Byatt G, Dalrymple-Alford JC (1996) Both anteromedial and anteroventral thalamic lesions impair radial-maze learning in rats. Behav Neurosci 110: 1335–1348.

Chen LL, Lin LH, Green EJ, Barnes CA, McNaughton BL (1994) Head direction cells in the posterior cortex I Anatomical distribution and behavioural modulation. Exp Brain Res 101: 8–23.

Cho J, Sharp PE (2001) Head direction place and movement correlates for cells in the rat retrosplenial cortex. Behav Neurosci 115: 3–25.

Chudasama Y, Bussey TJ, Muir JL (2001) Visual attention in the rat: A role for the prelimbic cortex and thala-mic nuclei. Behav Neurosci 115: 417–428.

Chudasama Y, Muir JL (2001) Effects of selective thalamic and prelimbic cortex lesions on two types of visual discrimination and reversal learning. Eur J Neurosci 14: 1009–1020.

Clarke S, Assal G, Bogousslavsky J, Regli F, Townsend DW, Leenders KL, Blecic S (1994) Pure amnesia after unilateral left polar infarct: topographic and sequential neuropsychological and metabolic (PET) correlations. J Neurol Neurosurg Psychiat 57: 27–34.

Cooper BG, Mizumori SYJ (1999) Retrosplenial cortex inactivation selectively impairs navigation in the dark. Neuro Report 10: 625–630.

Cooper BG, Mizumori SYJ (2001) Temporary inactivation of the retrosplenial cortex causes transient reorganization of spatial coding in the hippocampus. J Neurosci 21: 3986–4001.

Cruce JAF (1975) An autoradiographic study of the projections of the mammillothalamic tract in the rat. Brain Res 85: 211–219.

Delay J, Brion S (1969) Le syndrome de Korsakoff. Paris: Masson and Cie.

Davila MD, Shear PK, Lane B, Sullivan EV, Pfefferbaum A (1994) Mammillary body and cerebellar shrinkage in chronic alcoholics: an MRI and neuropsychological study. Neuropsychology 8: 433–444.

Dudchenko PA, Taube JS (1997) Correlation between head direction cell activity and spatial behavior on a radial arm maze. Behav Neurosci 111: 13–19.

Dusoir H, Kapur N, Brynes DP, McKinstry S, Hoare RD (1990) The role of diencephalic pathology in human memory disorder. Brain 113: 1695–1706.

Eichenbaum H, Otto T, Cohen NJ (1994) Two functional components of the hippocampal memory system. Behav Brain Sci 17: 449–518.

Friedman HR, Janas JD, Goldman-Rakic PS (1990) Enhancement of metabolic activity in the diencephalon of monkeys performing working memory tasks: a 2-deoxyglucose study in behaving rhesus monkeys. J Cogn Neurosci 2: 18–31.

Frohardt RJ, Marcroft JL, Taube JS (2001) Lesion of the anterior thalamus impair path integration performance on a food carrying task. Soc Neurosci Abstr 27: 315.11.

Gabriel M (1993) Discriminative avoidance learning: a model system. In BA Vogt and M Gabriel, eds., Neurobiology of Cingulate Cortex and Limbic Thalamus, Boston: Birkhauser, pp. 478–523.

Gabriel M, Foster K, Orona E (1980) Interaction of laminae of the cingulate cortex with the anteroventral thalamus during behavioral learning. Science 208: 1050–1052.

Gabriel M, Cuppernell C, Shenk JI, Kubota Y, Henzi V, Swanson D (1995) Mammillothalamic tract transection blocks anterior thalamic training—induced neuronal plasticity and impairs discriminative avoidance behavior in rabbits. J Neurosci 15: 1437–1445.

Gaffan D (1992) The role of the hippocampus-fornix-mammillary system in episodic memory. In LR Squire and N Butters, eds., Neuropsychology of Memory, New York: The Guildford Press, pp. 336–346.

Gainotti G, Aimonti S, Di Betta AM, Silveri MC (1998) Retrograde amnesia in a patient with retrosplenial tumour. Neurocase 4: 519–526.

Gamper E (1928) Zur Frage der Polioencephalitis der chronischen Alkoholiker Anatomische Befunde beim chronischem Korsakow und ihre Beziehungen zum klinischen Bild. Dtsch Z Nervenheilkd 102: 122–129.

Gentilini M, de Renzi E, Cris G (1987) Bilateral parmedian thalamic artery infarcts: report of eight cases. J Neurol Neurosurg Psychiat 50: 900–909.

Golob EJ, Stackman RW, Wong AC, Taube JS (2001) On the behavioural significance of head direction cells: neural and behavioural dynamics during spatial memory tasks. Behav Neurosci 115: 285–304.

Golob EJ, Wolk DA, Taube JS (1998) Recordings of postsubicular head direction cells following lesions of the laterodorsal thalamic nucleus. Brain Res 780: 9–19.

Goodridge JP, Taube JS (1997) Interaction between the postsubiculum and anterior thalamus in the generation of head direction cell activity. J Neurosci 17: 9315–9330.

Gray JA, McNaughton N (1983) Comparison between the behavioural effects of septal and hippocampal lesions: a review. Neurosci Biobehav Rev 7: 119–188.

Gudden H (1896) Klinishe und anatomische Beitraege zur Kenntniss der multiplen Alkoholneuritis nebst Bemärkungen über die Regenerationsvorgänge in peripheren Nervensystem. Archiv Psychiat Nerven 28: 643–741.

Harding A, Halliday G, Caime D, Kril J (2000) Degeneration of anterior thalamic nuclei differentiates alcoholics with amnesia. Brain 123: 141–154.

Harker KT, Whishaw IQ (2002) Impaired spatial performance in rats with retrosplenial lesions: importance of the spatial problem and the rat strain in identifying lesion effects in a swimming pool. J Neurosci 22: 850–860.

Harper DN, McLean AP, Dalrymple-Alford J (1994) Forgetting in rats following medial septum or mammillary body damage. Behav Neurosci 198: 1–12.

Hasselmo M, Cannon RC, Koene R (2002) A simulation of parahippocampal and hippocampal structures guiding spatial navigation of a virtual rat in a virtual environment: a functional framework for theta theory. In M Witter and F Wouterlood, eds., The Parahippocampal Region, Oxford: Oxford Unversity Press, pp. 139–161.

Hildebrandt H, Muller S, Bussmann-Mork B, Goebel S, Eilers N (2001) Are some memory deficits unique to lesions of the mammillary bodies? J Clin Exp Neuropsychol 23: 490–501.

Holdstock JS, Shaw C, Aggleton JP (1995) The performance of amnesic subjects on tests of delayed matching-to-sample and delayed matching-to-position. Neuropsychologia 33: 1583–1596.

Holmes EJ, Jacobson S, Stein BM, Butters N (1983a) Ablations of the mammillary nuclei in monkeys: effects on postoperative memory. Exp Neurol 81: 97–113.

Holmes EJ, Jacobson S, Stein BM, Butters N (1983b) An examination of the effects of mammillary body lesions on reversal learning sets in monkeys. Physiol Psychol 11: 159–165.

Jaffard R, Beracochea D, Cho Y (1991) The hippocampal-mamillary system: anterograde and retrograde amnesia. Hippocampus 1: 275–278.

Kahn EA, Crosby EC (1972) Korsakoff's syndrome associated with surgical lesions involving the mammillary bodies. Neurology 22: 117–125.

Kapur N, Crewes H, Wise R, Abbott P, Carter M, Millar J, Lang D (1998) Mammillary body damage results in memory impairment but not amnesia. Neurocase 4: 509–517.

Kapur N, Scholey K, Moore E, Barker S, Mayes A, Brice J, Fleming J (1994) The mammillary bodies revisited: their role in human memory functioning. In L Cermak, ed., Neuropsychological Explorations of Memory and Cognition: Essays in Honour of Nelson Butters, New York: Plenum Press, pp. 159–189.

Kapur N, Thompson S, Cook P, Lang D, Brice J (1996) Anterograde but not retrograde memory loss following combined mammillary body and medial thalamic lesions. Neuropsychologia 34: 1–8.

Kirk IJ (1998) Frequency modulation of hippocampal theta by the supramammillary nucleus and other hypothalamo-hippocampal interactions: Mechanisms and functional implications. Neurosci Biobehav Rev 22: 291–302.

Kirk IJ, Mackay JC (2003) The role of theta-range oscillations in synchronising and integrating activity in distributed mnemonic networks. Cortex 39: 993–1008.

Kirk IJ, Oddie SD, Konopacki J, Bland BH (1996) Evidence for differential control of posterior hypothalamic supramammillary and medial mammillary theta related cellular discharge by ascending and descending pathways. J Neurosci 16: 5547–5554.

Kocsis B, Vertes RP (1994) Characterization of neurons of the supramammillary nucleus and mammillary body that discharge rhythmically with hippocampal theta in the rat. J Neurosci 14: 7040–7052.

Knierim JJ, Kudrimoti HS, McNaughton BL (1995) Place cells head direction cells and the learning of landmark stability. J Neurosci 15: 1648–1659.

Kopelman MD (1995) The Korsakoff syndrome. Br J Psychiat 166: 154–173.

Kriekhaus EE (1964) Decrements in avoidance behavior following mammillothalamic tractotomy in cats. J Neurophys 27: 753–767.

Kriekhuas EE, Chi CC (1966) Role of freezing and fear in avoidance decrements following mammillothalamic tractotomy in cat: I Two-way active avoidance. Psychonom Sci 4: 263–266.

Krieckhaus EE, Coons EE, Greenspon T, Weiss J, Lorenz R (1968) Retention of choice behavior in rats following mammillothalamic tractotomy. Physiol Behav 3: 125–131.

Krieckhaus EE, Lorenz R (1968) Retention and relearning of lever-press avoidance following mammillothalamic tractotomy. Physiol Behav 3: 433–438.

Maguire EA (2001a) Neuroimaging studies of autobiographical event memory. Philos Trans Roy Soc Lond B 356: 1441–1451.

Maguire EA (2001b) The retrosplenial contribution to human navigation: a review of lesion and imaging findings. Scand J Psychol 42: 225–238.

Mair RG (1994) On the role of thalamic pathology in diencephalic amnesia. Rev Neurosci 5: 105–140.

Mair WGP, Warrington EK, Weiskrantz L (1979) Memory disorder in Korsakoff's psychosis. Brain 102: 749–783.

Mandler G (1980) Recognizing: The judgment of previous occurrence. Psych Rev 87: 252–271.

Mayes AR, Meudell PR, Mann D, Pickering A (1988) Location of lesions in Korsakoff's syndrome: neuropathological data on two patients. Cortex 24: 367–388.

Mizumori SJY, Miya DY, Ward KE (1994) Reversible inactivation of the lateral dorsal thalamus disrupts hippocampal place representation and impairs spatial learning. Brain Res 644: 168–174.

Mizumori SJY, Williams JD (1993) Directionally selective mnemonic properties of neurons in the lateral dorsal nucleus of the thalamus of rats. J Neurosci 13: 4015–4028.

Neave N, Nagle S, Aggleton JP (1997) Evidence for the involvement of the mammillary bodies and cingulum bundle in allocentric spatial processing by rats. Eur J Neurosci 9: 941–955.

Paller KA, Acharya A, Richardson BC, Plaisant O, Shimamura AP, Reed BR, Jagust WJ (1997) Functional neuroimaging of cortical dysfunction in alcoholic Korsakoff's syndrome. J Cogn Neurosci 9: 277–293.

Parker A, Gaffan D (1997a) Mammillary body lesions in monkeys impair object-in-place memory: functional unity of the fornix-mamillary system. J Cogn Neurosci 9: 512–521.

Parker A, Gaffan D (1997b) The effect of anterior thalamic and cingulate cortex lesions on object-in-place memory in monkeys. Neuropsychologia 35: 1093–1102.

Pearce JM, Roberts ADL, Good M (1998) Hippocampal lesions disrupt navigation based on cognitive maps but not heading vectors. Nature 396: 75–77.

Perfect TJ, Mayes AR, Downes JJ, Van Eijl R (1996) Does context discriminate recollection from familiarity in recognition memory? Quart J Exp Psych 49A: 797–813.

Rémy M (1942) Contribution à l'étude de la maladie de Korsakov. Etude anatomo-clinique Monatsschrift Psychiat Neurol 106: 128–144.

Ridley RM, Maclean CJ, Young FM, Baker HF (2002) Learning impairments in monkeys with combined but not separate excitotoxic lesions of the anterior and mediodorsal thalamic nuclei. Brain Res 950: 39–51.

Rigges HE, Boles RS (1944) Wernicke's encephalopathy: clinical and pathological studies of 42 cases. Quart J Stud Alcohol 5: 361–370.

Rosenstock J, Field TD, Greene E (1977) The role of the mammillary bodies in spatial memory. Exp Neurol 55: 340–352.

Rudge P, Warrington EK (1991) Selective impairment of memory and visual perception in splenial tumours. Brain 114: 349–360.

Santin LJ, Rubio S, Begaga A, Arias JL (1999) Effects of mammillary body lesions on spatial reference and working memory tasks. Behav Brain Res 102: 137–150.

Saravis S, Sziklas V, Petrides M (1990) Memory for places and the region of the mammillary bodies in the rat. Eur J Neurosci 2: 556–564.

Schnider A, Gutbrod K, Hess CW, Schroth G (1996) Memory without context: amnesia with confabulation after infarction of the right capsular genu. J Neurol Neurosurg Psychiatr 61: 186–193.

Seki M, Zyo K (1984) Anterior thalamic afferents from the mammillary body and the limbic cortex in the rat. J Comp Neurol 229: 242–256.

Shibata H (1992) Topographic organization of subcortical projections to the anterior thalamic nuclei in the rat. J Comp Neurol 323: 117–127.

Squire LR, Amaral DG, Zola-Morgan S, Kritchevsky M, Press G (1989) Description of brain injury in the amnesic patient NA based on magnetic resonance imaging. Exp Neurol 105: 23–35.

Stackman RW, Taube JS (1998) Firing properties of rat lateral mammillary single units: Head direction head pitch and angular head velocity. J Neurosci 18: 9020–9037.

Sutherland RJ, Hoesing JM (1993) Posterior cingulate cortex and spatial memory: a microlimnology analysis. In BA Vogt and M Gabriel, eds., Neurobiology of Cingulate Cortex and Limbic Thalamus: A Comprehensive Treatise, Boston: Birkhauser, pp. 461–477.

Sutherland RJ, Rodriguez AJ (1989) The role of the fornix/fimbria and some related subcortical structures in place learning and memory. Behav Brain Res 32: 265–277.

Sutherland RJ, Whishaw IQ, Kolb B (1988) Contributions of the cingulate cortex to two forms of spatial learning and memory. J Neurosci 8: 1863–1872.

Sziklas V, Petrides M (1993) Memory impairments following lesions to the mammillary region. Eur J Neurosci 5: 525–540.

Sziklas V, Petrides M (1998) Memory and the region of the mammillary bodies. Prog Neurobiol 54: 55–70.

Sziklas V, Petrides M (1999) The effects of lesions to the anterior thalamic nuclei on object-place associations in rats. Eur J Neurosci 11: 559–566.

Sziklas V, Petrides M (2000) Selectivity of the spatial learning deficit after lesions of the mammillary region in rats. Hippocampus 10: 325–328.

Stackman RW, Taube JS (1998) Firing properties of lateral mammillary single units: head direction head pitch and angular head velocity. J Neurosci 18: 9020–9037.

Takahashi N, Kawamura M, Shiota J, Kasahata N, Hirayama K (1997) Pure topographic disorientation due to a right retrosplenial lesion. Neurology 49: 464–469.

Tanaka Y, Miyazawa Y, Akaoka F, Yamada T (1997) Amnesia following damage to the mammillary bodies. Neurology 48: 160–165.

Taube JS (1995) Head direction cells recorded in the anterior thalamic nuclei of freely moving rats. Journal of Neuroscience 15: 70–86.

Taube JS, Goodridge JP, Golob EJ, Dudchenko PA, Stackman RW (1996) Processing the head direction Signal: A review and commentary. Brain Res Bull 40: 477–486.

Taube JS, Kesslak JP, Cotman CW (1992) Lesions of the rat postsubiculum impair performance on spatial tasks. Behav Neural Biol 57: 131–143.

Torvik A (1987) Topographic distribution and severity of brain lesions in Wernicke's encephalopathy. Clin Neuropathol 6: 25–29.

Valenstein E, Bowers D, Verfaillie M, Heilman KM, Fay A, Watson RT (1987) Retrosplenial amnesia. Brain 110: 1631–1646.

Van der Werf YD, Scheltens P, Lindeboom J, Witter MP, Uylings HBM, Jolles J (2003) Deficits of memory executive functioning and attention following infarctions in the thalamus; a study of 22 cases with localised lesions. Neuropsychologia 41: 1330–1344.

Van der Werf YD, Witter MP, Uylings HBM, Jolles J (2000) Neuropsychology of infarctions in the thalamus: a review. Neuropsychologia 38: 613–627.

Van Groen T, Vogt BA, Wyss JM (1993) Interconnections between the thalamus and retrosplenial cortex in the rodent brain. In BA Vogt and Meds Gabriel, eds., Neurobiology of Cingulate Cortex and Limbic Thalamus: A Comprehensive Handbook, Boston: Birkhauser, pp. 123–150.

Van Groen T, Wyss JM (1992) Projections from the laterodorsal nucleus of the thalamus to the limbic and visual cortices in the rat. J Comp Neurol 324: 427–448.

Van Groen T, Kadish I, Wyss JM (2002a) Role of the anterodorsal and anteroventral nuclei of the thalamus in spatial memory in the rat. Behav Brain Res 132: 19–28.

Van Groen T, Kadish I, Wyss JM (2002b) The role of the laterodorsal nucleus of the thalamus in spatial learning and memory in the rat. Behav Brain Res 136: 329–337.

Vann SD, Aggleton JP (2004a) Mammillary bodies: Two memory systems in one? Nature Rev Neursci 5: 35–44.

Vann SD, Aggleton JP (2004b) Testing the importance of the retrosplenial guidance system: Effects of different sized retrosplenial lesions on heading direction and spatial working memory. Behav Brain Res 155: 97–108.

Vann SD, Aggleton JP (2002) Extensive cytotoxic lesions of the rat retrosplenial cortex reveal consistent deficits on tasks that tax allocentric spatial memory. Behav Neurosci 116: 85–94.

Vann SD, Aggleton JP (2003) Evidence of a spatial encoding deficit with lesions of the mammillary bodies or mammillothalamic tract. J Neurosci 23: 3506–3514.

Vann SD, Brown MW, Aggleton JP (2000) Fos expression in the rostral thalamic nuclei and associated cortical regions in response to different spatial memory tests. Neurosci 101: 983–991.

Vann SD, Wilton LAK, Muir JL, Aggleton JP (2003) Testing the importance of the caudal retrosplenial cortex for spatial memory in rats. Behav Brain Res 140: 107–118.

Victor M (1988) The irrelevance of mammillary body lesions in the causation of the Korsakoff amnesic state. Int J Neurol 21: 51–57.

Victor M, Adams RD, Collins GH (1971) The Wernicke-Korsakoff Syndrome. Philiadelphia: F A Davis.

Vogt BA, Peters A (1981) Form and distribution of neurons in rat cingulate cortex: areas 32, 24 and 29. J Comp Neurol 195: 603–625.

Vogt BA, Finch DM, Olson CR (1992) Functional heterogeneity in cingulate cortex: the anterior executive and posterior evaluative regions. Cereb Cortex 2: 435–443.

Von Cramon DY, Hebel N, Schuri U (1985) A contribution to the anatomical basis of thalamic amnesia. Brain 108: 993–1008.

Von Cramon DY, Schuri U (1992) The septo-hippocampal pathways and their relevance to human memory: a case report Cortex 28: 411–422.

Warburton EC, Aggleton JP (1999) Differential deficits in the Morris water maze following cytotoxic lesions of the anterior thalamus and fornix transaction. Behav Brain Res 98: 27–38.

Warburton EC, Aggleton JP, Muir JL (1998) Comparing the effects of selective cingulate cortex and cingulum bundle lesions on a spatial navigation task. Eur J Neurosci 10: 622–634.

Warburton EC, Baird AL, Aggleton JP (1997) Assessing the magnitude of the allocentric spatial deficit associated with complete loss of the anterior thalamic nuclei in rats. Behav Brain Res 87: 223–232.

Ward-Robinson J, Wilton LAK, Muir JL, Honey RC, Vann SD, Aggleton JP (2002) Sensory preconditioning in rats with lesions of the anterior thalamic nuclei: Evidence for intact nonspatial 'relational' processing. Behav Brain Res 133: 125–133.

Whishaw IQ, Maaswinkel H, Gonzalez CLR, Kolb B (2001) Deficits in allocentric and ideothetic spatial behaviour in rats with posterior cingulate cortex lesions. Behav Brain Res 118: 67–76.

Wilton LAK, Baird AL, Muir JL, Honey RC, Aggleton JP (2001) Loss of the thalamic nuclei for "head direction" impairs performance on spatial memory tasks in rats. Behav Neurosci 115: 861–869.

Yasuda Y, Watanabe T, Tanaka H, Tadashi I, Akiguchi I (1997) Amnesia following infarction in the right retrosplenial region. Clin Neurol Neurosurgery 99: 102–105.

Yonelinas AP (2002) The nature of recollection and familiarity: A review of 30 years of research. J Memory Lang 46: 441–517.

Zola-Morgan S, Squire LR, Amaral DG (1989) Lesions of the hippocampal formation but not lesions of the fornix or the mammillary nuclei produce long lasting memory impairment in monkeys. J Neurosci 9: 898–913.

IV NEURAL MECHANISMS OF SPATIAL ORIENTATION IN NONHUMAN PRIMATES AND HUMANS

14 Head Direction and Spatial View Cells in Primates, and Brain Mechanisms for Path Integration and Episodic Memory

Edmund T. Rolls

The aims of this chapter are to show that there are head direction cells in primates as well as in rats; to describe their properties; to show that a new class of cells found in the primate hippocampus—spatial view cells—are different from head direction cells and from rat place cells; to show the utility of spatial view cells in forming episodic memories; to show how a single network can associate both discrete representations about objects and continuous spatial representations to form episodic memories; and to show how path integration may be performed in continuous attractor networks to update their spatial representations by idiothetic (self-motion) cues in the dark.

Head direction cells are described in the presubiculum of the monkey, *Macaca mulatta*, used as a model of what is likely to be present in humans. The firing rate of these cells is a function of the head direction of the monkey, with a response that is typically 10 to 100 times larger to the optimal as compared to the opposite head direction. The mean half-amplitude width of the tuning of the cells was 76°. The response of head direction cells in the presubiculum was not influenced by where the monkey was located, there being the same tuning to head direction at different places in a room, and even outside the room. The response of these cells was also independent of the spatial view observed by the monkey, and also the position of the eyes in its head. The average information about head direction was 0.64 bits, about place was 0.10 bits, about spatial view was 0.27 bits, and about eye position was 0.04 bits. The cells maintained their tuning for periods of at least several minutes when the view details were obscured or the room darkened.

This representation of head direction could be useful, together with the hippocampal spatial view cells and whole body motion cells found in primates in such spatial and memory functions as path integration and episodic memory. It is shown that discrete and continuous attractor networks can be combined so that they contain both object and spatial information, and thus provide a model of episodic memory. Self-organizing continuous attractor neural networks that can perform path integration from velocity signals (e.g., head direction from head velocity, place from whole-body motion, and spatial view from eye- and whole-body motion) are described.

Head Direction Cells in Primates

While making recordings of spatial view cells (which respond to a location in space being viewed by the monkey, and are described in the following paragraphs) in the actively locomoting monkey (Rolls, 1999; Rolls et al., 1997, 1998; Robertson et al., 1998; Georges-François et al., 1999), we discovered (Robertson et al., 1999) a population of cells not previously found in primates, which we call head direction cells. We call these cells head direction cells because they have many similarities to head direction cells in rats. Rat head direction cells have a firing rate that is a simple function of head direction in the horizontal plane (see Taube et al., 1996; Muller et al., 1996). The firing does not depend on the rat's location. The cells in the rat are found in the dorsal presubiculum (also referred to as the postsubiculum), and also in some other brain structures including the anterior thalamic nuclei (Taube et al., 1996; chapter 1 by Sharp). The rat head direction cells can apparently be influenced by vestibular (and/or other self-motion related) input, in that they maintain and update their tuning even when the rat is in darkness. The cells can be reset by visual landmarks. The discovery of head direction cells in primates is of interest, because it provides useful evidence with which to develop hypotheses of primate hippocampal function in the context of what is encoded in the primate hippocampus in terms of spatial view.

To perform the experiments, we arranged for the monkey to see positions in space with different head directions, with different eye positions, and when the monkey was located at different positions in the laboratory. The recordings were made both during active locomotion, with the monkey walking (on all four feet in a baby walker), and when the monkey was still for a few seconds and visually exploring the environment by eye movements. The neuronal activity for a cell was sorted according to each hypothesis to be tested (head direction, allocentric view, place, and eye position), and an ANOVA was performed to determine whether the cell had significantly different firing rates when sorted according to each of the hypotheses. In addition, we calculated the quantitative measure of the information about the different hypotheses that was available in the firing rate of the cell. We were able to show, for example, that these cells convey much more information about head direction than about spatial view, the place where the monkey is, or about eye position. The transmitted information about the stimuli carried by neuronal firing rates was computed using techniques that have previously been fully described (e.g., Rolls et al., 1997; Rolls and Treves, 1998; Rolls et al., 1997).

An example of a head direction cell recorded in a macaque is shown in figure 14.1. The data for this diagram were obtained with the monkey stationary in the positions shown at

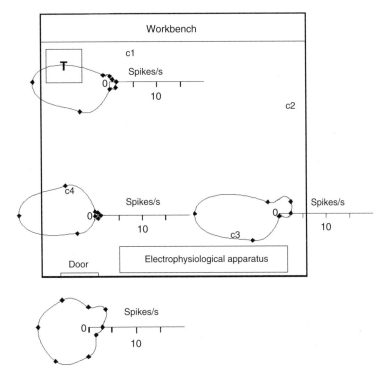

Figure 14.1
The responses of a head direction cell (AV070). Polar response plots of the firing rate (in spikes/s) when the monkey was stationary at different positions (shown at the 0 on the firing rate scale) in (and one outside) the room are shown. The monkey was rotated to face in each direction. The mean response of the cell from at least four different firing rate measurements in each head direction in pseudorandom sequence is shown. Cups to which the monkey could walk on all fours to obtain food are shown as c1, c2, c3, and c4. Polar firing rate response plots are superimposed on an overhead view of the square room to show where the firing for each plot was recorded. The plot at the lower left was taken outside the room, in the corridor, where the same head direction firing was maintained.

the 0 on the firing rate scale. The mean response of the cell from at least four different firing rate measurements in each head direction is shown. The polar firing rate response plot shows that the cell had its maximum firing rate when the monkey was facing west. The polar response plots were remarkably similar for three different positions in the room. A one-way ANOVA for the different head directions showed highly significantly different firing for the different head directions ($F(1,7) = 51.1$, $P < 0.0001$) (see table 14.1). The average information over the eight head directions was 0.58 bits, and the maximal information about any one head direction was 2.26 bits (see table 14.1). The cell showed the same head direction tuning outside the laboratory in the corridor (see figure 14.1), a place where the monkey had never previously walked at floor level. When the data for the cell were cast to show how much information the cell firing provided about the place where

Table 14.1
Head direction cells (The average information, and the maximum information about any one condition [Imax] with the data cast according to head direction, allocentric view, eye position and place)

Cell	Head direction			Allocentric View			Eye Position			Place		
	Information (bits)	I_{max} (bits)	Anova F (df) P	Information (bits)	I_{max} (bits)	Anova F (df) P	Information (bits)	I_{max} (bits)	Anova F (df) P	Information (bits)	I_{max} (bits)	Anova F (df) P
av070	0.58	2.26	51.1 (7) $<10^{-4}$	0.08	0.08	0.776 (1) 0.391		n.a.		0.16	0.49	1.78 (3) 0.153
av115	0.62	2.59	23.5 (7) $<10^{-4}$	0.09	0.10	2.91 (1) 0.103		n.a.		0.03	0.05	1.08 (2) 0.342
av195	1.11	1.67	59.21 (23) 3×10^{-16}	0.55	1.74	49.31 (14) 0.0001	0.03	0.08	3.56 (7) 0.001	0.16	0.19	26.12 (2) 0.0001
az080	0.41	1.14	19.26 (23) 3×10^{-13}	0.32	0.54	40.78 (7) 0.0001	0.01	0.21	2.17 (12) 0.011	0.05	0.12	10.36 (4) 0.0001
av192	0.38	0.99	13.98 (7) $<10^{-4}$	0.28	0.29	0.077 (1) 0.784	0.03	0.89	1.88 (14) 0.024	0.12	0.15	8.01 (2) 0.001
AVG	0.64	1.71		0.27	0.55		0.02	0.39		0.10	0.20	

Note: Further details are provided by Robertson et al. (1999).

the monkey was located, the information was low (0.16 bits), and the ANOVA across different places was not significant (see table 14.1). The neuron conveyed little information about spatial view (0.08 bits), in that the firing rate of the cell was very similar inside and outside the room even though the spatial views were completely different. The cell was located in the presubiculum (see figure 14.3).

The results of an experiment in which the firing of a head direction cell was recorded for many minutes while the room was completely obscured by ceiling-to-floor curtains is shown in figure 14.2, curve *b* (cell av115c3). The head direction tuning was very similar when the curtains were closed with the monkey in situ (compare to figure 14.2, curve *a* with the curtains open). When the room lights were subsequently extinguished so that the square space enclosed by the curtains (which could provide a minimal reference frame) was no longer visible, a head direction tuning curve was still present, though with no visual anchor at all, the peak of the tuning did drift a little during five minutes in darkness, as shown in figure 14.2, curve *c*. This is consistent with the hypothesis that visual cues can reset the cells and prevent them from drifting over long periods. This is similar to the hypothesis for head direction cells in rats (see Taube et al., 1996; Muller et al., 1996).

The results over all head direction cells that were fully tested are shown in table 14.1, and in table 14.2, which summarizes the half-amplitude tuning widths of the cells, and the

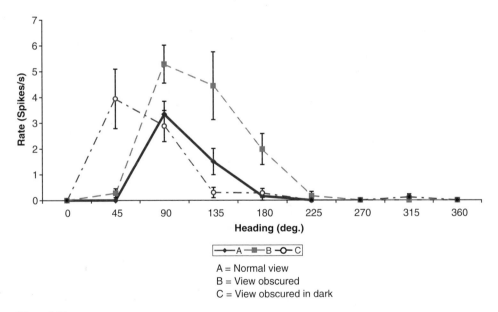

Figure 14.2
(A) The firing of a head direction cell recorded with the normal view of the room. (B) The firing rate when the room was completely obscured by ceiling-to-floor curtains. (C) The responses of the same cell recorded not only with the blackout curtain, but also with the lights off. The mean and standard error of the mean response is shown.

Table 14.2
Head direction cells: firing rates

Location	Cell Number	Peak Rate (spikes/s)	$\frac{1}{2}$ Amplitude Width (deg.)	Null Rate (Spikes/s)
Presubiculum	(1) AV070c2	17.2	72	0.8
Presubiculum	(2) AV115c3	4.3	54	0.0
Presubiculum	(3) AV195	29.1	89	0.9
Presubiculum	(4) AZ080	2.3	90	0.0
	Mean	13.2	76.3	0.4
Parahippocampal gyrus	(5) AV192c4	15.7	139	2.2

peak firing rates. For cells av070 and av115, data were not available (n.a.) for eye position. The first four cells in table 14.1 were recorded in the presubiculum, and were among a set of 12 different cells analyzed in the presubiculum. The individual head direction cells shown in table 14.1 had highly significant head direction tuning, as shown.

It was also shown that the information about head direction increased approximately linearly as the number of cells in the sample was increased from one to four (Robertson et al., 1999). Thus, up to this number of cells, approximately independent information was conveyed by the neurons. (The application of information theory to analyzing neuronal responses is described by Rolls and Treves, 1998, and by Rolls and Deco, 2002.)

The sites in the brain where the head direction cells were located are shown in figure 14.3. All the cells had low spontaneous firing rates (mean = 0.8 spikes/s, interquartile range 0–1.0). The peak firing rates were also relatively low (mean 10.0 spikes/s, interquartile range 6–13). These characteristics, together with the large amplitude and broad action potentials indicate that these neurons are likely to be pyramidal cells. Four cells were in the presubiculum, and in addition, three neurons with head direction cell properties were recorded in the primate parahippocampal gyrus. (Further details about the population of cells analyzed are provided by Robertson et al., 1999.) We have not so far found head direction cells in the hippocampus itself (CA3 and CA1), or in the dentate gyrus.

The head direction cells are very different from the spatial view cells (later described in more detail), which are found in the primate hippocampus and parahippocampal gyrus. For example, for a given head direction, if the monkey is moved to different places in the environment where the spatial view is different, spatial view cells give different responses. In contrast, the response of head direction cells remains constant for a given head direction, even when the spatial view is very different, as the data shown in figure 14.1 and the tables show. To provide a simple concept to emphasize the difference, one can think of head direction cells as responding like a compass attached to the top of the head, which will signal head direction even when the compass is in different locations, including in a totally different, and even novel, spatial environment, as illustrated in figure 14.1.

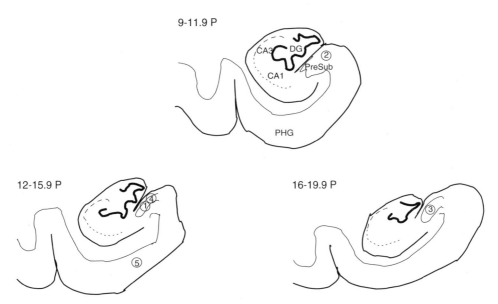

Figure 14.3
The hippocampal and parahippocampal sites at which different head direction cells were recorded. Coronal sections at different distances in mm posterior (P) to the sphenoid reference are shown. The number inside each circle corresponds to the cell number shown in table 14.1. CA3, CA3 hippocampal pyramidal cell field; CA1, CA1 hippocampal pyramidal cell field; DG, dentate gyrus; PHG, parahippocampal gyrus; PreSub, presubiculum.

A hypothesis that can be tested in primates is whether eye position affects the responses of head direction cells. They might respond to compass-related head direction, or to compass-related eye gaze (i.e., the direction of the eye, taking into account head direction and eye position in the head). The evidence we have so far indicates that their firing rate for a given head direction does not depend on eye position (see Robertson et al., 1999). Moreover, they carried little information about eye position (table 14.1). Thus, the evidence so far available suggests that the cells signal head direction rather than (allocentric or compass-related) eye-gaze angle. However, because the tuning of the head direction cells is relatively broad, the range of possible eye positions might not move the firing to a part of the head direction tuning where the effect of differences in eye position (in the head) would make a significant difference to the (allocentric) eye-gaze angle. It will be of interest in future research to explore this further, when the head direction is set to the steepest part of the head direction tuning of a cell.

Taken in the context of evidence on the neurophysiology and functions of the primate (including human) hippocampal system, head direction cells could perform a number of functions. One would be as part of a memory system. By remembering the compass bearing (head direction) and distance traveled, it is possible to find one's way back to the origin, even with a number of sectors of travel, and over a number of minutes. This is referred to as path integration, and can occur even without a view of the environment. Head direction cells provide part of the information to be remembered for such spatial memory functions. Complementary information also required for this is available in the whole-body motion cells that we have described in the primate hippocampus (O'Mara et al., 1994). These cells provide information, for example, about linear translation, or axial whole-body rotation. Part of the way in which head direction cell firing could be produced is by taking into account axial movements, which are signaled by some of these whole-body motion cells (O'Mara et al., 1994). It is an interesting hypothesis that this function is performed by some of the structures related to the hippocampal system, such as the pre-subiculum. Spatial memory and navigation can also benefit from visual information about places being looked at, which can be used as landmarks, and spatial view cells added to the head direction cells and whole-body motion cells would provide the basis for a good memory system, which is useful in navigation. Another possibility is that primate head direction cells are part of a system for computing during navigation which direction to head next. This would require not only a memory system of the type just described and elaborated elsewhere (Rolls, 1989, 1996, 1999; Treves and Rolls, 1994; Rolls and Treves, 1998) that can store spatial information of the type found in the hippocampus, but also an ability to use this information to compute what bearing would be needed next. Such a system might be implemented using a hippocampal memory system that grouped together spatial views, whole-body motion, and head direction information. The system would be different from that in the rat (Burgess et al., 1994; McNaughton et al., 1996), in that spatial view is represented in the primate hippocampus.

Spatial View Cells in Primates

In the rat, many hippocampal pyramidal cells fire when the rat is in a particular place, as defined, for example, by the visual spatial cues in an environment such as a room (O'Keefe 1990, 1991; Kubie and Muller, 1991). It has been discovered that in the primate hippocampus, many spatial cells have responses not related to the place where the monkey is, but instead related to the place the monkey is looking (Rolls, 1999; Rolls et al., 1997, 1998; Robertson et al., 1998; Georges-François et al., 1999; Rolls and O'Mara, 1995). These are called "spatial view cells", an example of which is shown in figure 14.4. These cells encode information in allocentric (world-based, as contrasted with egocentric, body-related) coordinates (Georges-François et al., 1999; Rolls et al., 1998). In some cases they can respond to remembered spatial views because they respond when the view details are obscured, and use idiothetic (self-motion) cues, including eye position and head direction, to trigger this memory recall operation (Robertson et al., 1998). Another idiothetic input that drives some primate hippocampal neurons is linear and axial whole-body motion (O'Mara et al., 1994).

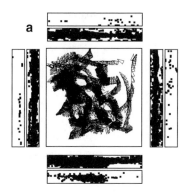
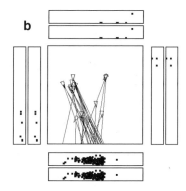

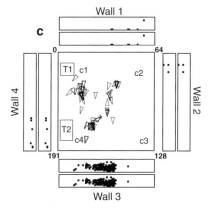

Figure 14.4

Examples of the firing of a hippocampal spatial view cell when the monkey was walking around the laboratory. (a) The firing of the cell is indicated by the spots in the outer set of four rectangles, each of which represents one of the walls of the room. There is one spot on the outer rectangle for each action potential. The base of the walls is toward the center of the diagram. The positions on the walls fixated during the recording sessions are indicated by points in the inner set of four rectangles, each of which also represents a wall of the room. The central square is a plan view of the room, with a triangle printed every 250 ms to indicate the position of the monkey, thus showing that many different places were visited during the recording sessions. (b) A similar representation of the same recording sessions as in (a), but modified to indicate some of the range of monkey positions and horizontal gaze directions when the cell fired at more than 12 spikes/s. (c) A similar representation of the same recording sessions as in (a), but modified to indicate more fully the range of places (and head directions) when the cell fired. The triangle indicates the current position of the monkey, and the line projected from it shows which part of the wall is being viewed at any one time while the monkey is walking. One spot is shown for each action potential. The neuron fires when the monkey looks at a particular position on the walls, even if to look at that position the monkey adopts a different head direction because of the place of the monkey in the room. (After Georges-Francois et al., 1999.)

Part of the interest of spatial view cells is that they could provide the spatial representation required to enable primates to perform object-place memory, for example, remembering where they saw a person or object, which is an example of an episodic memory. Indeed, similar neurons in the hippocampus respond in object-place memory tasks (Rolls et al., 1989). Associating such a spatial representation with a representation of a person or object could be implemented by an autoassociation network implemented by the recurrent collateral connections of the CA3 hippocampal pyramidal cells (Rolls, 1989, 1996; Treves and Rolls, 1994; Rolls and Treves, 1998). Some other primate hippocampal neurons respond in the object-place memory task to a combination of spatial information and information about the object seen (Rolls et al., 1989). Further evidence for this convergence of spatial and object information in the hippocampus is that in another memory task for which the hippocampus is needed—learning where to make spatial responses conditional on which picture is shown—some primate hippocampal neurons respond to a combination of which picture is shown, and where the response must be made (Miyashita et al., 1989; Cahusac et al., 1993).

These primate spatial view cells are thus unlike place cells found in the rat (O'Keefe, 1979, 1990, 1991; Kubie and Muller, 1991; Wilson and McNaughton, 1993). Primates, with their highly developed visual and eye movement control systems, can explore and remember information about what is present at places in the environment without having to visit those places. Such spatial view cells in primates would thus be useful as part of a memory system, since they would provide a representation of a part of space that would not depend on exactly where the monkey or human was, and which could be associated with items that might be present in those spatial locations. An example of the utility of such a representation in humans would be remembering where a particular person had been seen. The primate spatial representations would also be useful in remembering trajectories through environments, of use, for example, in short-range spatial navigation (O'Mara et al., 1994; Rolls and Deco, 2002).

The representation of space in the rat hippocampus, which concerns the place where the rat is located, may be related to the fact that with a visual system that is less developed than the primate's, the rat's representation of space may be defined more by the olfactory and tactile and distant visual cues present, and may thus tend to reflect the place where the rat is. An interesting hypothesis concerning how this difference could arise from essentially the same computational process in rats and monkeys is as follows (Rolls, 1999; De Araujo et al., 2001): The starting assumption is that in both the rat and the primate, the dentate granule cells and the CA3 and CA1 pyramidal cells respond to combinations of the inputs received. In the case of the primate, a combination of visual features in the environment will, because of the fovea providing high spatial resolution over a typical viewing angle of perhaps $10°$ to $20°$, result in the formation of a spatial view cell, the effective trigger for which will thus be a combination of visual features within a relatively small part of space. In contrast, in the rat, given the extensive visual field subtended by the rodent retina, which may extend over 180–270, a combination of visual features formed over such a wide visual angle would effectively define a position in space that is a place. The actual processes by which the hippocampal formation cells would come to respond to feature combinations could be similar in rats and monkeys, involving, for example, competitive learning in the dentate granule cells, autoassociation learning in CA3 pyramidal cells, and competitive learning in CA1 pyramidal cells (Treves and Rolls, 1994; Rolls and Treves, 1998). Thus, the selective properties of spatial view cells in primates and place cells in rats might arise by the same computational process but be different in that primates are foveate and view a small part of the visual field at any one time, whereas the rat has a very wide visual field (for details see de Araujo et al., 2001). Although the representation of space in rats may therefore be in some ways analogous to the representation of space in the primate hippocampus, the difference does have implications for theories, and modeling, of hippocampal function.

In rats, the presence of place cells has led to theories that the rat hippocampus is a spatial cognitive map, and can perform spatial computations to implement navigation through spatial environments (O'Keefe and Nadel, 1978; O'Keefe, 1991; Burgess et al., 1994, 1996). The details of such navigational theories could not apply in any direct way to what is found in the primate hippocampus. Instead, what is applicable to both the primate and rat hippocampal recordings is that hippocampal neuronal activity represents space (for the rat, primarily where the rat is, and for the primate primarily of positions "out there" in space), which is a suitable representation for an episodic memory system. In primates, this would enable one to remember, for example, where an object was seen. In rats, it might enable memories to be formed of where particular objects (for example those defined by olfactory, tactile, and taste inputs) were found. Thus, at least in primates, and possibly also in rats, the neuronal representation of space in the hippocampus may be appropriate for forming memories of events (which usually in these animals have a spatial component). Such memories would be useful for spatial navigation, for which—according to the present hypothesis—the hippocampus would implement the memory component but not the spatial computation component. Evidence that what neuronal recordings have shown is represented in the nonhuman primate hippocampal system may also be present in humans is that regions of the hippocampal formation can be activated when humans look at spatial views (Epstein and Kanwisher, 1998, O'Keefe et al., 1998).

Attractor Networks that Combine Continuous (e.g., Spatial) with Discrete (Object) Information, and Episodic Memory

A class of network that can maintain the firing of its neurons to represent any location along a continuous physical dimension such as spatial position, head direction, etc is called a continuous attractor neural network (CANN) (see chapter 18; Rolls and Deco, 2002; and references provided later in this chapter.) It uses excitatory recurrent collateral connections with associative modifiability between the neurons to reflect the distance between the neurons in the state space of the animal (e.g., head direction space). These networks can maintain the packet or bubble of neural activity constant for long periods, wherever it is started, to represent the current state (head direction, position, etc.) of the animal, and are likely to be involved in many aspects of spatial processing and memory, including spatial vision. Global inhibition (implemented by feedback inhibitory interneurons) is used to keep the number of neurons in a bubble or packet of actively firing neurons relatively constant, and to help to ensure that there is only one activity packet. Continuous attractor networks may be thought of as very similar to autoassociation or discrete attractor networks (Rolls and Treves, 1998; Rolls and Deco, 2002) and have the same architecture, as illustrated in figure 14.5. The main difference is that the patterns stored in a CANN are continuous patterns, with each neuron having broadly tuned firing that decreases, for example, with a Gaussian function, as the distance from the optimal firing location of the cell is varied, and with different neurons having tuning that overlaps throughout the space. Such tuning is illustrated in figure 14.6, together with the examples of discrete (separate) patterns (each pattern implemented by the firing of a particular subset of the neurons), with no continuous distribution of the patterns throughout the space, which are useful for

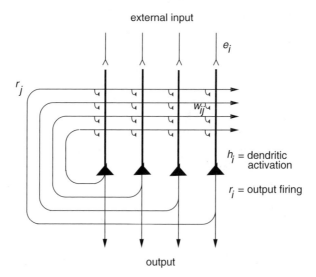

Figure 14.5
The architecture of a continuous attractor neural network (CANN). Recurrent collateral axons with associatively modifiable synaptic connections make contact with the excitatory pyramidal cells in the network. The vertical lines are the dendrites, the cell bodies are triangles, and the axons extend out of the bottom of each cell body. The synaptic weight or strength for axon j to the dendrite of neuron i is w_{ij}. The external firing rate input to the network is conveyed by axons e_i. Feedback inhibitory interneurons are not shown. (For details see Rolls et al., 2002; Rolls and Deco, 2002.)

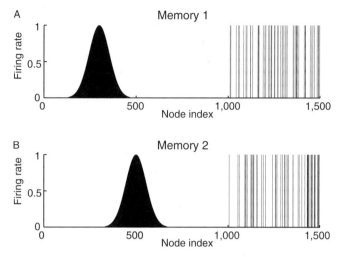

Figure 14.6
The types of firing patterns stored in continuous attractor networks are illustrated for the patterns present on neurons 1–1000 for Memory 1 (when the firing is that produced when the spatial state represented is that for location 300), and for Memory 2 (when the firing is that produced when the spatial state represented is that for location 500). The continuous nature of the spatial representation results from the fact that each neuron has a Gaussian firing rate that peaks at its optimal location. This particular mixed network also contains discrete representations that consist of discrete subsets of active binary firing rate neurons in the range 1001–1500. The firing of these latter neurons can be thought of as representing the discrete events that occur at the location. Continuous attractor networks by definition contain only continuous representations, but this particular network can store mixed continuous and discrete representations, and is illustrated to show the difference of the firing patterns normally stored in separate continuous attractor and discrete attractor networks. For this particular mixed network, during learning, Memory 1 is stored in the synaptic weights, then Memory 2, etc. Each memory contains part that is continuously distributed to represent physical space and part that represents a discrete event or object.

storing arbitrary events or objects. A consequent difference is that the CANN can maintain its firing at any location in the trained continuous space, whereas a discrete attractor or autoassociation network moves its population of active neurons towards one of the previously learned attractor states, and thus implements the recall of a particular previously learned pattern from an incomplete or noisy (distorted) version of one of the previously learned patterns.

It has now been shown that attractor networks can store both continuous patterns and discrete patterns, and can thus be used to store, for example, the location in (continuous, physical) space (e.g., the place "out there" in a room represented by spatial view cells) where an object (a discrete item) is present (Rolls et al., 2002; cf. Rolls, 1989, 1996). Such associations between an object and the place where it is located are prototypical of episodic or event memory, and may be implemented in the primate hippocampus (Rolls et al., 2005). In this network, when events are stored that have both discrete (object) and continuous (spatial) aspects, then the whole place can be retrieved later by the object, and the object can be retrieved by using the place as a retrieval cue. Such networks are likely to be present in parts of the brain, such as the hippocampus, which receive and combine inputs both from systems that contain representations of continuous (physical) space, and from brain systems that contain representations of discrete objects, such as the inferior temporal visual cortex. The combined continuous and discrete attractor network described by Rolls et al. (2002) shows that in brain regions where the spatial and object processing streams are brought together, a single network can represent and learn associations between both types of input. Indeed, in brain regions such as the hippocampal system, it is essential that the spatial and object-processing streams are brought together in a single network, for it is only when both types of information are in the same network that spatial information can be retrieved from object information, and vice versa, which is a fundamental property of episodic memory (Rolls and Treves, 1998; Rolls and Deco, 2002).

Continuous Attractor Networks and Path Integration

We have considered how spatial representations could be stored in continuous attractor networks, and how the activity can be maintained at any location in the state space in a form of short term memory when the external (e.g., visual) input is removed (Rolls and Deco, 2002). However, many networks with spatial representations in the brain can be updated by internal, self-motion (i.e., idiothetic), cues even when there is no external (e.g., visual) input. Examples are head direction cells in the post- and presubiculum of rats and macaques, place cells in the rat hippocampus, and spatial view cells in the primate hippocampus. The major question arises about how such idiothetic inputs could drive the activity packet in a continuous attractor network, and in particular, how such a system could be set up biologically by self-organizing learning.

One approach to simulating the movement of an activity packet produced by idiothetic cues (which executes a form of path integration whereby the current location is calculated from recent movements) is to employ a look-up table that stores (taking head direction cells as an example), for every possible head direction and head rotational velocity input generated by the vestibular system, the corresponding new head direction (Samsonovich and McNaughton, 1997). Another approach involves modulating the strengths of the recurrent synaptic weights in the continuous attractor on one, but not the other, side of a currently represented position, so that the stable position of the packet of activity, which requires symmetric connections in different directions from each node, is lost, and the packet moves in the direction of the temporarily increased weights, although no possible biological implementation was proposed as to how the appropriate dynamic synaptic weight changes might be achieved (Zhang, 1996). Another mechanism (for head direction cells) (Skaggs et al., 1995) relies on a set of cells, termed (head) rotation cells, which are coactivated by head direction cells and vestibular cells and drive the activity of the attractor network by anatomically distinct connections for clockwise and counterclockwise rotation cells, in what is effectively a look-up table. However, no proposal was made about how this could be achieved by a biologically plausible learning process; this has been the case until recently for most approaches to path integration in continuous attractor networks, which rely heavily on rather artificial pre-set synaptic connectivities.

Stringer et al. (2002a) introduced a proposal with more biological plausibility about how the synaptic connections from idiothetic inputs to a continuous attractor network can be learned by a self-organizing learning process. The essence of the hypothesis is described with figure 14.7. The continuous attractor synaptic weights w^{RC} are set up under the influence of the external visual inputs I^V (Rolls and Deco, 2002). At the same time, the idiothetic synaptic weights w^{ID} (in which the ID refers to the fact that they are in this case produced by idiothetic inputs, produced by cells that fire to represent the velocity of clockwise and anticlockwise head rotation), are set up by associating the change of head

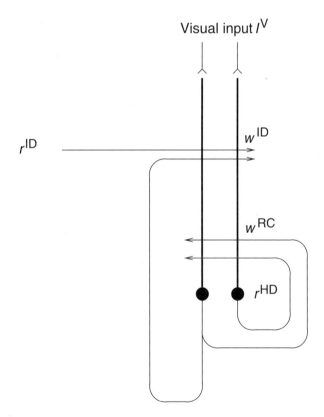

Figure 14.7
General network architecture for a one-dimensional continuous attractor model of head direction cells that can be updated by idiothetic inputs produced by head rotation cell firing (r^{ID}). The head direction cell firing is r^{HD}, the continuous attractor synaptic weights are w^{RC}, the idiothetic synaptic weights are w^{ID}, and the external visual input is I^V. (For details see Stringer et al., 2002a.)

direction cell firing that has just occurred (detected by a trace memory mechanism subsequently described) with the current firing of the head rotation cells r^{ID}. (Neurons that reflect head rotation are found in the primate hippocampus, O'Mara et al., 1994; and neurons influenced by head rotation are also found in the parietal cortex, Klam and Graf, 2003.) For example, when the trace memory mechanism incorporated into the idiothetic synapses w^{ID} detects that the head direction cell firing is at a given location (indicated by the firing r^{HD}) and is moving clockwise (produced by the altering visual inputs I^V) and there is simultaneous clockwise head rotation cell firing, the synapses w^{ID} learn the association, so that when that rotation cell firing occurs later without visual input, it takes the current head direction firing in the continuous attractor into account, and moves the location of the head direction attractor in the appropriate direction.

For the learning to operate, the idiothetic synapses onto head direction cell i with firing r_i^{HD} need two inputs: the short-term memory traced term from other head direction cells $\bar{r}_j^{HD}$ (which is just an average over, e.g., the preceding 1 s), and the head rotation cell input with firing r_k^{ID}; and the learning rule can be written

$$\delta \mathbf{W}_{ijk}^{ID} = k \mathbf{r}_i^{HD} \bar{\mathbf{r}}_j^{HD} \mathbf{r}_k^{ID} \tag{14.1}$$

where k is the learning rate associated with this type of synaptic connection.

After learning, the firing of the head direction cells would be updated in the dark (when $I_i^V = 0$) by idiothetic head rotation cell firing r_k^{ID} as follows

$$\tau \frac{dh_i^{HD}(t)}{dt} = -h_i^{HD}(t) + \frac{\phi_0}{C^{HD}} \sum_j (w_{ij}^{RC} - w^{INH}) r_j^{HD}(t) + I_i^V + \phi_1 \left(\frac{1}{C^{HD \times ID}} \sum_{j,k} w_{ijk}^{ID} r_j^{HD} r_k^{ID} \right). \tag{14.2}$$

The last term introduces the effects of the idiothetic synaptic weights w_{ijk}^{ID}, which effectively specify that the current firing of head direction cell i, r_i^{HD}, must be updated by the previously learned combination of the particular head rotation now occurring indicated by r_k^{ID}, and the current head direction indicated by the firings of the other head direction cells r_j^{HD} indexed through j. This makes it clear that the idiothetic synapses operate using combinations of inputs, in this case, of two inputs. Neurons that sum up the effects of such local products are termed Sigma-Pi neurons. Although such synapses are more complicated than the two-term synapses often used, such three-term synapses (with two axons connecting to the dendrite) appear to be useful to solve the computational problem of updating representations based on idiothetic inputs in the way described. Synapses that operate according to Sigma-Pi rules might be implemented in the brain by a number of mechanisms described by Koch (1999) and Stringer et al. (2002a), including having two inputs close together on a thin dendrite, so that local synaptic interactions would be emphasized.

Simulations demonstrating the operation of this self-organizing learning to produce movement of the location being represented in a continuous attractor network were described by Stringer et al. (2002a), and one example of the operation is shown in figure

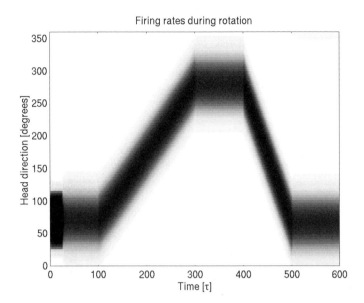

Figure 14.8
Idiothetic update of the location represented in a continuous attractor network. The firing rate of the cells with optima at different head directions (organized according to head direction on the ordinate) is shown by the blackness of the plot, as a function of time. The activity packet was initialized to a head direction of 75°, and the packet was allowed to settle without visual input. For t = 0 to t = 100 there was no rotation cell input, and the activity packet in the continuous attractor remained stable at 75°. For t = 100 to t = 300 the clockwise rotation cells were active with a firing rate of 0.15 to represent a moderate angular velocity, and the activity packet moved clockwise. For t = 300 to t = 400 there was no rotation cell firing, and the activity packet immediately stopped, and remained still. For t = 400 to t = 500 the counter-clockwise rotation cells had a high firing rate of 0.3 to represent a high velocity, and the activity packet moved counter-clockwise with a greater velocity. For t = 500 to t = 600 there was no rotation cell firing and the activity packet immediately stopped.

14.8. They also showed that, after training with just one value of the head rotation cell firing, the network showed the desirable property of moving the head direction being represented in the continuous attractor by an amount that was proportional to the value of the head rotation cell firing. Stringer et al. (2002a) also describe a related model of the idiothetic cell update of the location represented in a continuous attractor, in which the rotation cell firing directly modulates, in a multiplicative way, the strength of the recurrent connections in the continuous attractor in such a way that clockwise rotation cells modulate the strength of the synaptic connections in the clockwise direction in the continuous attractor, and vice versa.

It should be emphasized that although the cells are organized in figure 14.8 according to the spatial position being represented, there is no need for cells in continuous attractors that represent nearby locations in the state space to be close together, since the distance in the state space between any two neurons is represented by the strength of the connection between them, not by where the neurons are physically located. This enables continuous attractor networks to represent spaces with arbitrary topologies, as the topology is represented in the connection strengths (Stringer et al., 2002a, b, 2003). These path integration models have also been extended to deal with the update of rat hippocampal place cells by self-motion (Stringer et al., 2002b) and primate hippocampal spatial view cells by self-motion (see Rolls and Deco, 2002).

Conclusion

This chapter has described the discovery of head direction cells in the primate presubiculum, placed them in the context of spatial view cells found in the primate hippocampus, suggested a computational explanation for the presence of spatial view cells in the primate hippocampus but place cells in the rat hippocampus, shown how both spatial and discrete (e.g., object or event) representations could be combined in a single attractor network suitable for episodic memory, and shown how path integration might be implemented in self-organizing neural networks for head direction or spatial position in the brain.

Acknowledgments

This research was supported by the Medical Research Council, and by the Human Frontier Science Program.

References

Burgess N, O'Keefe J (1996) Neuronal computations underlying the firing of place cells and their role in navigation. Hippocampus 6: 149–762.

Burgess N, Recce M, O'Keefe J (1994) A model of hippocampal function. Neural Networks 7: 1065–1081.

Cahusac PMB, Rolls ET, Miyashita Y, Niki H (1993) Modification of the responses of hippocampal neurons in the monkey during the learning of a conditional spatial response task. Hippocampus 3: 29–42.

de Araujo IET, Rolls ET, Stringer SM (2001) A view model which accounts for the spatial fields of hippocampal primate spatial view cells and rat place cells. Hippocampus 11: 699–706.

Epstein R, Kanwisher N (1998) A cortical representation of the local visual environment. Nature 392: 598–601.

Georges-François P, Rolls ET, Robertson RG (1999) Spatial view cells in the primate hippocampus: allocentric view not head direction or eye position or place. Cereb Cortex 9: 197–212.

Hölscher C, Rolls ET, Xiang J-Z (2003) Perirhinal cortex neuronal activity related to long term familiarity memory in the macaque. Eur J Neurosci, 18: 2037–2046.

Klam F, Graf W (2003) Vestibular response kinematics in posterior parietal cortex neurons of macaque monkeys. Eur J Neurosci 18: 995–1010.

Koch C (1999) Biophysics of Computation, Oxford: Oxford University Press.

Kubie JL, Muller RU (1991) Multiple representations in the hippocampus. Hippocampus 1: 240–242.

Miyashita Y, Rolls ET, Cahusac PMB, Niki H, Feigenbaum JD (1989) Activity of hippocampal neurons in the monkey related to a conditional spatial response task. J Neurophysiol 61: 669–678.

McNaughton BL, Barnes CA, Gerrard JL, Gothard K, Jung MW, Knierim JJ, Kudrimoti H, Qin Y, Skaggs WE, Suster WE, Weaver KL (1996) Deciphering the hippocampal polyglot: the hippocampus as a path integration system. J Exp Biol 199: 173–185.

Muller RU, Ranck JB, Taube JS (1996) Head direction cells: properties and functional significance. Curr Opin Neurobiol 6: 196–206.

O'Keefe J, Nadel L (1978) The Hippocampus as a Cognitive Map. Oxford: Clarendon Press.

O'Keefe J (1979) A review of the hippocampal place cells. Prog Neurobiol 13: 419–439.

O'Keefe J (1990) A computational theory of the cognitive map. Prog Brain Res 83: 301–312.

O'Keefe J (1991) The hippocampal cognitive map and navigational strategies. In J Paillard, Ed., Brain and Space. Oxford: Oxford University Press, pp. 273–295.

O'Keefe J, Burgess N, Donnett JG, Jeffery KJ, Maguire EA (1998) Place cells, navigational accuracy, and the human hippocampus. Phil Trans Royal Soc, Lond B 353: 1333–1340.

O'Mara SM, Rolls ET, Berthoz A, Kesner RP (1994) Neurons responding to whole-body motion in the primate hippocampus. J Neurosci 14: 6511–6523.

Robertson RG, Rolls ET, Georges-François P. (1998) Spatial view cells in the primate hippocampus: Effects of removal of view details. J Neurophysiol 79: 1145–1156.

Robertson RG, Rolls ET, Georges-François P, Panzeri S (1999) Head direction cells in the primate pre-subiculum. Hippocampus 9: 206–219.

Rolls ET (1989) Functions of neuronal networks in the hippocampus and neocortex in memory. In JH Byrne and Wo Berry, eds., Neural Models of Plasticity: Experimental and Theoretical Approaches San Diego: Academic Press, chap. 13, pp. 240–265.

Rolls ET (1996) A theory of hippocampal function in memory. Hippocampus 6: 601–620.

Rolls ET (1999) Spatial view cells and the representation of place in the primate hippocampus. Hippocampus 9: 467–480.

Rolls ET, Deco G (2002) Computational Neuroscience of Vision. Oxford: Oxford University Press.

Rolls ET, O'Mara SM (1995) View-responsive neurons in the primate hippocampal complex. Hippocampus 5: 409–424.

Rolls ET, Robertson RG, Georges-François P (1997) Spatial view cells in the primate hippocampus. Eur J Neurosci 9: 1789–1794.

Rolls ET, Treves A (1998) Neural Networks and Brain Function. Oxford: Oxford University Press.

Rolls ET, Stringer SM, Trappenberg TP (2002) A unified model of spatial and episodic memory. Proc Royal Soc B 269: 1087–1093.

Rolls ET, Treves A, Tovee M (1997) The representational capacity of the distributed encoding of information provided by populations of neurons in the primate temporal visual cortex. Exp Brain Res 114: 149–162.

Rolls ET, Xiang JZ, Franco L (2005) Object, space and object-space representations in the primate hippocampus. In preparation.

Rolls ET, Treves A, Tovee M, Panzeri S (1997) Information in the neuronal representation of individual stimuli in the primate temporal visual cortex. J Comp Neurosci 4: 309–333.

Rolls ET, Treves A, Robertson RG, Georges-François P, Panzeri S (1998) Information about spatial view in an ensemble of primate hippocampal cells. J Neurophysiol 79: 1797–1813.

Rolls ET, Miyashita Y, Cahusac PMB, Kesner RP, Niki H, Feigenbaum J, Bach L (1989) Hippocampal neurons in the monkey with activity related to the place in which a stimulus is shown. J Neurosci 9: 1835–1845.

Samsonovich A, McNaughton B (1997) Path integration and cognitive mapping in a continuous attractor neural network model. J Neurosci 17: 5900–5920.

Skaggs WE, Knierim JJ, Kudrimoti HS, McNaughton BL (1995) A model of the neural basis of the rat's sense of direction. In G Tesauro, DS Touretzky, and TK Leen eds., Advances in Neural Information Processing System, vol. 7 Cambridge, MA: MIT Press, pp. 173–180.

Stringer SM, Trappenberg TP, Rolls ET, Araujo IET (2002a) Self-organizing continuous attractor networks and path integration:one-dimensional models of head direction cells. Network: Comp Neural Sys 13: 217–242.

Stringer SM, Rolls ET, Trappenberg TP, Araujo IET (2002b) Self-organizing continuous attractor networks and path integration. Two-dimensional models of place cells. Net Comp Neural Sys 13: 429–446.

Stringer SM, Rolls ET, Trappenberg TP (2003) Self-organising continuous attractor networks with multiple activity packets, and the representation of space. Neural Net 17: 5–27.

Taube JS, Goodridge JP, Golob EJ, Dudchenko PA, Stackman RW (1996) Processing the head direction signal: a review and commentary. Brain Res Bull 40: 477–486.

Treves A, Rolls ET (1994) A computational analysis of the role of the hippocampus in memory. Hippocampus 4: 374–391.

Wilson MA, McNaughton BL (1993) Dynamics of the hippocampal ensemble code for space. Science 261: 1055–1058.

Zhang K (1996) Representation of spatial orientation by the intrinsic dynamics of the head-direction cell ensemble: a theory. J Neurosci 16: 2112–2126.

15 Posterior Cortical Processing of Self-Movement Cues: MSTd's Role in Papez's Circuit for Navigation and Orientation

Charles J. Duffy, William K. Page, and Michael T. Froehler

Optic flow is the patterned visual motion seen by a moving observer; it is used to facilitate navigation and spatial orientation (Gibson, 1950). Optic flow is analyzed by cerebral cortex in the context of proprioceptive and vestibular signals that accompany self-movement. Somatic cues about self-movement are always available, but people moving in a lighted environment are greatly guided by vision.

The role of parietotemporal cortex in spatial orientation was recognized in studies of human traumatic brain injury (Holmes, 1918). Such observations were synthesized into a dichotomous view of extrastriate visual processing that assigned spatial analysis to dorsal areas and object analysis to ventral areas (Kleist, 1935). Since those early studies, these ideas have been developed into a foundation for modern research on the role of posterior cerebral cortex in spatial orientation (Mountcastle, 1976; Ungerleider and Mishkin, 1982).

Parallel developments in the functional analysis of cerebral archicortex, the hippocampus, and associated structures, lead to the recognition of a cortico-subcortical system for memory and emotion (Papez, 1937). Behavioral and lesion studies subsequently supported the notion that such a cortico-subcortical system might also be involved in cognitive mapping for navigation and orientation (Tolman, 1948), with a key role soon recognized for the hippocampus (O'Keefe and Nadel, 1978).

We now review studies on cortical sensory processing related to navigation and orientation, illustrate the nature of this work by detailing some of our related studies, and develop a case for extending Papez's notion of cortico-subcortical processing systems to this domain.

Self-Movement Analysis for Spatial Orientation

Visuospatial Processing in Parietotemporal Cortex
Occipitoparietal lesions impair self-movement control in humans (Paterson and Zangwill, 1944; Critchley, 1953) and monkeys (Ungerleider and Brody, 1977; Sugishita et al., 1978).

PET (de Jong et al., 1994; Dupont et al., 1994; Shipp et al., 1994; Cheng et al., 1995) and fMRI (Tootell et al., 1995; Sereno et al., 1995; Tootell and Taylor, 1995) studies confirm this localization showing optic-flow-induced activation in areas that are also active during visuospatial perception (Haxby et al., 1994) and spatial navigation (Aguirre and D'Esposito, 1997).

Posterior parietotemporal cortex processes visuospatial signals in a series of cortical areas that traverse the superior temporal sulcus (STS) and intraparietal cortex (IP) (figure 15.1). Posterior parietal area 7a neurons have large receptive fields (>40° × 40°) (Yin and Mountcastle, 1977) and respond to moving patterns without regard to their color, orientation, or shape (Robinson et al., 1978). Some 7a neurons are sensitive to radial patterns of motion around the fixation point, preferring object motion either in toward the fixation point or out from the fixation point. This opponent vector receptive field organization (Motter and Mountcastle, 1981) is combined with axial direction preferences and speed sensitivity that make these neurons potentially applicable to the analysis of self-movement (Motter et al., 1987; Steinmetz et al., 1987).

The posterior edge of the STS contains the middle temporal area (MT) with smaller visual receptive fields (approx. 10° × 10°). MT neurons are selective for the direction of object motion in a columnar map of direction preferences covering the contralateral visual field (Allman and Kaas, 1971; Dubner and Zeki, 1971). MT neurons project to the anterior bank of the STS in a zone between MT and 7a referred to as the medial superior

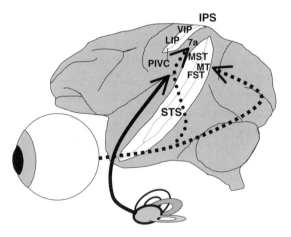

Figure 15.1
Lateral view of the macaque monkey brain highlighting regions within the parietotemporal cortex. The intraparietal sulcus (IPS) and the superior temporal sulcus (STS) have been opened to reveal PIVC, LIP, VIP, MT, MST and FST. These areas are at the junction of dorsal extrastriate visual motion processing, inferior parietal vestibular analysis, and the posterior parietal terminus of the colliculopulvinoparietal network for attention and orientation. We view this region as a center for the analysis of multisensory cues relevant to localization, spatial orientation, and navigation.

temporal area (MST). Dorsal MST (MSTd) neurons have large receptive fields, often including a quadrant of the visual field as well as a bilateral area around the fixation point. These neurons are most sensitive to large patterns of movement, with many being specific to radial or circular patterns of motion common in the optic flow that is seen during self-movement (Saito et al., 1986; Duffy and Wurtz, 1991; Orban et al., 1992; Graziano et al., 1994).

MSTd neurons prefer optic flow with foci of expansion (FOE) in a particular segment of the visual field (figure 15.2) (Duffy and Wurtz, 1995; Bremmer et al., 1997b), suggesting a role in self-movement direction discrimination that is supported by MST microstimulation effects on FOE perception (Britten and Van, 1998). These findings imply that MSTd may be intimately involved in converting the basic visual motion properties of the more posterior MT neurons into the "more explicitly spatial properties" of the more anterior 7a neurons. Neurons in the ventral inferior parietal area (VIP) respond to optic flow along with tactile stimulation of the face (Schaafsma and Duysens, 1996), leading to the suggestion that these neurons may be involved with processing movement in near-space whereas MST neurons may be involved with self-movement in the extra-personal space (Bremmer et al., 1997a). Thus, posterior parietal cortex may integrate self-movement cues

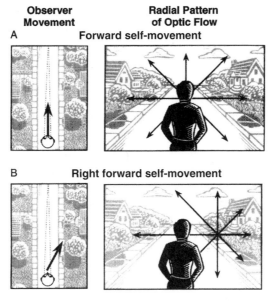

Figure 15.2
Optic flow is the visual motion resulting from the movement of an observer. The radial pattern of optic flow contains a focus of expansion that indicates the observer's direction of self-movement. (A) During forward self-movement in the direction of gaze (left), the observer sees a symmetric, radial pattern of optic flow in which the focus of expansion is at the fixation point (right). (B) During right forward self-movement with gaze maintained forward (left), the observer sees a radial pattern in which the focus of expansion is displaced to the right of gaze (right) indicating a rightward direction.

(Nakayama and Loomis, 1974) as part of a dorsal stream network for self-movement perception (Schaafsma and Duysens, 1996; Siegel and Read, 1997).

Gaze Orientation Effects in Parietotemporal Cortex

Parietotemporal neurons also respond to eye position: extrastriate areas V3A, area V6 and V6A (Galletti and Battaglini, 1989; Galletti et al., 1995; Nakamura et al., 1999) and posterior parietal 7a, LIP, VIP, MT, and MST (Sakata et al., 1980; Andersen and Mountcastle, 1983; Anderson et al., 1990; Bremmer et al., 1997b; Baader, 1991; Squatrito and Maioli, 1996, 1997; Duhamel et al., 1997; Read and Siegel, 1997; Siegel et al., 2003). Similarly, head position also modulates neural responses in 7a and LIP (Brotchie et al., 1995; Snyder et al., 1998). In general, these eye and head effects on gaze are proportionate to gaze position and modulate visual responses through a "gain field" (Andersen and Braunstein, 1985; Zipser and Andersen, 1988). These mixed modality responses are consistent with an intermediate layer in a conversion process from a retinal to motor frames of reference (Bremmer et al., 1998; Xing and Andersen, 2000; Pouget et al., 2000).

Parietotemporal cortex responds to eye and/or head velocity as well as position. Neurophysiological recordings indicate that many 7a (Kawano et al., 1984), VIP (Bremmer et al., 1997a); and MST (Komatsu and Wurtz, 1988a; Komatsu and Wurtz, 1988b; Erickson and Thier, 1991; Thier and Erickson, 1992; Kawano et al., 1994; Squatrito and Maioli, 1996, 1997; Bremmer et al., 1997b) neurons respond to pursuit eye movements. Many neurons in VIP appear to respond to either the acceleration, velocity, or position of the head (Klam and Graf, 2003).

Dynamic gaze shifts during ocular, cranial, or combined pursuit movements alter the retinal pattern of optic flow. MSTd neurons appear to partially compensate for certain directions of smooth pursuit eye movements (Bradley et al., 1996) depending on pursuit speed (Shenoy et al., 2002). We have shown that individual MSTd neurons do not compensate for pursuit, but the MSTd neuronal population can accurately reconstruct real self-movement heading despite pursuit in any direction (Page and Duffy, 1999; Upadhyay et al., 2000; Ben Hamed et al., 2003). MSTd (Shenoy et al., 1999) and VIP (Duhamel et al., 1997) neurons with visual responses that are modulated by eye and head position and velocity show a range of effects during gaze shifts that may contribute to transforming heading representation from retinal/ocular to orbital/cranial/somatic reference frames.

Whole-Body Movement Responses in Parietotemporal Cortex

Vestibular signals about self-movement activate neurons in a number of parietal cortical areas, particularly area 2v (Fredrickson et al., 1966; Schwarz and Fredrickson, 1971), 7a (Kawano et al., 1980; Ventre and Faugier-Grimaud, 1988; Faugier-Grimaud and Ventre, 1989) and the parietoinsular and retroinsular areas (Guldin et al., 1992; Guldin and

Grüsser, 1998; Akbarian et al., 1994). Semicircular canal input is evident in neuronal responses to body rotation in MST (Erickson and Thier, 1992), 7a (Kawano et al., 1980; Snyder et al., 1998), VIP (Bremmer et al., 2002; Thier and Erickson, 1992) and the adjacent superior temporal polysensory area (Hietanen and Perrett, 1996). In addition, a number of studies now find evidence of vestibular otolith input during real translational acceleration in MSTd (Duffy, 1998; Bremmer and Lappe, 1999) and the adjacent area VIP (Schlack et al., 2002).

The most parsimonious view of navigational cue interactions is that performance is best supported by experience in the modality to be used in the task (Kearns et al., 2002; Lambrey et al., 2002). Humans can navigate by using both optic flow and vestibular cues during self-movement (Pavard and Berthoz, 1977; Israel and Berthoz, 1989). They also can navigate with earth-stationary objects, but they chiefly rely on optic flow when it is available (van den Berg and Brenner, 1994; Warren et al., 2001). Moving observers integrate visual and nonvisual cues about self-movement, but it is still unclear how and where in cortex visual, vestibular and eye and head signals are transformed from sensory specific frames of reference to motor. Efforts to understand how signals are integrated at the neuronal level have met with limited success because investigators have been able to test only a limited number of stimulus types and a limited number of directions.

Optic flow and vestibular signals are integrated during self-movement (Cornilleau-Peres and Droulez, 1994; Regan and Vincent, 1995; Israel et al., 1996). Translational acceleration has little impact on robust responses to optic flow in both MST (Duffy, 1998; Bremmer and Lappe, 1999) and adjacent ventral intraparietal cortex (VIP) (Bremmer et al., 2002). However, when the optic flow and movement stimuli signal different directions of movement, robust interactions emerge in MST (Duffy, 1998) and VIP (Schlack et al., 2002). Although individual MST neurons respond to optic flow, real movement (vestibular), and gaze shifts, limited studies have incorporated all three stimuli. Shenoy et al. (1999) rotated the head and/or eyes while the animal was viewing optic flow and found that MST neurons partially compensate for gaze shifts. We have studied the neuronal responses of MSTd neurons to naturalistic optic flow stimuli as well as to whole-body translational movement. Our studies lead us to conclude that MSTd is involved in the processing of self-movement cues for the representation of self-movement direction to support navigation and orientation. The studies described later in this chapter support this view and show how MSTd might contribute to spatial perception, cognition, and behavior.

MSTd Neuronal Responses to Self-Movement

These studies are based on over 200 neurons recorded in four rhesus monkeys (Page and Duffy, 2003). Three experiments are described: (1) linear translational movement with gaze-fixed, (2) linear translational movement with landmark pursuit eye movements, and (3) circular translational movement with gaze fixed.

Single neurons were recorded using microelectrodes passed through a transdural guide tube mounted in a recording grid in the cylinder. MSTd neurons were identified by their physiologic characteristics as previously described, briefly: large receptive fields ($>20° \times 20°$), which included the fixation point, a preference for large moving patterns rather than moving bars or spots, and direction selective responses (Komatsu and Wurtz, 1988b; Duffy and Wurtz, 1991; Duffy and Wurtz, 1995). Histologic analysis confirmed that the neurons studied were located in MSTd on the anterior bank of the superior temporal sulcus.

Linear Translational Movement with Gaze Fixed

The monkey chair, eye coil, and video display systems were mounted on a 1×2 m platform on a double-rail drive apparatus (figure 15.3A). Platform movements were controlled with position feedback from the drive motors. In linear translation trials, the platform was position 60 cm from the center of the room to one of eight starting positions. The platform then moved on a straight path through the center to stop after a total excursion of 120 cm. During these movements, the platform accelerated at 30 cm/s^2 for 1 s, maintained a constant velocity of 30 cm/s for 3 s, and then decelerated at 30 cm/s^2 for 1 s (figure 15.3C). During movement in light trials, a wall-mounted light array was illuminated. It contained 600 small, white lights uniformly distributed across a 322 cm $\times$ 168 cm wall that was 220 cm from the monkey's centered position. These lights were stationary, so any visual motion was the result of observer movement. All of the lights were always in the monkey's field of view, although the array subtended different horizontal angles depending on the distance of the sled from the wall.

We assessed the influence of vestibular cues on self-movement responses by recording MSTd neuronal activity during translational movement with gaze fixed straight ahead on a target that moved with the sled. Figure 15.4A (top) shows the directional responses of a neuron with transient activation during left-forward acceleration (0–1 s) that reversed to a right-backward preference during deceleration (4–5 s). This reversal suggests an underlying vestibular mechanism. That neuron did not respond significantly to optic flow simulating the same eight directions of self-movement (figure 15.4A, middle). Nevertheless, translational movement in light, which combined vestibular and visual stimulation, yielded a much stronger response than that obtained in darkness but had the same directionality and directional reversals seen in darkness (figure 15.4A, bottom).

A very different set of findings was obtained from the neuron illustrated in figure 15.4B, which shows movement in darkness responses that build up across the steady speed and

Figure 15.3
MSTd neurons were recorded during translational self-movement while the monkey maintained fixed gaze. (A) The two-axis monkey sled moved across the room in eight directions; right-forward movement is illustrated. The monkey continuously viewed the far wall that was covered by 600 small white lights while maintaining neutral gaze throughout the movement by fixating a target that moved to remain directly in front on the animal. (B) The retinal patterns of optic flow are shown as schematic drawings for the eight directions of movement (boxes; black

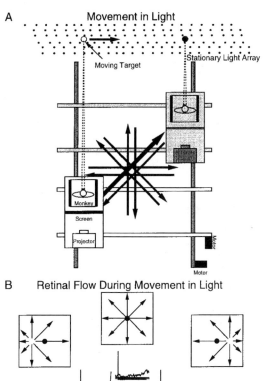

A   Movement in Light

Moving Target

Stationary Light Array

Monkey

Screen

Projector

Motor

Motor

B   Retinal Flow During Movement in Light

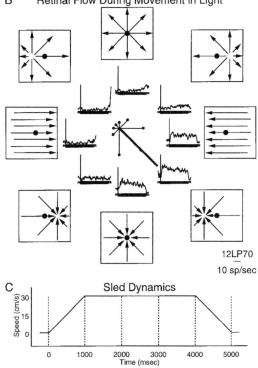

12LP70

10 sp/sec

C   Sled Dynamics

Speed (cm/s)

30

15

0

0   1000   2000   3000   4000   5000

Time (msec)

circles are gaze fixation points). The corresponding neuronal responses are shown as spike density histograms (SDHs) averaging responses to six repetitions of the 5 s self-movement stimuli in the direction indicated by the SDH's position relative to the center of the figure. The polar plot (center) illustrates the relevant self-movement stimulus direction as radial limb direction and response amplitude as radial limb length, with significant responses indicated by a filled ball, and the net vector shown by a heavy line. (C) The speed profile of sled movement for all eight directions included 1 s of acceleration, 3 s of steady-speed movement, and 1 s of deceleration.

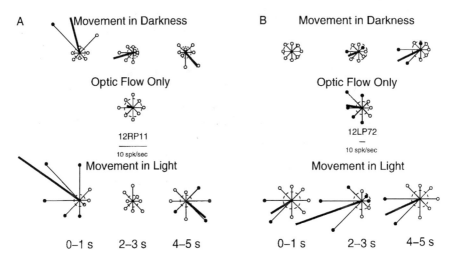

Figure 15.4
The time-course of MSTd neuronal responses to gaze fixed self-movement. (A, B) Directional responses for two neurons shown as polar plots for the acceleration, steady-state and deceleration stimulus intervals. These plots show the relevant self-movement stimulus direction as radial limb direction and response amplitude as radial limb length, with significant responses indicated by a filled ball, the net vector shown by a heavy line, and control activity indicated by a dashed circle. (A) A neuron showing transient responses to acceleration and deceleration. Acceleration evokes left-forward direction selectivity during the first 1 s of movement in darkness, while deceleration evokes right-backward direction selectivity in the fifth 1 s of movement. These responses are consistent with activation by acceleration, likely transduced by the vestibular otoliths. Simulated optic flow alone resulted in minimal responses (middle) yet the movement responses were enhanced during gaze-fixed movement in the light (bottom). (B) A neuron showing responses with increasing left-backward direction selectivity for the 5 s of movement in darkness. The optic-flow-alone responses show a leftward preference (middle). When the stimuli were combined in the gaze-fixed movement in light condition, the neuron responded more vigorously and with shorter latency than in the dark condition.

deceleration phases of the movement with increasing left-backward direction selectivity (figure 15.4B, top). The presentation of optic flow simulating the self-movement scene yielded moderately left-forward direction selectivity (figure 15.4B, middle). Combining vestibular and visual stimulation, using gaze fixed translational movement in light, yielded strong responses that began during the acceleration phase, peaked during the steady speed movement, and declined during deceleration (figure 15.4B, bottom).

The varying time-course of these responses, and their reversal of preferred direction during deceleration, support the vestibular origin of the responses to movement in darkness. Overall, optic flow alone evoked larger responses than movement in darkness, with a substantial increase in the number of responsive neurons from 59% in darkness to 87% (95/109) in light. There were far more sustained responses in light, and almost all of the responses began at stimulus onset, during the acceleration period. Movement in light showed a wide range of effects that in some cases reflected the vestibular influences, in other cases reflected the visual influences, and often showed a dynamic

A   Movement in Darkness   B   Movement in Light

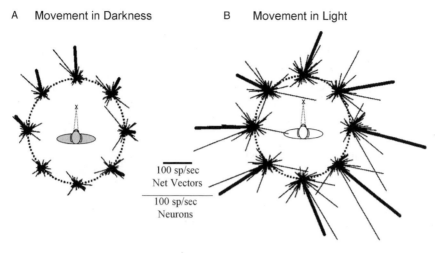

100 sp/sec
Net Vectors

100 sp/sec
Neurons

Figure 15.5
Population responses to gaze fixed movement in darkness (A) and to movement in light (B). Each cluster corresponds to one of the eight stimulus self-movement directions and each thin line indicates the contribution from one neuron. The direction of this vector indicates the neuron's preferred direction and the length is proportionate to the neuronal response to that stimulus. The population net vector for each direction (bold lines) is the vector sum for the 109 neurons tested in these studies. The population vectors more closely approximate the stimulus direction during movement in light.

interaction of vestibular and visual influences across the 5 s period of the movement in light stimulus.

Summing the vector responses of all 109 neurons to all eight directional stimuli derived population responses to self-movement with gaze fixed (Georgopoulos et al., 1986). In darkness, these responses were of relatively low amplitude but maintained a generally veridical representation of self-movement direction, especially during forward movement (figure 15.5A). When the light array was illuminated, the population responses showed the same dramatic increase in response amplitude that was typical among the single neurons (figure 15.5B). In addition, light also greatly improved the accuracy of the population net vector's indication of the self-movement direction in all stimuli. Thus, MSTd neurons appear capable of representing self-movement in darkness and in light, but the population responses are stronger and more accurate during movement in light.

Translational Movement with Pursuit Eye Movements
The significance of visual contributions to self-movement perception has been disputed since the recognition that concurrent pursuit eye movements distort the retinal image of optic flow (Longuet-Higgins and Prazdny, 1980). To test the impact of pursuit on MSTd neuronal responses to self-movement, we combined the previously described self-movement stimuli with naturalistic pursuit eye movements (Page and Duffy, 2003). These

eye movements were induced by having the monkey fixate a central earth-fixed point so that it would have to use pursuit eye movements to maintain fixation as it moved around the room (figure 15.6A). The pattern of eye movements (figure 15.6) distorted the retinal image of the optic flow field (figure 15.6B).

Neuronal responses to movement in light with landmark pursuit often appeared to be the vector sum of the responses to movement in light with gaze fixed and the responses to pursuit eye movements simulating those occurring during landmark pursuit. Figure 15.7A (top) shows the directional responses of a neuron with transient activation during the steady-speed interval of right-backward movement in light, with gaze fixed. This neuron responded vigorously to pursuit like that occurring during movement to the left while fixating an earth-fixed landmark (figure 15.7A, middle). These responses combined during movement in light with landmark pursuit to create a left-backward preference, which seemed to weigh the pursuit response more than the response to movement in light with gaze fixed (figure 15.7A, bottom).

Other neurons showed a greater influence of the movement in light with gaze fixed responses. The neuronal responses illustrated in figure 15.7B show strong responses throughout movement in light with gaze fixed showing a right-backward self-movement direction preference (top). This neuron showed only weak responses to pursuit, preferring pursuit like that occurring during rightward movement in light while fixating an earth-fixed landmark (figure 15.7B, middle). This neuron responded vigorously to movement in light with landmark pursuit, showing a stronger right-backward self-movement direction preference which seemed to weigh responses to the movement in light with gaze fixed more than the response to pursuit (figure 15.7B, bottom).

The examples given above typify the two types of responses commonly seen with movement in light during landmark pursuit. About 70% of the neurons showed stronger movement in light responses with gaze fixed than during landmark pursuit. For these neurons, the gaze fixed self-movement direction preferences tended to be the opposite of their pursuit-only response preferences. This created vector subtraction when these stimuli were combined, and hence the landmark pursuit responses were smaller than the gaze fixed

Figure 15.6
MSTd neuronal responses during landmark pursuit movement. (A) During the landmark pursuit condition, the monkey maintained its gaze on an earth-fixed target by making smooth pursuit eye movements. (B) The retinal patterns of optic flow during landmark pursuit are shown as schematic drawings for the eight directions of movement (boxes). The open arrows represent the direction of landmark pursuit eye movements in each of the stimulus conditions. (When moving directly forward of backward, there is no landmark pursuit.) The corresponding neuronal responses are shown as spike density histograms, which average responses to six repetitions of the 5 s self-movement stimuli and are plotted in the direction of self-movement. The polar plot (center) illustrates the self-movement directions as thin radial limbs in the stimulus direction and response amplitude as radial limb length. The vector sum of these limbs creates the overall response net vector (heavy line). (C) Horizontal eye movements during landmark pursuit. Forward and backward movement required steady gaze (flat lines). Lateral movements required symmetric movements of intermediate amplitude, while oblique movements required greater deviation of the eyes when the animal was nearer the wall.

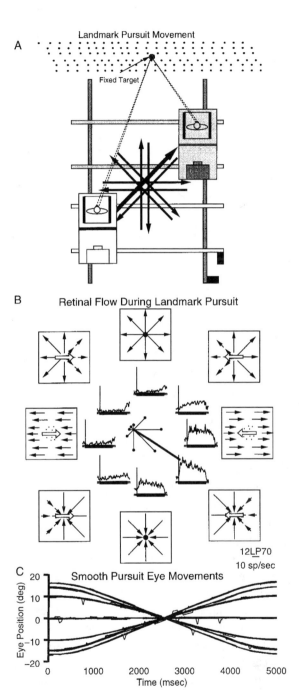

A   Landmark Pursuit Movement

Fixed Target

B   Retinal Flow During Landmark Pursuit

12LP70
10 sp/sec

C   Smooth Pursuit Eye Movements

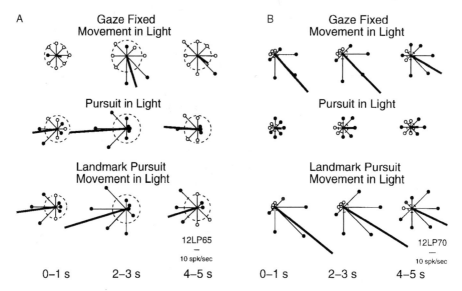

Figure 15.7
Polar responses of responses to landmark pursuit movement in light (bottom) combine the effects of gaze-fixed movement in light (top) and pursuit in light (middle) for the corresponding self-movement directions. (A) Directional responses of a neuron that shows a backward response to the 2–3 s interval of movement, yet a strong response to pursuit in light simulating leftward self-movement during all intervals. When the stimuli are combined in the landmark pursuit condition, the direction appears to be dominated by the leftward pursuit response with some backward deviations during the middle interval, possibly resulting from the self-movement. (B) Directional responses of a second neuron that shows a strong response to right-backward movement in light. This neuron shows a weak but consistent rightward response in the pursuit only condition. Landmark pursuit evokes an enhanced right-backward response that shows a systematically rightward shift that may be due to the influence of the pursuit response.

responses. About 30% of the neurons showed stronger movement in light responses during landmark pursuit than with gaze fixed. These neurons had similar self-movement direction preferences in the gaze-fixed condition and to pursuit alone. This created vector summation when these stimuli were combined, and hence the landmark pursuit responses were larger than the gaze-fixed responses.

Population net vectors were derived for responses to self-movement during landmark pursuit. In darkness, these responses were of relatively low amplitude with broadly veridical self-movement directions (figure 15.8A). Notably, these population responses were somewhat larger than those obtained during movement in darkness with gaze fixed, suggesting that a single earth-fixed point may provide an important visual cue about relative self-movement. In light, the population response during landmark pursuit showed the same high amplitude and accurate directionality seen during movement in light with gaze fixed (figure 15.8B). Thus, contrary to theoretical predictions (Longuet-Higgins and Prazdny, 1980), visual information about self-movement is not made unreliable by concurrent pursuit eye movements. It appears that extraretinal pursuit signals can be used to adjust

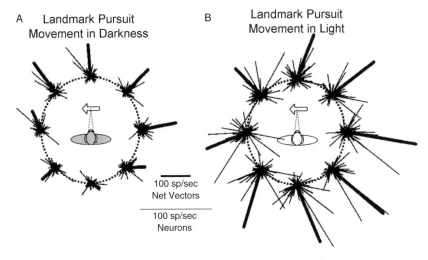

Figure 15.8
Population responses to landmark pursuit movement in darkness (A) and to movement in light (B). Each cluster corresponds to one of the eight stimulus self-movement directions and contains a vector for each neuron (thin lines). The direction of this vector indicates the neuron's preferred direction and the length is proportionate to the neuronal response to the stimulus. The population net vector for each direction (bold lines) is the sum of the vectors for 109 neurons tested in these studies. The population vectors approximate the stimulus direction in both light and dark conditions, although the amplitude of the response is enhanced in the movement in light, especially when moving backward.

the population response for the distorting effects of pursuit on the retinal image of optic flow.

These findings are summarized in figure 15.9, showing that the population net vector direction reflects the self-movement direction in movement in darkness and in light, with gaze fixed, or during landmark pursuit. When moving in light, the responses are larger and more accurate. When pursuit is superimposed, the responses remain large and accurate. Alternative population response analyses (Ben Hamed et al., 2003) show that these effects might yield accuracy at or exceeding that of human performance. This supports the view that MSTd neurons are well-suited to contribute to the estimation of self-movement direction in a variety of naturalistic conditions.

Circular Translational Movement with Gaze Fixed

Naturalistic self-movement consists of sequences of self-movement directions that define paths between places in the environment. Place specificity is commonly seen in hippocampal neurons and in some related structures. Place selectivity might well influence the processing of self-movement cues by creating a locational context based on movement history and goals. The potential for such influences of self-movement context prompted us to test whether the heading selective responses of MSTd neurons might show evidence of such effects (Froehler and Duffy, 2002).

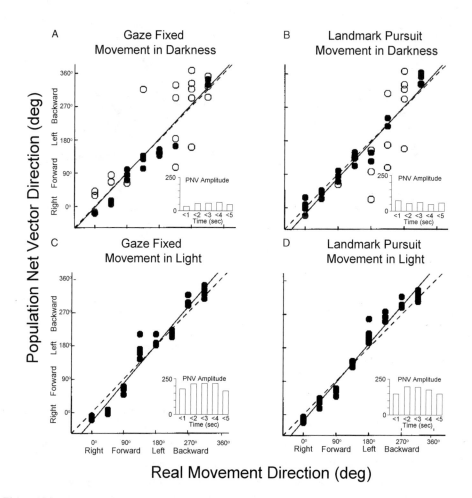

Figure 15.9
Population vector accuracy and amplitude across five 1 s stimulus periods based on the combined responses to all four basic types of self-movement. Each scatter plot shows the population vectors for one of the four basic self-movement conditions, and each point shows the direction of the population vector for the five movement intervals (ordinate) in relation to the direction in that movement stimulus (abscissa). Filled points represent significant net vectors (Z value of the circular distribution with p < .05) and the solid line indicates the least squares linear regression used to fit these points. The accompanying bar graphs show the average amplitude of the population net vectors (ordinate) for each of the five 1 s stimulus intervals (abscissa). (A) The population vectors for gaze fixed movement in darkness show a clear relationship between the population vector direction and the movement direction ($r^2 = .79$, slope = 1.03) but with relatively small population vector amplitudes in all intervals. (B) Landmark pursuit movement in darkness shows similar effects especially with backward movements ($r^2 = .84$, slope = 1.07). (C) Population vectors for gaze-fixed movement in light show a more consistent relationship between population vector direction and movement directions ($r^2 = .96$, slope = 1.14) with much larger population vector amplitudes. (D) Landmark pursuit movement in light shows similar effects ($r^2 = .97$, slope = 1.15).

In circular translation trials, the platform was positioned at one of four points along a circle 120 cm in diameter. The platform then moved on a clockwise (CW) or counterclockwise (CCW) circular path to travel 360° in eight seconds with an additional 0.5 s of gradual deceleration. Throughout all stimulus trials, the monkey maintained neutral gaze by fixating a red spot that was projected onto the facing wall at eye height and moved to remain directly in front of the monkey. We presented translational self-movement on CW and CCW circular paths through the room (figure 15.10A). Each trial consisted of a complete circuit around the path covering all self-movement directions with the reverse sequence of self-movement directions on the CW and CCW paths. MSTd neurons showed similar self-movement direction selective responses to these stimuli as they had to linear translation. However, these neurons showed substantial differences in their responses to the same self-movement directions occurring on the CW and CCW paths. Figure 15.10B illustrates the self-movement direction tuning curve of a neuron that preferred forward self-movement directions but showed much stronger responses when those directions were presented in CW path than in the CCW path. The difference between the preferred self-movement direction responses on the CW and CCW paths is shown as a contrast ratio for each of the 63 neurons studied with these stimuli (figure 15.9C). Forty percent of the neurons showed a twofold difference between responses from the two paths, with equal numbers preferring CW and CCW. This path selectivity may reflect the sequence of self-movement directions that is unique for each path. Alternatively, path selectivity may reflect the co-incidence of the preferred self-movement directions with other stimulus features that are unique to a location in the room and the directions used to get to that location.

Path selectivity was not the only new effect seen in these studies. We also found that some MSTd neurons showed a complete reversal of their preferred self-movement directions on the CW and CCW paths. These neurons formed a unique class distinct from the self-movement, direction selective neurons because their direction preferences changed depending on the path. They are also not included among the path selective neurons because they yielded equally strong responses on both the CW and CCW paths. The reversal of the self-movement direction preferences of these neurons on the two paths meant that they were responding as the monkey moved past the same place in the room on both paths; all places having opposite headings during CW and CCW movement. Twenty percent of the neurons showed such place selective responses.

The effects of particular places in the room on MSTd neurons are also seen in their activity while the monkey was in a stationary position. Between movement trials, the animals were positioned at four different locations in the room. Many neurons showed differences in their resting activity depending on the animal's position in the room. Figure 15.11A shows such an effect for an MSTd neuron that was more active when the animal was at the right-front of the room and least active when the animal was at the left-rear of the room. We compared these sites of stationary location preference to the sites of moving place preference in all neurons that showed both effects (figure 15.11B). There was a high

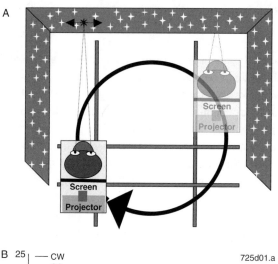

A

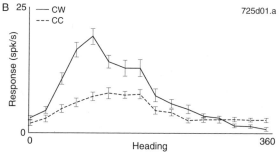

B   25
— CW
--- CC
725d01.a

Response (spk/s)

0
0
Heading
360

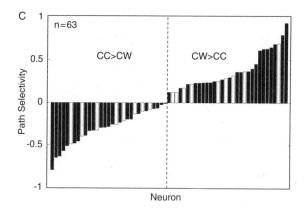

C   1
n=63

Path Selectivity

0.5

CC>CW   CW>CC

0

-0.5

-1
Neuron

Figure 15.10
Movement on a curved path evokes path-selective responses. (A) The monkey was moved on a motorized sled along clockwise (CW) and counterclockwise (CC) circular paths. The room was illuminated by arrays of small lights on the facing wall and two visible side walls. The monkey maintained neutral gaze by fixating a projected LED that tracked sled movement, and always remained oriented toward the facing wall. (B) One neuron's response to continuous directions on the CW (solid) and CC (dashed) paths, averaged over 24 trials. This neuron shows path-dependent direction selectivity for the CW path. (C) Path selectivity was measured as the contrast ratio between peak responses on the CW and CC paths (ordinate) for each neuron (abscissa). Filled bars indicate the 73% of neurons that had a significantly directional response (Z-statistic) on at least one path. There is a continuum of path effects across the sample of neurons recorded.

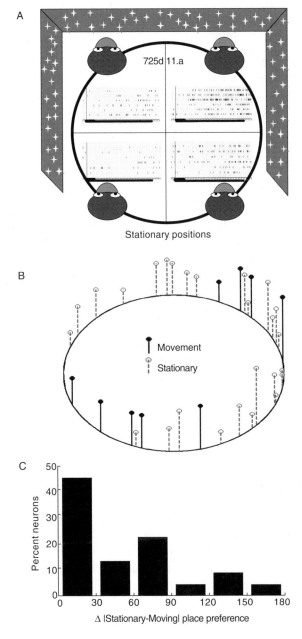

Figure 15.11
Place-selective responses with and without movement. (A) The monkey was moved to one of four stationary locations in the room and remained gaze-fixed and motionless for 8.5 s. The rasters show one neuron's activity at each stationary position, revealing a preference for the right-forward location. (B) Shown are the preferred places during stationary positioning (open, n = 26) and translational movement along the circular path (filled, n = 9) for significant responses. There is a range of preferred places, with no relationship to fixation-distance. (C) Place-selective neurons respond to their preferred place whether the monkey is moving or stationary. The bar graph shows the angular distance between the preferred place during sled movement and stationary location trials for the 46 neurons with place effects. The predominance of small differences reflects the similarity of preferred locations in movement and stationary trials.

rate of concordance between these effects with most neurons tending to have their preferred stationary location near their preferred movement place (figure 15.11C).

Thus, MSTd neurons not only encode instantaneous self-movement direction, but they also show specific responses to the path of self-movement and the location of the animal in that environment. Together, these findings suggest that MSTd might play an important role in processing sensory information to support spatial orientation and navigation.

Conclusions and Inferences

Sensory-Motor Integration of Self-Movement Direction Cues

MSTd neurons respond to vestibular, as well as visual, signals about self-movement (Duffy, 1998). This is consistent with vestibular projections to dorsal extrastriate visual areas that might mediate self-movement responses in darkness.

Gaze-fixed movement in darkness responses showed several characteristics suggestive of their vestibular origin. First, they showed clear direction selectivity such that they responded more strongly to movement in one preferred direction in the ground plane, with smaller responses evoked by movement in other directions. Second, their time course showed a clear relationship to the acceleration phase of movement, suggesting a link to the accelerometer function of the vestibular otoliths, rather than a link to visual or oculomotor events that did not influence the responses that we have recorded during translational movement. Third, their direction selectivity often reversed in the deceleration phase of a movement stimulus, suggesting that these responses reflect the direction of the movement force, which reverses from acceleration to deceleration during a particular direction of movement.

Light often seems to simply accentuate the neuronal responses seen during movement in darkness, but the effects are usually more complex. The time course of movement in light responses has more rapid onset with significant activation at the very beginning of movement acceleration. Light responses also tended to be more sustained, commonly being maintained throughout the entire movement stimulus. The direction preferences of light responses also differ from those obtained during movement in darkness. Although a number of neurons have similar direction preferences during gaze-fixed movement in light and in darkness, those responses mostly occurred in neurons with stronger vestibular than visual directionality. In most MSTd neurons, the relative strength and direction preferences of vestibular and visual responses interacted in a nonadditive manner across the acceleration, steady-speed, and deceleration phases of our movement stimuli.

At this time, we see no compelling case to be made for a systematic relationship between vestibular and visual direction preferences in individual MSTd neurons. Neither do we see a compelling justification why such a relationship should be expected: The independently distributed representation of vestibular and visual directionality may support the maintenance of veridical self-movement direction estimation in naturalistic circumstances in which head rotation, gaze position, and self-movement direction are variably aligned. If vestibular and visual directionalities were aligned in individual neurons, then specific combinations of head rotation and gaze position might be required for accurate estimation of self-movement direction. The independence of vestibular and visual direction preferences obviates the implementation of such a restrictive neuronal architecture.

Pursuit eye movements during translational self-movement have been thought to disrupt self-movement direction estimation by optic flow analysis (Longuet-Higgins and Prazdny, 1980). We studied MSTd neuronal responses to self-movement in the naturalistic condition that we refer to as landmark pursuit—the dynamic, pursuit eye movements required by a moving observer to maintain fixation on an earth-fixed point. In single neurons, pursuit responses interact with visual and vestibular effects to create a complex spectrum of response properties. These effects are evident during landmark pursuit in darkness. Landmark pursuit in light shows the complex three-way interactions between vestibular, visual, and pursuit effects.

These diverse single neuron response properties may be more readily understood from the perspective of population responses in MSTd (figure 15.12A). We have taken the approach of population vector summation for self-movement direction estimation in MSTd. This method illustrates that vestibular responses support veridical self-movement representation, even with the small numbers of neurons recorded in this study. In addition, MSTd's population response shows the substantial enhancement of self-movement direction estimation during movement in light. Naturalistic self-movement occurs in a great many conditions that are intermediate between darkness and light. Corresponding parametric changes in the relative strength of visual and vestibular signals in MSTd might alter the population response to adapt to those effects.

MSTd's population response was also assessed during self-movement in the landmark pursuit condition. Contrary to theoretical predictions, the population response maintained its veridical representation of self-movement direction both in darkness and in light. These findings support the idea that cortical neurons combine vestibular, visual, and oculomotor signals to estimate self-movement direction (Berthoz and Viaud-Delmon, 1999; Hartley et al., 2000). Thus, MSTd might integrate visual and vestibular sensory modalities, and serve sensory and oculomotor functions, to support navigation and spatial orientation.

MSTd's Role in Papez's Circuit for Navigation

Studies using circular patterns of translational self-movement revealed new properties of MSTd's self-movement responses. Many neurons showed the same self-movement direction selective responses regardless of whether the preferred direction was encountered on a CW or CCW path. Other neurons showed path-dependent direction selectivity with stronger responses to the preferred self-movement direction on either the CW or CCW path.

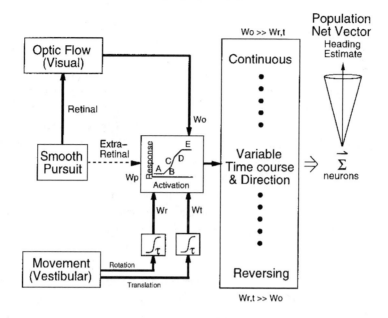

A Multi-modal Interactions in MST

B A Papez's Circuit for Navigation

Figure 15.12
Model summary of self-movement direction estimation in MSTd. (A) The visual and vestibular responses interact in a manner that is influenced by the time-course of the vestibular effects and its directional alignment with the visual effects. The summation is governed by non-additive response dynamics, here characterized as a sigmoidal activation-response curve that yields sub-additive effects (A, E), additive effects (B, D), and superadditive effects (C). These signals vector sum to provide a population representation of self-movement direction in darkness and light. (B) Schematic drawing of Papez's circuit for navigation. Arrows indicate direction of spatial information transfer: posterior parietal cortex (PPC), parahippocampal areas (Para Hippo), hippocampus (Hippo), anterior thalamus (AT), posterior cingulate cortex (area 23), retrosplenial cortex (RS).

Path-dependent self-movement direction selectivity can be interpreted as the combining of direction selectivity with other stimulus attributes that may distinguish the opposite parts of the room at which the preferred self-movement direction occurs on the CCW or CW paths. Path dependence may also reflect temporal summation effects across the sequence of directions that occur in reverse order on the CCW and CW paths. Finally, path dependence can be a consequence of interactions between direction selectivity and the monkey's awareness of its position in the room, especially with respect to the start/stop location at which a reward will be delivered. All of these mechanisms may play some role in the diverse response properties observed in these studies, and further studies are underway to characterize these factors.

Some neurons showed a reversal of their preferred self-movement direction between CCW and CW paths such that they preferred one direction on one path and the opposite direction on the other path. This corresponds to neurons being most active when the animal passes through a certain place in the room. Further evidence of such place selectivity was obtained when the monkeys were held at four different stationary positions in the room. Many neurons showed a preference for one of those positions over the others, and that preference showed a good correspondence with the place in the room that evoked the strongest responses during circular translational movement.

These studies suggest that MSTd neurons not only represent the instantaneous self-movement direction, but also can provide a neural basis for deriving the path of movements that led to the current direction, and even the location at which those self-movements might occur. The latter attributes are particularly reminiscent of the place cell responses recorded from hippocampal pyramidal neurons (O'Keefe and Dostrovsky, 1971; McNaughton et al., 1983; Muller et al., 1994). MSTd might interact with the hippocampus to form a distributed neural system for navigation and orientation (McNaughton et al., 1989).

Such a cortical-subcortical system would form a dorsal limb of Papez's circuit (Papez, 1937). This dorsal limb would integrate limbic and posterior cingulate mechanisms serving the control of navigation and spatial orientation. It would be analogous to the ventral limb that Papez described for limbic and anterior cingulate integration serving the control of emotion (Vogt et al., 1992). This limbic-cingulate dichotomy (Baleydier and Mauguiere, 1980) may be analogous to the dorsal/ventral visual dichotomy (Ungerleider and Mishkin, 1982) as it describes parallel subdivisions within a functional system that possesses other unifying properties.

Papez's circuit for navigation (figure 15.12B) might be thought of as beginning in dorsal extrastriate visual-cortical areas that combine visual, vestibular, and other signals relevant to self-movement perception and spatial orientation (Schaafsma and Duysens, 1996; Siegel and Read, 1997; Bremmer et al., 2002). These parietotemporal areas are reciprocally connected with parahippocampal cortices (Jones and Powell, 1970; Van Hoesen, 1982; Kosel et al., 1982; Anderson et al., 1990; Clower et al., 2001; Lavenex et al., 2002; Ding et al., 2003) that then connect reciprocally with the hippocampus (Mesulam et al., 1977; Amaral et al., 1983; Cavada and Goldman-Rakic, 1989; Rockland and Van Hoesen, 1999). The resulting spatial activity in the hippocampus may produce its place neuron responses (O'Keefe and Nadel, 1978; McNaughton et al., 1994; Nishijo et al., 1997).

Parahippocampal and subicular areas project to the anterior and lateral dorsal thalamus via the fornix and the mammillothalamic tract (Aggleton et al., 1986) that might contribute head direction sensitivity and related spatial response properties. Reciprocal projections from the anterior and lateral dorsal thalami to posterior cingulate and retrosplenial cortical areas (Baleydier and Mauguiere, 1980; Mufson and Pandya, 1984; Morris et al., 1999) engage these cortical areas in spatial processing (Whishaw et al., 2001). They, in turn, project reciprocally to posterior parietal cortical areas (Baleydier and Mauguiere, 1980; Pandya et al., 1981; Morris et al., 1999; Leichnetz, 2001), completing the corticosubcortical circuit.

Two related points should be emphasized regarding this Papez's circuit for navigation. First, there is additional spatial input to posterior parietal cortex from the colliculo-pulvinoparietal visual system (Trevarthan, 1968) that maintains a source of visuospatial information parallel to the geniculocalcarine input (Pasik and Pasik, 1972; Sanders et al., 1974). Second, this corticosubcortical circuit includes a rich feedback system based on its extensive reciprocal connections, so that it should be thought of as a substrate for bidirectional information flow supporting navigation and spatial orientation.

It is tempting to speculate that particular routes through such a circuit might play special roles in the parietal cortical response properties observed in our studies. Multisensory integration may result from the converging output of geniculocalcarine, colliculopulvinar, and adjacent vestibular cortices that project to MSTd. MSTd might then transmit integrated self-movement signals to temporal lobe parahippocampal areas that are extensively interconnected with the hippocampus. The time-course integration that contributes to MSTd's path-dependent responses might reflect direct temporal lobe feedback, whereas place/location effects in MSTd might be linked to the action of the long loop pathway through the Papez's circuit. This is consistent with lesion studies that implicate hippocampal-anterior thalamic connections in spatial memory (Aggleton and Mishkin, 1985; Aggleton et al., 1995). We consider this scheme to be a theoretical framework for guiding further investigations.

References

Aggleton JP, Desimone R, Mishkin M (1986) The origin, course, and termination of the hippocampothalamic projections in the macaque. J Comp Neurol 243: 409–421.

Aggleton JP, Mishkin M (1985) Mamillary-body lesions and visual recognition in monkeys. Exp Brain Res 58: 190–197.

Aggleton JP, Neave N, Nagle PR, Hunt PR (1995) A comparison of the effects of anterior thalamic, mamillary body and fornix lesions on reinforced spatial alteration. Behav Brain Res 68: 91–101.

Aguirre GK, D'Esposito M (1997) Environmental knowledge is subserved by separable dorsal/ventral neural areas. J Neurosci 17: 2512–2518.

Akbarian S, Grusser OJ, Guldin WO (1994) Corticofugal connections between the cerebral cortex and brainstem vestibular nuclei in the macaque monkey. J Comp Neurol 339: 421–437.

Allman JM, Kaas JH (1971) A representation of the visual field in the caudal third of the middle temporal gyrus of the owl monkey (Aotus trivirgatus). Brain Res 31: 85–105.

Amaral DG, Insausti R, Cowan WM (1983) Evidence for a direct projection from the superior temporal gyrus to the entorhinal cortex in the monkey. Brain Res 275: 263–277.

Andersen GJ, Braunstein ML (1985) Induced self-motion in central vision. J Expl Psychol: Human Percept Perf 11: 122–132.

Andersen RA, Mountcastle VB (1983) The influence of the angle of gaze upon the excitiability of the light-sensitive neurons of the posterior parietal cortex. J Neurosci 3: 532–548.

Anderson RA, Asanuma C, Essick G, Siegel RM (1990) Corticocortical connections of anatomically and physiologically defined subdivisions within the inferior parietal lobule. J Comp Neurol 296: 65–113.

Baader A (1991) Simulation of self-motion in tethered flying insects: an optical flow field for locusts. J Neurosci Meth 38: 193–199.

Baleydier C, Mauguiere F (1980) The duality of the cingulate gyrus in monkey. Neuroanatomical study and functional hypothesis. Brain 103: 525–554.

Ben Hamed S, Page WK, Duffy CJ, Pouget A (2003) MSTd neuronal basis functions for the population encoding of heading direction. J Neurophys 90: 549–558.

Berthoz A, Viaud-Delmon I (1999) Multisensory integration in spatial orientation. Curr Opin Neurobiol. 9: 708–712.

Bradley DC, Maxwell M, Andersen RA, Banks MS, Shenoy KV (1996) Mechanisms of heading perception in primate visual cortex. Science 273: 1544–1549.

Bremmer F, Duhamel J-R, Hamed SB, Graf W (1997a) The representation of movement in near extra-personal space in the macaque ventral intraparietal area (VIP). In P Their, and HO Karnath eds., Parietal Lobe Contributions to Orientation in 3D Space. Heidelberg: Springer-Verlag, pp. 619–630.

Bremmer F, Duhamel JR, Ben H, Graf W (2002) Heading encoding in the macaque ventral intraparietal area (VIP). Euro J Neurosci 16: 1554–1568.

Bremmer F, Ilg UJ, Thiele A, Distler C, Hoffmann KP (1997b) Eye position effects in monkey cortex. I. visual and pursuit-related activity in extrastriate area MT and MST. J Neurophys 77: 944–961.

Bremmer F, Lappe M (1999) The use of optical velocities for distance discrimination and reproduction during visually simulated self motion. Exp Brain Res 127: 33–42.

Bremmer F, Pouget A, Hoffmann KP (1998) Eye position encoding in the macaque posterior parietal cortex. Eur J Neurosc 10: 153–160.

Britten KH, Van W (1998) Electrical microstimulation of cortical area MST biases heading perception in monkeys. Nature Neurosci 1: 59–63.

Brotchie PR, Andersen RA, Snyder LH, Goodman SJ (1995) Head position signals used by parietal neurons to encode locations of visual stimuli. Nature 375: 232–235.

Cavada C, Goldman-Rakic PS (1989) Posterior parietal cortex in rhesus monkey: I. Parcellation of areas based on distinctive limbic and sensory corticocortical connections. J Comp Neurol 287: 393–421.

Cheng K, Fujita H, Kanno I, Miura S, Tanaka K (1995) Human cortical regions activated by wide-field visual motion: an $H_2{}^{15}O$ PET study. J Neurophys 74: 413–427.

Clower DM, West RA, Lynch JC, Strick PL (2001) The inferior parietal lobule is the target of output from the superior colliculus, hippocampus, and cerebellum. J Neurosci 21: 6283–6291.

Cornilleau-Peres V, Droulez J (1994) The visual perception of three-dimensional shape from self-motion and object-motion. Vis Res 34: 2331–2336.

Critchley M (1953) The Parietal Lobes. New York: Hafner Publishing.

De Jong BM, Shipp S, Skidmore B, Frackowiak RSJ, Zeki S (1994) The cerebral activity related to the visual perception of forward motion in depth. Brain 117: 1039–1054.

Ding SL, Morecraft RJ, Van H (2003) Topography, cytoarchitecture, and cellular phenotypes of cortical areas that form the cingulo-parahippocampal isthmus and adjoining retrocalcarine areas in the monkey. J Comp Neurol 456: 184–201.

Dubner R, Zeki SM (1971) Response properties and receptive fields of cells in an anatomically defined region of the superior temporal sulcus. Brain Res 35: 528–532.

Duffy CJ (1998) MST neurons respond to optic flow and translational movement. J Neurophys 80: 1816–1827.

Duffy CJ, Wurtz RH (1991) Sensitivity of MST neurons to optic flow stimuli. I. A continuum of response selectivity to large-field stimuli. J Neurophys 65: 1329–1345.

Duffy CJ, Wurtz RH (1995) Response of monkey MST neurons to optic flow stimuli with shifted centers of motion. J Neurosci 15: 5192–5208.

Duhamel JR, Bremmer F, BenHamed S, Graf W (1997) Spatial invariance of visual receptive fields in parietal cortex neurons. Nature 389: 845–848.

Dupont P, Orban GA, De Bruyn B, Verbruggen A, Mortelmans L (1994) Many areas in the human brain respond to visual motion. J Neurophys 72: 1420–1424.

Erickson RG, Thier, PA (1991) neuronal correlate of spatial stability during periods of self-induced visual motion. Exp Brain Res 86: 608–616.

Erickson RG, Thier P (1992) Responses of direction-selective neurons in monkey cortex to self-induced visual motion. In B Cohen, DL Tomko and F Guedry eds., Sensing and Controlling Motion: Vestibular and Sensorimotor Function. New York: New York Academy of Science, pp. 766–774.

Faugier-Grimaud S, Ventre J (1989) Anatomic connections of inferior parietal cortex (area 7) with subcortical structures related to vestibulo-ocular function in a monkey (Macaca fascicularis). J Comp Neurol 280: 1–14.

Fredrickson JM, Figge U, Scheid P, Kornhuber HH (1966) Vestibular nerve projection to the cerebral cortex of the rhesus monkey. Exp Brain Res 2: 318–327.

Froehler MT, Duffy CJ (2002) Cortical neurons encoding path and place: where you go is where you are. Science 295: 2462–2465.

Galletti C, Battaglini PP (1989) Gaze-dependent visual neurons in area V3A of monkey prestriate cortex. J Neurosci 9: 1112–1125.

Galletti C, Battaglini PP, Fattori P (1995) Eye position influence on the parieto-occipital area PO (V6) of the macaque monkey. Eur J Neurosci 7: 2486–2501.

Georgopoulos AP, Schwartz AB, Kettner RE (1986) Neuronal population coding of movement direction. Science 233: 1416–1419.

Gibson JJ (1950) The Perception of the Visual World. Boston: Houghton Mifflin.

Graziano MSA, Andersen RA, Snowden RJ (1994) Tuning of MST neurons to spiral motion. J Neurosci 14: 54–67.

Guldin WO, Akbarian S, Grüsser OJ (1992) Cortico-cortical connections and cytoarchitectonics of the primate vestibular cortex: A study in squirrel monkeys (Saimiri sciureus). J Comp Neurol 326, 375–401.

Guldin WO, Grüsser OJ (1998) Is there a vestibular cortex? Trends Neurosci 21: 254–259.

Hartley T, Burgess N, Lever C, Cacucci F, O'Keefe J (2000) Modeling place fields in terms of the cortical inputs to the hippocampus. Hippocampus 10: 369–379.

Haxby JV, Horwitz B, Ungerleider LG, Maisog JM, Pietrini P, Grady CL (1994) The functional organization of human extrastriate cortex: A PET-rCBF study of selective attention to faces and locations. J Neurosci 14: 6336–6353.

Hietanen JK, Perrett DI (1996) A comparison of visual responses to object- and ego-motion in the macaque superior temporal polysensory area. Exp Brain Res 108: 341–345.

Holmes G (1918) Disturbances of vision by cerebral lesions. Brit J Ophthalm 2: 353–384.

Israël I, Berthoz A (1989) Contribution of the otoliths to the calculation of linear displacement. J Neurophysiol 62, 247–263.

Israël I, Bronstein AM, Kanayama R, Faldon M, Gresty MA (1996) Visual and vestibular factors influencing vestibular "navigation." Exp Brain Res 112: 411–419.

Jones EG, Powell TPS (1970) An anatomical study of converging sensory pathways within the cerebral cortex of the monkey. Brain 93: 793–820.

Kawano K, Sasaki M, Yamashita M (1980) Vestibular input to visual tracking neurons in the posterior parietal association cortex of the monkey. Neurosci Letters 55–60.

Kawano K, Sasaki M, Yamashita M (1984) Response properties of neurons in posterior parietal cortex of monkey during visual-vestibular stimulation. I. Visual tracking neurons. J Neurophys 51: 340–351.

Kawano K, Shidara M, Watanabe Y, Yamane S (1994) Neural activity in cortical area MST of alert monkey during ocular following responses. J Neurophys 71: 2305–2324.

Kearns MJ, Warren WH, Duchon AP, Tarr MJ (2002) Path integration from optic flow and body senses in a homing task. Perception. 31: 349–374.

Klam F, Graf W (2003) Vestibular response kinematics in posterior parietal cortex neurons of macaque monkeys. Eur J Neurosci. 18: 995–1010.

Kleist K (1935) Uber Form und Orstsblindheit bei Verletzungen des Hinterhautlappens. Deutsch Z Nervenheilk 138: 206–214.

Komatsu H, Wurtz RH (1988a) Relation of cortical areas MT and MST to pursuit eye movements. I. Localization and visual properties of neurons. J Neurophys 60: 580–603.

Komatsu H, Wurtz RH (1988b) Relation of cortical areas MT and MST to pursuit eye movements. III. Interaction with full-field visual stimulation. J Neurophys 60: 621–644.

Kosel KC, Van H, Rosene DL (1982) Non-hippocampal cortical projections from the entorhinal cortex in the rat and rhesus monkey. Brain Res 244: 201–213.

Lambrey S, Viaud-Delmon I, Berthoz A. (2002) Influence of a sensorimotor conflict on the memorization of a path traveled in virtual reality. Cog Brain Res 14: 177–186.

Lavenex P, Suzuki WA, Amaral DG (2002) Perirhinal and parahippocampal cortices of the macaque monkey: projections to the neocortex. J Comp Neurol 447: 394–420.

Leichnetz GR (2001) Connections of the medial posterior parietal cortex (area 7m) in the monkey. Anat Rec 263: 215–236.

Longuet-Higgins HC, Prazdny K (1980) The interpretation of a moving retinal image. Proc R Soc Lond B 208: 385–397.

McNaughton BL, Barnes CA, O'Keefe J (1983) The contributions of position, directon, and velocity to single unit activity in the hippocampus of freely-moving rats. Exp Brain Res 52: 41–49.

McNaughton BL, Leonard B, Chen LL (1989) Cortical-hippocampal interactions and cognitive mapping: A hypothesis based on reintegration of the parietal and inferotemporal pathways for visual processing. Psychobiol 17: 230–235.

McNaughton BL, Mizumori SJY, Barnes CA, Leonard BJ, Marquis M, Green EJ (1994) Cortical representation of motion during unrestrained spatial navigation in the rat. Cereb Cortex 4: 27–39.

Mesulam MM, Van Hoesen GW, Pandya DN, Geschwind N (1977) Limbic and sensory connections of the inferior parietal lobule (area PG) in the rhesus monkey: a study with a new method for horseradish peroxidase histochemistry. Brain Res. 136(3): 393–414.

Morris R, Petrides M, Pandya DN (1999) Architecture and connections of retrosplenial area 30 in the rhesus monkey (Macaca mulatta). Eur J Neurosci 11: 2506–2518.

Motter BC, Mountcastle VB (1981) The functional properties of the light-sensitive neurons of the posterior parietal cortex Studies in waking monkeys: foveal sparing and opponent vector organization. J Neurosci 1: 3–26.

Motter BC, Steinmetz MA, Duffy CJ, Mountcastle VB (1987) Functional properties of parietal visual neurons: Mechanisms of directionality along a single axis. J Neurosci 7: 154–176.

Mountcastle VB (1976) The world around us: neural command functions for selective attention. The F. O. Schmitt Lecture in Neuroscience for 1975. Neurosci Res Progr Bull 14: 2–47.

Mufson EJ, Pandya DN (1984) Some observations on the course and composition of the cingulum bundle in the rhesus monkey. J Comp Neurol 225: 31–43.

Muller RU, Bostock E, Taube JS, Kubie JL (1994) On the directional firing properties of hippocampal place cells. J Neurosci 14: 7235–7251.

Nakamura K, Chung HH, Graziano MS, Gross CG (1999) Dynamic representation of eye position in the parieto-occipital sulcus. J Neurophys 81: 2374–2385.

Nakayama K, Loomis JM (1974) Optical velocity patterns, velocity-sensitive neurons, and space perception: a hypothesis. Perception 3: 63–80.

Nishijo H, Ono T, Eifuku S, Tamura R (1997) The relationship between monkey hippocampus place-related neural activity and action in space. Neurosci Lett 226: 57–60.

O'Keefe J, Dostrovsky J (1971) The hippocampus as a spatial map. Preliminary evidence from unit activity in the freely moving rat. Brain Res 34: 171–175.

O'Keefe J, Nadel L (1978) The Hippocampus as a Cognitive Map. Oxford: *Clarendon* Press.

Orban GA, Lagae L, Verri A, Raiguel S, Xiao D, Maes H, Torre V (1992) First-order analysis of optical flow in monkey brain. PNAS 89: 2595–2599.

Page WK, Duffy CJ (1999) MST neuronal responses to heading direction during pursuit eye movements. J Neurophys 81: 596–610.

Page WK, Duffy CJ (2003) Heading representation in MST: sensory interactions and population encoding. J Neurophys 89: 1994–2013.

Pandya DN, Van H, Mesulam MM (1981) Efferent connections of the cingulate gyrus in the rhesus monkey. Exp Brain Res 42: 319–330.

Papez JW (1937) A proposed mechanism of emotion. Archives of Neurology and Psychiatry 38: 725–743.

Pasik P, Pasik T (1972) Extrageniculostriate vision in the monkey. V. Role of accessory optic sytem. Brain Res 450–428.

Paterson A, Zangwill OL (1944) Disorders of visual space perception associated with lesions of the right cerebral hemisphere. Brain 67: 331–358.

Pavard B, Berthoz A (1977) Linear acceleration modifies the perceived velocity of a moving scene. Perception 6(5), 529–540.

Pouget A, Dayan P, Zemel R (2000) Information processing with population codes. [Review] Nature Revi Neurosci 1: 125–132.

Read HL, Siegel RM (1997) Modulation of responses to optic flow in area 7a by retinotopic and oculomotor cues in monkey. Cereb Cortex 7: 647–661.

Regan D, Vincent A (1995) Visual processing of looming and time to contact throughout the visual field. Vis Res 35: 1845–1857.

Robinson DL, Goldberg ME, Stanton GB (1978) Parietal association cortex in the primate: Sensory mechanisms and behavioral modulations. J Neurophys. 41: 910–932.

Rockland KS, Van Hoesen GW (1999) Some temporal and parietal cortical connections converge in CA1 of the primate hippocampus. Cerebral Cortex 9: 232–237.

Saito H, Yukie M, Tanaka K, Hikosaka K, Fukada Y, Iwai E (1986) Integration of direction signals of image motion in the superior temporal sulcus of the macaque monkey. J Neurosci 6: 145–157.

Sakata H, Shibutani H, Kawano K (1980) Spatial properties of visual fixation neurons in posterior parietal association cortex of the monkey. J Neurophysiol 43: 1654–1672.

Sanders MD, Warrington EK, Marshall J, Wieskrantz L (1974) "Blindsight": vision in a field defect. Lancet 7860: 707–708.

Schaafsma SJ, Duysens J (1996) Neurons in the ventral intraparietal area of awake macaque monkey closely resemble neurons in the dorsal part of the medial superior temporal area in their responses to optic flow. J Neurophysiol 76: 4056–4068.

Schlack A, Hoffmann KP, Bremmer F (2002) Interaction of linear vestibular and visual stimulation in the macaque ventral intraparietal area (VIP). Eur J Neurosci 16: 1877–1886.

Schwarz DWF, Fredrickson JM (1971) Rhesus Monkey vestibular cortex: A bimodal primary projection field. Science 172: 280–281.

Sereno MI, Dale AM, Reppas JB, Kwong KK, Belliveau JW, Brady TJ, Rosen BR, Tootell RBH (1995) Borders of multiple visual areas in humans revealed by functional magnetic resonance imaging. Science 268: 889–893.

Shenoy KV, Bradley DC, Andersen RA (1999) Influence of gaze rotation on the visual response of primate MSTd neurons. J Neurophys 81: 2764–2786.

Shenoy KV, Crowell JA, Andersen RA (2002) Pursuit speed compensation in cortical area MSTd. J Neurophys 88: 2630–2647.

Shipp S, deJong BM, Zihl J, Frackowaik RSJ, Zeki S (1994) The brain activity related to residual motion vision in a patient with bilateral lesions of V5. Brain 117: 1023–1038.

Siegel RM, Raffi M, Phinney RE, Turner JA, Jando G (2003) Functional architecture of eye position gain fields in visual association cortex of behaving monkey. J Neurophys 90: 1279–1294.

Siegel RM, Read HL (1997) Analysis of optic flow in the monkey parietal area 7a. Cereb Cortex 7: 327–346.

Snyder LH, Batista AP, Andersen RA (1998) Change in motor plan, without a change in spatial locus of attention, modulates activity in posterior parietal cortex. J Neurophysiol 79: 2814–2819.

Squatrito S, Maioli MG (1996) Gaze field properties of eye position neurones in areas MST and 7a of the macaque monkey. Vis Neurosci 13: 385–398.

Squatrito S, Maioli MG (1997) Encoding of smooth pursuit direction and eye position by neurons of area MSTd of macaque monkey. J Neurosci 17: 3847–3860.

Steinmetz MA, Motter BC, Duffy CJ, Mountcastle VB (1987) Functional properties of parietal visual neurons: Radial organization of directionalities within the visual field. J Neurosci 7: 177–191.

Sugishita M, Ettlinger G, Ridley RM (1978) Disturbance of cage-finding in the monkey. Cortex 14: 431–438.

Thier P, Erickson RG (1992) Vestibular input to visual-tracking neurons in area MST of awake rhesus monkeys. Ann NY Acad Sci 656: 960–963.

Tolman EC (1948) Cognitive maps in man and animals. Psychol Rev 55: 189–208.

Tootell RB, Taylor JB (1995) Anatomical evidence for MT and additional cortical visual areas in humans. Cereb Cortex 5: 39–55.

Tootell RBH, Reppas JB, Kwong KK, Malach R, Born RT, Brady TJ, Rosen BR, Belliveau JW (1995) Functional analysis of human MT and related visual cortical areas using magnetic resonance imaging. J Neurosci 15: 3215–3230.

Trevarthan C (1968) Two mechanisms of vision in primates. Psychol Forschung 31: 229–337.

Ungerleider LG, Brody BA (1997) Extrapersonal spatial orientation: The role of the posterior parietal, anterior frontal, and inferotemporal cortex. Exp Neurol 56: 265–280.

Ungerleider LG, Mishkin M (1982) Two cortical visual systems. In DJ Ingle, MA Goodale, and RJW Mansfield eds., Analysis of Visual Behavior. Cambridge, MA: MIT Press, 549–586.

Upadhyay UD, Page WK, Duffy CJ (2000) MST responses to pursuit across optic flow with motion parallax. J Neurophys 84: 818–826.

Van den Berg AV, Brenner E (1994) Humans combine the optic flow with static depth cues for robust perception of heading. Vis Res 34: 2153–2167.

Van Hoesen GW (1982) The parahippocampal gyrus: New observations regarding cortical connections in the monkey. Trends Neurosci 5: 345–350.

Ventre J, Faugier-Grimaud S (1988) Projections of the temporo-parietal cortex on vestibular complex in the macaque monkey (*Macaca fascicularis*). Exp Brain Res 72: 653–658.

Vogt BA, Finch DM, Olson CR (1992) Functional heterogeneity in cingulate cortex: the anterior executive and posterior evaluative regions. Cereb Cortex 2: 435–443.

Warren WH, Kay BA, Zosh WD, Duchon AP, Sahuc S (2001) Optic flow is used to control human walking. Nature Neurosci 4: 213–216.

Whishaw IQ, Maaswinkel H, Gonzalez CL, Kolb B (2001) Deficits in allothetic and idiothetic spatial behavior in rats with posterior cingulate cortex lesions. Behav Brain Res 118: 67–76.

Xing J, Andersen RA (2000) Models of the posterior parietal cortex which perform multimodal integration and represent space in several coordinate frames. J Cogn Neurosci 12: 601–614.

Yin TC, Mountcastle VB (1997) Visual input to the visuomotor mechanisms of the monkey's parietal lobe. Science 197: 1381–1383.

Zipser D, Andersen RA (1988) A back-propagation programmed network that simulates response properties of a subset of posterior parietal neurons. Nature 331: 679–684.

16 Vestibular, Proprioceptive, and Visual Influences on the Perception of Orientation and Self-Motion in Humans

Isabelle Israël and William H. Warren

As people move about, they perceive changes in their orientation and position in the environment, and can update these values with respect to significant locations in space. Analytically, self-motion can be decomposed into two components: (1) observer rotation, which has a direction (pitch, yaw, roll), an angular speed, and a total angular displacement; and (2) observer translation, which also has a direction of motion (or heading), a linear speed, and a total linear displacement. However, the problem of perceiving self-rotation and translation is complicated by the fact that the human form is not a rigid body, but a hierarchy of segments consisting of mobile eyes in a mobile head on a mobile trunk on a pair of legs.

To determine the attitude and motion of each segment, a family of perceptual systems comes into play. The orientation of the eye in the head may be determined from extraretinal signals such as efference to or proprioception from the extraocular muscles. The motion of the head in three-dimensional-space can be determined via the vestibular organs, including semicircular canals sensitive to angular acceleration and otoliths sensitive to linear acceleration, including gravity. Temporal integration of these signals can yield information about head velocity and displacement. The orientation of the head on the trunk is specified by neck proprioception, and the trunk's position and motion with respect to the ground by podokinetic or substratal information, a compound of proprioceptive and efferent signals from the legs and feet. In principle, these body-based senses allow for a chain of coordinate transformations between reference frames for each segment, but as we will show, they appear to be relied upon in a task-specific manner. Finally, the visual system may detect rotation and translation of the eye with respect to environmental objects on the basis of optic flow or the displacements of landmarks, bypassing such coordinate transformations.

In the present chapter, we review psychophysical and behavioral evidence regarding the perception of rotation and orientation, briefly describe the perception of translation and heading, and discuss the combination of the two in path integration.

Perceiving Rotation and Orientation

Vestibular and Proprioceptive Systems

The semicircular canals are the only sensors that are stimulated specifically and exclusively by angular head motion, so it can be claimed that they are dedicated to the detection of self-rotation. Indeed the vestibulo-ocular reflex (VOR) works properly only when the semicircular canals and the corresponding neural networks are intact. However, there is no conscious percept of vestibular stimulation, and we become aware of this sense only when we experience motion sickness, inner ear pathology, or postrotatory sensations. On the other hand, the semicircular canals are never stimulated in isolation, leading many researchers to investigate vestibular interactions with other senses and the multisensory perception of self-motion.

The perception of self-rotation from vestibular and proprioceptive information has been investigated psychophysically using estimates of either angular velocity or angular displacement. The latter has been achieved by obtaining retrospective estimates of the total angular displacement after a rotation—or concurrent estimates of one's change in orientation during a rotation—which we will describe in turn. Studies of vestibular thresholds for rotational velocity and acceleration have also been performed, but will not be reviewed here (see Benson et al., 1989; Benson and Brown, 1989).

Retrospective Estimates of Angular Displacement   One method for testing the vestibular perception of angular displacement is by comparing it with the performance of the vestibulor-ocular reflex (VOR). When a normal human subject is briefly turned in total darkness while trying to fixate a target in space, the VOR produces slow-phase compensatory eye movements that tend to hold the eyes on target. While this response is generally too weak for accurate compensation, it seems to be corrected by supplementary saccades in the compensatory direction (Segal and Katsarkas, 1988), even in the dark (VOR + saccade). To measure the perceived angular displacement, a retrospective estimate can be obtained using the vestibular memory–contingent saccade (VMCS) paradigm (Bloomberg et al., 1988), in which, after a brief passive whole-body rotation in the dark, the participant must saccade to a previously seen target based on a vestibular estimate of the total rotation. Bloomberg et al. (1991) found that the VMCS response measured after rotation was indeed indistinguishable from the combined VOR + saccade response measured during rotation, even when the latter was adaptively modified by prolonged visual-vestibular conflict (Bloomberg et al., 1991a). Israël et al. (1991) repeated the VMCS paradigm with different delays between the end of body rotation and the saccade. They found that vestibular information about the rotation amplitude can be stored without significant distortion for 1 min, longer than the time constant of the semicircular canals. The retrospective performance thus probably involves storing an estimate of the angular displacement in spatial memory.

Israël et al. (1993) compared these two measures during yaw and pitch rotations. They found, first, a strong correlation between VMCS + saccade and the VOR responses, with a slightly greater accuracy in the former (figure 16.1). The finding that a concurrent response (VOR) is less accurate than a retrospective one (VMCS) is well known in subjective magnitude estimation (Young, 1984), and it is classically attributed to the concurrent task that is interfering with the perception being estimated (Guedry, 1974; Stevens, 1960). Second, a greater accuracy was observed with yaw than with pitch rotation, consistent with thresholds for angular motion perception (Clark and Stewart, 1970), despite the fact the imposed rotations were well above threshold. Third, there was an unexplained greater accuracy for rotations that did not stimulate the otoliths.

The perception of angular displacement from neck proprioception has been investigated in a paradigm similar to VMCS. Nakamura and Bronstein (1993) assessed the perception of trunk rotation about a stationary (earth-fixed) head by having participants make eye saccades in the direction of trunk orientation. Normal subjects could accurately identify trunk orientation independent of trunk velocity and total displacement. The authors concluded that trunk orientation is perceived veridically and that neck-spinal afferents carry a tonic signal that is accessible by the ocular motor system. Mergner et al. (1998) had participants saccade to a previously seen target following passive rotations of the head and/or trunk. Saccades based on vestibular input from full-body rotation fell short at low

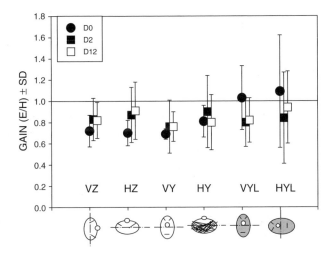

Figure 16.1
VOR and VMCS for rotations on the Z (body vertical) and Y (interaural) axes. The gain is the ratio of the eye saccades amplitude (E) over the head rotation angle (H). D0, VOR; D2, delay of 2 s before the saccade (in the VMCS); D12, delay of 12 s; V, subject's head in the vertical plane before the rotation; H, in the horizontal plane; Z, Y, rotation axes; L, low acceleration (gray pictograms). The only trials without otoliths stimulation are those at the left (VZ) and right (HYL) extremities. (Adapted from Israël et al., 1993, with permission.)

stimulus frequencies, but the addition of neck proprioception, produced by passive rotation of the head on an earth-fixed trunk, improved response accuracy.

It is well known that the prefrontal cortex (PFC) plays a primary role in visual spatial memory (Funahashi et al., 1993). To determine whether this role extends to vestibular spatial memory, Israël et al. (1995) recorded VMCS (as well as visual memory-guided saccades) in patients with various cortical lesions. It was found that (1) the PFC is involved in the memorization of saccade goals encoded in spatiotopic (absolute spatial) coordinates, whether stimuli are visual or vestibular, (2) the supplementary eye field but not the frontal eye field is involved in the control of the vestibular-derived, goal-directed saccades, and (3) the parietotemporal cortex (i.e., the vestibular cortex) but not the posterior parietal cortex is involved in the control of such saccades. Therefore it was concluded, first, that the role of the PFC includes both visual and vestibular spatial memory, and second that two different cortical networks are respectively involved in the latter and in the control of memory-guided saccades made to visual targets. These networks have only the PFC in common, which could control VMCS. This provides a physiological basis for distinguishing the cognitive processing of ego- and exocentric space.

However, in the classical VMCS paradigm the initially viewed target is directly in front of the subject, so that the expected saccade is a simple reproduction of the head or body rotation in the reverse direction. It was subsequently found that the saccade accuracy greatly decreases when the target is eccentric rather than straight ahead (Blouin et al., 1995, 1995a, 1997, 1998, 1998a). The data suggest that these errors stem not only from an underestimation of rotation magnitude, but also from an inability to use passive vestibular signals to update an internal representation of the target position relative to the body. Neck proprioception is more effective in this task.

Intrigued by this result, Israël et al. (1999) studied memory-guided saccades in three conditions: visual-memory guided saccades (the visual target was at 10° or 20°, right or left), saccades to the remembered spatiotopic position of the same visual target after whole-body rotation, and saccades to the remembered retinotopic position of the visual target after whole-body rotation. Visual feedback presented after each trial allowed eye position correction, as in Bloomberg et al.'s experiments. The results extend those of Blouin et al., and indicate that vestibular information contributes to updating the spatial representation of target position when visual feedback is provided.

Extending such target manipulations, Mergner et al. (2001) thoroughly examined the interactions between visual, oculomotor, vestibular, and proprioceptive signals for updating the location of visual targets in space after intervening eye, head, or trunk movements. They presented subjects in the dark with a target at various horizontal eccentricities, and after a delay in darkness asked them to point a light spot (with a joystick) to the remembered target location. In the "visual-only" condition, pointing accuracy was close to ideal (the slope of the estimation curve was close to unity). In the "visual-vestibular" condition, subjects were rotated during the delay; after a 0.8 Hz (28.8°/s) rotation, pointing was close to ideal, but after a 0.1 Hz (3.6°/s) rotation, the slopes of the estimation curves were below unity, indicating underestimation of body rotation (figure 16.2). The eccentricity of the target further reduced the slopes. In the "visual-vestibular-neck" condition, different combinations of vestibular and neck stimuli were administered during the delay (head fixed on the rotating body, head fixed in space on the rotating body, and synergistic and antagonistic vestibular-neck combinations). As long as these rotations were fast (0.8 Hz), the mean accuracy was close to ideal, but with 0.1 Hz rotations of the trunk about a stationary head, a shift toward the trunk occurred (i.e., the slope decreased), whereas head rotation on the stationary trunk yielded slopes close to unity irrespective of the frequency, suggesting that the effects summed and the errors cancelled each other. Variability of the responses was always lowest for targets presented straight-ahead. The authors concluded that, (1) subjects referenced "space" to prerotatory straight-ahead, and (2) they used internal estimates of eye, head, and trunk displacements with respect to space to match current target position with its remembered position—in effect inverting the physical coordinate transformations produced by the displacements. While Mergner et al. (2001) developed a descriptive model of human orientation in space, they specifically admitted that the model could not reproduce the drop in performance with eccentric targets found by Blouin et al., which was partly attributed to the low frequency components of Blouin's vestibular stimulation.

Estimates of angular displacement and angular velocity have been used interchangeably to characterize vestibular perception of self-rotation, on the assumption that the two estimates are equivalent because perceived displacement is simply the time integral of perceived velocity. Mergner et al. (1996) tested this hypothesis by directly comparing displacement and velocity estimates. Participants were presented with whole-body yaw rotations in the dark, with one group estimating peak velocity and the other group estimating total displacement. Experimenters then used the velocity estimates to predict the displacement estimates by assuming that the velocity signal decayed exponentially from the reported peak value (reflecting the dynamics of vestibular mechanisms) and mathematically integrating it. Predicted and reported displacements were similar for a time constant of 20 s, in good agreement with earlier studies. The authors concluded that displacement estimates can indeed be considered equivalent to velocity estimates of self-rotation over the range of stimulus parameters tested.

However, Becker et al. (2000) found that the vestibular perception of angular velocity and displacement are differentially affected by seated or standing posture. Sinusoidal rotations in the horizontal plane were delivered to subjects sitting in a rotating chair or standing on a rotating platform, and judgments were obtained by retrospective magnitude estimation. While displacement estimates did not depend on posture, velocity estimates were more accurate for sitting than for standing, particularly with large amplitude stimuli. Posture had no effect upon the vestibular detection threshold. This demonstrates that perceived displacement does not always equal the time integral of perceived velocity. In addition, the persistence of nearly veridical displacement estimates at constant velocities

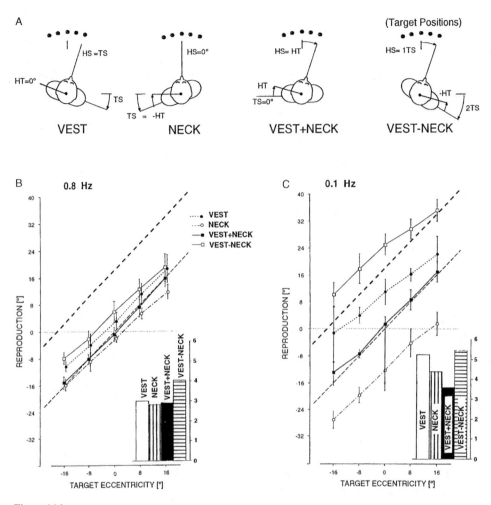

Figure 16.2
Visual-vestibular-neck interactions in delayed pointing after passive rotation. Superimposed in each panel are the results for the four stimulus combinations: VEST (solid circles), NECK (open circles), VEST + NECK (solid squares), and VEST-NECK (open squares). Thin dashed 45° lines, "ideal" performance. Heavy dashed 45° lines, hypothetical performance of subjects with absent vestibular function (applies only to VEST). (A) Pictographic representation of the four vestibular-neck stimulus combinations used (view of subject from above). (B) Stimuli of 18° at 0.8 Hz. (C) Stimuli of 18° at 0.1 Hz. Note that the estimation curves for VEST + NECK fall very close to the ideal 45° lines, both at 0.8 Hz and 0.1 Hz, while those for VEST-NECK show the largest offset from these lines. Insets give across-trials standard deviation (in degrees) for the four stimulus combinations (averaged across all target eccentricities). (VEST, whole-body rotation (the orientation of the head-in-space, HS, equals that of trunk-in-space, TS). NECK; trunk rotation with head kept stationary (stimulus, head-to-trunk, HT). VEST + NECK, head rotation on stationary trunk. VEST-NECK, head and trunk rotation in space in same direction, but trunk with double amplitude to maintain HT constant). (Adapted from figure 4 of Mergner et al., 2001, with permission.)

over extended durations (when vestibular signals have stopped) suggests the intervention of cognitive processes.

Concurrent Perception of Angular Displacement   When investigating multisensory self-motion perception, the kinematics of motion and response characteristics of the different sensory channels should also be taken into account. This is why concurrent self-rotation perception tests are also frequently used.

As we have noted earlier, in order to determine trunk motion in space, the vestibular signal of head motion in space must be combined with neck proprioception about the trunk-to-head excursion. Mergner et al. (1991) studied the vestibular-neck interaction with a concurrent tracking task, in which the subjects manipulated both a head-pointer and a trunk-pointer to indicate their perceived rotation during passive sinusoidal yaw rotations of the trunk and/or head in the dark. For the perception of trunk rotation in space, rotation was underestimated with vestibular stimulation alone (whole-body rotation) and with neck stimulation alone (trunk rotation under an earth-fixed head). The gains were low, only about 0.7 at 0.4 Hz and decreasing at lower frequencies. Judgments were similarly erroneous for other vestibular-neck combinations, with one noticeable exception: during head rotation on a stationary trunk, subjects veridically perceived the trunk as stationary. For the perception of head rotation in space, vestibular stimulation yielded the same frequency characteristics as for the trunk. Neck stimulation (trunk rotation under a stationary head) induced an illusion of the head rotating in space, but with head rotation on a stationary trunk, perception became almost veridical. The neck contribution reflected the sum of two components: the nonideal neck signal that contributed to the perception of "trunk in space," and the nearly ideal neck signal produced by head rotation on a stationary trunk.

Mergner et al. (1993) investigated the interaction of vestibular signals and leg proprioception in seated subjects. Stimulation consisted of sinusoidal and transient whole-body rotations in space (vestibular stimulation) and rotations of the feet relative to the trunk, induced by a moving platform (leg proprioception). Responses were obtained with a pointing procedure similar to that described above, in which the subject manipulated both a feet-pointer and a trunk-pointer. First, the perception of relative motion between feet and trunk was veridical across the frequencies tested and had a low detection threshold (0.2°/s). Rotation of the feet under the stationary trunk evoked an illusion of trunk turning, which reached a considerable magnitude at low frequencies. Second, the perception of trunk rotation from vestibular stimulation was underestimated, especially at low frequencies, with a detection threshold close to 1.0°/s. Third, with combinations of vestibular stimulation and leg proprioception, perception varied monotonically as a function of both inputs. Rotation was underestimated except during trunk rotation about stationary feet, when it was approximately veridical and the threshold dropped to 0.2°/s, suggesting that it was essentially determined by leg proprioception.

To elucidate the role of the "starting point" in perceiving angular displacement, Israël et al. (1996) passively rotated subjects on a motor-driven turntable. Subjects then had to return to the starting point by using a joystick to control the direction and velocity of the turntable in total darkness. The starting point could be defined prior to rotation by an earth-fixed, visual target, or given by the initial body orientation. Subjects succeeded in returning to the starting point in all conditions, but had lower variability when the target was visually presented. The larger scatter in the other conditions was directly related to variations in the peak return velocity, whereas there was no relationship between return amplitude and velocity with the visual target. These results suggest that visual presentation of an earth-fixed starting point facilitates real time integration, improving accuracy during self-controlled motion in the dark.

A related observation was reported by Israël et al. (1995a), who instructed subjects to use push buttons to rotate the turntable through angles of ±90°, 180°, or 360° (outward), and then to rotate back to the initial position (return), in complete darkness. On average, participants undershot the specified angle on the outward rotation, but the variability was lower on the return rotation. (No corrective rotation was imposed prior to the return.) The data suggest that subjects maintained an internal representation of the starting point (the initial body orientation), which served as a clearer goal (for the return) than did a specified rotation angle (for the outward rotation), in an environment devoid of any spatial reference.

Yardley et al. (1998, 1999) sought to determine whether significant attentional resources are required to monitor vestibular information for changes in body orientation. To provide interference, participants either counted backwards during rotation (Yardley et al., 1998) or performed a dual-task paradigm (Yardley et al., 1999). The results indicate that a small but significant degree of attention or cognitive effort is necessary to accurately monitor the direction and amplitude of self-rotation, during both passive and active locomotion.

To investigate the role of gaze stabilization during the control of whole-body rotation, Siegler and Israël (2002) tested subjects seated on a mobile robot that they could control with a joystick. They were asked to perform 360° rotations in the dark while maintaining their gaze, when possible, on the position of a visible (at the beginning of the rotation) or imagined (after about 110° rotation) earth-fixed target. This required active head rotations. Subjects performed better on a 360° whole-body rotation in the dark when asked to stabilize gaze in space than when no specific instruction was given. Furthermore, performance was significantly related to head stabilization in space. These results revealed the importance of head-free gaze control for spatial orientation, insofar as it involves spatial reference cues and sensory signals of different modalities, including efferent copy and neck proprioceptive signals. The benefits of free head movements amply confirm the findings of Mergner et al. (1991; 2001) about the role of neck proprioception on self-rotation estimate.

When subjects actively step about the vertical axis without vision, there are two sources of information about the angular displacement: the vestibular signal and the podokinetic or substratal signals. To investigate the podokinetic contribution, Jürgens et al. (1999) had participants either stand passively on a rotating platform (vestibular) or actively step about their vertical axis on a stationary platform (podokinetic and vestibular). Rotations consisted of short acceleration epochs followed by constant velocity periods, which participants had also learned to produce when actively turning. Perceived displacement was either verbally estimated or indicated by stopping when a specified displacement had been reached. The results showed that perception of angular displacement is more precise during active turning (see also Yardley et al., 1998), and that the intention to achieve a specified displacement modifies the perception of passive rotation but not that of active turning.

Becker et al. (2002) investigated how vestibular and podokinetic signals are fused in the perception of angular displacement. They compared three conditions: (1) passive rotation, standing at the center of a rotating platform (vestibular only); (2) treadmill stepping opposite to the rotating platform, so that the body remained fixed in space (podokinetic only); and (3) active turning, stepping around the stationary platform (vestibular and podokinetic). Angular velocity varied across trials (15–60°/s) but was constant within a trial. Participants signaled when they thought they had reached a previously specified angular displacement, ranging from 60° to 1080°. The error was smaller during active turning than during passive rotation and treadmill stepping. The authors found this to be compatible with the idea that vestibular and podokinetic signals are averaged, but only for the case of fast rotation. Finally, participants could estimate large angular displacements surprisingly well during passive rotation, even though the duration of motion far exceeded the conventional vestibular time constant of 20 s. This indicates that the initial velocity estimate based on the vestibular signal can be maintained long after the signal itself has decayed (a result similar to that found by Becker et al., 2000).

Mittelstaedt and Mittelstaedt (1996) and Mittelstaedt (1995) also investigated the perception of angular displacement over long time intervals. Participants were positioned in darkness face forward or backward on a rotating platform, at radial distances of $r = 0$–1.6 m, and accelerated to a constant angular velocity ($w = 0.35$–0.87 rad/s or 20–50°/s) within 0.8 s. They successively indicated when they felt they had turned through another 180°. Fairly veridical at first, these reports lagged progressively as though perceived velocity declined exponentially to zero. When $r = 0$, the data revealed idiosyncratic time constants (20–90 s) that were independent of disk velocity, confirming the results of Becker et al. (2002) for passive rotation. But at other radial distances the time constants increased with $r*w$, and hence depended on centrifugal force. After at least 2 min, the rotation was stopped and participants continued to indicate 180° turns at successive intervals as before. The deceleration force induced a postrotatory aftereffect with time constants that were independent of radius and disk velocity, as would be expected if the prolonged time constants during rotation were due to the added orthogonal (centrifugal) force.

Illusions Multisensory illusions have also been used as tools to increase our understanding of the mechanisms of self-motion perception.

Gordon et al. (1995) and Weber et al. (1998) exposed participants to between 30 min and 2 h of walking on the perimeter of a rotating platform, such that the body remained fixed in space. After adaptation, participants were blindfolded and asked to walk straight ahead on firm ground. However they generated walking trajectories that were curved, and continued to do so, with gradually decreasing curvature, over the next half hour (figure 16.3). The angular velocities associated with these trajectories were well above vestibular threshold, yet all participants consistently perceived themselves as walking straight ahead. On the other hand, when the blindfolded participants were asked to propel themselves in a straight line in a wheelchair, postadaptation trajectories showed no change from before adaptation. Thus, sensory-motor adaptation appears to have been limited to the podokinetic components of gait. Such findings may have implications for the diagnosis and rehabilitation of locomotor and vestibular disorders.

Jürgens et al. (1999a) asked whether this podokinetic after-rotation (PKAR) is due to (1) an intersensory recalibration triggered by the conflict between the visual signal of stationarity and the somatosensory signal of feet-on-platform rotation, or (2) an adaptation of the somatosensory afferents to prolonged unilateral stimulation, irrespective of the visual stimulation. Participants turned about their vertical axis for 10 min on a stationary or a counterrotating platform (so they remained fixed in space), under visual conditions of either darkness, optokinetic stimulation consistent with body rotation, or a head-fixed optical pattern consistent with no rotation. After adaptation, they tried to step in place on a stationary platform without turning, while in darkness. All adaptation conditions that included active stepping without optokinetic stimulation yielded the PKAR effect. With consistent optokinetic stimulation during adaptation, PKAR increased, indicative of an optically induced afterrotation (oPKAR) that summed with the standard PKAR. This oPKAR could also be demonstrated in isolation, by passively rotating subjects in front of the optokinetic pattern, yielding an afterrotation in the contralateral direction. Not unexpectedly, when the optokinetic pattern was illuminated, the PKAR was rapidly and totally suppressed because subjects could control a straight course on the basis of visual information. Surprisingly, however, when darkness was restored, PKAR smoothly resumed, and within about 1 min appeared to continue the course it had been following prior to illumination. This report therefore extends the previous observations by showing: (1) that PKAR follows any situation involving prolonged unilateral podokinetic circling, (2) that it cannot be "discharged" by brief periods of straight stepping under visual control, and (3) that a second type of oPKAR is induced by optokinetic stimulation. The authors concluded that PKAR does not result from an adaptation to sensory conflict, but occurs because the somatosensory flow of information partially habituates to long-lasting unilateral stimulation, so that asymmetrical stimulation is taken to correspond to straight stepping.

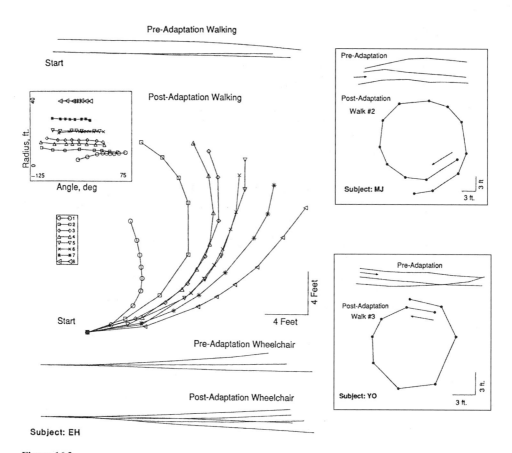

Figure 16.3
Adaptation to 2 h walking on the perimeter of a rotating disc. Locomotor trajectories of three subjects. Top lines show the trajectories of pre-adaptation attempts at walking "straight ahead" with eyes blindfolded. Representative of all subjects, roughly straight trajectories were achieved. In marked contrast, the central set of curved lines and data points shows a complete set of post-adaptation trajectories for subject EH. The actual starting points of trials were in different locations of the room, but for the purpose of illustration they are superimposed. The top left inset plots calculated radial distances of individual points on a given curve from the calculated "best center" of curvature, against angular deviation of these radii from that of the starting point. The close approximation to straight horizontal lines indicates the constancy of trajectory curvature. The progressive increase of average radius from one trajectory to the next illustrates the trend of readaptation to normal conditions. Bottom lines reproduce trajectories of straight line attempts in the self-propelled wheelchair pre- and postadaptation. Characteristically, there were no significant postadaptation changes in these trajectories. Selected postadaptation trajectories from two additional subjects are shown on the right side, exemplifying attempts which could not be completed due to approaching physical obstructions. (Adapted from figure 1 in Gordon et al., 1995, with permission.)

Many studies have investigated whether the self-movement signals that serve to stabilize gaze are also sent upstream to inform perceptual systems. Howard et al. (1998) measured postrotatory ocular nystagmus and sensations of body rotation in standing subjects after 3 min of adaptation in the following conditions, all in the dark: (1) passive rotation about the vertical axis (vestibular only), (2) active turning (vestibular and podokinetic), and (3) stepping about the vertical axis on a counterrotating platform, so body orientation remained fixed in space (podokinetic only). Following passive rotation, slow phase postrotatory nystagmus occurred in the same direction as the rotation (i.e., sensations of self-rotation were opposite to the direction of previous movement), and after active turning it was reduced in velocity. Surprisingly, after stepping in the absence of body rotation, nystagmus also appeared and was in the opposite direction of intended turning, an effect known as the antisomatogyral illusion. Rieser et al. (1995) also showed that humans rapidly adjust the calibration of their motor actions to changing circumstances. Siegler et al. (2000) examined whether postrotatory effects alter the perception of self-motion and eye movements during a subsequent rotation. Blindfolded participants seated on a mobile robot first experienced a passive whole-body rotation about the vertical axis, and then reproduced the displacement angle by controlling the robot with a joystick. The reproduction began either immediately after the passive rotation (no delay), or after the subjective postrotatory sensations had ended (free delay). Participants accurately reproduced the displacement angles in both conditions, though they did not reproduce the stimulus dynamics. The peak velocities produced after no delay were higher than those after the free delay, suggesting that postrotatory effects biased the perception of angular velocity in the no-delay condition. Postrotatory nystagmus did not reflect the postrotatory sensations, consistent with the results of Mittelstaedt and Jensen (1999) for 2D rotations.

DiZio et al. (1987a, 1987b) sought to determine whether gravitoinertial force magnitude influences oculomotor and perceptual responses to coriolis, cross-coupled stimulation (making head movements about an axis other than that of rotation elicits a complex pattern of stimulation of the vestibular system known as coriolis, cross-coupled stimulation). During the free-fall and high-force phases of parabolic flight, blindfolded participants were passively rotated about the yaw axis at constant velocity while they made standardized head movements. The characteristics of horizontal nystagmus and the magnitude of experienced self-motion were measured. Both responses were less intense during the free-fall periods than during the high force periods. Although the slow phase velocity of nystagmus reached the same initial peak level in both force conditions, it decayed more quickly in zero G during free fall. These findings demonstrate that the response to semicircular canal stimulation depends on the background level of gravitoinertial force.

During natural movements, visual and vestibular information are complementary. Cue conflict experiments help to understand the relative importance of these signals and how they are combined. As illusions, sensory conflicts have been used as tools to help understanding the mechanics of self-motion perception. The vestibular-ocular reflex (VOR) and perception of angular displacement were compared by Ivanenko et al. (1998) before and after adaptation to inconsistent visual-vestibular stimulation. During adaptation, participants were exposed to 45 min of repeated passive whole-body rotations of 180°, combined with visual rotations of only 90° in a virtual reality display of a room. In postadaptation tests in the dark, large inter-individual variability was observed for both the VOR gain and estimates of angular displacement. The individual VOR gains were not correlated with perceived angles of rotation either before or after adaptation. Postadaptation estimates of angular displacement decreased by 24% when compared with preadaptation estimates, while the VOR gain did not change significantly. These results show that adaptive plasticity in VOR and in self-rotation perception may be independent of one another.

With two participants who had demonstrated a great capacity for adaptation in this last experiment (symmetrical visual-vestibular stimulation), Viaud-Delmon et al. (1999) examined adaptation to asymmetrical incoherent visual-vestibular stimulation. The authors sought to obtain separate (and different) adaptation to right and left stimulations. The test was similar to that mentioned earlier, but to achieve a 90° rotation in the virtual room the subject had to be rotated by 180° to the right, or by 90° to the left. Strikingly, after 45 min of asymmetrical left-right stimulation, perception of angular displacement in dark decreased equally for rotations to the right and to the left. This finding indicates that the calibration of vestibular input for spatial orientation did not undergo a directionally specific control.

In this section we have seen that the vestibular contribution to perceived rotation is accurate only in the simplest situations: when the head is rotated on the stationary upright trunk, with no distracting visual targets and no trunk or leg movements. However, in more complex situations estimates are much better when the vestibular system works in concert with the proprioceptive system. These sensory systems are typically coactivated, both on earth and in weightlessness, and they display a similar frequency dependence under rotation. Both convey only internal idiothetic information, and are thus susceptible to illusions, i.e., erroneous interpretations of the motion of the mobile segments of the head, trunk, and legs hierarchy. Vestibular and proprioceptive contributions to spatial orientation are thus highly sensitive to other influences from the visual, motor, and cognitive systems.

Visual System

A rotation of the observer's eye in a visible environment generates a global pattern of motion on the retina, known as the rotational component of retinal flow. Specifically, yaw or pitch produces a parallel lamellar flow pattern (see figure 16.4b), whereas roll about the line of sight produces a rotary flow pattern. The direction of flow is opposite the direction of observer rotation, and its angular velocity is equivalent to the observer's rotation rate, independent of environmental depth. Thus, the observer's rotation in a stationary

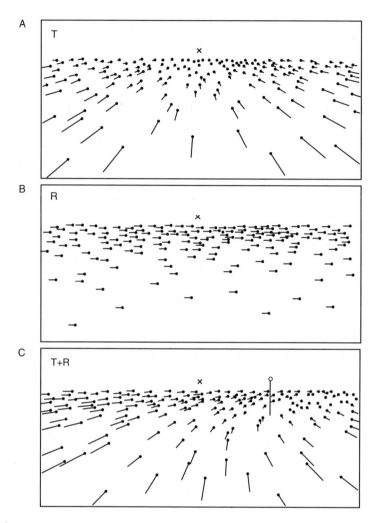

Figure 16.4
The instantaneous retinal velocity field for self-motion over a ground plane. Each vector represents the retinal velocity of a point on the ground plane, where the point is the tail of the vector. (A) Translational component: radial flow field produced by observer translation toward the "X," parallel to the ground plane. "X" denotes the focus of expansion. (B) Rotational component: lamellar flow field produced by observer rotation to the right about a vertical axis. (C) Rotation and translation: flow field produced by translation toward the "X" while rotating about a vertical axis to fixate the "O", which is attached to the ground plane. This field is the vector sum of (A) and (B). Note that the same velocity field can be produced by travel on a circular path.

environment is fully specified by the retinal flow. Here we focus on yaw rotation about a vertical axis, because it is most relevant to spatial orientation in terrestrial animals.

Circular Vection and Angular Velocity   Consistent with the facts of optic flow, a large-field display of lamellar motion, such as that produced by a cylindrical drum rotating about a stationary observer at a constant velocity, can induce a strong sensation of self-rotation in the opposite direction known as circular vection. The latency for the onset of circular vection (CV) is typically about 2–3 s (Brandt et al., 1973), whereas complete vection, in which the rotating drum appears stationary and all motion is attributed to self-rotation, is often not achieved until 8–12 s. Presumably, the latency is due to a conflict between optic flow and the absence of vestibular stimulation at the onset of drum rotation, which indicates that no angular acceleration occurred; complete vection might then be achieved only after a delay related to the vestibular time constant, the duration ordinarily required for the canals to stabilize after acceleration to a constant velocity and the vestibular signal to decay. The delay is reduced by simultaneous vestibular stimulation, either smooth or impulsive acceleration of the observer platform in a direction opposite the visual motion (Brandt et al., 1974). This finding suggests that brief vestibular stimulation is sufficient to specify angular acceleration at the onset of self-rotation, which can then be sustained by constant-velocity optic flow. Conversely, platform acceleration in the same direction as visual motion eliminates vection (Young et al., 1973), even though the subject is actually rotating! Thus, the two sources of information can cancel each other. The delay to achieve complete vection also depends on the initial optical acceleration of the rotating drum. With accelerations below $5°/s^2$ vection is complete at onset, whereas at higher visual accelerations there is an increasing delay (Melcher and Henn, 1981). Such findings are consistent with the view that the optokinetic response has low-pass characteristics and is sensitive to constant-velocity stimulation, whereas the vestibular signal has high-pass characteristics and is sensitive to acceleration or initial velocity, but not to sustained velocity, with a time constant of around 20 s (Young, 1981; Howard, 1986).

The perceived speed of circular vection corresponds closely to that of the visual display over a wide range of speeds, consistent with the fact that the optic flow rate specifies the speed of self-rotation. This relationship is linear up to a saturation velocity of about 120°/s, whereupon perceived speed levels off (Brandt et al., 1973). Surprisingly, Wist et al. (1975) reported that perceived speed increases with the perceived distance of the display, despite the fact that angular velocities do not vary with distance. They suggest that yaw rotation may be partially interpreted as lateral translation, for which the speed of self-motion does increase with distance, due to the similarity of their corresponding flow patterns. As the rotating drum is accelerated, Melcher and Henn (1981) found that perceived speed closely tracks the visual velocity at low accelerations ($\leq 2°/s^2$), but it initially lags the display at high accelerations ($10°/s^2$). Conversely, with vestibular stimulation provided by a rotating chair in darkness, perceived speed corresponds to the actual speed at high accelerations, but increasingly underestimates the actual velocity at lower accelerations. With a rotating chair in the light, however, perceived and actual speeds are linearly related with a gain near 1 up to 60°/s at all accelerations tested. This result again reflects the complementary frequency responses of the visual and vestibular systems, such that their combined performance yields accurate estimates over a wide range.

Restricting the field of view in such experiments has shown that a smaller visual angle of stimulation reduces the subjective strength and perceived speed of both circular and roll vection (Brandt et al., 1973; Held et al., 1975; Allison et al., 1999). This finding is consistent with Gibson's (1950) observation that a global transformation of the optic array corresponds to self-motion, whereas local transformations tend to correspond to the motion of objects. However, vection can also be induced with small fields of view, less than 15° in diameter (Andersen and Braunstein, 1985; Howard and Heckmann, 1989). A case in point is the train illusion, in which an observer looking out the window of a stationary train experiences self-motion when the train on the adjacent track begins to move. Note that, in this case, the motion is produced by a more distant surface within a small, bounded region of the array.

Subsequent research has found that such foreground-background relationships have a strong influence on vection. Self-motion generally occurs within a stationary environmental frame of reference, and thus generates optic flow from background surfaces. In contrast, moving objects generally move in front of a stationary environmental background (Gibson, 1968). Brandt et al. (1975) originally reported that presenting stationary bars in front of a moving pattern had little effect on circular vection, but greatly reduced vection when they were perceived as being in the background. This result was confirmed by Ohmi et al. (1987), who monocularly presented two layers of dots moving in opposite directions, which spontaneously reversed their order in depth. The pattern that was perceived to be in the background determined the direction of circular vection. Howard and Heckmann (1989) tested a central display that was either nearer or farther than a surround display, as specified by binocular disparity. They concluded that the effect of motion is greater when it is in the background than the foreground, and that both visual field size and depth order influence vection. Note that Zugaro et al. (2001) similarly observed that background cues preferentially anchor head direction cells (see chapter 4). It has also been observed that the presence of a stationary foreground enhances the vection produced by a moving background (Howard and Howard, 1994; Nakamura and Shimojo, 1999). This is likely due to relative motion with the foreground increasing the perceived speed of the background, thereby enhancing vection.

It was originally believed that the retinal locus of stimulation also influenced vection; specifically, that the periphery dominated the perception of self-motion, whereas central vision dominated the perception of object motion (Brandt et al., 1973; Dichgans and Brandt, 1978). However, it has subsequently been shown that both circular and linear vection can be induced in central vision, and that there are no differences in the subjective strength or perceived speed of circular vection once central and peripheral stimulation are equated for area (Andersen and Braunstein, 1985; Post, 1988; Howard and Heckmann, 1989).

To investigate how visual and vestibular signals are combined, Mergner et al. (2000) obtained verbal estimates and pointer indications of perceived self-rotation in three viewing conditions. Subjects were presented with sinusoidal yaw rotations of an optokinetic pattern alone or in combination with rotations of a Barany chair. With pure optokinetic stimulation, specific instructions yielded different perceptual states: (1) when normal subjects were primed with induced motion (i.e., the illusory motion of a stationary target, opposite to the direction of the real motion of the inducing stimulus; thus normal subjects were primed with a stationary target superimposed upon the optokinetic moving display), the gain of circular vection was close to unity up to frequencies of 0.8 Hz, followed by a sharp decrease at higher frequencies; (2) when they were instructed to "stare through" the optokinetic pattern into far space, CV was absent at higher frequencies, but increasingly developed below 0.1 Hz; and (3) when they tracked the moving pattern with eye movements, vection was usually absent. In patients with loss of vestibular function, vection showed similar dynamics to those of normal subjects in the primed condition, independent of instructions. With vestibular stimulation alone (rotation in darkness), self-rotation judgments in normal subjects showed high-pass characteristics, falling from a maximum at 0.4 Hz to zero at 0.025 Hz. With combined visual and vestibular stimulation, perception of self-rotation in the "stare through" condition showed a clear modulation in association with the optokinetic stimulus, and therefore it did not correspond to the actual body rotation at low frequencies; this modulation was reduced in the tracking condition. The authors concluded that self-motion perception normally takes the visual scene as a reference, and vestibular input is simply used to verify the kinematic state of the scene. If the scene appears to be moving with respect to an earth-fixed reference frame, the visual signal is suppressed and perception is based on the vestibular signal (see also Berthoz et al., 1975).

Angular Displacement and Orientation   If the velocity of vection can be accurately perceived, then in principle the total angle of displacement could be visually determined by mathematically integrating the optic flow over time. Alternatively, in an environment with distinctive stable landmarks, the angle of self-rotation is given by the angular displacement of the landmarks, and one's current spatiotopic orientation is defined by the directions of visible landmarks.

To investigate the perception of active angular displacement, Bakker et al. (1999) asked participants at the center of a rotating platform to turn through a specified angle (in increments of 45°) either by stepping or by using an automated manipulandum. With optic flow alone, presented in a head-mounted display of a three-dimensional forest of trees (24° H × 18° V), target angles were greatly undershot with a gain factor of about 0.6. With vestibular information alone, the gain was about 0.7, and with vestibular plus podokinetic information, turning was most accurate, about 0.9 (see also Jürgens et al., 1999; Yardley et al., 1998). Chance et al. (1998) similarly observed that learning object locations in a virtual environment was more accurate when participants actively turned (visual, vestibular and podokinetic information) than when they were passively presented with a visual display.

This undershooting of total displacement with vision alone suggests that angular speed may have been overestimated. The suggestion that such errors stem from a small, head-mounted display seems unlikely because small fields of view tend to reduce, not increase, the perceived speed of rotation (Brandt et al., 1973). Schulte-Pelkum et al. (2003) tested a larger random-dot field on a cylindrical screen ($86°\,H \times 64°\,V$) and found that target angles were still undershot, but with a higher gain of 0.85. These findings suggest that temporal integration of optic flow tends to underestimate the total angular displacement.

Jürgens et al. (2003) examined the perception of angular displacement during passive rotation over a much wider range, up to 900°. Participants on a platform in a large-field rotating drum experienced a brief acceleration followed by three different velocities, and reported when a target angle had been reached. There was a linear relationship between the perceived and target displacement and the average performance was quite accurate: a gain near 1.06 with vision alone, 0.94 with vestibular alone, and 1.02 with both, with lower variability in the visual conditions. However, in the vision alone condition, target angles were greatly undershot at the low rotation rate (15°/s), suggesting that speed was overestimated, while angles were overshot at the high rotation rate (60°/s), suggesting that speed was underestimated. Similar effects were observed when the lights were turned off after the first 90° and subjects pushed a button to signal each successive 90° rotation. Interestingly, the angular estimates did not depend upon a subjective experience of vection. The authors concluded that the temporal integration system can extrapolate the initial perceived velocity, based on early visual and/or vestibular information, in order to determine the total angular displacement. They also proposed that the perceived velocity is biased toward the mean of recent experienced or expected velocities. They argue that the vision-based undershoot reported by Bakker et al. (1999) may result from their head-mounted display being less "potent" than a rotating drum, but this seems contrary to the fact that it apparently induced higher perceived speeds. Alternatively, the undershoot might be due to the relatively low rotation velocity of about 9°/s generated by the participants in the Bakker et al. (1999) study.

Becker at al. (2002a) investigated circular vection using four viewing conditions of an optokinetic drum, turning at 15, 30 or 60°/s: participants (1) attentively followed the visual details of the moving optokinetic pattern (FOL) (similar to the "tracking with eye movements" instruction of Mergner et al., 2000), (2) stared at the pattern (STA) (similar to the stare through instruction), (3) voluntarily suppressed their optokinetic reflex (SUP) (maintaining gaze at an imaginary stationary point), or (4) suppressed the optokinetic reflex by fixating a stationary fixation point (FIX). To quantify CV, subjects pressed a button to indicate each successive perceived rotation of 90°. The total apparent angular displacement increased gradually in the order FOL < STA < SUP < FIX; vection latency (5 to 55 s) decreased in the same order. Slow eye velocity (ranging from 3 to 50°/s; measured to confirm that subjects followed the viewing instruction and to quantify the retinal slip) was the same in FOL and STA, but lower during SUP. The authors concluded that (1) the influence of eye movements on circular vection depends on whether these are intentional (FOL) or not (STA); (2) the increase in circular vection (cumulated 90° indications) during voluntary suppression of the optokinetic reflex (SUP) suggests that afferent motion cues such as retinal slip are processed with larger gain than efferent motion cues such as eye-movement signals; hence (3) the enhancement of circular vection during fixation (FIX) is not, or not solely, due to induced motion of the fixation point opposite the direction of optic flow (see Mergner et al., 2000).

Thus, estimates of angular displacement from integrating optic flow appear to be approximately veridical, but are subject to influences of rotation velocity, fixation, and possibly display size and distance. On the other hand, an environment containing visual landmarks may permit quite accurate orientation judgments. Riecke et al. (2002) presented a virtual display of Tübingen's market square on a cylindrical screen and trained participants to locate 22 target objects. They were then physically rotated to random orientations and asked to point to unseen target objects, yielding mean absolute errors of only 16.5° (variability 17°). Removing vestibular information did not significantly affect performance when landmarks were available, but reduced performance when optic flow had to be integrated. This indicates that spatial orientation can rely on salient visual landmarks, bypassing the temporal integration of optic flow.

Perceiving Translation and the Direction of Self-Motion

Vestibular and Proprioceptive Systems

There is an extensive literature on the sensitivity of the vestibular system to linear acceleration, often investigated with centrifuges so as to avoid linear space limitations (Anastasopoulos et al., 1996; Angelaki, 2003; Bles and Degraaf, 1993; Young, 1981; Böhmer and Mast, 1999; Clarke and Engelhorn, 1998; Furman and Baloh, 1992; Merfeld et al., 2001; Seidman et al., 2002; Tribukait, 2003; Wearne et al., 1999) as well as other protocols (Angelaki and McHenry, 1999; Baloh et al., 1988; Benson and Brown, 1989; Berthoz et al., 1975; Bles et al., 1995; Bronstein and Gresty, 1988; Gianna et al., 1997; Glasauer, 1995; Glasauer and Israël, 1995; Golding and Benson, 1993; Harris et al., 2000b; Hlavacka et al., 1996; Melvill-Jones and Young, 1978; Paige et al., 1998; Pavard and Berthoz, 1977; Walsh, 1961; Wertheim et al., 2001). In this section we merely highlight some recent work on the perceived displacement and direction of translational motion, as it ties in with our closing discussion of path integration.

Linear Displacement   The magnitude of linear displacement can be quite accurately determined over short distances from otolith signals. Israël and Berthoz (1989) applied the VMCS paradigm with lateral body displacements along the interaural axis in darkness. Although the linear VOR per se was very small, subjects could stabilize their gaze on a previously seen straight-ahead target with VOR + saccades. When subjects were instructed not to move their eyes during self-motion (VMCS), most of them could still correctly reproduce the head movement amplitude with saccades. This indicates that linear head displacement was perceived and stored with the adequate metrics and could be used to drive the saccadic system. Bilabyrinthectomized patients could not perform any adequate gaze stabilization, showing that the observed performance required vestibular signals.

Over longer distances, Berthoz et al. (1995), Israël et al. (1997), and Grasso et al. (1999), found that participants who are passively accelerated through a target distance along the anterior-posterior (AP) axis can accurately replicate that distance when traveling at a different acceleration (all without vision). This suggests that vestibular information allows consistent within-modality estimates of linear displacement. During active walking, participants are highly accurate at reproducing a travel distance as long as the walking speeds on the target and test paths are the same (Mittelstaedt and Mittelstaedt, 2001). They can also accurately walk to a static visual target without vision, and estimate this distance on the basis of either vestibular or podokinetic information alone, as long as they travel at a normal walking speed, step length, and frequency. This suggests that the path integration system is calibrated for normal walking. As observed for angular displacement, podokinetic signals are the most accurate and appear to be dominant during linear displacement.

Direction of Heading   Telford et al. (1995) compared vestibular, podokinetic, and visual judgments of the direction of self-motion, or heading. The participants were passively transported at an acceleration above the otolith threshold, actively walked from a standstill with a sub-threshold acceleration, and/or viewed optic flow from a three-dimensional array of vertical rods in a head-mounted display. The task was to align the head in the perceived direction of self-motion. Visual judgments were an order of magnitude more precise than podokinetic or vestibular judgments. When the visual heading and the vestibular heading were misaligned by 30°, pointing judgments were completely determined by optic flow; when the visual and podokinetic headings were misaligned by 30°, judgments were in between them (Ohmi, 1996). Thus, it appears that heading direction can be determined in any modality, but optic flow allows for the most precise judgments. Vestibular heading estimates are highly variable and strongly dominated by visual information. (See Duffy, et al., this volume, for more on visual and vestibular influences on the neural estimation of heading.)

Visual System

Translation of the observer's eye through the environment generates a radial pattern of motion known as the *translational component* of retinal flow (see figure 16.4a). The *focus of expansion* in this flow pattern corresponds to the current direction of heading (Gibson, 1950). The radial structure of the pattern depends solely on the observer's direction of heading, whereas the rate of flow depends upon both the observer's speed and the distance of environmental surfaces.

Linear Vection   The characteristics of *linear vection* are quite similar to those of circular vection. In this case, an experience of self-translation, usually along the AP axis, is induced by lamellar flow presented laterally (Berthoz et al., 1975) or radial flow presented in the frontal plane (Lishman and Lee, 1973). The latency for linear vection is about 1–2 s, and it has low-pass characteristics with a frequency cutoff of 0.5 Hz and a time constant of about 1 s (Berthoz et al., 1975; Berthoz and Droulez, 1982). In contrast, the otolith system has high-pass characteristics, with sensitivity to linear acceleration only at frequencies above 1 Hz (Melvill-Jones and Young, 1978). This is again consistent with a division of labor between the visual and vestibular systems.

Linear Displacement   Perceiving the total displacement from optic flow is more problematic during translation than rotation, because the flow rate is inversely proportional to the distance of environmental surfaces. Thus, determining one's speed or displacement from optic flow depends on perceived distance. With a display of a moving grating at a fixed distance, the speed of linear vection has been found to be linear up to a saturation velocity of over 90°/s (Berthoz et al., 1975; Carpenter-Smith et al., 1995).

In experiments on perceived displacement, Bremmer and Lappe (1999) asked participants to judge whether a display of self-motion over a textured ground plane depicted a greater travel distance than a standard display, while they held eye height and depth structure constant. They obtained a gain of 0.98, even when the speed of self-motion was varied between standard and test. Frenz et al. (2003) determined that such relative judgments remain reasonably accurate despite variation of the visually specified eye height and viewing angle of the ground plane, leading them to conclude that distance estimates are based on the perceived speed of self-motion through the environment rather than simply on proximal image velocities. Interestingly, when asked to reproduce the travel distance in a sample display by controlling optical speed with a joystick, most participants regenerate the velocity profile of the sample display (constant velocity, sinusoidal, or a sequence of velocity plateaus) (Bremmer and Lappe, 1999). A similar pattern has been observed for the vestibular-based reproduction of passive displacements (Berthoz et al., 1995; Israël et al., 1997), suggesting that self-motion may be encoded as a velocity history rather than as a temporally integrated distance value.

On the other hand, Harris et al. (2000a, b) reported large misestimates of travel distance using a static visual target in a virtual corridor. Subjects first viewed a target, then experienced visual stimulation (motion presented in a head-mounted display) or vestibular stimulation (passive mechanical displacement in the dark) corresponding to acceleration down the corridor, and were asked to indicate when they passed the target. With visual stimulation alone, performance was quite accurate (distance gain of 1.04), but with vestibular stimulation alone subjects undershot the target distance (gain of 0.5), as previously reported by Israël et al. (1993a). In contrast, when the target was first specified by mechanically accelerating the subject through the target distance, judgments were accurate with vestibular stimulation of the same or a different acceleration (distance gain of 0.96), but they greatly overshot the target distance with visual stimulation (gain of 4.3). These results suggest that visual and vestibular estimates of travel distance are not well-calibrated, so that visual distance is underestimated and vestibular distance is overestimated relative to one another. Subsequently, Redlick et al. (2001) found that judgments of visually determined travel distance actually depend on the acceleration of the visual display: subjects undershot a static target with accelerations less than $0.1 \, \text{m/s}^2$ (including constant velocities) whereas gains were close to 1 at accelerations above $0.2 \, \text{m/s}^2$ (which is above the vestibular threshold). However, it is difficult to interpret this set of results, because the displays contained no binocular disparity and were presented at optical infinity, had stripes on the walls but no texture on the floor, and were simulated with an unusually low eye height—any of which could have led to errors in perceived distance and hence in perceived self-motion.

There is thus some difference of opinion regarding the perception of linear displacement from optic flow. Relative judgments of travel distance over a ground surface appear to be quite good, but there may be errors at low accelerations or miscalibration with respect to vestibular estimates.

Direction of Heading   The instantaneous direction of translation is specified by the radial optic flow pattern, in which the focus of expansion (FOE) corresponds to the heading direction. The location of the FOE in relation to environmental landmarks thus provides information about the orientation of the locomotor path in the environment. We briefly describe some basic findings on the perception of heading (for recent reviews, see Lappe et al., 1999; Warren, 2004; and chapter 15 by Duffy et al., in this volume).

Observers can judge their direction of translation from random-dot displays of radial flow with an accuracy of 1° of visual angle (Warren et al., 1988). Accuracy is similar in various three-dimensional environments, such as a ground plane, a frontal plane, or a cloud of dots, but decreases as the number of dots is reduced. Such results indicate that the visual system spatially integrates local motion signals to estimate the heading direction (Warren et al., 1991; Burr et al., 1998).

However, the perception of heading is complicated by the fact that the eye can also rotate during translation, a common occurrence when one fixates a point in the world during locomotion. If the eye is simultaneously translating and rotating in space, the flow pattern on the retina is the sum of the rotational (lamellar) and translational (radial) components, and can be quite complex (see figure 16.4c). To determine the instantaneous heading, the visual system must somehow analyze the translational and rotational components.

There are two general approaches to this *rotation problem*. First, it is possible that extraretinal signals about the rotation of the eye and head are used to estimate the rotational component of self-motion, which is then subtracted from the retinal flow to recover the translational component of self-motion (Banks et al., 1996). Second, it is theoretically possible that heading can be determined from the retinal flow alone, because motion parallax in the flow pattern corresponds to observer translation, whereas common lamellar motion corresponds to observer rotation. Thus, the visual system might (1) determine the heading directly from motion parallax (Rieger and Lawton, 1985; Royden, 1997), (2) first estimate observer rotation from the lamellar flow and subtract it to determine the heading (Perrone, 1992), or (3) possess templates for the set of flow patterns produced by combinations of translation and rotation (Lappe and Rauschecker, 1993; Perrone and Stone, 1994).

The psychophysical evidence on the rotation problem is mixed. Warren and Hannon (1988; 1990) initially reported that heading judgments were similarly accurate with an actual eye rotation (flow and extra-retinal signals specify rotation) and a display that simulated the optical effects of an eye rotation (flow specifies rotation, extra-retinal signals specify no rotation), indicating that heading can be perceived from retinal flow alone, even when it is in conflict with extra-retinal signals. However, the simulated rotation rates in these experiments were low (<1°/s). Royden et al. (1992) and Banks et al. (1996) subsequently found that heading judgments were increasingly inaccurate at faster rotations (1 to 5°/s), with errors in the direction of simulated rotation, consistent with the extra-retinal hypothesis. Royden (1994) argued that observers actually based their judgments on a perceived curved path of self-motion rather than on the instantaneous heading direction. Observers are more accurate under conditions designed to elicit estimates of the instantaneous heading: (1) when judging the direction they are skidding while traveling on a circular path (Stone and Perrone, 1997), (2) when asked to base heading judgments on the illusory motion of the fixation point during simulated rotation (van den Berg, 1996), or (3) when asked to judge heading in short displays (<500 ms) of simulated rotation (Grigo and Lappe, 1999). These results suggest that the visual system can estimate instantaneous heading, although observers tend to judge their perceived path of self-motion.

Such observations raise the question of how the visual system recovers the path of self-motion over time from complex retinal flow patterns, which is known as the *path problem*.

The problem is that the flow field is ambiguous with respect to the observer's path: the same instantaneous flow field can be generated by a straight path of self-motion with an eye rotation about the vertical axis, or by a circular path of self-motion (see figure 16.4c). This ambiguity can be resolved in more realistic environments with distinct objects. Li and Warren (2000; 2002) found that when displays contain reference objects, path judgments are quite accurate, even at high simulated rotation rates (see also Cutting et al., 1997; Wang and Cutting, 1999). They proposed that the visual system determines the instantaneous heading with respect to objects in the environment (the *object-relative heading*), and then recovers the path of self-motion by tracking the object-relative heading over time. For example, if the path is straight, the heading point will remain fixed in the scene, whereas if the path is curved, it will shift relative to objects over time.

The data thus indicate that both retinal flow and extra-retinal signals contribute to detecting the path of self-motion. This may account for the mixed results in the heading literature. Crowell and Andersen (2001) reported that the role of extra-retinal signals is merely to gate the interpretation of the lamellar component of flow from a three-dimensional scene as being due to an eye rotation or to a curved path of self-motion. With distinct objects in the scene, the retinal flow appears to dominate extra-retinal signals in determining the path of self-motion (Li and Warren, 2000). The direction of the locomotor path in the environment can thus be determined whether or not the eye is simultaneously rotating.

Combining Rotation and Translation in Path Integration

The literature we have reviewed shows that, considered individually, estimates of angular displacement, linear displacement, and the direction of locomotion are all quite veridical, at least at normal walking speeds under full-cue conditions or within a single modality. Given that this is the case, one might expect that a path integration system could combine these linear and angular estimates to perform accurate navigation. A number of models of path integration describe how linear and angular displacements might be combined (Maurer and Seguinot, 1995), enabling an observer to return to their starting location in a homing task. One approach continuously updates a *homing vector* that preserves only the direction and distance to the home location (Fujita et al., 1990); alternatively, a record of the traveled paths or velocity profiles may be preserved (Fujita et al., 1993). It is thus somewhat surprising that path integration in humans appears to be rather coarse, with large constant and variable errors.

To examine interactions between angular and linear displacements in the vestibular system, Ivanenko et al. (1997) had blindfolded participants undergo passive whole-body motion in the horizontal plane, including pure rotations in place, corner-like trajectories, and arcs of a circular trajectory. Stimulation of the semicircular canals was the same for all trajectories, but was accompanied by otolith stimulation during the arc motion. When subjects used a pointer to reproduce the total angular displacement after the motion, they consistently overestimated their rotation angle on all trajectories. However, when they continuously pointed toward a distant unseen target during the motion, pointing was highly accurate and matched the dynamics of angular motion. It was concluded that (1) the brain can distinguish and memorize the angular component of complex two-dimensional motion, despite a large inter-individual variability; (2) in the range of linear accelerations used, no effect of otolith-canal perceptual interaction was shown; and (3) angular displacements can be dynamically transformed into matched pointing movements.

In a similar experiment, Ivanenko et al. (1997a) tested passive rotation in place, passive linear motion, and a semicircular trajectory. Body orientation in the horizontal plane was controlled independently of the trajectory, so that different combinations of otolith and canal stimulation were produced. Participants had to point toward a previously seen target during the motion, and in a second session had to make a drawing of the perceived trajectory at the end of the movement. The movement of the pointer closely matched the dynamics of the rotational component of the planar motion. This suggests that, in the range of linear accelerations tested, there was no interference of otolith input on canal-mediated perception of angular motion. The curvature of the drawn paths could largely be explained by the input to the semicircular canals, without taking into account the directional dynamics of the otolith input during passive motion. Thus, the reconstruction of the trajectory in space does not appear to involve integrating the linear and angular components of the motion into a unified two-dimensional representation. This result suggests that rotational and translational motions may not be accurately combined to recover one's path (also see chapter 17 by Hicheur et al.).

One test of path integration that combines linear and angular displacements is a homing task such as *triangle completion*. The participant starts at a home location, travels actively or passively along two specified legs of a triangle, and is then asked to return home along the third leg of the triangle. Loomis et al. (1993) found that blindfolded subjects with only vestibular and podokinetic information performed triangle completion with surprisingly poor accuracy. Absolute (unsigned) errors were 24° for the final turn toward home, and 1.68 m for the length of the return path, or about 30% of the triangle's third leg, on average. Constant (signed) errors revealed a compression in the range of responses, such that participants tended to overshoot on short legs and undershoot on long legs, and overturn small angles and slightly underturn large angles. The authors suggested that this regression toward the mean of a set of tested triangles is consistent with a path integration system that preserves some record of traveled paths rather than simply updating the homing vector. With optic flow alone, Péruch et al. (1997) found even less accurate triangle completion performance in subjects using a joystick in a simple virtual environment. In contrast to active walkers, their subjects consistently underturned all final angles.

Surprised by these results, Nico et al. (2002) submitted blindfolded subjects to passive linear displacements along the two equal sides of a triangular path. Subjects were then oriented toward the starting point and asked to complete the triangle by driving straight to the starting point, either blindfolded or with full vision in a small (7 × 6 m) or a large (38 × 38 m) room. Room dimensions exerted a significant effect on performance: in the smaller room blindfolded responses were always too short, although subjects correctly reached the starting point when visual feedback was allowed (figure 16.5). In contrast, in the larger room, subjects correctly responded while blindfolded but drove significantly farther than required with full vision. These data show that vestibular navigation is highly sensitive to both stored (knowledge of environment) and current visual information.

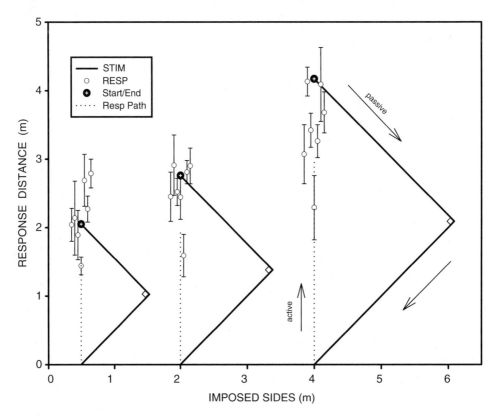

Figure 16.5
Triangle completion with self-driven transport while seated on a mobile robot. The circles containing plus signs indicate the starting and expected arrival points. Triangle legs (black solid lines) show the passively traveled trajectories in darkness (stimulus), before the actively controlled straight transport in light (response: dotted lines). The empty dots (±SD) each show subject's responses; subjects had not seen the start/end point. These data are from the smaller experimental room used. Responses were too long (overshoots) when the same task (with the same "stimulus dark-response visual" condition) was performed in the larger room, and too short (undershoot) when executed in darkness ("stimulus dark-response dark" condition).

In order to compare optic flow and vestibular/podokinetic information in the same setup, Kearns et al. (2002) tested triangle completion in a large virtual environment. Participants walked freely within a 12-m by 12-m area while wearing a head-mounted display (60° H × 40° V). To test optic flow alone, a seated observer steered with a joystick in a virtual texture-mapped arena, which resulted in large variable errors in final angle (SD = 33°) and path length (SD = 1.5 m, 28% of the required path length). Constant errors reflected under-turning of most final turns, similar to Péruch et al. (1997), as well as undershooting of long legs and slight overshooting of short legs. When participants actively walked in the virtual environment, performance was more consistent and exhibited a different pattern of constant errors, with or without optic flow. Variable errors in final angle (SD = 20°) and path length (SD = 1 m, 22% of the required length) were somewhat smaller, whereas constant errors reflected consistent overturning of the final angle rather than underturning. This pattern of results indicates that observers can perform path integration using optic flow if necessary, but they rely predominantly on vestibular/podokinetic information during active walking.

Kearns (2003) measured the relative contribution of visual and vestibular/podokinetic information by selectively manipulating the visual gain of the translational or rotational flow during active walking. Thus, for a given walked distance, the observer appeared to travel through a greater (150%) or shorter (67%) visual distance in the virtual arena; turning angles were manipulated similarly. The relative contribution of vestibular/podokinetic information to triangle completion performance was about 85% overall, but there was a significant contribution of about 15% from optic flow. It thus appears that the temporal integration of optic flow makes a small but reliable contribution to path integration, even during active walking. Overall, however, the large errors in triangle completion suggest that relatively veridical estimates of rotational and translational displacements are not accurately combined during path integration.

On the other hand, when Kearns (2003) added five landmarks near the two outbound legs, accuracy improved dramatically, and the visual contribution increased to 50% for the translational gain and 60% for the rotational gain. The landmarks appear to provide a visual reference frame within which the observer can update position more accurately than by integrating the optic flow. Yet there still remains a strong contribution of vestibular/podokinetic information to updating position. However, when landmarks are positioned near a target location, subjects completely rely on them as beacons for navigation (Foo et al., in press) (figure 16.6). During triangle completion, if a landmark near the home location is surreptitiously shifted as the subject walks the first two legs of the triangle, the change goes unnoticed and elicits corresponding deviations in the final turn. It has recently been found that this is the case for shifts of as much as 28°, well above the resolution of vestibular/podokinetic path integration (Foo et al., 2004). This suggests that the visual system relies heavily on local landmarks, when available, rather than path integration mechanisms in order to remain oriented in the environment.

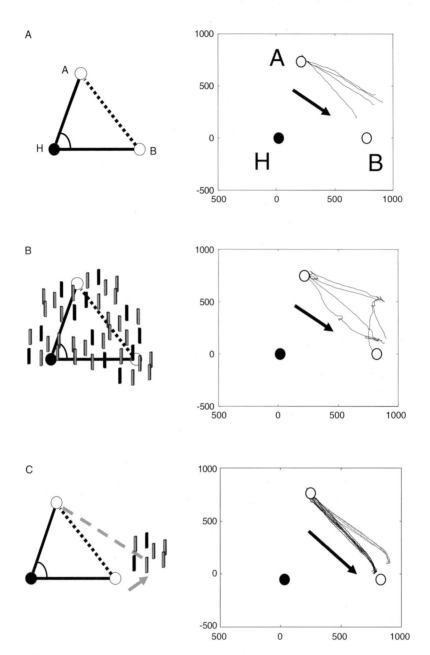

Figure 16.6
Shortcuts between two learned locations in human walking. During training (left panels), subjects repeatedly walked from home (H) to location A and back, turned through angle H, and walked from home to location B and back. They were then tested on the novel short-cut from A to B (right panels). Traces represent individual trials from a representative subject. (a) Desert world: With no visual landmarks (only a textured ground plane), accumulating errors are characteristic of path integration. (b) Forest world: With a random array of colored posts, errors accumulate until local landmark configuration is visible, then subjects home in on target location. (c) Local landmarks: When landmarks near the target location are shifted by 9° on catch trials (gray traces), subjects follow them completely. Complete dominance of local landmarks also occurs with shifts up to 28° in a continuous triangle completion task. (Adapted from Foo et al., in press.)

Conclusion

The results reviewed in this chapter point to the conclusion that whole-body rotation and translation at typical locomotor speeds, including angular and linear displacements, are veridically perceived and reported on the basis of visual, vestibular, and podokinetic information. These abilities allow for the accurate control of self-motion, and should in principle provide a reliable sensory basis for maintaining one's orientation to the environment and for path integration over longer paths of locomotion. Yet paradoxically, path integration performance in a simple task such as triangle completion is quite unreliable and inaccurate. These observations imply that difficulties may reside in combining estimates of angular and linear displacement to determine a complex path, a process that deserves further study. Fortunately, it appears that the visual system has developed an alternative orientation system based on visual landmarks, which allows for highly accurate and precise orientation and navigation within a heterogeneous environment. In the absence of distinctive landmarks, the system can fall back on a coarse path integration system, which may suffice to bring the observer within range of another landmark.

References

Allison RS, Howard IP, Zacher JE (1999) Effect of field size, head motion, and rotational velocity on roll vection and illusory self-tilt in a tumbling room. Perception 28: 299–306.

Anastasopoulos D, Gianna C, Bronstein A, Gresty MA (1996) Interaction of linear and angular vestibulo-ocular reflexes of human subjects in response to transient motion. Exp Brain Res 110: 465–472.

Andersen GJ, Braunstein ML (1985) Induced self-motion in central vision. J Exp Psychol Human Percept Perf 11: 122–132.

Angelaki DE (2003) Three-dimensional ocular kinematics during eccentric rotations: evidence for functional rather than mechanical constraints. J Neurophysiol 89: 2685–2696.

Angelaki DE, McHenry MQ (1999) Short-latency primate vestibuloocular responses during translation. J Neurophysiol 82: 1651–1654.

Bakker NH, Werkhoven P, Passenier PO (1999) The effects of proprioceptive and visual feedback on geographical orientation in virtual environments. Presence 8: 36–53.

Baloh RW, Beykirch K, Honrubia V, Yee RD (1988) Eye movements induced by linear acceleration on a parallel swing. J Neurophysiol 60: 2000–2013.

Banks MS, Ehrlich SM, Backus BT, Crowell JA (1996) Estimating heading during real and simulated eye movements. Vis Res 36: 431–443.

Becker W, Jürgens R, Boss T (2000) Vestibular perception of self-rotation in different postures: a comparison between sitting and standing subjects. Exp Brain Res 131: 468–476.

Becker W, Nasios G, Raab S, Jurgens R (2002) Fusion of vestibular and podokinesthetic information during self-turning towards instructed targets. Exp Brain Res 144: 458–474.

Becker W, Raab S, Jurgens R (2002a) Circular vection during voluntary suppression of optokinetic reflex. Exp Brain Res 144: 554–557.

Benson AJ, Brown SF (1989) Visual display lowers detection threshold of angular, but not linear, whole-body motion stimuli. Aviat Space Environ Med 60: 629–633.

Benson AJ, Hutt EC, Brown SF (1989) Thresholds for the perception of whole body angular movement about a vertical axis. Aviat Space Environ Med 60: 205–213.

Berthoz A, Pavard B, Young LR (1975) Perception of linear horizontal self motion induced by peripheral vision (linear-vection): basic characteristics and visual-vestibular interactions. Exp Brain Res 23: 471–489.

Berthoz A, Droulez J (1982) Linear self motion perception. In AH Wertheim, WA Wagenar, and HW Leibowitz, eds., Tutorials on Motion Perception New York: Plenum Press, pp. 157–199.

Berthoz A, Israël I, Georges-François P, Grasso R, Tsuzuku T (1995) Spatial memory of body linear displacement: what is being stored? Science 269: 95–98.

Bles W, de Graaf B (1993) Postural consequences of long duration centrifugation. J Vestib Res 3: 87–95.

Bles W, Jelmorini M, Bekkering H, de Graaf B (1995) Arthrokinetic information affects linear self-motion perception. J Vestib Res 5: 109–116.

Bloomberg JJ, Melvill Jones G, Segal BN, McFarlane S, Soul J (1988) Vestibular-contingent voluntary saccades based on cognitive estimates of remembered vestibular information. Adv OtoRhinoLaryngol 40: 71–75.

Bloomberg JJ, Melvill Jones G, Segal BN (1991) Adaptive plasticity in the gaze stabilizing synergy of slow and saccadic eye movements. Exp Brain Res 84: 35–46.

Bloomberg JJ, Melvill Jones G, Segal BN (1991a) Adaptive modification of vestibularly perceived rotation. Exp Brain Res 84: 47–56.

Blouin J, Gauthier GM, Van Donkelaar P, Vercher JL (1995) Encoding the position of a flashed visual target after passive body rotations. NeuroReport 6: 1165–1168.

Blouin J, Gauthier GM, Vercher JL (1995a) Failure to update the egocentric representation of the visual space through labyrinthine signal. Brain Cogn 1: 1–22.

Blouin J, Gauthier GM, Vercher JL (1997) Visual object localization through vestibular and neck inputs. 2: Updating off-mid-sagittal-plane target positions. J Vestib Res 7: 137–143.

Blouin J, Labrousse L, Simoneau M, Vercher JL, Gauthier GM (1998) Updating visual space during passive and voluntary head-in-space movements. Exp Brain Res 122: 93–100.

Blouin J, Okada T, Wolsley C, Bronstein A (1998a) Encoding target-trunk relative position: cervical versus vestibular contribution. Exp Brain Res 122: 101–107.

Böhmer A, Mast F (1999) Chronic unilateral loss of otolith function revealed by the subjective visual vertical during off center yaw rotation. J Vestib Res 9: 413–422.

Brandt T, Dichgans J, Koenig E (1973) Differential effects of central versus peripheral vision on egocentric and exocentric motion perception. Exp Brain Res 16: 476–491.

Brandt T, Dichgans J, Buchele W (1974) Motion habituation: inverted self-motion perception and optokinetic after-nystagmus. Exp Brain Res 21: 337–352.

Brandt T, Wist ER, Dichgans J (1975) Foreground and background in dynamic spatial orientation. Percept Psychophys 17: 497–503.

Bremmer F, Lappe M (1999) The use of optical velocities for distance discrimination and reproduction during visually simulated self-motion. Exp Brain Res 127: 33–42.

Bronstein A, Gresty MA (1988) Short latency compensatory eye movement responses to transient linear head acceleration: a specific function of the otolith-ocular reflex. Exp Brain Res 71: 406–410.

Burr DC, Morrone MC, Vaina LM (1998) Large receptive fields for optic flow detection in humans. Vis Res 38: 1731–1743.

Carpenter-Smith TR, Futamura RG, Parker DE (1995) Inertial acceleration as a measure of linear vection: an alternative to magnitude estimation. Percept Psychophys 57: 35–42.

Chance SS, Gaunet F, Beall AC, Loomis JM (1998) Locomotion mode affects the updating of objects encountered during travel: the contribution of vestibular and proprioceptive inputs to path integration. Presence 7: 168–178.

Clark B, Stewart JD (1970) Thresholds for the perception of angular acceleration about the three major body axes. Acta Otolaryngol (Stockh) 69: 231–238.

Clarke AH, Engelhorn A (1998) Unilateral testing of utricular function. Exp Brain Res 121: 457–464.

Crowell JA, Andersen RA (2001) Pursuit compensation during self-motion. Perception 30: 1465–1488.

Cutting JE, Vishton PM, Flückiger M, Baumberger B, Gerndt JD (1997) Heading and path information from retinal flow in naturalistic environments. Percept Psychophys 59: 426–441.

Dichgans J, Brandt T (1978) Visual-vestibular interaction: Effects on self-motion percepton and postural control. In H Leibowitz and H-L Teuber, eds., Handbook of Sensory Physiology New York: Springer-Verlag, pp. 755–804.

DiZio P, Lackner JR, Evanoff JN (1987a) The influence of gravitoinertial force level on oculomotor and perceptual responses to Coriolis, cross-coupling stimulation. Aviat Space Environ Med 9 Pt 2: A218–223.

DiZio P, Lackner JR, Evanoff JN (1987b) The influence of gravitoinertial force level on oculomotor and perceptual responses to sudden stop stimulation. Aviat Space Environ Med 58: A224–230.

Foo P, Warren WH, Duchon A, and Tarr MJ (in press) Do humans integrate routes into a cognitive map? Map vs. landmark-based navigation of novel shortcuts. J Exp Psych: Learn Mem Cog

Foo P, Harrison M, Duchon AP, Warren WH, Tarr MJ (2004) Humans follow landmarks over path integration. In: Vision Science Society. Sarasota, FL.

Frenz H, Bremmer F, Lappe M (2003) Discrimination of travel distances from "situated" optic flow. Vis Res 43: 2173–2183.

Fujita N, Klatzky RL, Loomis JM, Golledge RG (1993) The encoding-error model of pathway completion without vision. Geograph Anal 25: 295–314.

Fujita N, Loomis JM, Klatzky RL, Golledge RG (1990) A minimal representation for dead-reckoning navigation: updating the homing vector. Geograph Anal 22: 326–335.

Funahashi S, Bruce CJ, Goldman-Rakic P (1993) Dorsolateral prefrontal lesions and oculomotor delayed-response performance: evidence for mnemonic "scotomas" J. Neurosci 13: 1479–1497

Furman JM, Baloh RW (1992) Otolith-ocular testing in human subjects. Ann NY Acad Sci 656: 431–451.

Gianna C, Gresty MA, Bronstein A (1997) Eye movements induced by lateral acceleration steps—effect of visual context and acceleration levels. Exp Brain Res 114: 124–129.

Gibson JJ (1950) Perception of the Visual World. Boston: Houghton Mifflin.

Gibson JJ (1968) What gives rise to the perception of motion? Psychol Rev 75: 335–346.

Glasauer S (1995) Linear acceleration perception: Frequency dependence of the hilltop illusion. Acta Otolaryngol (Stockh) 115 Suppl 520 PT 1: 37–40.

Glasauer S, Israël I (1995) Otolithic thresholds influence the perception of passive linear displacement. Acta Otolaryngol (Stockh) 115 Suppl 520 PT 1: 41–44.

Golding JF, Benson AJ (1993) Perceptual scaling of whole-body low frequency linear oscillatory motion. Aviat Space Environ Med 7: 636–640.

Gordon CR, Fletcher WA, Melvill Jones G, Block EW (1995) Adaptive plasticity in the control of locomotor trajectory. Exp Brain Res 102: 540–545.

Grasso R, Glasaver S, Georges-François P, Israël I (1999) Replication of passive whole body linear displacements from inertial cues. Facts and mechanisms. Ann NY Acad Sci 871: 345–366.

Grigo A, Lappe M (1999) Dynamical use of different sources of information in heading judgments from retinal flow. J Opt Soc Amer A 16: 2079–2091.

Guedry FE (1974) Psychophysics of vestibular sensation. In HH Kornhuber, eds., Handbook of Sensory Physiology, vol. VI/2. Berlin: Springer Verlag, pp. 3–154.

Harris LR, Jenkin M, Zikovitz DC (2000a) Visual and non-visual cues in the perception of linear self motion. Exp Brain Res 135: 12–21.

Harris LR, Jenkin M, Zikovitz DC (2000b) Vestibular capture of the perceived distance of passive linear self motion. Arch Ital Biol 138: 63–72.

Held R, Dichgans J, Bauer J (1975) Characteristics of moving visual scenes influencing spatial orientation. Vision Res 15: 357–365.

Hlavacka F, Mergner T, Bolha B (1996) Human self-motion perception during translatory vestibular and proprioceptive stimulation. Neurosci Lett 210: 83–86.

Howard IP (1986) The perception of posture, self-motion, and the visual vertical. In KR Boff, L Kaufman and JP Thomas, eds., Handbook of Perception and Human Performance, pp. 18–11 to 18–62. New York: John Wiley.

Howard IP, Heckmann T (1989) Circular vection as a function of the relative sizes, distances, and positions of two competing visual displays. Perception 18: 657–665.

Howard IP, Howard A (1994) Vection: the contributions of absolute and relative visual motion. Perception 23: 745–751.

Howard IP, Zacher JE, Allison RS (1998) Post-rotatory nystagmus and turning sensations after active and passive turning. J Vestib Res 8: 299–312.

Israël I, Berthoz A (1989) Contribution of the otoliths to the calculation of linear displacement. J Neurophysiol 62: 247–263.

Israël I, Bronstein A, Kanayama R, Faldon M, Gresty MA (1996) Visual and vestibular factors influencing vestibular "navigation." Exp Brain Res 112: 411–419.

Israël I, Fetter M, Koenig E (1993) Vestibular perception of passive whole-body rotation about horizontal and vertical axes in humans: goal-directed vestibulo- ocular reflex and vestibular memory-contingent saccades. Exp Brain Res 96: 335–346.

Israël I, Chapuis N, Glasauer S, Charade O, Berthoz A (1993a) Estimation of passive horizontal linear whole-body displacement in humans. J Neurophysiol 70: 1270–1273.

Israël I, Grasso R, Georges-François P, Tsuzuku T, Berthoz A (1997) Spatial memory and path integration studied by self-driven linear displacement. I. Basic properties. J Neurophysiol 77: 3180–3182.

Israël I, Rivaud S, Gaymard B, Berthoz A, Pierrot-Deseilligny C (1995) Cortical control of vestibular-guided saccades in man. Brain 118: 1169–1183.

Israël I, Rivaud S, Pierrot-Deseilligny C, Berthoz A (1991) "Delayed VOR": an assessment of vestibular memory for self motion. In L Requin and GE Stelmach, eds., Tutorials in Motor Neuroscience, Netherlands: Kluwer Academic Publishers, pp. 599–607.

Israël I, Sievering D, Koenig E (1995a) Self-rotation estimate about the vertical axis. Acta Otolaryngol (Stockh) 115: 3–8.

Israël I, Ventre-Dominey J, Denise P (1999) Vestibular information contributes to update retinotopic maps. NeuroReport 10: 3479–3483.

Ivanenko YP, Grasso R, Israël I, Berthoz A (1997) Spatial orientation in humans: perception of angular whole-body displacements in two-dimensional trajectories. Exp Brain Res 117: 419–427.

Ivanenko YP, Grasso R, Israël I, Berthoz A (1997a) The contribution of otoliths and semicircular canals to the perception of two-dimensional passive whole-body motion in humans. J Physiol (Lond) 502: 223–233.

Ivanenko YP, Viaud-Delmon I, Siegler I, Israël I, Berthoz A (1998) The vestibulo-ocular reflex and angular displacement perception in darkness in humans: adaptation to a virtual environment. Neurosci Lett 241: 167–170.

Jürgens R, Boss T, Becker W (1999a) Podokinetic after-rotation does not depend on sensory conflict. Exp Brain Res 128: 563–567.

Jürgens R, Boss T, Becker W (1999) Estimation of self-turning in the dark: comparison between active and passive rotation. Exp Brain Res 128: 491–504.

Jürgens R, Nasios G, Becker W (2003) Vestibular, optokinetic, and cognitive contribution to the guidance of passive self-rotation toward instructed targets. Exp Brain Res 151: 90–107.

Kearns MJ, Warren WH, Duchon AP, Tarr M (2002) Path integration from optic flow and body senses in a homing task. Perception 31: 349–374.

Kearns MJ (2003) The roles of vision and body senses in a homing task: the visual environment matters. Ph.D. Dissertation Brown University, Providence, RI USA.

Lappe M, Rauschecker JP (1993) A neural network for the processing of optic flow from ego-motion in man and higher mammals. Neur Comp 5: 374–391.

Lappe M, Bremmer F, van den Berg AV (1999) Perception of self-motion from visual flow. Trends Cog Sci 3: 329–336.

Li L, Warren WH (2000) Perception of heading during rotation: sufficiency of dense motion parallax and reference objects. Vis Res 40: 3873–3894.

Li L, Warren WH (2002) Retinal flow is sufficient for steering during simulated rotation. Psychol Sci 13: 485–491.

Lishman JR, Lee DN (1973) The autonomy of visual kinesthesis. Perception 2: 287–294.

Loomis JM, Klatzky RL, Golledge RG, Cicinelli JG, Pellegrino JW, Fry PA (1993) Nonvisual navigation by blind and sighted: assessment of path integration ability. J Exp Psych: Gen. 122: 73–91.

Maurer R, Seguinot V (1995) What is modeling for? A critical review of the models of path integration. J Theor Biol 175: 457–475.

Melcher GA, Henn V (1981) The latency of circular vection during different accelerations of the optokinetic stimulus. Percept Psychophys 30: 552–556.

Melvill-Jones G, Young LR (1978) Subjective detection of vertical acceleration: a velocity-dependent response. Acta Otolaryngol. 85: 45–53.

Merfeld DM, Zupan LH, Gifford CA (2001) Neural processing of gravito-inertial cues in humans. II. Influence of the semicircular canals during eccentric rotation. J Neurophysiol 85: 1648–1660.

Mergner T, Hlavacka F, Schweigart G (1993) Interaction of vestibular and proprioceptive inputs. J Vestib Res 3: 41–57.

Mergner T, Nasios G, Anastasopoulos D (1998) Vestibular memory-contingent saccades involve somatosensory input from the body support. NeuroReport 9: 1469–1473.

Mergner T, Rumberger A, Beckert W (1996) Is perceived angular displacement the time integral of perceived angular velocity? Brain Res Bull 40: 467–470.

Mergner T, Nasios G, Maurer C, Becker W (2001) Visual object localisation in space—interaction of retinal, eye position, vestibular and neck proprioceptive information. Exp Brain Res 141: 33–51.

Mergner T, Schweigart G, Müller M, Hlavacka F, Becker W (2000) Visual contributions to human self-motion perception during horizontal body rotation. Arch Ital Biol 138: 139–166.

Mergner T, Siebold C, Schweigart G, Becker W (1991) Human perception of horizontal trunk and head rotation in space during vestibular and neck stimulation. Exp Brain Res 85: 389–404.

Mittelstaedt ML, Glasauer S (1992) The contribution of inertial and substratal information to the perception of linear displacement. In H Krejcova and J Jerabek, eds., Proceedings of XVIIth Barany Society Meeting Czechoslovakia: Castle Dobris. pp. 102–105.

Mittelstaedt ML (1995) Influence of centrifugal force on angular velocity estimation. Acta Otolaryngol (Stockh) 115 Suppl. 520 PT 2: 307–309.

Mittelstaedt ML, Jensen W (1999) Centrifugal force affects perception but not nystagmus in passive rotation. Ann NY Acad Sci 871: 435–438.

Mittelstaedt ML, Mittelstaedt H (1996) The influence of otoliths and somatic graviceptors on angular velocity estimation. J Vestib Res 6: 355–366.

Mittelstaedt ML, Mittelstaedt H (2001) Idiothetic navigation in humans: estimation of path length. Exp Brain Res 139: 318–332.

Nakamura T, Bronstein A (1993) Perception of neck rotation assessed by "remembered saccades." NeuroReport 4: 237–239.

Nakamura S, Shimojo S (1999) Critical role of foreground stimuli in perceiving visually induced self-motion (vection). Perception 28: 893–902.

Nico D, Israël I, Berthoz A (2002) Interaction of visual and idiothetic information in a path completion task. Exp Brain Res 146: 379–382.

Ohmi M (1996) Egocentric perception through interaction among many sensory systems. Cognitive Brain Research 5: 87–96.

Ohmi M, Howard IP, Landolt JP (1987) Circular vection as a function of foreground-background relationships. Perception 16: 17–22.

Paige GD, Telford L, Seidman SH, Barnes GR (1998) Human vestibuloocular reflex and its interactions with vision and fixation distance during linear and angular head movement. J Neurophysiol 80: 2391–2404.

Pavard B, Berthoz A (1977) Linear acceleration modifies the perceived velocity of a moving visual scene. Perception 6: 529–540.

Perrone JA (1992) Model for the computation of self-motion in biological systems. J Opt Soc Am A 9: 177–194.

Perrone JA, Stone LS (1994) A model of self-motion estimation within primate extrastriate visual cortex. Vision Research 34: 2917–2938.

Péruch P, May M, Wartenberg F (1997) Homing in virtual environments: effect of field of view and path layout. Perception 26: 301–311.

Post RB (1988) Circular vection is independent of stimulus eccentricity. Perception 17: 737–744.

Redlick FP, Jenkin M, Harris LR (2001) Humans can use optic flow to estimate distance of travel. Vision Res 41: 213–219.

Riecke BE, von der Heyde M, Bülthoff HH (2002) Spatial updating in virtual environments: What are vestibular cues good for? J Vis 2(7): 421a.

Rieger JH, Lawton DT (1985) Processing differential image motion. J Opt Soc Am A 2: 354–360.

Rieser JJ, Pick HL, Ashmead DH, Garing AE (1995) Calibration of human locomotion and models of perceptual-motor organization. J Exp Psychol Hum Percep Perf 21: 480–497.

Royden CS (1994) Analysis of misperceived observer motion during simulated eye rotations. Vis Res 34: 3215–3222.

Royden CS (1997) Mathematical analysis of motion-opponent mechanisms used in the determination of heading and depth. J Opt Soc Am A 14: 2128–2143.

Royden CS, Banks MS, Crowell JA (1992) The perception of heading during eye movements. Nature 360: 583–585.

Schulte-Pelkum J, Riecke BE, von der Heyde M, Bülthoff HH (2003) Screen curvature does influence the perception of visually simulated ego-rotations. J Vis 3(9): 411a.

Segal BN, Katsarkas A (1988) Goal-directed vestibulo-ocular function in man: gaze stabilization by slow-phase and saccadic eye movements. Exp Brain Res 70: 26–32.

Seidman SH, Paige GD, Tomlinson RD, Schmitt N (2002) Linearity of canal-otolith interaction during eccentric rotation in humans. Exp Brain Res 147: 29–37.

Siegler I, Israël I (2002) The importance of head-free gaze control in humans performing a spatial orientation task. Neurosci Lett 333: 99–102.

Siegler I, Viaud-Delmon I, Israël I, Berthoz A (2000) Self-motion perception during a sequence of whole-body rotations in darkness. Exp Brain Res 134: 66–73.

Stevens SS (1960) The psychophysics of sensory function. Am Sci 48: 226–253.

Stone LS, Perrone JA (1997) Human heading estimation during visually simulated curvilinear motion. Vis Res 37: 573–590.

Telford L, Howard IP, Ohmi M (1995) Heading judgments during active and passive self-motion. Exp Brain Res 104: 502–510.

Tribukait A (2003) Human vestibular memory studied via measurement of the subjective horizontal during gondola centrifugation. Neurobiol Learn Mem 80: 1–10.

Van den Berg AV (1996) Judgements of heading. Vis Res 36: 2337–2350.

Viaud-Delmon I, Ivanenko YP, Grasso R, Israël I (1999) Non-specific directional adaptation to asymmetrical visual-vestibular stimulation. Cog Brain Res 7: 507–510.

Walsh EG (1961) Role of the vestibular apparatus in the perception of motion on a parallel swing. J Physiol (Lond) 155: 506–513.

Wang RF, Cutting JE (1999) Where we go with a little good information. Psychol Sci 10: 71–75.

Warren WH (2004) Optic flow. In LM Chalupa and JS Werner, eds., The Visual Neurosciences. Cambridge, MA: MIT Press, p. 1247–1259.

Warren WH, Hannon DJ (1988) Direction of self-motion is perceived from optical flow. Nature 336: 162–163.

Warren WH, Hannon DJ (1990) Eye movements and optical flow. Opt Soc Am A 7: 160–169.

Warren WH, Morris MW, Kalish M (1988) Perception of translational heading from optical flow. J Exp Psychol Hum Percep Perf 14: 646–660.

Warren WH, Blackwell AW, Kurtz KJ, Hatsopoulos NG, Kalish ML (1991) On the sufficiency of the velocity field for perception of heading. Biol Cybernet 65: 311–320.

Wearne S, Raphan T, Cohen B (1999) Effects of tilt of the gravito-inertial acceleration vector on the angular vestibuloocular reflex during centrifugation. J Neurophysiol 81: 2175–2190.

Weber KD, Fletcher WA, Gordon CR, Melvill Jones G, Block EW (1998) Motor learning in the "podokinetic" system and its role in spatial orientation during locomotion. Exp Brain Res 120: 377–385.

Wertheim AH, Mesland BS, Bles W (2001) Cognitive suppression of tilt sensations during linear horizontal self-motion in the dark. Perception 30: 733–741.

Wist ER, Diener HC, Dichgans J, Brandt T (1975) Perceived distance and the perceived speed of self-motion: linear vs. angular velocity? Perception and Psychophysics 17: 549–554.

Yardley L, Higgins M (1998) Spatial updating during rotation: the role of vestibular information and mental activity. J Vestib Res 8: 435–442.

Yardley L, Gardner M, Lavie N, Gresty MA (1999) Attentional demands of perception of passive self-motion in darkness. Neuropsychologia 37: 1293–1301.

Young LR (1984) Perception of the body in space: Mechanisms. In I Darian-Smith, ed., Handbook of Physiology, sec. 1: The Nervous System, v. III: Sensory Processes, pt. 2 Bethesda: American Physiological Society, pp. 1023–1066.

Young LR, Dichgans J, Murphy R, Brandt T (1973) Interaction of optokinetic and vestibular stimuli in motion perception. Acta Otolaryngol (Stockh) 76: 24–31.

17 Head Direction Control during Active Locomotion in Humans

Halim Hicheur, Stefan Glasauer, Stéphane Vieilledent, and Alain Berthoz

As humans walk along curved trajectories (or turn around a corner), they involuntarily and unconsciously turn their head in advance of body rotations, an anticipatory head orientation mechanism (Glasauer et al., 1995, 2002; Grasso et al., 1996, 1998a; Takei et al., 1996, 1997). In this chapter, we will examine this "directionality" behavior.

The first section will present data from studies in human subjects, which summarize knowledge about the anticipatory head orientation as well as preliminary results that provide new insights about the modulation of the anticipatory head orientation by the variations in the geometrical form of the locomotor path. In the second section of the chapter, we will provide some evidence for the existence of separate mechanisms for the control of direction and distance during human locomotion, which is accurately predicted by a descriptive statistical model.

We will discuss our results in relation to some neurophysiological evidence providing a neural basis for a sense of directional orientation in animals.

Head Orientation Anticipates Future Walking Direction

Navigational Planning
Navigating in the environment requires the brain to update information about the orientation and the position of the body on the basis of both spatial memory and sensory inputs arising from the environment (or transmitted from the body itself) during the displacement. In the case of human navigation, locomotion toward a desired goal requires not only coordinated movements of the lower and upper limbs, but also planning and following an appropriate trajectory.

Trajectories in the form of simple shapes, such as circles, ellipses or triangles, can be easily recognized when they are visually presented to human subjects. However, path identification by human subjects may depend upon different parameters related to perception and action mechanisms. Among them, the viewpoint from which the shape is observed has been extensively studied (Amorim et al., 1998; Wexler et al., 2001) as has the perceived geometry of shapes of curved paths (Viviani and Stucchi, 1989, 1992). As a result, when subjects plan to walk along a path with a given geometry, the body trajectory may be a composite, resulting from interactions between the biomechanical properties of the locomotor apparatus and the cognitive representation of the shape to be followed, and this may profoundly differ from the desired path shape (Vieilledent et al., 2003).

Multisensory Contributions to the Control and Perception of the Body Displacement

It has been demonstrated that during blindfolded locomotion, human subjects can reach a previously seen visual target several meters away on the floor (Thomson, 1983) even after a number of detours. This result, replicated by several groups, indicates that information about step length derived from proprioceptive or outflow motor command signals, as well as vestibular signals, could contribute to the updating of the mental representation of the subject's location in space (Mittelstaedt and Glasauer, 1991). Although the possible contribution of proprioceptive or motor outflow signals has been amply documented, the contribution of vestibular cues has been under debate (Rieser et al., 1995). Vestibular (inertial) measurement of a locomotor trajectory can be performed by "path integration", namely, the integration of linear and angular head acceleration signals provided by the vestibular organs (the canals measure angular head rotation and the otoliths measure head linear acceleration and head tilt). The contribution of the vestibular system to the orientation and localization of the body in space after a displacement, in both animals and humans, has long been suggested (Beritoff, 1965; Potegal, 1982).

During blindfolded navigation and trajectory planning in relation to internal references (Bove et al., 2001), there is a major contribution of vestibular (Gordon et al., 1995) and proprioceptive information. However, in many situations where vision is available, the CNS tends to preferentially depend upon visual information (Kennedy et al., 2003). This enables stable locomotor displacements without veering (Boyadjian et al., 1999; Millar, 1999; Vuillerme et al., 2002). Visual signals, when available to the subjects, play different roles in the control of human locomotion, such as implementing avoidance strategies critical for regulation of dynamic stability, anticipating adjustments necessary to accommodate different constraints in the travel path, and route planning (Patla, 1997). Thus, vision provides instantaneous information about the near and far surroundings which allows the subject to specifically regulate different aspects of locomotion in a predictive fashion. Nevertheless, the quality of visual information largely depends upon the control and stabilization of the head. In this context, heading appears to be a key parameter for assuring the efficiency of locomotion. Heading has been considered as the direction the body faces during forward displacements (Beall and Loomis, 1996). It is important to distinguish the direction toward which we are looking from the direction in which we are moving (Regan and Beverley, 1982), although often heading corresponds to the direction of self motion. Since the head contains both vestibular and visual systems and is linked to the remaining parts of the body by the neck, which contains proprioceptive sensors, the continuous control of head motion is likely to play a key role in the necessary coordination of the entire set of body segments during locomotion.

Visual Control of Locomotion

Gibson (1958) first proposed that the center of the optic flow pattern during forward movement of the animal indicates the direction of movement. Since then, the properties of optic flow have been extensively studied, showing that this assumption remains true only under certain conditions. Straightforward locomotion with negligible eye movements produces a radial pattern of optic expansion that is symmetrical around the direction of heading and, in this particular case, the focus of expansion of the flow field indicates the locomotor heading. However, as soon as the eyes rotate in the head and the gaze direction shifts away from the direction of travel, the focus of expansion no longer specifies the direction of the locomotor displacement (see chapter 15 by Duffy et al.). This could potentially lead the subjects to mistake their linear trajectory as a curvilinear one. Since the flow pattern on the retina usually consists of a combination of self-movement and eye movement components, the question is still under debate as to whether the direction of heading can be recovered only from the retinal flow or if additional "extraretinal" information (vestibular, proprioceptive, and an efference copy of the motor command to turn the head) is necessary for human subjects (Crowell et al., 1998; Schubert et al., 2003). Direction of self-motion could be perceived from the optical flow (Warren and Hannon, 1988; Stone and Perrone, 1997), and artificial neural networks have been built in order to simulate retinal flow fields that could be experienced during movements over a ground plane (Perrone and Stone, 1994; Lappe and Rauschecker, 1994; Crowell, 1997; Perrone and Stone, 1998). In contrast, Wann et al. (2000; 2003) proposed that it may not be necessary to recover heading from optic flow in the control of curved locomotion. Rather, they emphasized the role of extraretinal information in the active control of steering when taking curved paths.

Furthermore, it was recently shown that, in subjects wearing prism spectacles, optic flow and the scene structure (for example, the ground texture) do not always contribute to the control of locomotion (Perrone and Stone, 1998; Harris and Bonas, 2003). However, other experiments performed in virtual reality confirmed that both optical flow and the visual direction of a target are relevant cues for the control of locomotion (Fajen and Warren, 2000; Warren et al., 2001). According to these authors, the "visual control law" for steering toward a goal in the environment is a linear combination of these two variables with different weights, according to the task's demands. Thereby, the relative modulation of flow and directional cues would allow human subjects to have a robust control of locomotion under different environmental conditions. Since the head can steer

locomotion, Lappe et al. (1999) argued that the future motion path is often more important than the current instantaneous heading. Bertin et al. (2000), adapted a passive transportation paradigm of blindfolded subjects in the real world (Ivanenko et al., 1997a;
Ivanenko et al., 1997b) to sighted subjects in a virtual environment, and showed that head
orientation is a critical variable for perceiving a bidimensional trajectory (over a horizontal ground plane). Although knowledge of the paths already travelled is certainly necessary, the path to be travelled has to be anticipated to insure not only the control of
locomotion but also the efficiency of navigation.

Head Motion during Human Locomotion

Head and gaze stabilization in space have been observed for several different locomotor
tasks (Pozzo et al., 1990; 1991). These authors suggested that the head plays the role of
an inertial guidance platform allowing human subjects to acquire visual as well as vestibular information from a coherent and stable perceptual base. Gaze was also analyzed in subjects required to step on regularly or irregularly spaced tracks of footprints, over a 10 m
distance (Patla and Vickers, 2003). Distinguishing between gaze fixations at the tracks and
at the direction of travel, the authors showed that the latter is dominant and is not influenced by the regularity of the footprint pattern. Some footprint fixations briefly occurred
before the foot landed on the ground targets (800–1000 ms). The authors suggested that
travel direction gaze fixation facilitates the acquisition of environmental and self-motion
information, while footprint gaze fixation allows subjects to regulate their gait patterns.

   Grasso et al. (1996; 1998b) were the first to describe gaze and head anticipation during
human locomotion around a corner, that is, when the direction of locomotion is changing
over time. These authors showed that during locomotion along curved paths, the eyes and
head deviate toward the future direction of curved trajectories. They suggested that such
anticipatory orienting synergies help to prepare a stable reference frame for intended action
(Grasso et al., 1998b). This deviation begins with the head and is followed by the trunk
reorientation and by the change in direction of the trajectory of the centre of mass of the
walker. This can be deeply modified when the head is artificially immobilized relative to
the trunk (Hollands et al., 2001), or when steering is potentially compromised by unexpected head yaw movements (Vallis et al., 2001). Imai et al. (2001) then showed that the
body, head and eyes tend to be aligned with the changes in the gravitoinertial acceleration
vector, which corresponds to the sum of linear accelerations acting on the head. In normal
conditions, before and after the turn, gaze is predominantly aligned with environmental
features lying in the plane of progression, but just prior to changing the direction of their
displacement, subjects produce saccadic eye movements and heading changes which align
gaze with the end point of the required travel path. These recent findings are consistent
with the notion that aligning the head with the intended direction provides the
CNS with an allocentric "reference frame" for the control the movement of the body
in space.

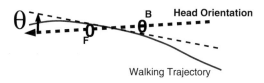

Figure 17.1
Illustration of the method for calculating anticipatory angle θ. The helmet (bold line) was placed on the subject's head so that the midpoint between the two first markers was aligned with the head yaw rotation axis. Thus the line that indicates the head orientation passed through these two markers (Head Forward F and Behind B). A third marker corresponded to the movement of a fixed point on the head. This marker was placed exactly at the middle of the segment linking the two first markers. For each point M of the walking trajectory, we calculated the equations of the tangent line (thin dashed line). We then calculated the angle θ as the angle between the tangent to the walking trajectory and the head orientation. Thus this angle (arrow) is a difference between the head and walking direction (instantaneous head orientation relatively to the current direction of the walking trajectory). Positive θ values correspond to the head oriented toward the left side of the trajectory and negative ones correspond to the head turned to the right.

Anticipatory head orientation is defined here as the orientation of the head relative to the tangent to head trajectory during walking. The anticipatory head orientation is represented as θ which is quantified as the angle between the current walking direction and the instantaneous head orientation relative to the walking trajectory (see figure 17.1 for details of calculation).

Circular Paths

We investigated the anticipation of head orientation when subjects are asked to walk around a circular path either with vision or blindfolded (Takei et al., 1997; Grasso et al., 1998b; Grasso et al., 1998a). Experiments were carried out in a large room (5.1 × 6.2 × 3.4 m length/width/height). A two-camera ELITE system measured head motion in three dimensions.

For head position and direction measurements, subjects wore helmets equipped with two infra-red reflecting markers in the mid-sagittal plane (their midpoint was in the head yaw rotation axis). The mean of the x, y coordinates of all successive positions p_t occupied by the head corresponds to the barycenter of the trajectory executed. The mean of the instantaneous distances from the barycenter to all successive positions p_t was taken as an approximation of the average trajectory radius.

Subjects' stepping rates were computed by means of Fourier analysis of vertical head displacement. Real-time matching between head orientation and trajectory direction was quantitatively assessed in the frequency domain by means of cross spectral analysis. The averaged cross spectrum of pairs of variables was computed by using a standard fast Fourier transform (FFT). Details of the mathematical procedure can be found elsewhere (Grasso et al., 1996; Takei et al., 1996). In order to quantify anticipatory head movements during walking, the magnitude squared coherence function (MSC) was calculated. This is analogous to the squared correlation coefficient in linear regression: it ranges from 0 to 1 and indicates the correlation between synchronous sinusoidal fluctuations (if any) in a given pair of parameters. This provides a coherence value for each frequency present in the signal, the phase shift Φ and the transfer function gain G. From Φ, a corresponding anticipatory time delay can be calculated by applying the formula: delay = $\Phi/(2*\pi*f)$, where f is the frequency at which the phase shift Φ is estimated.

Subjects were trained to walk with eyes open (counterclockwise, CCW) at a comfortable speed along a circular trajectory marked on the floor until they felt confident in reproducing the path without looking. The experiment consisted of reproducing the memorized trajectory in three conditions: (1) eyes open (LIGHT), (2) blindfolded (DARK), and (3) while reading aloud from a newspaper held in their hands (READ). The READ condition was intended to impede visual pursuit, impose a mental work load, and modify the biomechanical properties of the head-neck system by locking the head to the arms and stiffening the neck, thereby impeding rotatory movements.

All participants walked quite accurately along tracks of three circles of different radii in all conditions. However, the trajectories were never completely smooth, more closely resembling curved polygons because of the biomechanics of bipedal gait. All participants also displayed fluctuations of head direction in the horizontal plane (which we call "yawing" oscillations). The results of this experiment demonstrate two main phenomena concerning the head orientation during the steering of locomotion:

1. Head yawing oscillations are coupled with the stepping cycle and are anticipatory with respect to the corresponding walking direction changes. This behavior strongly suggests the presence of an eye-head coordinated nystagmus as has been observed in the monkey (Solomon and Cohen, 1992), and in humans (Bles et al., 1984) running along circular paths both in light and in darkness: its origin has been attributed to a velocity storage mechanism (related to the velocity of the body in space), excited by multisensory (visual, vestibular, and proprioceptive) inputs. In the human, as in the monkey, such a nystagmus continues when the platform along which subjects are running is counterrotated to null angular motion in space, confirming its nonvestibular origin (see chapter 16 by Israël & Warren).

2. There is a constant deviation of mean head orientation θ toward the interior of the circular trajectory. This is probably of visual origin, because it disappears when visual pursuit of environmental cues is suppressed (in the DARK and READ conditions respectively). Such head orientation oscillations exhibited three typical characteristics: a) they had half the frequency of the stepping rate, that is, the frequency of the whole locomotor cycle; b) they were always smaller than the synchronous oscillations of walking direction (gain G = 0.38 ± 0.028 in LIGHT, 0.46 ± 0.014 in DARK and 0.47 ± 0.030 in READ) and, finally c) they systematically anticipated (100–200 ms) the correlated fluctuations of the walking direction in all conditions. This phasic anticipation was longer when the radius was shorter ($p < 0.05$). In the LIGHT condition the head was tonically oriented toward the inner part

of the circle: $\theta = 18.3° \pm 3.5°$ (mean $\pm$ SEM), while it tended to align with the direction of trajectory when vision was impeded or distracted by the concurrent task ($\theta = 4.5° \pm 4.8°$ in DARK and $0.8° \pm 3.2°$ in READ).

On the basis of these observations, Grasso et al. (1996) proposed that mechanisms of anticipatory phasic head orientation with respect to turns during walking are related to the vestibular and optokinetic nystagmus that are also expected to occur during such tasks. Indeed, the rapid phases of nystagmic eye movements, which are biased opposite to the direction of the displacement of the visual field, are now known to function not only as resetting movements but to also comprise genuine anticipatory orienting reactions (Grasso et al., 1998b).

The anticipatory time interval of the head orientation oscillations (120–200 ms) has been recently confirmed by Courtine et al. (2003) for locomotion along arcs of circles. There were no significant differences between intervals in tests with and without vision. Imai et al. (2001) observed that the head orientation could lead the walking direction change by up to 25°. These authors attributed this to tilts of the gravitoinertial acceleration (GIA) vector. Patients with central vestibular and cerebellar disease were unable to anticipate or rapidly compensate for the tilt of the GIA. This is likely to explain their instability in gait when turning corners. In this case "the central vestibular system may not be able to generate appropriate head tilts to smoothly steer the turn" (Imai et al., 2001 p. 16).

Locomotion along a Trajectory with Variable Curvature The dependence of the phasic anticipation on circles with different radii, reported earlier led us to further investigate anticipatory head orientation in a complex trajectory with a continuously varying radius of curvature along a large perimeter. Some preliminary results are presented concerning continuous modulation of anticipatory head orientation when the trajectory varies successively from a CCW to a clockwise (CW) direction. Subjects (using vision) walked along a lemniscate (a shape resembling a figure eight, but with clearly identifiable straight components, see figure 17.2) drawn on the ground along a perimeter of 20.0 m. Subjects were required to perform three trials, each consisting of five successive repetitions (or laps). The volunteer subjects (n = 9) wore helmets equipped with three infrared reflecting markers placed in the midsagittal plane, and analyses were similar to the previous experiments.

As illustrated for two typical subjects (figure 17.2) the head remains aligned with the body trajectory in the straight parts of the path near the center of the lemniscate. The head ceases to be aligned with the direction of locomotion just prior to the beginning of the curves and continues to anticipate until the end of each bend. The head alternates from deviations to the left relative to the tangent to the walking trajectory when the subjects walk in the CCW direction, and turning to the right when the subjects walk in the CW direction.

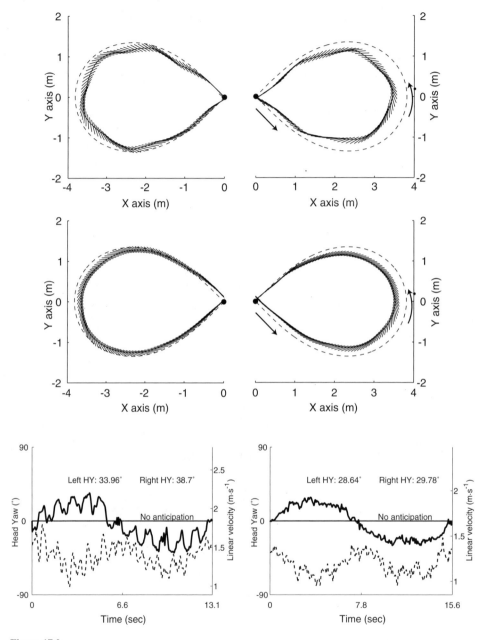

Figure 17.2
Top view of the head orientation during locomotion along a lemniscate for two typical subjects (S6, subject 6; S2, subject 2). The subjects started in the middle of the shape and walked the right loop first (arrows) before walking along the left loop in the CW direction. The ideal path drawn on the ground that the subjects had to follow is represented as a dashed line. (bottom) For each of the subjects, the time courses of θ, the head orien-

The analysis of the time course of θ reveals that the magnitude of the angular difference between the direction of the head and the direction of locomotion averages 30° for each loop of the lemniscate (as illustrated in figure 17.2, bottom). The time course of the head yaw angle corresponds to that of the tangential velocity of the subjects. There were some discrepancies between the shape of the path marked on the ground and the actual trajectory walked by the subjects. Preliminary analyses suggest that the head is anticipatively oriented toward its actual future position rather than toward the ideal future position along the viewed path. This suggests that some of the subjects used an anchoring strategy. Such an anticipation of future directional changes in the locomotor path would act to stabilize the body-centered reference frame. The results for all subjects showed that the anticipative head orientation mechanism is a continuous process for steering along curved paths in humans (when walking on the straighter part of the trajectory, no anticipation is observed, see figure 17.2, top).

Several factors can be proposed to explain this modulation of this "head directionality" anticipatory mechanism. Indeed, vision, gait biomechanics, proprioceptive, and vestibular information may each play a role in the elaboration of this anticipatory behaviour. The fact that anticipatory head orientation is also observed without vision (Courtine et al., 2003) indicates that visual perception of direction changes cannot totally explain this mechanism. The phasic component of the anticipatory head orientation depends partly on the biomechanics of locomotion. This effect is manifested by the high frequency oscillations corresponding to step frequency (see the time course of θ for subject 2, figure 17.2). This corresponds to the fact that the head's lateral oscillations are coupled to the mass transfer of the body from one side to the other. But as is shown for two typical subjects, this mechanical effect is not systematically observed (see subject 6), while the overall profile of the θ(t) plot remains similar for all subjects. Indeed, in the θ(t) plot, the two loops of the locomotor path are easily identifiable, revealing the concomitant oscillations of the anticipatory head orientation with the varying curvature of the path. Mechanical factors induced by stepping are insufficient to explain the tonic component of the anticipatory head orientation.

Vallis et al. (2003) showed that the anticipatory head orientation is not observed when subjects had to avoid an obstacle in the travel path. They explained this observation by noting differences in the goals of the two respective locomotor tasks: steering tasks versus locomotor postural adjustments where the primarily goal is to maintain balance in order to not bump into the obstacle. Thus, the results presented here apply only to certain locomotor behaviours, such as steering tasks.

tation with respect to the trajectory (dark line), and of the tangential walking velocity (pale line) are displayed (bottom). Left RY and right HY correspond respectively to the maximal angular head excursion during locomotion along the left and right loops of the lemniscate. The kinematics variables (3D spatial coordinates of markers located on a helmet) were recorded at a sampling rate of 60 Hz using an optoelectronic video motion capture device (Vicon V8, Oxford Metrics Ltd.) including 13 cameras.

Separate Control of Distance and Direction during Human Locomotion

In this section we present evidence for separate control of the distance and the direction during human locomotion. Anatomical, physiological, and psychophysical studies have suggested that the brain has distinct mechanisms to process direction and distance information separately (e.g., the head direction cell system). This dissociation between these two parameters of human locomotor paths was first suggested by our group (Berthoz et al., 1999; Glasauer et al., 2002) and is now confirmed by a descriptive model developed by one of the authors (S.G.).

Dissociation of distance and direction has been shown in many motor tasks, e.g., reaching to nearby targets (e.g., Soechting and Flanders, 1989) and is also found for coding of targets in visuospatial working memory (Chieffi and Allport, 1997; McIntyre et al., 1998). This is supported by neurophysiological studies, which show movement-direction tuning of neurons in the primary motor cortex (Georgopoulos et al., 1982) and premotor areas (Caminiti et al., 1991) or amplitude tuning in the premotor cortex (Kurata, 1993) and subthalamic nucleus (Georgopoulos et al., 1983). A related dissociation can be expected in locomotor reaching tasks, where both the direction of walking and the distance to a goal are of importance for successful performance. Head direction cells in the postsubiculum (Taube et al., 1990) fire if the head of the rat is oriented in a specific direction with respect to the external world, while place cell activity in the hippocampus is related to the location of the animal (McNaughton et al., 1996).

To study whether such a dissociation can be found in controlling locomotion along curved trajectories, blindfolded subjects were asked to walk along a previously seen triangular path and return to the starting point, as described in detail elsewhere (Glasauer et al., 2002). In the following, we re-examine these data quantitatively to evaluate whether there is a dissociation of distance and direction in locomotion, or, in other words, whether the linear and angular components of a walked two-dimensional trajectory are independent of each other. To predict the distribution of the corner points at each corner of the triangle, we developed a descriptive statistical model from the errors in distance and direction. The model is based on three basic assumptions: (1) subjects memorize correctly the previously seen trajectory, (2) subjects believe they stay on the desired trajectory throughout their walk; hence, a subject turns when she or he assumes to be at the respective corner, and (3) the errors subjects make can be attributed to distance and direction independently. The second and third assumptions were already proposed to descriptively model triangle completion ("error encoding," Fujita et al., 1993). Our model includes several possible sources for errors, which are described in detail in later paragraphs. To study whether the vestibular system is relevant for walking two-dimensional trajectories, we included five labyrinthine-defective subjects (LDs) in our experiment. The importance of the vestibular system for direction processing was suggested from previous experiments on locomotor pointing (Glasauer et al., 1994) and by computational models on navigation

(Wan et al., 1994) and has now been confirmed experimentally for the head direction cell system (Stackman and Taube, 1997; see also chapter 7 by Stackman and Zugaro, this volume) and also for navigational abilities in the rat (Wallace et al., 2002).

A detailed description of the experiment and the data is given in Glasauer et al. (2002). Briefly, seven normal subjects (all male, aged 18–36 years) and five patients with vestibular loss (two patients with complete unilateral and three with complete bilateral vestibular loss, four females and one male, aged 27–65) participated in the study. Note that vestibular loss includes both otoliths and semicircular canals. All of the patients were well compensated, i.e., their symptoms, such as dizziness, vertigo, and nystagmus, had disappeared at least several months before the study. The subjects were asked to walk unguided a previously seen triangular path without vision and as accurately as possible without pausing. The path, marked on the ground by a cross at each corner, consisted of a right triangle with two 3-m-long segments (second corner 135°). The task was performed in alternating CW and CCW directions, but always approaching the right angle of the triangle first. The subjects were asked to walk the path three times in both directions. No feedback about performance was given. Each subject wore a helmet (equipped with noise-emitting headphones and black goggles) with three infrared-reflective markers located above the head in approximately the sagittal plane. The three-dimensional trajectories of the infrared-reflective markers fixed on the helmet were recorded using a video-based motion analysis system (Elite^{TM}) and analyzed afterward (figure 17.3). In the following, only the translational components in the horizontal plane are considered.

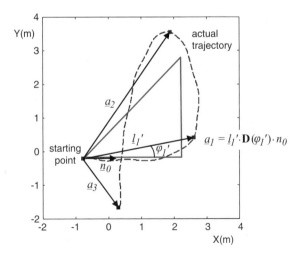

Figure 17.3
Example of a normal subject's trajectory (dashed line) during a counterclockwise walk along the triangle (fine solid line) in a map view. The corner points of the subject's trajectory are shown as black squares. The arrows from the starting point (left lower corner) show the vectors used in the descriptive model: n_0 is the initial walking direction to corner 1, a_1 the first corner point given by the length l_1' and the walking direction φ_1' of segment 1. a_2 and a_3 give the second and third corners (see text).

The corner points (corresponding to a minimum of tangential velocity, Glasauer et al., 1995, 2002) of each walk were calculated from the head trajectory by means of an interactive graphics software package. The length of each segment of the triangle walked and the angle turned from one segment to the next were computed from the corner points of each walk. Distance errors were determined as the difference between required length of a segment and the distance walked. Direction errors were determined as the difference between the required angle and the actual angle between two segments. Thus, cumulative effects have been excluded from the errors. For the first segment, the angular deviation from the required straight-ahead direction was determined. Since the previous analysis did not show directional differences CW and CCW walks were pooled for further analysis.

To reveal the causes of errors made and the differences between subject groups, a descriptive model was devised to analyze the errors made by the subjects. The model, based on the hypotheses described above, makes the following assumptions:

1. Random distance errors made on each segment i are proportional to the required length: d_i

2. Systematic distance errors made during the total walk are proportional to the required length: d_0

3. Random direction errors made on each segment i are due to not holding the straight-ahead direction (veer): α_i

4. Random direction errors made on each segment i are proportional to the angle of the previous turn: β_i

5. Systematic direction errors made during each walk are proportional to the angle of turn: β_0

Errors 1 and 2 reflect distance errors, which are assumed to be proportional to the required distance. This assumption is based on experimental results on straight walking (e.g., Rieser et al., 1990). Error 3 is a directional error made during straight walking due to veering. Errors 4 and 5 are directional errors made during a turn; they are assumed to be proportional to the required turning angle. Errors 2 and 5 correspond to a systematic over- or undershoot in distance or direction within one walk, while all other errors randomly change for each segment of the triangle. All errors are assumed to be normally distributed in the model.

The most important prerequisites of the model follow directly from the model equations described in the appendix:

1. Equal SDs for *relative* distance errors at each segment (eq. 17.2)

2. Equal correlation coefficients for each distance error correlation (eq. 17.3)

3. No correlation between direction errors at segment 1 and all others

4. No correlation between distance and direction errors

Thus, if the model is suitable for describing the observed errors, these prerequisites have to be met by the experimental data. The hypothesis of dissociation of distance and direction errors, is reflected in 3 and 4, while 1 and 2 follow from the assumption that distance errors are proportional to the walked distance, as shown by previous work on reaching a target (e.g., (Rieser et al., 1990)).

For further evaluation of the model, 200,000 simulations were performed using the parameters derived from the subject data (see Results). A two-dimensional histogram with 30×30 bins was calculated from the distributions of the model simulation and used to compute the confidence regions of the endpoints of each segment (figure 17.4). Subsequently, the position of each data point in model distribution was computed by nearest-neighbor interpolation of the two-dimensional histogram as the probability with which a specific corner point would be expected. For example, we would expect 10% of all points to lie outside of the 10% confidence region drawn in figure 17.4. The resulting diagram, a probability-probability plot, is shown in the lower panels of figure 17.4. To determine whether the distribution of the experimental data results from the predicted model distribution, we performed the Chi^2-test for distributions using a histogram with five bins. Comparison of variances between subject groups was done using the F-test. To account for the three walks per subject per direction, we used the number of walks divided by three as number of observations for the comparison of variances and significance of correlation coefficients. P-values smaller than 0.05, were regarded as significant. The model simulations and computations were done using the MATLAB software package.

The experimental data shown as corner points (endpoints of each segment) of all walks of normal and LD subjects are depicted in figure 17.4, together with the predicted confidence regions from the model simulations (see below).

Distance and Directional Errors

Table 17.1 shows the relative distance errors (error divided by the required length of the segment) and the direction errors for all subjects. Distance errors are given as relative errors since the relative distance errors are expected to exhibit the same standard deviation for all segments, as explained above in Methods.

The relative distance errors are close to zero for both subject groups and all segments. For normals, the variance of the relative distance error of segment 1 is significantly lower than that at segment 3 [$F(13, 13) = 3.07$, $p = 0.026$]. The variances of LDs neither differ from each other, nor from those of normals. The correlation coefficients for distance errors between segments are all significantly different from zero for normals (normals $r_{12} = 0.67$, $r_{13} = 0.74$, $r_{23} = 0.83$, all $p < 0.01$), but not for LDs ($r_{12} = 0.37$, $r_{13} = 0.57$, $r_{23} = 0.51$, n.s.).

For the direction errors, the expected increase in SD is found from segments 1 to 3 due to the increasing angle of turn. It is expected, since we assume that direction errors are approximately proportional to the angle turned. They are not due to a cumulative effect, since the errors are given as the difference between actual angle, as determined from the

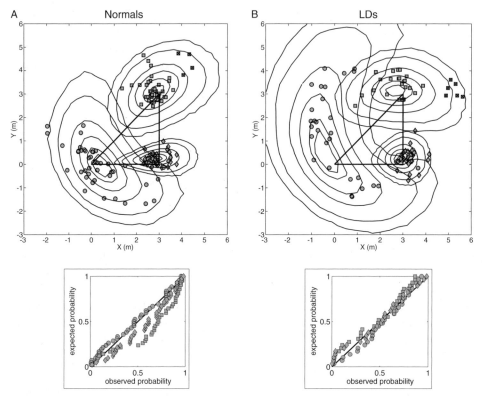

Figure 17.4
The top plots show the experimental data and model distributions in a map view. The starting point is the lower left corner of the triangle. The corner points determined from the data at the three corners are shown as symbols (1, diamonds, 2, squares, 3, circles) for normal (A, left) and LD subjects (B, right). Darker squares in the right upper corner are interpolated corner points from walks that went outside the field of view of the cameras. The confidence regions for distributions of endpoints (from outer to innermost line: 99%, 95%, 75%, 50%, 25%, 10%) are computed from simulations of the descriptive model. Below are shown the corresponding probability-probability plots: expected and observed probabilities of all data points for normal (left) and LD (right) subjects. Symbols denote corner points as in the main plots. Values below the diagonal are closer to the center of the model distribution than expected, those above are farther away. Thus, the model would provide a perfect prediction if all data points were on the diagonal line.

corner points, and required angle between segments. The variances of direction errors are significantly different between normals and LDs for segment 2 only [$F(13,9) = 4.56$, $p < 0.01$]. As explained in the appendix (Eq. 17.4a), the derived variances $C'\{\Delta\varphi_i^2\}$ on segments 2 and 3 should be equal. Using the direction error SDs from table 17.1 to compute these variances, it turns out that they do not differ between segments 2 and 3 for both groups [normals $F(13,13) = 1.97$, $p = 0.12$; LDs $F(9,9) = 2.0$, $p = 0.16$]. Hence, one more test for our assumptions about direction errors is met. The correlation coefficients for direction errors between segments of normals ($r_{12} = 0.04$, $r_{13} = 0.22$, $r_{23} = 0.61$) show no cor-

Table 17.1
Relative distance errors (±SD) and direction errors (in degrees, ±SD) for all subjects and segments of the triangle

	Normal subjects (n = 42 walks)		787 LD patients (n = 29 walks)	
	rel. distance error ± SD	direction error (deg) ± SD	rel. distance error ± SD	direction error (deg) ± SD
Segment 1 ($l_1 = 3$ m, $\varphi_1 = 0$ deg)	−0.031 ± 0.137	4.79 ± 4.50	0.086 ± 0.110	4.66 ± 6.87
Segment 2 ($l_2 = 3$ m, $\varphi_2 = 90$ deg)	0.028 ± 0.205	−4.48 ± 8.12	0.059 ± 0.136	−1.50 ± 17.39
Segment 3 ($l_3 = 4.51$ m, $\varphi_3 = 135$ deg)	0.072 ± 0.240	7.08 ± 14.92	0.014 ± 0.117	−13.31 ± 18.29

Note: The length of each segment and the angle to turn is given in the first column.

relation between segment 1 and all others, while those of segments 2 and 3 are correlated (p = 0.02). For LDs, however, all correlation coefficients are around r = 0.5 ($r_{12} = 0.61$, $r_{13} = 0.49$, $r_{23} = 0.55$, n.s.), suggesting a veering tendency, which is not independent for each segment but holds throughout one walk.

The model predicts no correlation between distance and direction errors. Indeed, for normals, the correlation never exceeded |r| = 0.3 (r = −0.3 for the correlation between distance error at segment 1 and direction error at segment 2). For LDs as well as for normals, the highest correlation coefficient was between distance error at segment 1 and direction error at segment 2 (r = −0.60, n.s.); no other exceeded |r| = 0.5. If these coefficients were significant in a larger sample of subjects, this would indicate an interaction between distance and direction errors. For example, subjects who perceive having walked past corner 1 may take this into account and correct for this error by changing the angle of turn toward corner two. Such an error correction mechanism could occur because most subjects made rounded trajectories at the corners inside of the triangle even with eyes open (see Glasauer et al., 2002).

Model Parameters

The model parameters computed from the data according to eqs. 17.2 through 17.5 (see appendix) are given in table 17.2. These parameters were applied to the model simulations, along with the means of direction errors (see table 17.1) and yielded the distributions shown in figure 17.4. A comparison of model parameters between normals and LDs reveals that the most significant difference is found for the direction error on each turn; this varies significantly more for LDs than for normals. While the SDs for the distance errors d_0 within one walk turned out to be even smaller for LD subjects, all SDs of direction errors were higher for LDs, leading to the much larger confidence regions of the distributions shown in figure 17.4.

Table 17.2
Model parameters (see text) for normal and LD subjects

	Normals	LDs	p-Values (F-Test)
SD of distance error on each segment d_i	0.107	0.102	0.42, n.s
SD of distance error for walk d_0	0.168	0.096	0.03
SD of direction error for straight walk α_i (rad)	0.079	0.120	0.10, n.s.
SD of direction error on each turn β_i	0.048	0.096	0.02
SD of direction error for walk β_0	0.078	0.120	0.10, n.s.

Note: All parameters are unit-free standard deviations (SD) of relative errors, except for parameter α_i which is the SD of the direction error at segment one—see Table 17.1—given in radians. Column 3 shows the p-values of the F-test ($F(9,13)$ or $F(13,9)$) comparing the squared SDs (variances) of normals and LDs.

The lower panels in figure 17.4 show the probability-probability plot of the corner points. If data would be taken randomly from the model distribution, they would lie close to the diagonal. For normals, the deviation from the expected distribution is significant only for corner 2 (chi^2 test, $p < 0.01$), because more values than expected lay close to the center of the distribution (see figure 17.4). For LDs, all data lay close to the diagonal, and the deviations were not significant for any of the corners.

The results of the present data analysis and the model predictions support the hypothesis of a dissociation of distance and direction during walking of two-dimensional trajectories: (1) distance and direction errors are not (or only weakly) correlated, similar to the absence of correlation between angle and distance in blindfolded circular walking (Takei et al. 1997), and (2) the descriptive model based on this dissociation describes the final arrival errors adequately. All three corners could be successfully described for LD patients. Normal subjects, however, walked more accurately to corner 2 than predicted by the model. This is due to their low SD of the relative distance error for segment 1 compared to the other segments. An explanation may be the simplification of the trajectory used in the model: real trajectories (see figure 17.3 and Glasauer et al. 2002) are curved between corners and not straight lines with distinct turning points, as assumed for the model.

A comparison of both groups of subjects shows that LDs have a significantly higher SD of error of direction than normals at corner 2, while normals show a higher SD of walked distance for segments 2 and 3 (see table 17.1). The latter finding may indicate that normals need not control their distance as accurately as LDs, because accurate directional control in normals is sufficient for a good overall performance.

The differences in model parameters computed from the data illustrate the differences in subject groups again (see table 17.2) and provide even more information. For distance errors, the variation on each segment of a walk does not differ between groups, while the variation of distance error within one walk, i.e., the tendency to consistently under- or overshoot each segment of a walk, is larger for normal subjects. The crucial parameters determining the width of the distribution of corner points are, however, the direction errors.

The variances of the respective model parameters are all larger for LDs than for normals, the significant difference being the variance of direction error at each turn. This parameter strongly suggests that LD subjects cannot negotiate the desired change of walking direction as well as normals. The other, not significantly different, parameters reflect the differences between walks: the veering due to not holding the straight-ahead direction and the tendency to over- or undershoot turns within one walk. Thus, the main source of directional errors in LDs is not veering on a segment or a consistent over- or undershooting of turns, but the inability to accurately perform a desired turn. In animals, a comparable inability has been demonstrated: frogs with unilateral lesions of the vestibular nerve are unable to turn toward a prey as desired, they largely overshoot their target (King and Straka, 1998). Since a comparable overshoot is not found in escape turns, the authors conclude that in frogs vestibular information plays a role only if accuracy of turning is required.

The differences between normals and LDs thus suggest that the semicircular canals are an important structure facilitating accurate turning around corners and also for maintaining a straight-ahead direction. This does not, in our view, contradict findings on normal subjects exhibiting curved trajectories after adaptation to walking on a rotating platform (Gordon et al., 1995). The semicircular canals are, in our experiment, neither required for walking straight nor to perform turns, but they aid in holding a direction or turning toward a goal. This suggests that proprioceptive and vestibular signals are averaged in some way to produce a more accurate estimate of turning. If one signal is missing, the noise level increases but not the mean outcome. Such averaging of proprioceptive and vestibular signals has been proposed, based on the results of perception of afterrotation after different paradigms involving passive turning, active turning, and walking in place on a rotating disc (Howard et al., 1998). Also, experiments on the perception of head and trunk rotation in different conditions showed that head-on-trunk and trunk-on-ground signals together already provide reliable estimates of head rotation (Mergner et al., 1991).

LDs show larger variations of over- or undershooting turns than normals, but on the average, they seem to be more careful about walking the required distance. Normals, in contrast, show smaller direction errors. Thus, as shown before (Glasauer et al., 1994), the vestibular system is apparently not involved in the computation of distance during active walking, but it enhances the ability to change the direction of locomotion as desired, as also suggested by a study on walking blindfolded along a circular trajectory (Takei et al., 1996). Nevertheless, since linear accelerations during walking can be taken into account by healthy subjects, as shown while walking on a rotating platform (Mittelstaedt and Glasauer, 1991), other sensors for linear acceleration such as the somatic graviceptors (Mittelstaedt and Mittelstaedt, 1996) may be involved.

Another question—which cannot be answered with the present data—is raised by the differences between predicted and actually found distribution of normals at corners 1 and 2. Do different mechanisms govern walking to a previously seen location and walking back to the starting point? Such a difference might be expected if an additional homing mechanism were used to walk back toward corner 3 (the starting point).

Discussion

The two sets of results presented in this study confirm the importance of head motion control during the generation of locomotor trajectories in humans (as suggested by Pozzo and Berthoz, 1990). The first section concerns how head orientation anticipates the future walking direction during steering tasks. This behavior demonstrates the capacity for the CNS to predict future directions (or curvature variations) of the locomotor path. It has been shown that this anticipation is first performed at the level of head and gaze movements. It was noted that mechanical factors might account for the high frequency oscillations related to stepping. The importance of directional signals has also been assessed during tasks in which human subjects had to walk along a memorized path. Labyrinthine-defective subjects showed significantly greater direction errors than normal subjects, revealing a likely role of vestibular information in the estimation of the direction of locomotor trajectory.

The Head Direction (HD) Cell System
The HD cell system likely belongs to a global network concerned with the representations of place and heading for navigation (McNaughton et al., 1996). Taube (1998) proposed that the anticipatory mechanism of head direction described here might be associated with the neurophysiological observation (in rats) of an anticipatory nature of head direction cells responses (see chapter 1 by Sharp for more information). Sensory inputs cannot easily account for such an anticipatory signal (Taube et al., 1996); rather (in rats), it is suggested that the motor efference copy inputs projecting to the head direction cells are related to this anticipatory mechanism. A motor-related input (rather than afferent vestibular or proprioceptive signals) could be involved in generating anticipatory head orientation, although we cannot infer whether this is achieved via HD cells (which have not yet been demonstrated in humans). However, head direction cells were found in the primate pre-subiculum (Robertson et al., 1999; see chapter 14 by Rolls). While the role of vestibular system in the generation of HD cell activity is still debated (Brown et al., 2002), there is evidence for this, since lesion studies showed that the directional responses are abolished in rats after an inactivation of labyrinthine inputs (Stackman and Taube, 1997). In our study with labyrinthine-defective subjects, the deficit in the evaluation of direction led to an altered perception and reproduction of their head angular movements in space, as shown in the turning task at the corners of the triangle. Assuming that these patients memorize correctly the previously seen "trajectory" (that is, they have a good representation of the intended path), the semicircular canals are of a crucial importance in holding a direction or turning towards a goal in the absence of vision. The fact that these patients correct their

deficits when vision is available is consistent with the fact that visual cues are the most reliable sensory input for estimating the motion direction (Kennedy et al., 2003). It is interesting to determine whether this deficit is mediated by vestibular-induced impairments of HD cells responses (if they actually exist in humans) or via other pathways. Repeating these experiments in neurological patients with damage to these respective pathways would test this. The following section presents evidence for possible neural substrates representing the spatial orientation of the head in humans.

Functional Imagery Studies of Spatial Orientation

Approaches using imagery methods (MRI or PET) combined with psychological tests provided new insights about brain mechanisms that permit humans to navigate in a given environment. Two types of navigational strategies are generally presented in the literature: they emphasize either a survey (or allocentric) or a route (or egocentric) processing. The first strategy is well illustrated by a subject trying to imagine a map of the environment and to mentally visualise the route on this map. On the other hand, while using a route strategy, subjects can try to remember the sequence of angular and linear displacements relative to visual landmarks as well as other cues or actions associated with the route. Both neurological lesions and imagery studies have allowed the localization of neuroanatomical areas, which are required or activated while subjects use one or the other strategy during navigation. Recently, Aguirre et al. (1999) reviewed this literature and proposed a taxonomy accounting for several spatial disorders present in patients with brain lesions. These authors emphasized the difficulty in identifying clearly the nature of the information (allocentric or egocentric) used by the subjects in order to solve a given navigational problem, as well as in localizing the associated recruitment of neuroanatomical structures during engagement of particular navigational strategies. However, evidence from an imagery study in humans showed that distinct cortical areas are activated when processing spatial information encoded either in allocentric or egocentric coordinates (Galati et al., 2000). Indeed, the right hemisphere-based frontoparietal network has been identified to be principally involved in egocentric processing while only a subset of these regions is activated during object-based (allocentric) processing. Lambrey et al. (2003) asked control and unilateral mediotemporal lobes resection patients (LTL or RTL) to navigate in a virtual environment and to memorize both the traveled path and the type (a chair, a tree, a man . . .) and location of seven landmarks. Their results showed that LTL patients were significantly impaired in the memory of the sequence of landmarks, and that RTL patients had an intermediate performance between the control group and RTL patients. Subsequently the authors proposed a distinct role of either the left or right mediotemporal lobes that would be activated, respectively, when humans use either a route or a survey strategy during navigation in their environment.

Moreover, a study by Iaria et al. (2003) using functional magnetic resonance imaging provided some evidence for the existence of a shift in the human brain activity when subjects change their strategies for navigating in space. When subjects used spatial landmarks to navigate in a virtual environment, the authors reported increased activity in the right hippocampus. At a later phase of training, the same subjects used a non-spatial strategy to navigate in the virtual environment, resulting in an increased activity of the caudate nucleus only. Other subjects who showed increased activity of the right hippocampus, both early and late, in training were found to have always used spatial landmarks to navigate. The study of Iaria et al. demonstrated the first direct evidence for the existence of plasticity in the cognitive strategies and in the corresponding activation of brain substrates in humans during spatial navigation.

Aguirre et al. (1999) proposed the term "heading disorientation" to illustrate the case of patients who are both able to recognize salient landmarks (which prove useful for normal subjects for spatial orientation) and to use route knowledge, but are unable to derive directional information from the landmarks they recognize (Takahashi et al., 1997). This inability reveals their loss of "sense of exocentric direction or heading within their environment" (Aguirre et al., 1999, p. 1620). In comparison with the activation of either the left or right mediotemporal lobes for the two types of navigational strategies (route vs survey), it is tempting to propose a distinct activation of a specific brain area (such as the retrosplenial or posterior cingulate region that is damaged in these patients) as responsible for a sense of direction in humans. However, the possible role of the retrosplenial region in heading perception remains rather speculative, since such deficits in spatial orientation are not systematically observed in patients suffering from retrosplenial amnesia (Rudge and Warrington, 1991). Thus, it would be judicious to limit our conclusions to affirming the existence of a large directional repertoire in humans allowing them to anticipate future changes in their travel direction. Indeed, it is not necessary to infer the existence of distinct corresponding neuroanatomical regions; further studies are required to test this hypothesis. Besides, it should be noted that the dissociated control between distance and direction presented earlier in this chapter also reinforces the existence of such a distinct directional control in human locomotion. In a review paper, Burgess et al. (2002) emphasize the role of the right hippocampus in memory tasks requiring allocentric processing of spatial location. These authors evoked a potential interaction of this processing with egocentric representations found in the parietal lobe. This interaction might consist of "translation of stored (hippocampal) allocentric information into the (parietal) egocentric representations required to guide movement or to support imagery of retrieval products" (p. 636). These propositions seem to be confirmed by a recent study of Ekstrom et al. (2003), which investigated the cellular networks underlying human spatial navigation. Burgess et al. also discussed the potential role of self-motion in the orientation of the spatial representation of an environment (i.e., according to the authors, this spatial representation can be characterized by the relative locations of objects in the environment but needs also to be correctly oriented with respect to that environment) and propose that idiothetic signals can be used to update this orientation, summarizing their proposals by suggesting the existence of an automatic process that updates internal representations to accommodate the consequences of action.

In line with the proposals of Burgess et al. (2002), we suggest here the necessary distinction between purely motor strategies and cognitive ones: the first strategies characterize a modulation of the locomotor activity considered here as local processes, while the second constitute global strategies that allow subjects to navigate in the environment. These two strategies might interact at some level in order to control the actual movement with respect to the spatial representation of the behavioral goal (in a comparable manner with the interaction between allocentric processing and egocentric representations required to guide movement, as proposed by Burgess). In our study, the anticipation of the future walking direction by head motion underpins the capacity for the subjects to correctly perceive and use (with or without vision) this future direction. Thus, a spatial cognitive simulation of the upcoming direction changes (or curvature changes) of the locomotor path may be combined with the actual head movement (motor inputs primarily, then associated with sensory information) in order to anticipate the future walking direction.

Acknowledgments

Some of the research reported here was supported by a grant from the French Ministry of Research (Programme Cognitique thème Action).

References

Aguirre GK, D'Esposito M (1999) Topographical disorientation: a synthesis and taxonomy. Brain 122(9): 1613–1628.

Amorim MA, Loomis JM, Fukusima SS (1998) Reproduction of object shape is more accurate without the continued availability of visual information. Perception 27: 69–86.

Beall AC, Loomis JM (1996) Visual control of steering without course information. Perception 25: 481–494.

Beritoff JS (1965) Neural mechanisms of higher vertebrate behavior. Transl.: WT Liberson. Boston: Little, Brown and Company.

Berthoz A, Amorim MA, Glasauer S, Grasso R, Takei Y, Viaud-Delmon I (1999) Dissociation between distance and direction during locomotor navigation. In RG Golledge, ed., Wayfinding Behavior Cognitive Mapping and Other Spatial Processes. Baltimore: Johns Hopkins University Press, pp. 328–348.

Bertin RJ, Israël I, Lappe M (2000) Perception of two-dimensional, simulated ego-motion trajectories from optic flow. Vis Res 40: 2951–2971.

Bles W, de Jong JM, de Wit G (1984) Somatosensory compensation for loss of labyrinthine function. Acta Oto-Laryngol 97(3–4): 213–221.

Bove M, Diverio M, Pozzo T, Schieppati M (2001) Neck muscle vibration disrupts steering of locomotion. J Appl Physiol 91: 581–588.

Boyadjian A, Marin L, Danion F (1999) Veering in human locomotion: the role of the effectors. Neurosci Lett 265: 21–24.

Brown JE, Yates BJ, Taube JS (2002) Does the vestibular system contribute to head direction cell activity in the rat? Physiol Behav 77(4–5): 743–748.

Burgess N, Maguire EA, O'Keefe J (2002) The human hippocampus and spatial and episodic memory. Neuron 35(4): 625–641.

Caminiti R, Johnson PB, Galli C, Ferraina S, Burnod Y (1991) Making arm movements within different parts of space: the premotor and motor cortical representation of a coordinate system for reaching to visual targets. J Neurosci 11(5): 1182–1197.

Chieffi S, Allport DA (1997) Independent coding of target distance and direction in visuo-spatial working memory. Psychol Res 60(4): 244–250.

Courtine G, Schieppati M (2003) Human walking along a curved path. I. Body trajectory, segment orientation and the effect of vision. Eur J Neurosci 18: 177–190.

Crowell JA (1997) Testing the Perrone and Stone (1994) model of heading estimation. Vis Res 37: 1653–1671.

Crowell JA, Banks MS, Shenoy KV, Andersen RA (1998) Visual self-motion perception during head turns. Nat Neurosci 1(8): 732–737.

Ekstrom AD, Kahana MJ, Caplan JB, Fields TA, Isham EA, Newman EL, Fried I (2003) Cellular networks underlying human spatial navigation. Nature 425: 184–188.

Fajen BR, Warren WH (2000) Go with the flow. Trends Cogn Sci 4(10): 369–370.

Fujita N, Klatzky RL, Loomis JM (1993) The encoding-error model of pathway completion without vision. Geog Anal 25, 4: 295–314.

Galati G, Lobel E, Vallar G, Berthoz A, Pizzamiglio L, Le Bihan D (2000) The neural basis of egocentric and allocentric coding of space in humans: a functional magnetic resonance study. Exp Brain Res 133: 156–164.

Georgopoulos AP, DeLong MR, Crutcher MD (1983) Relations between parameters of step-tracking movements and single cell discharge in the globus pallidus and subthalamic nucleus of the behaving monkey. J Neurosci 3(8): 1586–1598.

Georgopoulos AP, Kalaska JF, Caminiti R, Massey JT (1982) On the relations between the direction of two-dimensional arm movements and cell discharge in primate motor cortex. J Neurosci 2(11): 1527–1537.

Gibson JJ (1958) Visually controlled locomotion and visual orientation in animals. Brit J Psych 49: 182–194.

Glasauer S, Amorim MA, Bloomberg JJ, Reschke MF, Peters BT, Smith SL, Berthoz A (1995) Spatial orientation during locomotion following space flight. Acta Astronautica 8, 12: 423–431.

Glasauer S, Amorim MA, Viaud-Delmon I, Berthoz A (2002) Differential effects of labyrinthine dysfunction on distance and direction during blindfolded walking on a triangular path. Exp Brain Res 145: 489–497.

Glasauer S, Amorim MA, Vitte E, Berthoz A (1994) Goal-directed linear locomotion in normal and labyrinthine-defective subjects. Exp Brain Res 98: 323–335.

Gordon CR, Fletcher WA, Melvill Jones G, Block EW (1995) Adaptive plasticity in the control of locomotor trajectory. Exp Brain Res 102: 540–545.

Grasso R, Assaiante C, Prevost P, Berthoz A (1998a) Development of anticipatory orienting strategies during locomotor tasks in children. Neurosci Biobehav Rev 22(4): 533–539.

Grasso R, Glasauer S, Takei Y, Berthoz A (1996) The predictive brain: anticipatory control of head direction for the steering of locomotion. NeuroReport 7: 1170–1174.

Grasso R, Prevost P, Ivanenko YP, Berthoz A (1998b) Eye-head coordination for the steering of locomotion in humans: an anticipatory synergy. Neurosci Lett 253(2): 115–118.

Harris JM, Bonas W (2003) Optic flow and scene structure do not always contribute to the control of human walking. Vis Res 42: 1619–1626.

Hollands MA, Sorensen KL, Patla AE (2001) Effects of head immobilization on the coordination and control of head and body reorientation and translation during steering. Exp Brain Res 140: 223–233.

Howard IP, Zacher JE, Allison RS (1998) Post-rotatory nystagmus and turning sensations after active and passive turning. J Vest Res 8: 299–312.

Iaria G, Petrides M, Dagher A, Pike B, Bohbot VD (2003) Cognitive strategies dependent on the hippocampus and caudate nucleus in human navigation: variability and change with practice. J Neurosci 23: 5945–5952.

Imai T, Moore ST, Raphan T, Cohen B (2001) Interaction of body, head, and eyes during walking and turning. Exp Brain Res 136: 1–18.

Ivanenko YP, Grasso R, Israël I, Berthoz A (1997a) Spatial orientation in humans: perception of angular whole-body displacements in two-dimensional trajectories. Exp Brain Res 117: 419–427.

Ivanenko YP, Grasso R, Israël I, Berthoz A (1997b) The contribution of otoliths and semicircular canals to the perception of two dimensional passive whole-body motion in humans. J Phys (Lond) 502: 223–233.

Kennedy PM, Carlsen AN, Inglis JT, Chow R, Franks IM, Chua R (2003) Relative contributions of visual and vestibular information on the trajectory of human gait. Exp Brain Res 153(1): 113–117.

King JR, Straka H (1998) Effects of vestibular nerve lesions on orientation turning in the leopard frog, *Rana pipiens*. Biol Bull 195(2): 193–194.

Kurata K (1993) Premotor cortex of monkeys: set- and movement-related activity reflecting amplitude and direction of wrist movements. J Neurophys 69(1): 187–200.

Lambrey S, Samson S, Dupont S, Baulac M, Berthoz A (2003) Reference frames and cognitive strategies during navigation: is the left hippocampal formation involved in the sequential aspects of route memory? International Congress Series 1250: 261–274.

Lappe M, Bremmer F, Van Den Berg AV (1999) Perception of self-motion from visual flow. Trends Cogn Sci 3(9): 329–336.

Lappe M, Rauschecker JP (1994) Heading detection from optic flow. Nature 369: 712–713.

McIntyre J, Stratta F, Lacquaniti F (1998) Short-term memory for reaching to visual targets: psychophysical evidence for body-centered reference frames. J Neurosci 18(20): 8423–8435.

Mcnaughton BL, Barnes CA, Gerrard JL, Gothard K, Jung MW, Knierim JJ, Kudrimoti H, Qin Y, Skaggs WE, Suster M, Weaver KL (1996) Deciphering the hippocampal polyglot: the hippocampus as a path integration system. J Exp Biol 199: 173–185.

Mergner T, Siebold C, Schweigart G, Becker W (1991) Human perception of horizontal trunk and head rotation in space during vestibular and neck stimulation. Exp Brain Res 85: 389–404.

Millar S (1999) Veering re-visited: noise and posture cues in walking without sight. Perception 28: 765–780.

Mittelstaedt ML, Glasauer S (1991) Idiothetic navigation in gerbils and humans. Zool Jb Physiol 95: 427–435.

Mittelstaedt ML, Mittelstaedt H (1996) The influence of otoliths and somatic graviceptors on angular velocity estimation. J Vest Res 6: 355–366.

Patla AE (1997) Understanding the roles of vision in the control of human locomotion. Gait Posture 5: 54–69.

Patla AE, Vickers JN (2003) How far ahead do we look when required to step on specific locations in the travel path during locomotion? Exp Brain Res 148: 133–138.

Perrone JA, Stone LS (1994) A model of self-motion estimation within primate extrastriate cortex. Vis Res 34(21): 2917–2938.

Perrone JA, Stone LS (1998) Emulating the visual receptive-field properties of MST neurons with a template model of heading estimation. J Neurosci 18(15): 5958–5975.

Potegal M (1982) Vestibular and neostriatal contributions to spatial orientations. In Spatial Abilities: Development and Physiological Foundations (New York: Academic Press).

Pozzo T, Berthoz A, Lefort L (1990) Head stabilization during various tasks in humans. I. Normal subjects. Exp Brain Res 82: 97–106.

Pozzo T, Berthoz A, Lefort L, Vitte E (1991) Head stabilization during various tasks in humans. II. Patients with bilateral peripheral vestibular deficits. Exp Brain Res 85: 208–217.

Regan D, Beverley KI (1982) How do we avoid confounding the direction we are looking and the direction we are moving? Science 215(4529): 194–196.

Rieser JJ, Ashmead DH, Talor CR, Youngquist GA (1990) Visual perception and guidance of locomotion without vision to previously seen targets. J Mot Behav 19: 675–689.

Rieser JJ, Pick HL, Ashmead DH, Garing AE (1995) Calibration of human locomotion and models of perceptual-motor organization. J Exp Psychol Hum Percep Perf 21: 480–497.

Robertson RG, Rolls ET, Georges-François P, Panzeri S (1999) Head direction cells in the primate presubiculum. Hippocampus 9: 206–219.

Rudge P, Warrington EK (1991) Selective impairment of memory and visual perception in splenial tumours. Brain 114 (Pt 1B): 349–360.

Schubert M, Bohner C, Berger W, Sprundel M, Duysens JE (2003) The role of vision in maintaining heading direction: effects of changing gaze and optic flow on human gait. Exp Brain Res 150(2): 163–173.

Soechting JF, Flanders M (1989) Sensorimotor representations for pointing to targets in three-dimensional space. J Neurophys 62: 582–594.

Solomon D, Cohen B (1992) Stabilization of gaze during circular locomotion in light. I. Compensatory head and eye nystagmus in the running monkey. J Neurophys 67(5): 1146–1157.

Stackman RW, Taube JS (1997) Firing properties of head direction cells in the rat anterior thalamic nucleus: dependence on vestibular input. J Neurosci 17: 4349–4358.

Stone LS, Perrone JA (1997) Human heading estimation during visually simulated curvilinear motion. Vis Res 37: 573–590.

Takahashi N, Kawamura M, Shiota J, Kasahata N, Hirayama K (1997) Pure topographic disorientation due to right retrosplenial lesion. Neurol 49: 464–469.

Takei Y, Grasso R, Amorim MA, Berthoz A (1997) Circular trajectory formation during blind locomotion: a test for path integration and motor memory. Exp Brain Res 115: 361–368.

Takei Y, Grasso R, Berthoz A (1996) Quantitative analysis of human walking trajectory on a circular path in darkness. Brain Res Bull 40: 491–496.

Taube JS (1998) Head direction cells and the neurophysiological basis for a sense of direction. Prog Neurobiol 55(3): 225–256.

Taube JS, Goodridge JP, Golob EJ, Dudchenko PA, Stackman RW (1996) Processing the head direction cell signal: a review and commentary. Brain Res Bull 40(5–6): 477–486.

Taube JS, Muller RU, Ranck JBJ (1990) Head-direction cells recorded from the postsubiculum in freely moving rats. I. Description and quantitative analysis. J Neurosci 10(2): 420–435.

Thomson JA (1983) Is continous visual monitoring necessary in visually guided locomotion? J Exp Psychol Hum Percep Perf 9(3): 427–443.

Vallis LA, Mcfadyen BJ (2003) Locomotor adjustments for circumvention of an obstacle in the travel path. Exp Brain Res 152(3): 409–414.

Vallis LA, Patla AE, Adkin AL (2001) Control of steering in the presence of unexpected head yaw movements. Influence on sequencing of subtasks. Exp Brain Res 138: 128–134.

Vieilledent S, Kosslyn SM, Berthoz A, Giraudo MD (2003) Does mental simulation of following a path improve navigation performance without vision? Brain Res Cogn Brain Res 16: 238–249.

Viviani P, Stucchi N (1989) The effect of movement velocity on form perception: geometric illusions in dynamic displays. Percept Psychophys 46, 3: 266–274.

Viviani P, Stucchi N (1992) Biological movements look uniform: evidence of motor-perceptual interactions. J Exp Psychol Hum Percep Perf 18, 3: 603–623.

Vuillerme N, Nougier V, Camicioli R (2002) Veering in human locomotion: modulatory effect of attention. Neurosci Lett 331: 175–178.

Wallace DG, Hines DJ, Pellis SM, Whishaw IQ (2002) Vestibular information is required for dead reckoning in the rat. J Neurosci 22: 10009–10017.

Wan HS, Touretzky DS, Redish AD (1994) Towards a computational theory of rat navigation. In Proceedings of the 1993 Connectionist models summer school. New York: Lawrence Erlbaum, pp. 11–19.

Wann JP, Land M (2000) Steering with or without the flow: is the retrieval of heading necessary? Trends Cogn Sci 4: 319–324.

Wann JP, Wilkie RM (2003) Eye-movements aid the control of locomotion. J Vision 3: 1–9.

Warren WH, Hannon DJ (1988) Direction of self-motion is perceived from optic flow. Nature 336: 162–163.

Warren WH, Kay BA, Zosh WD, Duchon AP, Sahuc S (2001) Optic flow is used to control human walking. Nat Neurosci 4(2): 213–216.

Wexler M, Panerai F, Lamouret I, Droulez J (2001) Self-motion and the perception of stationary objects. Nature 409: 85–88.

Appendix: Formal Description of the Model

The arrival point according to the model can be written in Cartesian coordinates as the vector $\underline{a}_3$ from the starting point to the endpoint of the walk (see figure 17.3):

$$a_3 = D(\varphi_1') \cdot [l_1' + D(\varphi_2') \cdot (l_2' + D(\varphi_3') \cdot l_3')] \cdot n_0 \qquad (17.1)$$

with $\underline{n}_0$ being the normalized vector of the initial straight ahead direction. $\varphi_i' = (1 + \beta_0 + \beta_i)\varphi_i + \alpha_i$ is the direction walked depending on the desired direction φ_i and $l_i' = (1 + d_0 + d_i)l_i$ the distance walked depending on the desired distance l_i at segment i. $D(\varphi)$ denotes the rotation matrix. Here, we have assumed zero mean of errors for simplicity. Several predictions of the model can be tested by determining the standard deviations (SD) and correlation coefficients (r) of the distance and direction errors for each segment. The model parameters are computed from these variables by resolving the following equations. The variances of distance errors are given as

$$C\{\Delta l_i^2\} = l_i^2 \cdot (\sigma_{d0}^2 + \sigma_{di}^2) \qquad (17.2)$$

with C denoting the covariance and σ^2 being the variance of the respective parameter according to the model. The correlation coefficients for distance errors are

$$r = \frac{\sigma_{d0}^2}{\sigma_{d0}^2 + \sigma_{di}^2} \qquad (17.3)$$

Hence, if only systematic distance errors d_0 occur, the correlation coefficient between segments would equal unity: a subject systematically overshooting the first segment by 10% would also overshoot segments 2 and 3 by 10%, thus resulting in correlated distance errors. Deviations from such a perfect correlation are modeled by the error d_i which changes from segment to segment.

For direction errors, the variances are

$$C\{\Delta \varphi_i^2\} = \varphi_i^2 \cdot (\varphi_{\beta 0}^2 + \sigma_{\beta i}^2) + \sigma_{\alpha i}^2 \qquad (17.4)$$

As can be seen for segment 1 where the preceding angle of turn φ_1 is zero, the variance reduces to the variance of the veer $\sigma_{\alpha i}^2$. The variances of segments 2 and 3 are expected to increase with the angle of turn φ_i. More specifically, it follows that the difference of the variance at segment i and the variance of the veering is proportional to the angle turned prior to segment i:

$$C'\{\Delta\varphi_i^2\} = (C\{\Delta\varphi_i^2\} - \sigma_{\alpha i}^2)\big/\varphi_i^2 = \sigma_{\beta 0}^2 + \sigma_{\beta i}^2 \qquad (17.4\text{a})$$

This new variance $C'\{\Delta\varphi_i^2\}$ should be equal for segments 2 and 3; this provides a test for whether the data fit our hypotheses on direction errors (see below).

The correlation between the direction of walk at segment 2 and segment 3 is

$$r = \frac{\varphi_2 \cdot \varphi_3 \cdot \sigma_{\beta 0}^2}{\sqrt{(\varphi_2^2 \cdot (\sigma_{\beta 0}^2 + \sigma_{\beta i}^2) + \sigma_{\alpha i}^2) \cdot (\varphi_3^2 \cdot (\sigma_{\beta 0}^2 + \sigma_{\beta i}^2) + \sigma_{\beta i}^2)}} \qquad (17.5)$$

V THEORETICAL STUDIES AND NEURAL NETWORK MODELS OF THE HEAD DIRECTION SYSTEM

18 Attractor Network Models of Head Direction Cells

David S. Touretzky

Head Direction and Short-Term Memory

While the head direction (HD) system appears to play an important part in rodents' spatial representation and navigation abilities, it can also be understood as a short-term memory system. Rats keep track of their heading with respect to some reference direction, even when directional cues are not available, such as when navigating in the dark. Drift in the alignment of the HD system when rats forage in a cylinder in the dark is evidence for this memory function, because the system does not drift right away, but only after several minutes of foraging, presumably as a result of cumulative error in integrating angular velocity (Knierim et al., 1993; McNaughton et al., 1994; Goodridge et al., 1998). If drift were never observed, one might suspect that the animal still had access to some sort of sensory cue indicating its direction.

Short-term memory mechanisms have been proposed for numerous brain areas. Regions in parietal cortex appear to store the coordinates of visual targets to which a monkey must make a saccade (Duhamel et al., 1992), while regions in frontal cortex appear to be involved in remembering objects in a delayed stimulus discrimination task (Deco and Rolls, 2003). The maintenance of eye position in goldfish is another example of a short-term neural memory mechanism (Aksay et al., 2001). A single mathematical formalism, *attractor dynamics*, has been applied to model all of these memory mechanisms and more.

This chapter presents the basic concepts of attractor neural networks, focusing on their application to modeling the head direction system. I will keep the mathematics simple and concentrate on how one can construct actual models, in Matlab, to gain hands-on experience with this important class of dynamical system.

Attractors and Attractor Networks

A *dynamical system* is a mathematical system whose state evolves over time. The state is an N-dimensional vector, and its evolution is described by a system of differential equations that are functions of the current state plus some external input. Formally, we can represent the state vector $\langle z_1(t), \ldots, z_N(t) \rangle$ by the variable $\bar{z}(t)$, where t denotes time. Differential equations $dz_i(t)/dt$ describe how the vector components change, as a function of $\bar{z}$ and the external input X_i. The rate of evolution of element z_i is governed by a time constant τ_i. Thus,

$$\tau_i \frac{dz_i}{dt} = f_i(\bar{z}, X_i)$$

This is a very general definition, with no constraints on the trajectory through state space that $\bar{z}$ can undergo. We will now impose some. For a dynamical system to be useful as a model of short-term memory, it should have a set of *stable states* to which it returns if slightly perturbed. These stable states are called *attractors*, and serve as the memories of the system. Whenever the system drifts away from one of its stable states due to noise or some other source of error, its behavior should bring it back to a stable state. Such a system is said to exhibit *attractor dynamics*.

The simplest type of attractor architecture utilizes point attractors, meaning the stable states are discrete points well separated from each other in state space. Point attractors are useful for modeling certain kinds of associative memory tasks, where the subject has to memorize a set of items and then retrieve one based on a partial cue. However, for modeling spatial location information, continuous attractors are preferable. These have an infinite number of stable states lying in a one- or two-dimensional subspace of the state space $\bar{z}$. For example, the eye position system can be modeled using a line attractor (Seung, 1996), meaning the stable states lie on a one-dimensional manifold embedded in the N-dimensional state space. The HD system is modeled using a ring attractor (Skaggs et al., 1995; Zhang, 1996), which is also one-dimensional but has a circular structure. Two-dimensional attractor models have been proposed for the superior colliculus (Droulez and Berthoz, 1991), hippocampus (Samsonovich and McNaughton, 1997), and motor cortex (Lukashin et al., 1996).

Attractor dynamics can be implemented in a neural network by identifying the state components $z_i(t)$ with the outputs of individual neuron-like units. Calling such a system a "neural network" means that the functions f_i computed by these units take a certain simple form. We will assume that a neuron's output decays exponentially toward zero in the absence of excitatory inputs; the $-z_i$ term in the following equation establishes this exponential decay. We will also assume that a neuron's net activation, a weighted linear combination of its inputs, is fed through a nonlinear function to produce its output. One of the simplest nonlinear functions used in neural networks is the semilinear threshold function, denoted $[x]_+$. It outputs x when $x > 0$, and otherwise outputs 0. We will further simplify things by assuming that all the z_i neurons use the same time constant, τ_E. Thus, we have

$$\tau_E \frac{dz_i(t)}{dt} = -z_i(t) + [netact]_+$$

We define neuron z_i's net activation to be a linear combination, using a weight matrix w_{ij}, of afferent inputs from all the z_j's, plus a constant inhibitory bias γ_E, a dynamic global inhibition term $u(t)$, and an external input $X_i(t)$. With coupling constants w_{EE} and w_{EI} governing the strength of recurrent excitation and inhibition, respectively (figure 18.1), this gives:

$$\tau_E \frac{dz_i(t)}{dt} = -z_i(t) + \left[\gamma_E + w_{EE}\sum_j w_{ij}z_j(t) + w_{EI} \cdot u(t) + X_i(t)\right]_+ \quad (18.1)$$

The stable states of this network take a specific form: they are bump-like patterns of activity across a set of contiguous elements, as shown in figure 18.2. Not all bump shapes are stable. But given a stable bump, different memories can be represented by shifting the bump through different locations in the array of z_i's.

What properties are necessary to ensure that a network has stable attractor states? First, the neurons should be saturating nonlinear functions. The semilinear threshold function $[x]_+$ satisfies this requirement, but other saturating nonlinear functions may also be used, such as tanh, or the sigmoid function $(1 + \exp(-x))^{-1}$.

Second, the coupling strengths w_{ij} between neurons must support the stable states, i.e., in order to form bumps, neurons should have strong excitatory connections to nearby

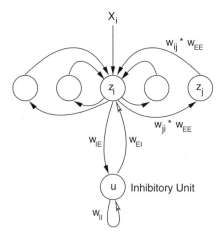

Figure 18.1
Connections to and from unit z_i in the network defined by equations 18.1 to 18.3.

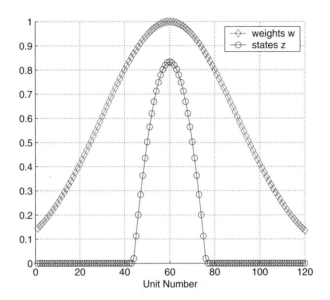

Figure 18.2
Top line shown the weights $w_{60,j}$ of the recurrent connections feeding into the 60th unit out of 120. Bottom line shows the states z_i of all units when the activity bump is centered over the 60th unit.

neighbors and weaker connections to more distant neighbors. We can achieve this by making the connection strength be a Gaussian function of the distance between units i and j. Assume N units organized in a ring, and let d_{ij} be the distance between units i and j on the ring. Then $d_{ii} = 0$ and $d_{ij} \leq N/2$ for all i, j. The *normalized* distance between two units $n_{ij} = d_{ij}/(N/2)$ ranges between 0 and 1. A suitable Gaussian weighting function that is independent of N is:

$$w_{ij} = \exp(-n_{ij}^2/2\sigma^2) \tag{18.2}$$

We use $\sigma = 0.5$, along with specific choices for the coupling constants discussed below, to give a bump width of approximately 25% of the ring. This matches the tuning curve widths of head direction cells, which are on the order of 90°–100°. Use of a different nonlinear function, such as tanh, would require a change to the standard deviation σ and other parameters in order to maintain the desired bump width. The shape of the bump is affected by, but not identical to, the shape of the recurrent excitatory weights. In this particular example, the shape of the weights is considerably broader than that of the resulting activity bump, but this need not always be the case (Compte et al., 2000).

The third condition for stability is that there be an appropriate source of dynamic inhibition to prevent runaway activation of all the z_i elements. We introduce an inhibitory interneuron with output $u(t)$ that receives excitation from all the exitatory neurons and makes inhibitory projections back to them and to itself. The inhibitory neuron is also governed by a differential equation, but with a different bias term γ_I and coupling constants w_{IE} and w_{II}, and a faster time constant $\tau_I < \tau_E$.

$$\tau_I \frac{du(t)}{dt} = -u(t) + \left[\gamma_I + w_{IE}\sum_i z_i(t) + w_{II} \cdot u(t)\right]_+ \tag{18.3}$$

It may seem odd to have only a single inhibitory neuron, but this illustrates the abstract nature of neural network models. If there were many inhibitory neurons, each receiving input from a random subset of the excitatory z_i's and projecting back to another random subset, their net effect would be the same as a single inhibitory neuron with uniform connectivity. For theories of the head direction system that make no distinctions among the inhibitory neurons found in those areas, one such neuron will suffice.

The fourth condition for stability is that there are constraints on the ratio of excitatory to inhibitory connection strengths that must be satisfied. These are expressed in terms of the coupling constants w_{EE}, w_{EI}, w_{IE}, and w_{II} and the time constants τ_E and τ_I. The details for the $N = 1$ neuron case, where the network consists of a single excitatory neuron plus one inhibitory neuron, are given by Tsodyks et al. (1997). For a more general solution, I'll simply give parameter values that have been found to work, and show how the model can be made independent of the number of neurons N over a wide range of values.

Computer simulations of dynamical systems are of necessity discrete approximations. The discrete approximations to the differential equations (18.1) and (18.3) using Euler's method, the simplest possible integration method, are:

$$z_i(t + \Delta t) = z_i(t) + \left(-z_i(t) + \left[\gamma_E + w_{EE}\sum_{j=1}^{N} w_{ij}z_j(t) + w_{EI} \cdot u(t) + X_i(t)\right]_+\right) \cdot \frac{\Delta t}{\tau_E} \tag{18.4}$$

$$u(t + \Delta t) = u(t) + \left(-u(t) + \left[\gamma_I + w_{IE}\sum_{j=1}^{N} z_i(t) + w_{II} \cdot u(t)\right]_+\right) \cdot \frac{\Delta t}{\tau_I} \tag{18.5}$$

More accurate integration methods, such as Runge-Kutta integration, could also be used. From equations (18.4) and (18.5), or their Runge-Kutta equivalents, it is straightforward to derive executable code.

Matlab Implementation of a Ring Attractor

We begin by defining N, the number of units in the attractor ring. We'll use 120 units as an example. The farthest distance between any two units on the ring is equal to the largest integer less than or equal to $N/2$.

```
N = 120;    halfN = floor(N/2);
```

Now we can calculate the matrix of distances d_{ij} between all pairs of units i and j around the ring. Note that $0 \leq d_{ij} \leq N/2$.

```
dij = abs(repmat(1:N,N,1) - repmat((1:N)',1,N));
dij(dij > halfN) = N - dij(dij > halfN);
```

If the Matlab code above seems obscure, trying out various subexpressions on the computer will make the meaning clear. We next compute the normalized distances n_{ij}, where $0 \leq n_{ij} \leq 1$:

```
nij = dij / halfN;
```

The weight between two units should be a Gaussian function of the distance between them. Because we're using normalized distance, the weight function scales automatically for any number of units N.

```
sigma = 0.5;
wij = exp(-nij.^2/(2*sigma^2));
```

All that remains is to fill in some parameter values. Note that the recurrent coupling constant w_{EE} and the coupling strength to the inhibitory unit w_{IE} must scale inversely with the number of neurons N in order to maintain consistent levels of excitatory input to each unit, independent of the ring size.

```
wEE = 45/N;          wIE = 60/N;
wEI = -6;            wII = -1;
gammaE = -1.5;       gammaI = -7.5;
tauE = 0.005;        tauI = 0.00025;

         deltaT = 0.0001;
```

For efficiency, we multiply the w_{ij} matrix by the coupling constant w_{EE} once, saving the result as w_{EEij}, so that we don't have to do it repeatedly with each update of $\bar{z}$. We can initialize $\bar{z}(0)$ to a crude bump shape by using one row of w_{EEij}, and the initial inhibition level $u(0)$ can be set to a value close to its stable state value. The external inputs X_i are initially zero, as is the time, t.

```
wEEij = wEE * wij;      % precompute scaled weight matrix
z = wEEij(:,halfN);     % initialize to a bump shape
u = 0.69;               % initialize inhibition
X = zeros(N,1);
t = 0;
```

The statements for updating the neuron states follow directly from equations 18.4 and 18.5. These are placed inside a loop to allow the system to settle to its stable state. Note that $[x]_+$ is implemented as max(0,x).

```
for i = 1 : 2000
  z = z + (-z + max(0, gammaE + wEEij*z + wEI*u + X)) *
(deltaT/tauE);
  u = u + (-u + max(0, gammaI + wIE*sum(z) + wII*u)) *
(deltaT/tauI);
  t = t + deltaT;
end
```

When the loop completes, we can plot a representative row of w_{ij}, and the output $\bar{z}$.

```
clf, hold on, grid on
plot(wij(:,halfN),'dm-')
plot(z,'o-')
```

The above code forms a complete Matlab program and will produce a plot similar to figure 18.2. The remaining plots in this chapter can be reproduced by initializing the external input vector X to the appropriate values. Readers are encouraged to also try out an interactive animation of the attractor bump available on the web (Touretzky, 2004), where external inputs can be specified with a mouse click, and the bump will move and change shape in real time in response to these inputs.

Properties of Attractor Networks

One of the essential properties of attractor networks is their resistance to noise, since noise is unavoidable (and in some circumstances, desirable) in neural systems. Figure 18.3 shows the effect of injecting continuously varying random noise in the interval [0, 0.5] into units whose activity forms a stable bump (top plot). After 2000 steps (right plot), the shape of the bump and the location of the peak are virtually unchanged due to the stability property of the attractor. In the absence of any external input the bump would gradually drift due to the cumulative effects of noise, and if one were to wait a sufficiently long time, it could be at a completely different location, but over shorter periods the stability is remarkable.

Figure 18.4 shows that a tonic input applied to one flank of the attractor bump (top plot) causes the bump to shift until it is centered over the input (bottom plot). The input X_i was calculated as $0.2 \cdot (w_{i,80})^8$. This is how information is stored in an attractor network memory: by setting the location of the attractor bump. Notice that the amplitude of the bump also increases as a result of the external input; it will decrease back to the level shown at the top once the external input is removed, but the bump will remain in its new position.

Figure 18.5 shows that the network will choose the larger of two inputs when they are presented on opposite flanks of the bump, while figure 18.6 shows that if the inputs are equal in magnitude, the bump will remain balanced between them. These properties

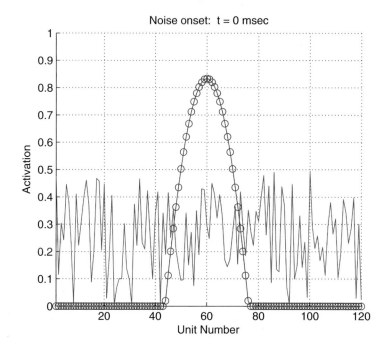

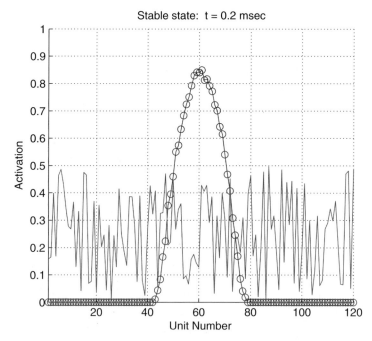

Figure 18.3
Noise resistance: when random noise in the interval [0, 0.5] is supplied at each time step as the external input to each unit (top), the bump retains both its general shape and the location of the peak (bottom). Note, however, that the perfectly smooth distribution of unit activations seen on the top is degraded slightly on the bottom.

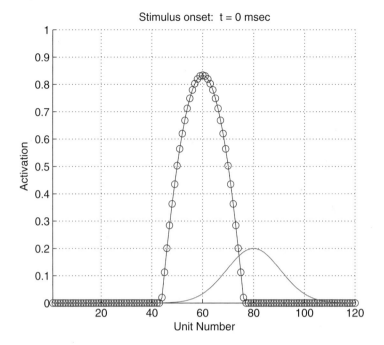

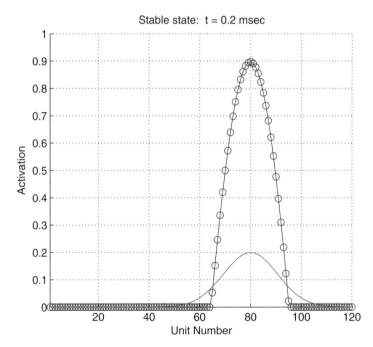

Figure 18.4
When an external input is applied to the flank of the bump (top), the bump shifts over until it is centered over the input (bottom).

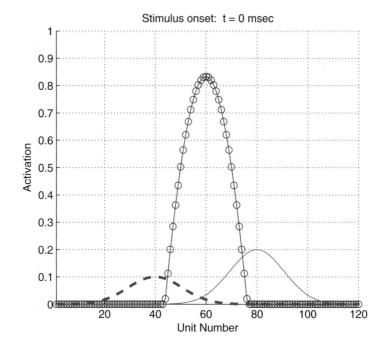

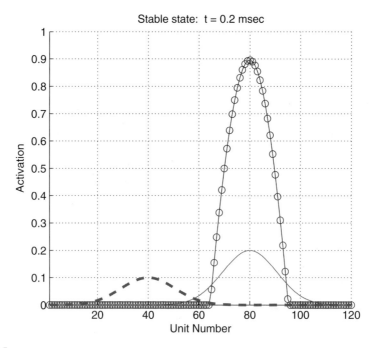

Figure 18.5
Choice behavior: When two conflicting external inputs are applied, one on either flank (top), the bump centers itself over the larger of the two (bottom).

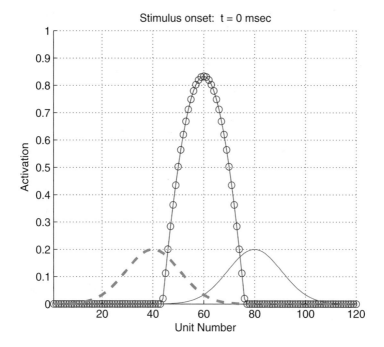

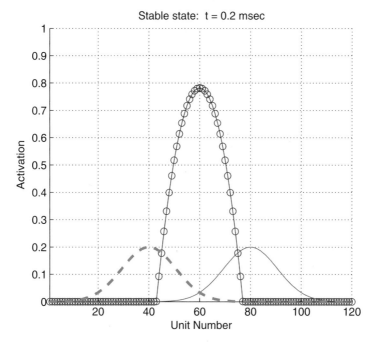

Figure 18.6
Equipotential point: When external inputs of equal magnitude are presented on opposite flanks of the bump (top), the bump retains its current position (bottom) rather than choosing arbitrarily between them. Note that the peak amplitude is slightly reduced, a result of increased activation of the inhibitory unit.

are crucial for integrating angular velocity in a model of the HD system, as we will see in the next section.

Figure 18.7 shows how addition gives rise to multiplication: applying a uniform external input $X_i = c$ to all units in the network alters the amplitude of the bump, but not its width or position (Salinas and Abbott, 1996). This property will also prove important for integrating angular velocity.

Figure 18.8 shows how the network automatically rejects outlier inputs, i.e., inputs not located on a flank of the bump, provided that they are weak. Sufficiently strong inputs will force a new bump to form at the input location and the existing bump to collapse due to recurrent inhibition. The effect on the bump of weak external input applied at different locations has been studied by several authors (Ben-Yishai et al., 1995; Tsodyks and Sejnowski, 1995; Hansel and Sompolisnky, 1998; Compte et al., 2000).

Figure 18.9 shows that when the network is presented with two inputs located on the same flank of the bump, it integrates them based on their relative activations rather than choosing one and ignoring the other. These two properties, outlier rejection and stimulus integration, help explain how input from multiple visual landmarks can be used to keep the HD system aligned with the environment.

A Survey of HD Models

The earliest model of the head direction system, by McNaughton et al. (1991), posited a linear associator that directly mapped current heading representation plus an angular velocity signal to a representation of future heading. This model captured the notion that heading could be updated as a function of angular velocity, but it could not account for the shapes of HD tuning curves or the differences in response properties of HD cells in different brain areas.

Subsequent models have been based on the *attractor hypothesis* first put forth by Skaggs et al. (1995), that the HD system is a ring attractor that integrates angular head velocity by moving the activation bump around the ring in a velocity-dependent fashion. No equations were provided in the Skaggs et al. paper, and there were no simulation results, but this seminal paper has given rise to a long line of models.

Zhang (1996) provided the first rigorous formulation of an HD attractor model, giving equations for a ring attractor in which bump motion resulted from varying a component of the recurrent connection weights. He presented simulations showing that with a proper choice of weight function, the shape of the bump could be preserved during motion. The shape resembled the tuning curve of an HD cell in postsubiculum.

Directly varying the matrix of connection weights is not a physiologically plausible mechanism by which angular velocity information could enter the HD system. The mechanism proposed by Skaggs et al., shown in figure 18.10, assumes another class of cells,

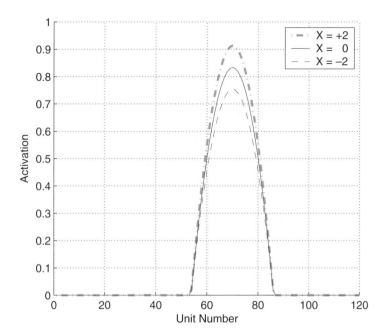

Figure 18.7
Amplitude modulation: When a uniform excitatory or inhibitory input is applied to all units, the height of the bump changes but the width does not. (After Salinas and Abbott, 1996.)

called turn-modulated head direction (TMHD) cells, whose firing rates are modulated by angular velocity. The head direction cells forming the large outer ring in the diagram are the attractor network; they drive two populations of TMHD cells shown as two inner rings. These populations exhibit activity bumps like the HD cells, but in one TMHD population the cells are more active for clockwise turns and less active for counterclockwise turns, relative to when the animal is not turning. In the other, the pattern is reversed. The cells in each of these populations project to corresponding HD cells, but with a slight offset based on their preferred turn direction. So a TMHD cell in the clockwise population, which becomes more active for turns in the clockwise direction, will project to HD cells whose preferred directions are offset clockwise from it, thus providing input on the clockwise flank of the HD activity bump. TMHD cells in the counterclockwise population provide their input on the counterclockwise flank.

When the animal is stationary, both TMHD populations have equal size activity bumps, so the input on both flanks of the HD bump is equal and the bump does not move (see figure 18.6). When the animal turns in the clockwise direction, the clockwise TMHD population becomes more active and the counterclockwise population becomes less active. Since the inputs on the two flanks are no longer in balance, the bump starts to shift in the

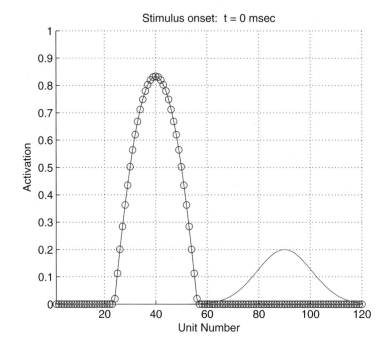

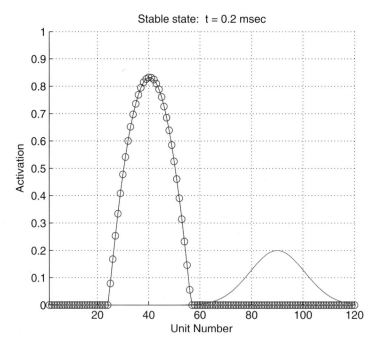

Figure 18.8
Outlier rejection: When an external input is applied far from the bump (top), it is ignored (bottom). The bump does not shift even after two thousand iterations of the update equations.

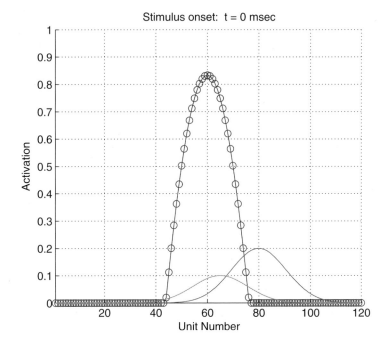

Stimulus onset: t = 0 msec

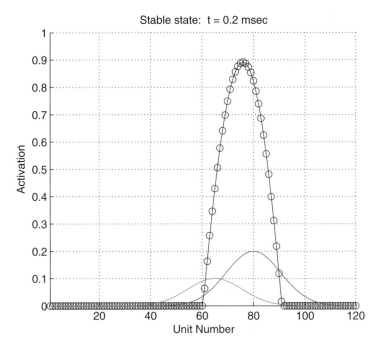

Stable state: t = 0.2 msec

Figure 18.9
Cue integration: When external inputs are close enough together to be mutually compatible (top), the bump positions itself based on their weighted average (bottom).

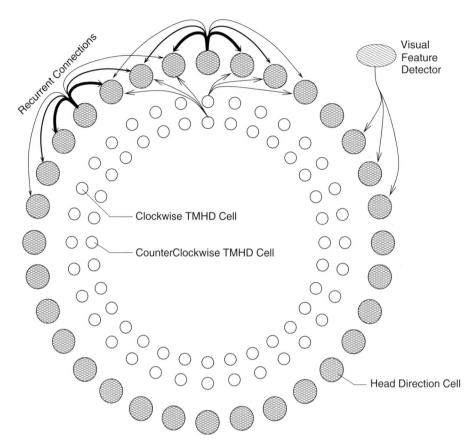

Figure 18.10
Head direction model from Touretzky and Skaggs, 2003, after Skaggs et al., 1995.

clockwise direction. But since the TMHD activity bumps track the HD bump, they will start to shift as well, and so the external input will remain located on the flank of the bump as it shifts, and the bump will therefore continue to shift around the ring for as long as the animal maintains its clockwise turning motion.

Blair and Sharp developed a shift register model of AD (the anterior dorsal nucleus of the thalamus), in which HD cells projected to their left and right neighbors (Blair, 1996; Sharp et al., 1996). Like the Skaggs et al. proposal, they postulated two populations of angular velocity-modulated HD cells in another brain area that made offset inhibitory connections back to the regular HD cells. But because this model lacked true attractor dynamics, the activity bump was a square wave, so HD cell tuning curves were not realistic. Angular velocity integration took place in AD, which had a one-way projection to PoS (postsubiculum). The anticipatory relationship of AD to PoS was attributed to conduction delay and synaptic integration time.

Redish et al. (1996) introduduced a "coupled attractor" model of PoS and AD in which each area was represented by a separate attractor network. PoS and AD are known to be reciprocally connected in the rat. In the model, PoS made three sets of projections to AD: a straight projection that kept the bumps aligned when the animal was at rest, plus clockwise and counterclockwise offset projections. There was also a straight projection from AD back to PoS. The strengths of the offset connections were dynamically modulated by angular head velocity, which avoided the need for TMHD cells. But the rapid modulation of connection strengths was a major weakness in terms of biological plausibility, as with Zhang's more abstract model. The Redish et al. model was able to integrate actual rat head trajectories with good accuracy, and since PoS projected to offset positions in AD, the AD bump anticipated the position of the PoS bump during turns. However, the assumption of an AD attractor network was not supported by the anatomy, as there are not thought to be any recurrent connections within AD.

Goodridge and Touretzky (2000) modeled the interactions of HD cells in three brain areas: PoS, AD, and LMN (lateral mammillary nucleus). Like the Skaggs et al. and Sharp et al. models, this model used angular velocity modulated HD cells. The TMHD cells were suggested to be LMN cells, because LMN cells do show direction-dependent velocity modulation (Stackman and Taube, 1998). PoS was modeled as an attractor network, but AD did not have attractor dynamics. LMN was modeled as two independent attractor networks, one excited by a clockwise angular velocity signal, the other by a counterclockwise signal. The angular velocity signals were projected uniformly to all the units in their respective networks, modulating the amplitude of the bumps as in figure 18.7. Whether LMN cells are actually modulated this way is less clear. Data from Stackman and Taube (1998) are compatible with amplitude modulation, but Blair et al. (1998) report that LMN cells may respond to velocity by changing the width of one flank of the bump rather than its overall amplitude.

The two populations of LMN cells in the Goodridge and Touretzky model made offset projections to AD. Depending on the degree of offset, the resulting activity bump in AD could have a bimodal appearance, and the height of the peak varied with angular velocity. Real AD cells do show velocity modulation (Blair and Sharp, 1995; Taube, 1995). Their tuning curves have been reported to distort with angular velocity, and their bimodality, described by Blair et al. (1997), is the basis for the Goodridge and Touretzky model. But it should be noted that the phenomena of AD tuning curve distortion and bimodality have been called into question by Taube and Muller (1998), who did not see these effects in their own experiments.

PoS cells in the Goodridge and Touretzky model had firing rates and tuning curve shapes that were independent of angular velocity. This was because of both the attractor properties of the PoS network and the way that the LMN inputs to AD were balanced: as one population became more active during a turn, the other became less active. AD therefore received a constant amount of excitation from LMN; only the spatial distribution of the input changed. AD combined the offset signals from the two LMN populations into a bimodal shape and then projected the result, a distorted bump, to PoS where the bump was cleaned up by the attractor dynamics. PoS then projected back to LMN to close the loop, keeping the TMHD bump location synchronized with the HD bump.

PoS does project to LMN in the rat, but reliance on this projection implies that the LMN bump should lag behind the PoS bump, when in reality it leads because of the greater anticipatory time interval (ATI). PoS cells have ATI values close to zero, while LMN cells have ATI values around +40 ms (Blair et al.) or +75 ms (Stackman and Taube). See the chapter by Sharp in this volume for a discussion of ATI values.

Blair and Sharp (2002; Sharp et al., 2001a) have proposed that integration of angular velocity takes place earlier in the HD system, in a recurrent loop between the dorsal tegmental nucleus (DTN) and LMN. DTN cells are GABAergic and are thought to make inhibitory projections to LMN cells. LMN in turn makes excitatory projections back to DTN. In Blair and Sharp's proposal, DTN HD cells play the role of TMHD cells, but rather than supplying an excitatory input to one flank of the LMN bump, they inhibit the opposite flank. DTN also contains angular velocity cells, some of which also show mild HD tuning (Bassett and Taube, 2001; Sharp et al., 2001b). These AV cells could be the source of velocity-dependent modulation of DTN HD cell firing rates. LMN cells, as observed by Blair and Sharp, show velocity modulation of their tuning curve widths rather than their firing rates (Blair et al., 1998). The mechanism modulating the tuning curve widths is unclear, but is perhaps a consequence of suppressing one flank of the bump. No simulations have been reported that replicate this phenomenon. It should be noted that Stackman and Taube's study of LMN cells did not report any modulation of tuning curve widths, but instead found differences in peak firing rate between clockwise and counterclockwise turns (Stackman and Taube, 1998).

Xie et al. (2002) described a "double-ring" network model, based on an idea originally put forth by Zhang (1996), that does not require a separate population of TMHD cells. Instead, the HD population is split into two rings, one of which receives a uniform angular velocity signal that increases for clockwise turns, while the other receives a signal that increases for counterclockwise turns. The two rings have asymmetric connections, e.g., a unit may receive excitation from only right neighbors on the same ring and left neighbors on the opposite ring. A significant contribution of this model is its ability to integrate a wide range of angular velocities using relatively slow time constants, consistent with NMDA or GABA$_B$ synapses. Previous models achieved accurate integration using unrealistically fast time constants.

Rubin et al. (2001) developed an even more physiologically realistic model using conductance-based, spiking neurons. In their model, thalamocortical relay (TC) cells excite thalamic reticular (RE) cells, which in turn inhibit the TC cells, which fire through post-inhibitory rebound. The model used a combination of local, strong $GABA_A$ inhibition and diffuse, weak $GABA_B$ inhibition to produce a stable bump shape.

Song and Wang (2003) constructed a head direction system model with attractor dynamics but without recurrent excitation, only inhibition. Following Blair and Sharp's proposal, they used three populations of units. Units in the excitatory population (LMN) projected to clockwise and counterclockwise angular velocity modulated inhibitory populations (DTN), which in turn projected back to the excitatory units with appropriate offsets, for example, a DTN unit that responded more strongly to clockwise turns would project to LMN units whose preferred directions were offset slightly counterclockwise from that of the DTN unit. So rather than an LMN unit providing recurrent excitation to its "neighbors" (cells with similar preferred directions), it drives two DTN populations which inhibit its rivals (cells with different preferred directions) via clockwise and counterclockwise offsets. Another interesting feature of Song and Wang's model is that it uses spiking neurons with a mixture of AMPA and NMDA synapses. NMDA synapses were found to enhance the stability of the attractor and prevent unwanted oscillations (Wang, 1999; Compte et al., 2000).

One difficulty facing all existing head direction system models is the difference in anticipatory time intervals (ATIs) among various HD areas. Blair and Sharp's proposal to locate the neural integrator in the LMN–DTN loop naturally accounts for LMN having a greater ATI than AD, to which it projects, or PoS, to which AD projects. But the difference in ATI values is considerably greater than can be explained by synaptic transmission delay. If LMN anticipates head direction by 40 ms or perhaps as much as 75 ms, it's not clear how cells in AD, which appear to lack recurrent connections, manage to anticipate by only 25 ms.

Another puzzle is the existence of symmetric angular head velocity cells in DTN. These cells show equal velocity modulation for turns in either direction. Bassett and Taube (2001) found a greater percentage of symmetric than asymmetric angular head velocity cells, but Sharp et al. (2001) did not report any symmetric cells. Current models of the HD system rely on the asymmetry of velocity modulation to shift the attractor bump in the appropriate direction. The purpose of symmetric angular velocity cells is unclear.

Using Landmarks to Correct Integration Error

Integrating angular velocity signals allows the rat to update its heading estimate in the absence of directional cues, but drift is inevitable due to cumulative integration error. Goodridge et al. reported drift in the cylindrical arena in the dark after only a few minutes (Goodridge et al., 1998).

To correct for drift, the rat must be able to derive heading information from sensory cues. The simplest example is a distant landmark (a North Star) whose allocentric bearing is the same from all viewing locations the rat might experience. The position of this land-mark on the retina provides direct confirmation of the animal's present heading. Skaggs et al. (1995) proposed a set of visual feature detectors sensitive to specific landmarks at specific egocentric bearings (figure 18.10), with Hebbian synapses onto HD cells. When a feature detector becomes active, its projections to currently active HD cells would be strengthened, thus binding the "feature at bearing" percept to a specfic heading. Later, if the HD system drifts out of alignment, the efferent projections from active feature detec-tors would fall more heavily on one flank of the bump and bring it back into proper registration with the visual environment. If multiple landmarks are present, the projec-tions from their respective feature detectors would combine to influence the bump, as in figure 18.9.

This simple proposal has some weaknesses. Feature detectors tuned to landmarks at par-ticular egocentric bearings have not yet been found in the rodent brain. Also, the mecha-nism works only for distal landmarks, whose allocentric bearings are unaffected by the rat's movements. Recovering heading information from the bearings of proximal land-marks is a more complex operation, requiring knowledge of the location from which the landmarks were being observed.

Discussion

Are attractors real? A growing body of physiological evidence from multiple memory systems supports the notion that short term memories have attractor-like properties. Although the precise way in which attractor dynamics is achieved in specific brain areas remains unclear, the increasing realism of the models, combined with parallel multi-unit recording techniques (Johnson et al., 2003), promises rapid answers.

Some current unanswered questions include where the disparities in ATI values across brain areas come from, and the mechanism by which LMN tuning curve widths are modulated. A much larger question, for which there are not yet satisfactory answers, is how ring attractor networks are constructed during the course of development. One recent proposal by Hahnloser (2003) has visual feature detectors tuned to specific egocentric bearings projecting onto two populations of HD cells. This provides a training signal that, along with another set of inputs encoding angular head velocity, induces formation of the necessary connection pattern for a double-ring attractor network (Xie et al., 2002).

Acknowledgments

Funded by National Institutes of Health MH 59932.

References

Aksay E, Gamkrelidze G, Seung HS, Baker R, Tank DW (2001) In vivo intracellular recording and perturbation of persistent activity in a neural integrator. Nature Neurosci 4(2): 184–193.

Bassett JP, Taube JS (2001) Neural correlates for angular head velocity in the rat dorsal tegmental nucleus. J Neurosci 21(15): 5740–5751.

Ben-Yishai R, Lev Bar-Or R, Sompolinksy H (1995) Theory of orientation tuning in visual cortex. Proc Natl Acad Sci USA 92: 3844–3848.

Blair HT, Sharp PE (1995) Anticipatory head direction signals in anterior thalamus: evidence for a thalamocortical circuit that integrates angular head motion to compute head direction. J Neurosci 15(9): 6260–6270.

Blair HT (1996) A thalamocortical circuit for computing directional heading in the rat. In DS Touretzky, MC Mozer, and ME Hasselmo eds., Advances in Neural Information Processing Systems 8, 152–158. Cambridge, MA: MIT Press.

Blair HT, Lipscomb BW, Sharp PE (1997) Anticipatory time intervals of head-direction cells in the anterior thalamus of the rat, implications for path integration in the head-direction circuit. J Neurophys 78(1): 145–159.

Blair HT, Cho J, Sharp PE (1998) Role of the lateral mammillary nucleus in the rat head-direction circuit: a combined single-unit recording and lesion study. Neuron 21: 1387–1397.

Blair HT, Sharp PE (2002) Functional organization of the rat head-direction circuit. In PE Sharp ed., The Neural Basis of Navigation, Boston: Kluwer, pp. 163–182.

Compte A, Brunel N, Goldman-Rakic PS, Wang X-J (2000) Synaptic mechanisms and network dynamics underlying visuospatial working memory in a cortical network model. Cereb Cortex 10: 910–923.

Deco G, Rolls ET (2003) Attention and working memory: a dynamical model of neuronal activity in the prefrontal cortex. Eur J Neurosci 18(8): 2374–2390.

Droulez. J, Berthoz A (1991) A neural network model of sensoritopic maps with predictive short-term memory properties. Proc Natl Acad Sci USA 88: 9653–9657.

Duhamel JR, Colby CL, Goldberg ME (1992) The updating of the representation of visual space in parietal cortex by intended eye movements. Science 255: 90–92.

Goodridge JP, Dudchenko PA, Worboys KA, Golob EJ, Taube JS (1998) Cue control and head direction cells. Behavioral Neurosci 112: 749–761.

Goodridge JP, Touretzky DS (2000) Modeling attractor deformation in the rodent head direction system. J Neurophys 83(6): 3402–3410.

Hahnloser RHR (2003) Emergence of neural integration in the head-direction system by visual supervision. Neuroscience 120: 877–891.

Hansel D, Sompolinksy H (1998) Modeling feature seletivity in local cortical circuits. In C Koch and I Segev eds., Methods in Neuronal Modeling: From Synapse to Networks, 2nd ed., chap. 13. Cambridge, MA: MIT Press.

Johnson A, Seeland KD, Redish AD (2003) Head-direction ensembles recorded from awake, behaving rats in an open field under cue-conflict situations. Soc Neurosci Abst 29: 289.6.

Knierim JJ, McNaughton BL, Duffield C, Bliss J (1993). On the binding of hippocampal place fields to the inertial orientation system. Soc Neurosci Abst 19: 795.

Lukashin AV, Amirikian BR, Mzhaev VL, Wilcox GL, Georgopoulos AP (1996) Modeling motor cortical operations by an attractor network of stochastic neurons. Biol Cybernet 74: 255–261.

McNaughton BL, Chen LL, Markus EJ (1991) Dead reckoning, landmark learning, and the sense of direction: a neurophysiological and computational hypothesis. J Cog Neurosci 3(2): 190–202.

McNaughton BL, Knierim JJ, Wilson MA (1994) Vector encoding and the vestibular foundations of spatial cognition: Neurophysiological and computational mechanisms. In M Gazzaniga ed., The Cognitive Neurosciences, Cambridge, MA: MIT Press, pp. 585–595.

Redish AD, Elga AN, Touretzky DS (1996) A coupled attractor model of the rodent head direction system. Network 7(4): 671–685.

Rubin J, Terman D, Chow C (2001) Localized bumps of activity sustained by inhibition in a two-layer thalamic network. J Comput Neurosci 10(3): 313–331.

Salinas E, Abbott LF (1996) A model of multiplicative neural responses in parietal cortex. Proc Natl Acad Sci USA 93: 11956–11961.

Samsonovich AV, McNaughton BL (1997) Path integration and cognitive mapping in a continuous-attractor neural network model. J Neurosci 17: 5900–5920.

Seung HS (1996) How the brain keeps the eyes still. Proc Natl Acad Sci USA 93: 13339–13344.

Sharp PE, Blair HT, Brown M (1996) Neural network modeling of the hippocampal formation spatial signals and their possible role in navigation: a modular approach. Hippocampus 6(6): 720–734.

Sharp PE, Blair HT, Cho J (2001a) The anatomical and computational basis of the rat head-direction cell signal. Trends Neurosci 24: 289–294.

Sharp PE, Tinkelman A, Cho J (2001b) Angular velocity and head direction signals recorded from the dorsal tegmental nucleus of Gudden in the rat: implications for path integration in the head direction cell circuit. Behav Neurosci 115(3): 571–588.

Skaggs WE, Knierim JJ, Kudrimoti HS, McNaughton BL (1995) A model of the neural basis of the rat's sense of direction. Advances in Neural Information Processing Systems 7: 173–180.

Song P, Wang X-J (2003) A three-population attractor network model of rodent head direction system without recurrent excitation. Soc Neurosci Abst 29: 939.3.

Stackman RW, Taube JS (1998) Firing properties of rat lateral mammillary single units: head direction, head pitch, and angular head velocity. J Neurosci 18: 9020–9037.

Taube JS (1995) Head direction cells recorded in the anterior thalamic nuclei of freely moving rats. J Neurosci 15(1): 1953–1971.

Taube JS, Muller RI (1998) Comparisons of head direction cell activity in the postsubiculum and anterior thalamus of freely moving rats. Hippocampus 8(2): 87–108.

Touretzky DS, Skaggs WE (2003) The rodent head direction system. In MA Arbib ed., Handbook of Brain Theory and Neural Networks, 2nd edn., Cambridge, MA: MIT Press, pp. 990–993.

Touretzky DS (2004) Attractor bump simulation program, implemented in Matlab. Available at <http://www.cs.cmu.edu/~dst/Matlab/bump>.

Tsodyks M, Sejnowski TJ (1995) Rapid switching in balanced cortical network models. *NETWORK* 6: 1–14.

Tsodyks MV, Skaggs WE, Sejnowski TJ, McNaughton BL (1997) Paradoxical effects of external modulation of inhibitory interneurons. J Neurosci 17(11): 4382–4388.

Wang X-J (1999) Synaptic basis of cortical persistent activity: the importance of NMDA receptors to working memory. J Neurosci 19(2): 9587–9603.

Xie X, Hahnloser RHR, Seung HS (2002) Double-ring network model of the head-direction system. Phy Rev E 66: 041902.

Zhang K (1996) Representation of spatial orientation by the intrinsic dynamics of the head-direction cell ensemble: a theory. J Neurosci 16(6): 2112–2126.

19 Head Direction Cells and Place Cells in Models for Navigation and Robotic Applications

Angelo Arleo and Wulfram Gerstner

For successful spatial behavior, both animals and autonomous artifacts must interact with their environments and process multimodal sensory information (e.g., visual, somatosensory, and inertial signals). Cognitive neuroscience defines navigation as the ability to determine and execute a trajectory from one place $\vec{p}$ to a desired location $\vec{p}_{goal}$ (Gallistel, 1990). To do this most efficiently, the navigator must select spatial information processes and the goal-directed strategies most appropriate to the requirements of the task.

Attaining a target position $\vec{p}_{goal}$ is simple if the latter is either directly visible or identified by a proximal visible cue (a beacon). In this case, an egocentric landmark-guidance behavior can be adopted to solve the task: orient toward the visible goal (or beacon) and approach it. This reactive strategy, named taxon navigation, can be understood in terms of simple Pavlovian stimulus-response associations (Trullier et al., 1997). If the trajectory to a hidden target can be identified by a sequence of sensory patterns (e.g., local visual cues), the navigator can learn a succession of stimulus-action associations to solve the task, namely, route navigation. However, true flexible goal-oriented behavior (e.g., allowing the subject to plan shortcuts) requires more complex information processing and the representation of the spatiotemporal properties of the environment by means of a topological or even a cognitive map (Tolman, 1948).

The hippocampal formation seems to exhibit such a spatial representation property. This brain area has been thought to mediate spatial coding ever since the experimental evidence for location-sensitive neurons (place cells) in the hippocampus of freely moving rats was found (O'Keefe and Dostrovsky, 1971). Hippocampal place (HP) cells in rats provide a spatial representation in allocentric (world centered) coordinates. Complementing this, neurons whose activity is tuned to the orientation of the head of the rat in the azimuthal plane have been observed in the hippocampal formation and other limbic regions (Ranck, 1984; Taube, 1998). These head direction (HD) cells have been proposed to endow the animal with an allocentric neural compass.

Place coding and directional sense are crucial for spatial learning, and this has led to the hypothesis that HP and HD cells may constitute the neural basis for cognitive spatial behavior of rats (O'Keefe and Nadel, 1978; McNaughton et al., 1996). Nonetheless, the issue of explicitly relating observations at the neuronal level (i.e., electrophysiological properties of HP and HD cells) to those at the behavioral level (i.e., the animal's capability to solve a spatial navigation task) remains an arduous task (Golob et al., 2001). The lack of experimental data concerning the intermediate levels (e.g., system level) is one of the factors that make it difficult to clearly identify the functional role of HP and HD cells.

It is one of the advantages of modeling that potential connections between findings on the neuronal level (e.g., HP and HD cells) and on the behavioral level (e.g., Morris water-maze task performance) can be explored systematically. Of course, models cannot prove that nature uses HP and HD cells for spatial cognition. Nevertheless, models can show that the information contained in these cells is indeed sufficient for navigation problems similar to the Morris water-maze task, if the place cell information is combined with learning triggered by reward signals that could, for example, be provided by dopaminergic neurons (Schultz et al., 1997).

This chapter reviews some neural network models for spatial learning and navigation and focuses on those that have been validated on robotic platforms. In particular, the chapter presents a class of models termed "neuromimetic," in the sense that their main principles take inspiration from behavioral, anatomo-functional, and neurophysiological findings. The chapter describes more extensively the approach by Arleo and Gerstner (2000, 2001, 2004) that stresses the importance of integrating multimodal sensory signals (e.g., vision and proprioceptive information) to maintain robust HP and HD representations. The model has been validated on a mobile robot, and shows that as long as the system is capable of maintaining the HP and HD representations stable over time, goal-oriented navigation can be performed effectively based on a reward-dependent learning scheme.

Toward Neuromimetic Spatial Learning in Robotics

The issue of designing autonomous navigating systems is still an open problem in robotics (Dorigo and Colombetti, 1998). The requirement of autonomy makes navigation particularly difficult. An autonomous artifact should have a self-contained control system to adapt its lifelong behavior to all possible situations it might face. In particular, the control system must be able to cope with previously unseen environments. In this section we review the state of the art in classical and neuro-inspired robotics.

From Classical to Behavior-Based Robotics
The classical artificial intelligence approach, based on predefined internal models of the world to endow robots with humanlike symbolic capabilities, has been recognized to be

unsuitable for navigation of fully autonomous systems (Brooks, 1991). First, real environments are often unpredictable, which makes it impossible to design a built-in knowledge base to associate an appropriate action to every possible sensory pattern. Second, the sensory-motor system is typically corrupted by noise whose distribution is often unknown (Thrun, 1998). For instance, because of wheel slippage, the execution of a given motor command leads the robot to a new position that cannot be predicted precisely. Third, predefined models are intrinsically biased because they reflect the anthropomorphic sensory worldview and inherit the structure of linguistic descriptions used to formulate them (Dorigo and Colombetti, 1998).

Autonomous robotics has moved towards a novel nonsymbolic approach termed behavior-based robotics (Brooks, 1991). The idea is to let the agent build up its own worldview by means of its own experience (i.e., learning). The principles for designing behavior-based robots often take inspiration from basic behavioral strategies observed in animals and from neurophysiological adaptive mechanisms such as neural plasticity. Most of the behavior-based learning frameworks, such as reinforcement learning (Sutton and Barto, 1998) and evolutionary techniques (Nolfi and Floreano, 2000), lead to reactive control policies without building any internal spatial models of the environment. Thus, the behavior-based learning paradigm can be employed to capture the functions undertaken by the taxon and route navigation systems of animals.

One of the principal current challenges for designing autonomous navigating artifacts consists in making the step from simple reactive behavior to more flexible cognitive navigation. On the other end of the scale, classical robotic architectures engineered so far are well suited for navigation in a fully known environment, but not as robust and adaptive as animals' spatial learning systems when exposed to changing or new environmental situations (e.g., Elfes, 1987; Kuipers and Byun, 1991; Thrun, 1998; Arleo et al., 1999). Therefore, similar to the rationale behind behavior-based robotics, moving towards a neuromimetic (i.e., biologically based) approach in modeling spatial cognition offers the attractive prospect of developing autonomous artifacts that emulate the navigation capabilities of animals.

Spatial Representation in Neurorobotics
An understanding of the functional role of spatial representations in neuromimetic agents may contribute to new developments and cross-disciplinary insights. Modeling biological solutions for spatial learning may lead to an applicational payoff in designing more flexible and robust autonomous artifacts. For instance, reproducing the ability of animals to acquire internal models incrementally and online according to the requirements of the given task-environment context may increase the degree of adaptiveness and robustness in current robotics. Conversely, the fact that artifacts are simpler and experimentally more explicit than biological organisms makes neurorobotics a useful tool to check new hypotheses concerning the underlying mechanisms of spatial behavior in animals. For

instance, synthesizing bio-inspired architectures may help to connect different levels explicitly (e.g., cellular, systemic, behavioral) and bridge the gap between the electro-physiological properties of HP and HD cells and their functional roles in spatial behavior.

Several neurorobotic approaches have addressed the issue of building internal spatial models suitable for supporting cognitive navigation (Schölkopf and Mallot, 1995; Burgess and O'Keefe, 1996; Arleo and Gerstner, 2000; Trullier and Meyer, 2000; Gaussier et al., 2002). These works focus on the properties of hippocampal place cells and head direction cells and investigate the two following issues: (1) How can animals establish appropriate allocentric place representations based on locally available sensory inputs? (2) How can HP and HD cells serve as a basis for goal-oriented navigation?

Burgess and O'Keefe put forth a model in which the visual information drives a neural layer of entorhinal cortical place cells, and then propagates through the network to form place fields in the hippocampus (CA1–CA3 regions) and in the subiculum (Burgess and O'Keefe, 1996). At the sensory level, the model stresses the importance of encoding the distance of the robot to salient visual cues. This information is then explicitly used to obtain location-sensitive neurons in the entorhinal cortex. Entorhinal cells project to the CA1–CA3 layer of the model through binary connections that are switched on by means of one-shot Hebbian learning (the term "one-shot" indicates that, once a binary connec-tion has been switched on, it cannot be further modified). Place selectivity is enhanced at the level of CA1–CA3 cells by applying a competitive learning scheme. The efferent pro-jections from CA1–CA3 to the subiculum are also activated by one-shot Hebbian learn-ing. Place selectivity is reduced at the subicular level, producing broader place fields than those in CA1–CA3. In order to explain the functional role of hippocampal place cells in navigation, Burgess and O'Keefe postulate a goal-memory system in which each target location is represented by a set of goal cells one synapse downstream from the subicular place cells. The goal cell activity estimates the allocentric vector (distance and direction) from the robot's position to the target. For instance, whenever the location of the robot $\vec{p}$ is north relative to the target $\vec{p}_{goal}$, the goal cell tuned to the north direction will fire pro-portionally to $\|\vec{p} - \vec{p}_{goal}\|$.

Schölkopf and Mallot propose a spatial learning model in which the robot builds a topo-logical view representation of the environment (Schölkopf and Mallot, 1995). The repre-sentation consists of a graph whose nodes correspond to local panoramic views while edges connect distinct views that are experienced by the robot in immediate temporal sequence (Muller et al., 1996). Place topology is encoded by labeling each arc of the graph by the egocentric movement (e.g., go left) that was necessary to move from one view to another. In this model, navigation is accomplished by planning a goal-directed path based on the view-graph representation. The robot explores "mentally" all experienced paths (as well as novel combinations of them) in order to determine the minimal-length sequence of movements leading from the current view to the one that corresponds to the target location.

Trullier and Meyer postulate that the hippocampus can be seen as an hetero-associative network that learns temporal relationships between successive configurations of stimuli (Trullier and Meyer, 2000). Thus, exploration is a process by which the robot experiences sequences of places, and stores these sequences onto a topological graph by transforming temporal relationships into spatial relationships. The direction of movement taken to travel between distinct places is used to label edges in the graph. Therefore, place units (nodes) form a recurrent neural network and the authors identify the CA3 hippocampal region as the anatomical locus for the topological graph. Each node is activated based on visual information, each place unit being tuned to the distance between the robot and a configuration of visual landmarks (e.g., wall corners). In order to achieve goal-oriented navigation, Trullier and Meyer extend the goal cell mechanism proposed by Burgess and O'Keefe (1996) and postulate the existence of "subgoal" cells, neurons that allow the robot to navigate toward a target by skirting around obstacles.

Gaussier and colleagues put forth a spatial learning model in which place recognition relies on the estimation of the allocentric azimuth of visual landmarks within a panoramic scene (Gaussier et al., 2002). During exploration, new place units are recruited, either when the robot encounters a novel or interesting place (e.g., a feeding location), or when it has executed an obstacle-avoidance behavior. The authors argue that these visual place cells find their anatomical counterpart in prehippocampal regions, where purely place coding takes place, whereas the hippocampus proper mediates the representation of transitions between places. In the model, CA3 pyramidal cells encode state transitions and CA1 cells participate in the selection of the most appropriate transition according to a specific motivation. Thus, a navigation map is learned that consists of a graph representing the topological relationships (edges) between state transitions (nodes).

The above neuromimetic models rely mainly upon visual information in order to establish a HP cell representation suitable for supporting the goal-directed behavior of a robot. Likewise, they assume an allocentric directional sense of the robot without modeling the rat's HD system explicitly. The rest of this chapter reviews a neurorobotic model that stresses the importance of combining different sensory modalities (e.g., vision and self-motion signals) to maintain stable head direction and place representations in two neural circuits that model HD and HP cells, respectively. These two neural systems are functionally coupled and interact with each other to form a unitary spatial learning system. For instance, inhibiting the HD circuit of the model would critically impair the capability of the robot to maintain a coherent place cell representation.

Integrating Multimodal Sensory Information for Robust Spatial Learning

Like animals, autonomous artifacts can sense their world via different sensory modalities and must use this information to locate themselves in an environment and select appropriate behavior.

The spatial information provided by a single sensory modality is often ambiguous or unstable over time. For instance, visual sensory aliasing (occurring when distinct areas of the environment are characterized by equivalent local visual patterns) can lead to singularities (i.e., ambiguous state representations) in a purely vision-based space coding (Sharp et al., 1990). On the other hand, integrating translational and rotational self-motion velocity signals over time, referred to as dead reckoning or path integration (Mittelstaedt and Mittelstaedt, 1980), is prone to systematic as well as nonsystematic errors that quickly disrupt purely idiothetic-based dynamics. Therefore, one solution for robust spatial learning is to employ a closed sensory processing loop in which idiothetic signals may disambiguate visual singularities and, conversely, visual information may be used to occasionally correct the drifts in the integrator of self-motion inputs.

Figure 19.1 shows a functional overview of the computational model described in the following paragraphs. The robot processes two sensory streams, visual and self-motion-related signals, to establish stable HD and HP representations. The combination of these two types of spatial information is achieved by means of unsupervised Hebbian learning. Goal-oriented navigation relies on a reinforcement learning scheme that maps places onto allocentric local actions based on reward-dependent signals.

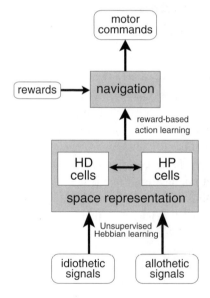

Figure 19.1
Functional overview of the spatial learning model. Allothetic and idiothetic signals are combined to establish stable HD and HP representations (see figures 19.3 and 19.8 for a more detailed description of the HD and HP models, respectively). Goal-oriented navigation is achieved by mapping places onto local actions based on reward-dependent learning.

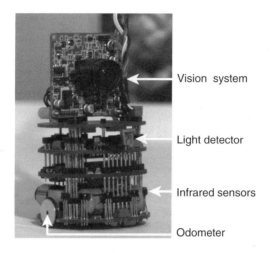

Vision system

Light detector

Infrared sensors

Odometer

Figure 19.2
The mobile Khepera miniature robot, a commercial platform produced and distributed by K-Team S.A. The Khepera has a cylindrical body with a diameter of 55 mm, and in the configuration used for the experiments is about 90 mm tall. Two DC motors drive two wheels independently providing the robot with nonholonomic motion capabilities. The robot's sensory system consists of a vision system, which includes a CCD black and white camera with an image resolution of 768×576 pixels and a view field covering about $90°$ in the horizontal plane and $60°$ in the vertical plane; eight infrared sensors that can detect obstacles within a distance of about 40 mm (six infrared sensors span the frontal $180°$ of the robot and two sensors cover approximately $100°$ of the posterior side); a light detector placed in the front of the robot; and wheel rotation encoders (odometers) to estimate both linear and angular displacements. (From Arleo, 2000.) See plate 5 for color version.

Figure 19.2 (see plate 5) shows the miniature mobile robot used for the experimental validation of the model. Exteroceptive sensory signals are provided by a two-dimensional vision system, eight infrared sensors to detect and avoid proximal obstacles (similar to rat whiskers), and a light detector. Idiothetic (self-motion related) signals are provided by wheel rotation encoders that estimate both the linear and the angular displacements of the robot (similar to proprioceptive and vestibular-derived signals in rodents).

Head Direction Cells

The robot is endowed with an internal sense of direction based upon a neural network model of the HD system (Arleo and Gerstner, 2001; Degris et al., 2004). The robot's HD circuit (figure 19.3) includes the postsubiculum (PoSC), the anterodorsal nucleus (ADN) of the thalamus, the lateral mammillary nucleus (LMN), and the dorsal tegmental nucleus (DTN) (see chapter 1 by Sharp and chapter 5 by Bassett and Taube for a description of the anatomofunctional circuit of the rat HD cells). Each anatomical region is modeled by a population of formal directional units with evenly distributed preferred directions ϑ_i relative to an absolute directional reference Φ.

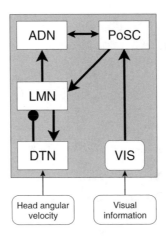

Figure 19.3
The HD model implemented on the robot. The circuit includes the postsubiculum (PoSC), the anterodorsal thalamic nucleus (ADN), the lateral mammillary nucleus (LMN), and the dorsal tegmental nucleus (DTN). Arrows and circles indicate excitatory and inhibitory projections, respectively. Head angular velocity signals enter the system via the DTN and are integrated over time by the DTN-LMN attractor-integrator network. Visual signals enter the system via a population of formal units (VIS) encoding the robot's egocentric bearing relative to a visual landmark. (Figure adapted from Goodridge and Taube, 1997, with permission.)

The dynamics of the system is primarily determined by self-motion signals that allow the robot to continuously estimate its allocentric heading $\vartheta(t)$ by integrating its angular velocity $\omega(t)$ over time. On the other hand, static visual information is employed to modify the intrinsic dynamics of the system, in order to prevent the angular velocity integrator from cumulative error, and polarize the directional representation whenever the robot enters a familiar environment.

In the model, DTN and LMN form a distributed attractor-integrator network (see chapter 18 by Touretzky for a description of the continuous attractor paradigm). This allows the system to bear, at any time t, a stable directional state ϑ corresponding to a Gaussian-shaped activity profile in which a subpopulation of LMN units with preferred directions $\vartheta_i \approx \vartheta$ discharge tonically, whereas the others exhibit a very low baseline frequency (figure 19.4). This attractor state persists in the absence of any sensory input, for instance when the robot is immobile in darkness.

During turns of the robot, the angular velocity signal $\omega(t)$ (provided by the wheel encoders) enters the circuit via DTN and is integrated over time through the DTN-LMN interaction. This yields a shift of the activity profile over the continuous attractor state space and provides an ongoing neural trace of the robot's orientation (Hahnloser, 2003).

The direction representation encoded by the LMN ensemble activity is transmitted to the PoSC via the ADN network. In the model, the PoSC constitutes the output interface of the HD system. In order to reconstruct the robot's current heading $\vartheta(t)$, a population

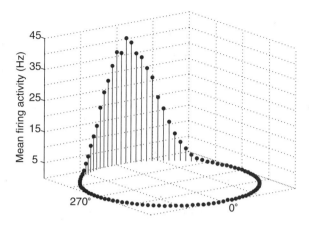

Figure 19.4
A sample of population activity pattern in the LMN layer of the model. Each cell has a specific preferred direction ϑ_i and the set of all preferred directions $\theta = \{ \vartheta_i \mid \forall i \in \text{LMN}\}$ covers the 360° uniformly. In the figure, each formal cell is represented by a black circle and the whole population forms a ring in the x-y plane. The mean firing rate of each formal HD cell is proportional to the height of the vertical bar below the black circle. Population vector coding is applied to estimate the robot's current heading $\vartheta(t) \approx 180°$ based on the ensemble cell activity. (Reprinted from Arleo and Gerstner, 2001 with permission from Elsevier. Copyright 2001.)

vector decoding scheme is applied (Georgopoulos et al., 1986). That is, the direction $\vartheta(t)$ is estimated by taking the center of mass $\vartheta'(t)$ of the PoSC activity profile.

The integration of the robot's angular velocity $\omega(t)$ is affected by a cumulative error which rapidly disrupts the HD coding. The gray area in figure 19.5 shows the mean deviation between the robot's actual heading $\vartheta(t)$ and the direction $\vartheta'(t)$ estimated by the HD system over time. The PoSC cells of the model receive visual information, which maintains the HD representation consistent over time. Let L denote a distal visual landmark and let VIS be a population of formal units encoding the robot's egocentric bearing $\alpha(t)$ relative to L. At any time t, the ensemble VIS activity is characterized by a Gaussian profile whose center of mass estimates the egocentric angle $\alpha(t)$. The synaptic projections from VIS to PoSC cells are established by means of LTP learning. That is, a Hebbian rule is employed to correlate the egocentric signal encoded by VIS cells with the allocentric HD representation encoded by PoSC cells. A corollary effect of applying this Hebbian rule is that only those visual cues that are perceived as stable by the robot can be strongly coupled with its internal directional representation (figure 19.6). The black area in figure 19.5 represents the mean HD reconstruction error when the system is calibrated by a stable visual input. In contrast to the purely idiothetic coding (gray area), the representation obtained by combining visual and self-motion signals displays an error that remains bounded over time. Finally, figure 19.7 shows the accuracy of the HD system in tracking the robot's current heading $\vartheta(t)$ over time.

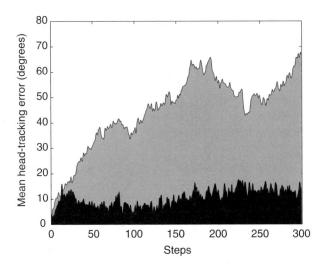

Figure 19.5
Mean error over time when estimating the robot's heading $\vartheta(t)$ based on the HD coding. The gray region in the diagram represents the cumulative deviation resulting from idiothetic-based dynamics alone, whereas the black area shows that the error remains bounded when visual signals are used to calibrate the HD system occasionally. (Reprinted from Arleo and Gerstner, 2001 with permission from Elsevier. Copyright 2001.)

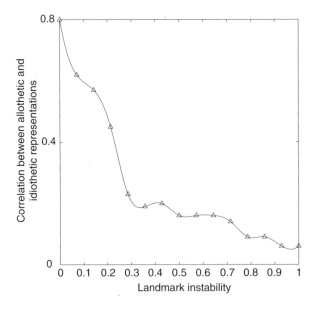

Figure 19.6
The diagram shows the strength of the correlation between visual and egomotion directional signals as a function of the (normalized) instability of a visual landmark during training. Due to Hebbian learning, the larger the instability, the smaller the correlational coupling. (Reprinted from Arleo and Gerstner, 2001 with permission from Elsevier. Copyright 2001.)

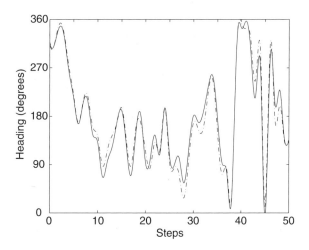

Figure 19.7
This example illustrates the ability of the HD system to track the robot's rotations over time. The solid line represents the robot's current heading $\vartheta(t)$, whereas the dashed line is the direction $\vartheta'(t)$ encoded by the HD cells. (From Arleo, 2000.)

Hippocampal Place Cells

The robot establishes and maintains two spatial representations in parallel: a vision-based representation, and an egomotion-based representation obtained by path integration. These two signals converge onto a model hippocampus and generate a large population of neurons with overlapping place fields similar to those found in CA3 and CA1. The goal of such a representation is two-fold: first, to cover space uniformly so as to form a continuous coarse coding representation (similar to a dense family of overlapping basis functions); and second, to use the place cell ensemble activity, rather than single cell activity, for self-localization (Arleo and Gerstner, 2000; Arleo et al., 2004). Figure 19.8 gives an overview of the hippocampal place cell model implemented on the robot.

Vision-Based Space Coding   Moving up the visual pathway anatomically (from the retina to the lateral geniculate nucleus, and then toward higher visual cortical areas), neurons become responsive to stimuli of increasing complexity, from orientation-sensitive cells (simple cells), to neurons responding to more complicated patterns (Hubel and Wiesel, 1962). In the model, low-level visual features are extracted by computing a vector of Gabor filter responses at the nodes of a sparse Log-polar retinotopic graph. Gabor filters are frequency- and orientation-selective filters providing a suitable mathematical model for simple cells in the visual cortex (Daugman, 1980). The magnitudes of the responses of the Gabor filters are taken as inputs to a population of view cells (VC), whose activity

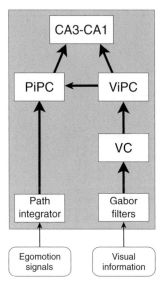

Figure 19.8
Overview of the hippocampal place cell model. The visual pathway includes a set of Gabor filters for image processing, a network of formal cells (VC) to encode views, and a population of vision-based place cells (ViPC). The idiothetic pathway includes the path integrator and a network of units (PiPC) encoding locations based on egomotion signals only. ViPC and PiPC are combined to form a stable space representation in the CA3-CA1 layer of the model.

becomes correlated to more complex spatial relationships between visual features. This allows the robot to recognize previously perceived views of the environment. Note that VC firing is a function of both the robot's gaze direction and position, and thus is not suitable for proper place discrimination.

The next step in the visual pathway of the model consists of applying unsupervised Hebbian learning to achieve allocentric spatial coding. A population of place units (vision-driven place cells; ViPC) is built incrementally one synapse downstream from the VC layer. At each location, the robot takes N views (forming a quasi-panoramic picture) and encodes them by the activity of N view cells. Then, the unsupervised learning scheme combines the gaze-dependent activity of the N view cells to drive ViPC cell activity. Due to the combination of multiple local views, ViPC cells become location selective and can discriminate places based only on vision. Figure 19.9a, b (see plate 6) shows two place fields obtained by recording two ViPC units when the robot was moving in a square arena after learning. The cell of figure 19.9a is maximally active only when the robot is in a localized region of the arena. Its firing rate decreases with a Gaussian-like law as the robot leaves that area. Due to visual aliasing, some cells can have multiple subfields, i.e., they cannot differentiate spatial locations effectively. For instance, the cell of figure 19.9b has

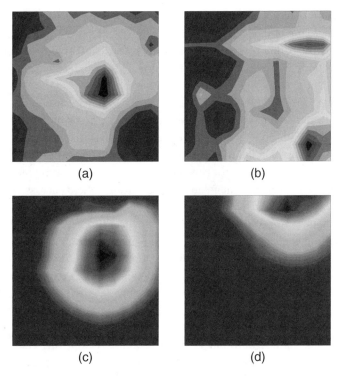

Figure 19.9
(a, b) Two samples of receptive fields obtained by recording from the vision-based place cell (ViPC) layer of the model. The squares represent overhead views of the environment. For each position $\bar{p}$ visited by the robot, the corresponding mean firing rate of the recorded cell is plotted. Red regions indicate high activity whereas dark blue regions denote low firing rates. The receptive field in (a) codes for a localized spatial location. The cell in (b) is maximally active at two different locations (multi-peak receptive field) because these purely vision-based representations are affected by the sensory aliasing problem. (c, d) Two typical place fields of cells in the CA3-CA1 layer of the model. Combining visual information and path integration yields stable place cell responses (single-peak receptive fields) that solve the visual aliasing problem. (From Arleo, 2000.) See plate 6 for color version.

a double-peak receptive field and encodes two distinct locations because they provide similar visual information.

The model postulates a role for the superficial layer of the lateral entorhinal cortex in allothetic space coding, suggesting it as a possible locus for the ViPC space representation. The entorhinal cortex constitutes the main "cortical gate" for the hippocampal formation, in the sense it receives highly processed inputs, via the perirhinal and parahippocampal cortices, from several neocortical associative areas (e.g., the parietal lobe) and conveys such information to the hippocampus via the perforant path (Witter, 1993).

Path Integration   The robot integrates its linear and angular displacements over time to generate an environment-independent representation of its position relative to a starting point $\vec{p}(t_0)$. Such a path integration mechanism is used to drive a set of place units PiPC, whose activity depends only on self-motion signals and provides idiothetic space coding.

PiPC units have preconfigured metric interrelations within an abstract allocentric reference frame S' which is mapped onto the physical space S according to the robot's entry position $\vec{p}(t_0)$ and the absolute directional reference Φ provided by HD cells. As discussed later, during spatial learning the robot couples the activity patterns of PiPC cells with the local views encoded by ViPC cells. This allows the system to learn a mapping function $S' \rightarrow S$ such that PiPC cells can maintain coherent firing patterns across different entries in a familiar environment. The vision-based representation ViPC is also employed to prevent the path integrator from accumulating errors over time (see section on Exploratory Behavior, later in this chapter).

The model proposes the superficial layer of the medial entorhinal cortex (MEC) as a possible anatomical locus for the PiPC representation. Indeed, experimental data suggest that the place field topology of location-sensitive cells in MEC does not change across different environments (Quirk et al., 1992).

Combining Visual and Egomotion Representations   During the robot-environment interaction, correlations between visually driven cells and path integration are processed by unsupervised Hebbian learning to build HP cell responses. ViPC and PiPC cells project to CA3–CA1 units by means of synapses established online by Hebbian learning. Thus, the activity of CA3–CA1 cells integrates allothetic and idiothetic signals to yield stable place selectivity. Figure 19.9c, d shows two typical place fields recorded in the CA3–CA1 layer of the model. Place fields are less noisy than those recorded from ViPC, and 97% of the recorded CA3–CA1 units do not exhibit multipeak fields, meaning that the system overcomes the sensory aliasing problem of purely vision-based representations.

As previously mentioned, the goal is to cover the environment by a large population of overlapping place fields to be used for the self-localization task. Such redundancy helps in terms of stability and robustness of the place code. Figure 19.10 (see plate 7) shows an example of CA3–CA1 population responses created by the robot after spatial learning. The two-dimensional space is covered by the CA3–CA1 place fields uniformly and densely. Note that place units are not topographically arranged within the CA3–CA1 layer of the model. That is, two cells i and j coding for two adjacent locations $\vec{p}_i$ and $\vec{p}_j$, respectively, are not necessarily neighboring neurons in the network. In the figure, CA3–CA1 cells are associated with their place field center only for monitoring purposes.

Population vector decoding (Georgopoulos et al., 1986; Wilson and McNaughton, 1993) is employed to reconstruct the robot's current position by computing the center of mass

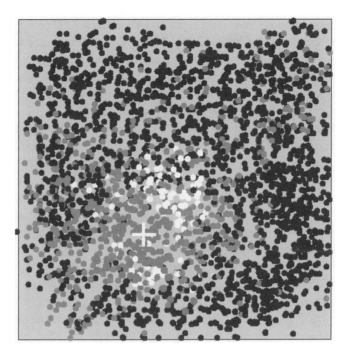

Figure 19.10
Sample of CA3-CA1 ensemble firing in the model. Each dot denotes the center of a place field. Red dots indicate highly active HP cells and dark blue dots denote silent neurons. The center of mass of the population activity (white cross) is used to reconstruct the robot's position. (From Arleo, 2000.) See plate 7 for color version.

of the ensemble CA3–CA1 firing pattern (white cross in figure 19.10). The estimated position $\vec{p}'(t)$ is near, but not necessarily identical, to the robot's actual location $\vec{p}(t)$. The approximation $\vec{p}'(t) \approx \vec{p}(t)$ is good for large neural populations covering the environment densely and uniformly (Salinas and Abbott, 1994).

Interrelation between Allothetic and Idiothetic Representations
In order to combine allothetic and idiothetic representations effectively, the system must maintain them coherently over time. This section describes how the robot aligns visual and self-motion signals during both the initial exploration of the environment and across different experimental sessions.

Exploratory Behavior and Path Integration Calibration   When the robot enters a novel environment, it must explore it to learn a place field representation incrementally, while maintaining allothetic and idiothetic spatial information coherent over time. Since the environment is unfamiliar, the robot starts by relying upon path integration only. The entry location $\vec{p}(t_0)$ becomes the origin (home) of the reference frame, relative to which the idiothetic space representation PiPC is built. The HD system provides the allocentric overall orientation of such spatial reference frame. As exploration proceeds, the local views encoded by the allothetic ViPC representation are mapped onto this spatial framework, such that vision and the path integrator can jointly participate in establishing a stable state space representation (see earlier section on Hippocampal place cells).

At the very beginning, exploration consists of short return trips (e.g., narrow loops) centered at the home location $\vec{p}(t_0)$ and directed toward evenly distributed radial directions. This behavior relies on the HD system and allows the robot to explore the home area exhaustively. Afterwards, the robot switches to an open-field exploration strategy. It starts moving in a random direction, recruiting a new subset of place units at each novel location. After a while, the path integrator has to be recalibrated; thus the robot stops creating place units and starts following its homing vector to return to the origin. As soon as it arrives and recognizes a previously visited location (not necessarily $\vec{p}(t_0)$), it utilizes the learned allothetic representation ViPC to realign the path integrator. Once vision calibrates the path integrator, the open-field exploratory behavior is resumed and the robot starts recruiting new place units again.

Such a loop-based exploratory pattern allows the robot to pursue exploration of the entire environment while keeping the dead reckoning error bounded over time (figure

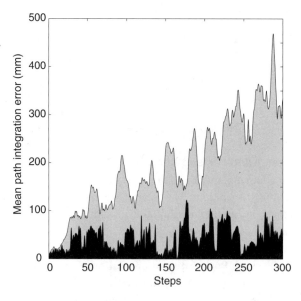

Figure 19.11
Uncalibrated (light gray curve) and calibrated (black curve) mean path integration error for loop-based exploration. (From Arleo et al., 2004, © 2004 IEEE.)

19.11). As a consequence of this loop-based behavior, the starting region is given great importance by the robot as it becomes familiar with a novel environment. Several behavioral studies have focused on the locomotor behavior of rodents in novel environments and have reported a typical exploratory pattern consisting of looped excursions centered at their starting home base (e.g., Drai et al., 2001). The model predicts that maintaining the path integrator and the vision-based representation mutually consistent over time might be one of the factors in such a loop-based exploratory behavior.

Intersession Coherence of the Spatial Representation   When entering a familiar environment, the robot needs to realign the components of its spatial representation (i.e., head direction, vision-based space code, and path integrator) in order to reactivate a coherent description of the environment. Failure of such a reinstantiating process might result in creating a new superfluous representation. Since the realigning procedure relies on the coupling between external and internal cues established during training by LTP correlational learning, impairing this mechanism would result in unstable intersession representations. This is consistent with experimental findings showing that animals with deficient LTP exhibit stable hippocampal maps within sessions, but exhibit unstable mapping between separate runs (Barnes et al., 1997).

In a first series of experiments, the constellation of visual cues is kept fixed during spatial learning. Thus, the system learns stable correlations between the idiothetic and allothetic components of the HD and HP representations. As a consequence, if the robot undergoes disorientation (disrupting the path integrator) before being placed back in the familiar environment, it can use visual information to polarize its HD representation, reset its path integrator, and reinstantiate the previously learned HP field representation properly. Figure 19.12a (see plate 8) shows three intersession responses of one HD cell and one HP cell from the PoSC and CA1–CA3 layers of the model, respectively. At the beginning of each session, the constellation of visual cues (whose centroid is represented by the asterisk in the figure) is rotated by 90°. Visual cues exert a strong control upon both directional and place representations: the HD and HP cells are anchored to the visual cues and their firing patterns rotate according to the visual reorientation. Importantly, the firing patterns of HD and HP cells are always updated consistently, suggesting a complete functional coupling between direction and place coding.

In a second series of experiments, the constellation of visual cues undergoes arbitrary rotations during spatial learning. Thus, the Hebbian learning scheme fails to establish stable correlations between idiothetic and allothetic inputs. As a consequence, when the robot is disoriented and put back in the explored environment, the HD and HP representations are not anchored to visual cues, and exhibit intersession remapping (figure 19.12b). These results are consistent with those reported by Knierim et al., (1995), from recordings of HD and HP cells in unrestrained rats.

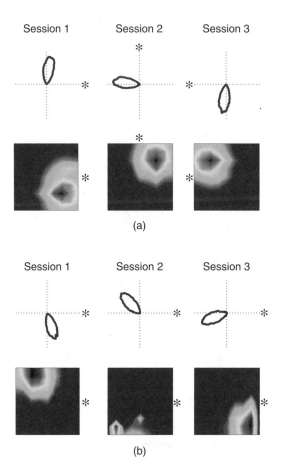

Figure 19.12
Intersession responses of one HD cell in the PoSC and one CA3-CA1 place cell of the model. At the beginning of each session the robot is disoriented. (a) During training the visual cue configuration (whose centroid is indicated by the asterisk) remains stable. Between probe sessions the constellation of visual cues undergoes a +90° rotation. Both the HD and the HP cell are controlled by the visual scene and reorient their receptive fields following the +90° intersession rotations. (b) The visual configuration is not stable during spatial learning. The data show that the disoriented robot fails to reactivate coherent representations across probe sessions, and remapping occurs. The directional and place selectivity does not maintain a fixed orientation relative to visual cues. See plate 8 for color version.

Action Learning: Goal-Oriented Spatial Behavior

The spatial learning system enables the robot to estimate its position in the environment based upon the ensemble firing of a population of HP cells. This section addresses the following question: how can the HP representation support goal-oriented navigation?

In the model, HP cells drive a downstream population of extra-hippocampal action cells whose ensemble activity mediates allocentric motor commands and guides the goal-oriented behavior of the robot (figure 19.1). Then, the navigation question is how to establish a mapping function $M: P \rightarrow A$ from the place cell activity space P to the action space A. A reinforcement learning scheme is employed to acquire M based on the robot's experience. The robot interacts with the environment and reward-dependent stimuli elicit the synaptic changes of the connections from place units to action units in order to learn the appropriate action-selection policy. After training, the system can relate any physical location to the most suitable local action to navigate toward the goal while avoiding obstacles. This results in an ensemble pattern of activity of the action units which provides a navigational map to support goal-directed behavior. Note that since the CA3–CA1 space coding presented (see section on Combining Visual and Egomotion Representations) solves the problem of ambiguous inputs or partially hidden states, the current state is fully known to the system and reinforcement learning can be applied in a straightforward manner.

Action learning consists of a sequence of training paths starting at random positions and ending either when the robot reaches the rewarding location $\vec{p}_{goal}$ or after a timeout. At the beginning of each trial, the robot determines its starting location and orientation based upon its HP and HD representations, respectively, (see section on Intersession Coherence of the Spatial Representation). Then, it starts searching for the goal while improving its action-selection policy. Temporal difference (TD) reinforcement learning (Sutton and Barto, 1998) is applied to allow the robot to learn to predict the outcome of its actions with respect to a given target. A prediction error $\delta(t)$ is used to estimate the difference between the expected and the actual future reward when, at a location $\vec{p}(t)$, the robot takes the action $a(t)$ and reaches the location $\vec{p}(t + 1)$ at time $t + 1$. Training enables the system to minimize this error locally. The convergence condition $\delta(t) \approx 0$ means that, given any state-action pair, the deviation between the predicted and the actual reward tends to zero.

Goal-learning performance is measured in terms of: (1) the mean search latency, i.e., the mean number of steps needed by the robot to find the target $\vec{p}_{goal}$, over training trials; (2) the generalization capabilities of the system, i.e., the ability to initiate goal-directed actions at locations never experienced during training. Figure 19.13a shows a navigation map learned by the robot when the rewarding location $\vec{p}_{goal}$ was in proximity of the upper left corner of a square environment. The map was acquired after only five training trials and enables the robot to navigate toward the goal from any position in the environment. The vector field representation of figure 19.13a has been obtained by rastering uniformly

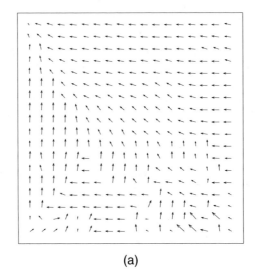

(a)

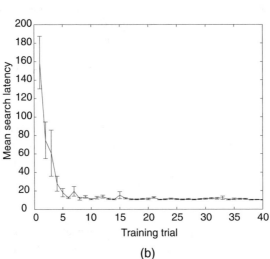

(b)

Figure 19.13
(a) Vector field representation of a navigation map learned by the robot after five training trials. The target location is near the upper left corner of the environment. Arrows represent the local motion directions encoded by the ensemble action cell activity after learning. (b) Mean search latency (i.e., mean number of steps needed by the robot to reach the target) as a function of training trials. The reward-based learning algorithm converges after approximately ten trials. (From Arleo et al., 2004, © 2004 IEEE.)

over the environment and computing, for each sampled position, the local action (arrow) encoded by the ensemble action cell activity. Many sampled locations were not visited by the robot during training; that is, the robot was able to associate appropriate goal-oriented actions to never experienced spatial positions. The mean amount of generalization, defined as the percentage of sampled positions that were not visited by the robot during training, is of about 45% for the map of figure 19.13a. This large generalization property is mainly a consequence of the coarse coding state representation provided by the CA3–CA1 place cells of the model. Figure 19.13b shows the mean search latencies as a function of training trials. The search latencies decrease rather rapidly and reach the asymptotic value (corresponding to appropriate goal-directed behavior) after approximately 10 trials. This convergence time is comparable to that of rats solving the reference memory task in the Morris water maze (Morris et al., 1982).

Figure 19.14 shows the navigation vector fields learned by the robot in the presence of one obstacle and two distinct types of rewarding locations, $\vec{p}_{goal}^{1}$ (simulating, for instance, a feeder position) and $\vec{p}_{goal}^{2}$ (simulating, for instance, the location of a water reservoir). Targets $\vec{p}_{goal}^{1}$ and $\vec{p}_{goal}^{2}$ are located at the bottom left and bottom right corners of the environment, respectively. First, the robot is trained to navigate towards $\vec{p}_{goal}^{1}$. Figure 19.14A represents the navigation map for $\vec{p}_{goal}^{1}$ learned by the robot after 30 training trials. While optimizing the navigation policy for $\vec{p}_{goal}^{1}$, the robot may encounter the rewarding location $\vec{p}_{goal}^{2}$ and start learning a partial navigation map for it, even if $\vec{p}_{goal}^{2}$ is not its current primary target. Figure 19.14B shows the knowledge about $\vec{p}_{goal}^{2}$ acquired by the robot while searching for $\vec{p}_{goal}^{1}$. Thus, when $\vec{p}_{goal}^{2}$ becomes the primary target, the robot does not start from zero knowledge and needs a short training period to learn an optimal policy to navigate toward $\vec{p}_{goal}^{2}$. Figure 19.14C displays the navigation map acquired by the robot after 10 training trials when searching for $\vec{p}_{goal}^{2}$.

Like the previous hypothesis by Brown and Sharp (1995), the model postulates that the anatomical interaction between the hippocampus and the ventral striatum, and in particular the fornix projection from the CA1 region to the nucleus accumbens, might be a part of the system where the reward-dependent action learning takes place. The nucleus accumbens seems involved in processing information concerning goal-oriented behavior (Tabuchi et al., 2000). Ventral striatal neurons receive space coding information from the hippocampal formation and are activated in relation to the expectation of rewards (Schultz et al., 1997). The presence of dopamine-dependent plasticity in the striatum suggests that dopamine responses might be involved in synaptic adaptation yielding, reward-based learning. In particular, dopamine neurons in the mammalian midbrain seem to encode the difference between expected and actual occurrence of reward stimuli (Schultz et al., 1997). Thus, the temporal difference error $\delta(t)$ used in the model to update the synaptic weights from CA3–CA1 cells to action cells may be thought of as a dopamine-like teaching signal.

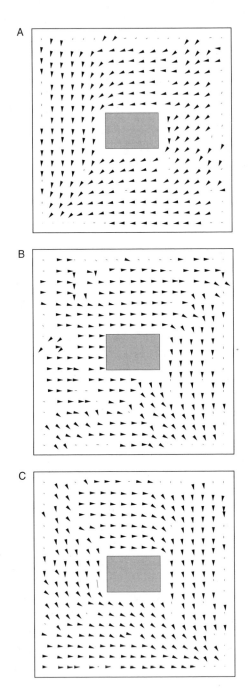

Figure 19.14

Navigation task in the presence of one obstacle (gray object) and two distinct targets, $\vec{p}_{goal}^{1}$ (nearby the bottom left corner) and $\vec{p}_{goal}^{2}$ (nearby the bottom right corner). (A) Navigation vector field learned by the robot after 30 trials when searching for $\vec{p}_{goal}^{1}$. (B) Partial navigation map for $\vec{p}_{goal}^{2}$ learned by the robot when focusing on $\vec{p}_{goal}^{2}$. (C) Final navigation map learned by the robot after 10 trials when searching for $\vec{p}_{goal}^{2}$. (From Arleo et al., 2004, © 2004 IEEE.)

Conclusions

What can we learn from models? As we have seen in this chapter, modeling allows us to illustrate the links between different levels of neuroscience. In particular, we have seen that a model that incorporates electrophysiological characteristics of head direction cells and place cells can be used for navigation in tasks akin to the Morris water maze and demonstrate effects on the behavioral level.

The model stresses the importance of the integration of different sensory modalities, in particular, a smart combination of proprioceptive and visual information for navigation. As a consequence, the model postulates that input to the hippocampus should consist of two streams (i.e., processing of proprioceptive and visual information) and suggests specific functional roles of the areas that provide inputs to hippocampus.

The involvement of the hippocampal formation in spatial navigation of animals has been investigated for a long time. Furthermore, very recent electrophysiological findings have shown the evidence for location-sensitive cells in the human hippocampus and parahippocampus (Ekstrom et al., 2003). Theoretical modeling and bio-inspired robotics may suggest one or several potential strategies of how animals and humans (could, in principle) solve the problem of navigation using the place cell information provided by the hippocampal formation. Also, neuromimetic models can provide hypotheses about the contribution of other nonhippocampal structures that might be critical for successful navigation. It will be the task of experiments to check whether the specific assumptions and predictions of a computational model are correct. The falsification of models may help toward further understanding.

References

Arleo A (2000) Spatial learning and navigation in neuro-mimetic systems, modeling the rat hippocampus. ISBN 3-89825-247-7, Verlag-dissertation.

Arleo A, Gerstner W (2000) Spatial cognition and neuro-mimetic navigation: a model of hippocampal place cell activity. Biol Cybern 83: 287–299.

Arleo A, Gerstner W (2001) Spatial orientation in navigating agents: Modeling head-direction cells. Neurocomputing 38–40: 1059–1065.

Arleo A, del R. Millán J, Floreano D (1999) Efficient learning of variable-resolution cognitive maps for autonomous indoor navigation. IEEE Trans Robotics and Automation 15: 990–1000.

Arleo A, Smeraldi F, Hug S, Gerstner W (2004) Cognitive navigation based on non-uniform Gabor space sampling, unsupervised growing networks, and reinforcement learning. IEEE Trans Neural Networks 15: 639–652.

Barnes CA, Suster MS, Shen J, McNaughton BL (1997) Multistability of cognitive maps in the hippocampus of old rats. Nature 388: 272–275.

Brooks RA (1991) Intelligence without representation. Artificial Intelligence 47: 139–159.

Brown MA, Sharp PE (1995) Simulation of spatial-learning in the Morris water maze by a neural network model of the hippocampal formation and nucleus accumbens. Hippocampus 5: 171–188.

Burgess N, O'Keefe J (1996) Neuronal computations underlying the firing of place cells and their role in navigation. Hippocampus 6: 749–762.

Daugman JG (1980) Two-dimensional spectral analysis of cortical receptive field profiles. Vision Research 20: 847–856.

Degris T, Sigaud O, Wiener SI, Arleo A (2004) Rapid response of head direction cells to reorienting visual cues: a computational model. Neurocomputing 58–60C: 675–682.

Dorigo M, Colombetti M (1998) Robot Shaping. Cambridge, MA: MIT Press.

Drai D, Kafkafi N, Benjamini Y, Elmer G, Golani I (2001) Rats and mice share common ethologically relevant parameters of exploratory behavior. Behav Brain Res 125: 133–140.

Ekstrom AD, Kahana MJ, Caplan JB, Fields TA, Isham EA, Newman EL, Fried I (2003) Cellular networks underlying human spatial navigation. Nature 425: 184–188.

Elfes A (1987) Sonar-based real-world mapping and navigation. IEEE J Robotics Automation 3: 249–256.

Gallistel CR (1990) The Organization of Learning. Cambridge, MA: MIT Press.

Gaussier P, Revel A, Banquet JP, Babeau V (2002) From view cells and place cells to cognitive map learning: processing stages of the hippocampal system. Biol Cybern 86: 15–28.

Georgopoulos AP, Schwartz A, Kettner RE (1986) Neuronal population coding of movement direction. Science 233: 1416–1419.

Golob EJ, Stackman RW, Wong AC, Taube JS (2001) On the behavioral significance of head direction cells: neural and behavioral dynamics during spatial memory tasks. Behav Neurosci 115: 285–304.

Goodridge JP, Taube JS (1997) Interaction between the postsubiculum and anterior thalamus in the generation of head direction cell activity. J Neurosci 17: 9315–9330.

Hahnloser RHR (2003) Emergence of neural integration in the head-direction system by visual supervision. Neuroscience 120: 877–891.

Hubel DH, Wiesel TN (1962) Receptive fields, binocular interaction and functional architecture in the cat's visual cortex. J Physiol 160: 106–154.

Knierim JJ, Kudrimoti HS, McNaughton BL (1995) Place cells, head direction cells, and the learning of landmark stability. J Neurosci 15: 1648–1659.

Kuipers BJ, Byun YT (1991) A robot exploration and mapping strategy based on a semantic hierarchy of spatial representations. Robot Auton Syst 8: 47–63.

McNaughton BL, Barnes CA, Gerrard JL, Gothard K, Jung MW, Knierim JJ, Kudrimoti H, Qin Y, Skaggs WE, Suster M, Weaver KL (1996) Deciphering the hippocampal polyglot: The hippocampus as a path integration system. J Exp Biol 199: 173–185.

Mittelstaedt ML, Mittelstaedt H (1980) Homing by path integrator in a mammal. Naturwissenschaften 67: 566–567.

Morris RG, Garrud P, Rawlins JN, O'Keefe J (1982) Place navigation impaired in rats with hippocampal lesions. Nature 297: 681–683.

Muller RU, Stead M, Pach J (1996) The hippocampus as a cognitive graph. J Gen Physiol 107: 663–694.

Nolfi S, Floreano D (2000) Evolutionary robotics. The Biology, Intelligence, and Technology of Self-Organizing Machines. Cambridge, MA: MIT Press.

O'Keefe J, Dostrovsky J (1971) The hippocampus as a spatial map. Preliminary evidence from unit activity in the freely-moving rat. Brain Res 34: 171–175.

O'Keefe J, Nadel L (1978) The Hippocampus as a Cognitive Map. Oxford: Clarendon Press.

Quirk GJ, Muller RU, Kubie JL, Ranck JB, Jr. (1992) The positional firing properties of medial entorhinal neurons: description and comparison with hippocampal place cells. J Neurosci 12: 1945–1963.

Ranck JB Jr (1984) Head-direction cells in the deep cell layers of dorsal presubiculum in freely moving rats. Society for Neuroscience Meeting 10: 599.

Salinas E, Abbott LF (1994) Vector reconstruction from firing rates. J Comput Neurosci 1: 89–107.

Schölkopf B, Mallot HA (1995) View-based cognitive mapping and path planning. Adap Behav 3: 311–348.

Schultz W, Dayan P, Montague PR (1997) A neural substrate of prediction and reward. Science 275: 1593–1599.

Sharp PE, Kubie JL, Muller RU (1990) Firing properties of hippocampal neurons in a visually symmetrical environment: contributions of multiple sensory cues and mnemonic processes. J Neurosci 10: 3093–3105.

Sutton RS, Barto AG (1998) Reinforcement Learning, an Introduction. Cambridge, MA: MIT Press-Bradford Books.

Tabuchi ET, Mulder AB, Wiener SI (2000) Position and behavioral modulation of synchronization of hippocampal and accumbens neuronal discharges in freely moving rats. Hippocampus 10: 717–728.

Taube JS (1998) Head direction cells and the neurophysiological basis for a sense of direction. Prog Neurobiol 55: 225–256.

Thrun S (1998) Learning maps for indoor mobile robot navigation. Artificial Intelligence 99: 21–71.

Tolman EC (1948) Cognitive maps in rats and men. Psychol Rev 55: 189–208.

Trullier O, Meyer JA (2000) Animat navigation using a cognitive graph. Biol Cybern 83: 271–285.

Trullier O, Wiener SI, Berthoz A, Meyer JA (1997) Biologically based artificial navigation systems: review and prospects. Prog Neurobiol 51: 483–544.

Wilson MA, McNaughton BL (1993) Dynamics of the hippocampal ensemble code for space. Science 261: 1055–1058.

Witter MP (1993) Organization of the entorhinal-hippocampal system: a review of current anatomical data. Hippocampus 3: 33–44.

20 Head Direction Cells and Neural Bases of Spatial Orientation: Synthesis and Future Perspectives

Sidney I. Wiener

This chapter will attempt to place into perspective some of the unresolved issues raised in the preceding chapters about the neural bases of spatial orientation. Relevant points will be revisited to provide context for assembling a synthetic view of the function of these systems, integrating observations made in the previous chapters. In the process, attention will be drawn to some elements that still need clarification. This will aim to help chart out directions for future research. The discussion will include several themes: vestibular role in the origin and elaboration of the head direction signal; selectivity of head direction cells for the orientation in the horizontal plane only; distinct multiple brain systems for processing head orientation signals; landmark familiarity and memory in polarizing directional responses; the influences of maze shape; reconciling signals of voluntary motor command, motor efferent collateral, and proprioceptive information; effects of tight restraint on neural orienting systems; brain mechanisms for navigation in humans; relations with EEG; and the question why so many brain areas have HD cells? (See the cited chapters for bibliographic citations.)

Vestibular Role in the Origin and Elaboration of the Head Direction Signal

The head direction (HD) signal is dependent upon inputs originating in the vestibular end organs. Stackman and Taube (1997; see chapter 7) demonstrated that sodium arsanilate-induced vestibular lesions lead to a suppression of directional responses in HD cells of the anterodorsal thalamic nucleus (ADN). Even after the rats recovered postural stability (and presumably stable gaze as well) the cells' activity showed no directional modulation, even after four days. After unilateral or bilateral vestibular lesions, background activity in the vestibular nuclei becomes abnormal, but this returns to normal within three days, permitting the behavioral recovery that Stackman and Taube observed in their animals. However, the background vestibular signal was not sufficient to permit directional responses to return, nor did exposure to visual cues. The latter is remarkable because HD cells are more powerfully influenced by visual signals than by idiothetic cues, including vestibular stimulation. Vestibular signals must hence play a particularly vital role. Why is this input, which has a relatively modest contribution in the intact animal, so crucial?

One possible explanation builds upon the popular hypothesis that the head direction signal is generated in the DTN-LMN (dorsal tegmental nucleus of Gudden–lateral mammillary nucleus) feedback circuit which functions as a dynamic attractor network (chapters by Sharp, Rolls and Touretzky). Such a dynamic neural architecture would permit the persistence of head direction cell activity over prolonged periods of time while the head remains stationary in one orientation. The robustness of such a network could be characterized in neurophysiological experiments under conditions when HD responses, and hence the attractors, break down (e.g., during tight restraint, observations of erratic response in dark reviewed by Knierim, or Taube's descriptions of the absence of directional responses in rats walking on the ceiling, and in hypogravity during parabolic flight). Neurons of the DTN receive inputs from the vestibular nuclei via the nucleus prepositus hypoglossi, and discharge as a function of head velocity in the horizontal plane. A new hypothesis, then, is that it is the absence of acceleration-triggered vestibular signals during head movement that leads to the disruption of the velocity responses of the DTN neurons, which then would interfere with the functioning of the DTN-LMN attractor-generating network. To verify this, velocity responses in DTN neurons could be tested after vestibular lesions. Such an experiment could be performed during the period of compensation and adaptive learning following a vestibular deficit, when optic field flow and proprioceptive information would gradually replace vestibular-based velocity information. These two signals also feed into the vestibular nuclei (which are thus named rather inappropriately). A related study could be made in human patients during compensation from vestibular lesions or after surgical neurectomy. Since vestibular lesions suppress HD cell activity, studies of these patients should be reevaluated in terms of characterizing the orientation and navigation capacities that are lost or retained in the absence of head direction cell responses, similar to the logic applied by Aggleton in chapter 13.

After the head direction signal emerges within the brainstem DTN and diencephalic LMN circuitry, it ascends through ADN, retrosplenial cortex, and postsubiculum (Pos) to the hippocampus, which then projects back to Pos, which in turn projects to the mammillary nuclei (chapter 2 by Hopkins). In chapter 1, Sharp reviewed several differences in the head direction signals in recordings of successively more rostral brain structures. One of these was that in the left and right LMN, directional response curves are narrower for ipsiversive turns (as opposed to contraversive ones). This is no longer found in the next structure in the pathway, the ADN, presumably because, as Hopkins notes, the projection from LMN to ADN is bilateral. This indicates that even though the postsubiculum receives this bilaterally influenced signal, the descending projections to LMN do not correct the directional asymmetry of the tuning curve widths in the LMN. The issue of how hippocampal outputs might affect the head direction system will be further discussed below.

Why Are Head Direction Cells Selective for the Orientation Only in the Horizontal (yaw) Plane?

The vestibular origin for HD signals likely provides the basis for their exclusive selectivity for the horizontal plane. The HD system shares elements of the vestibulo-oculomotor circuitry (including vestibular nucleus and nucleus prepositus hypoglossi (NPH). This system distinguishes signals from the three orthogonally positioned semicircular canals (see figure 6.1). In effect, signals from the horizontal canals are transmitted along a specific pathway leading to lateral rectus muscles for the vestibulocular reflex in the horizontal plane.

Thus, the oculomotor and head direction systems likely share some common substrates, particularly those isolating horizontal plane angular displacement signals (as reviewed by Glasauer in chapter 6). Even though areas in these pathways receive inputs from eye muscles, there is no evidence of eye position having any influence on head direction responses (as shown by Rolls's recordings in monkeys; chapter 14). It would be interesting to precisely determine the complete extent of the vestibulo-oculomotor infrastructure shared by HD pathways, and to identify where the latter branch off. Perhaps this could be tested with markers of activity, such as early genes. Eye position and motor command signals must be subtracted from the retinal image in order to give signals in head coordinates rather than retinal coordinates (see Duffy et al., chapter 15). At the level of the vestibular nuclei, there are already the vestibular-only (VO) neurons (Gdowski and McCrea, 1999; see chapter 6), which respond to the rotation of the head in space independently of eye movements. Surprisingly, they respond for passive whole body rotation, but are mostly insensitive to active neck rotation of the head on the trunk (Roy and Cullen, 2001, 2004; see chapter 6), despite the fact that active head movement on a stationary trunk stimulates the semicircular canals. It remains to be determined if these vestibular nucleus neurons have a privileged connectivity with the head direction system. It is noteworthy, however, that other brain systems are not restricted to representing head angle only in the horizontal plane. For example, vertical semicircular canals feed into a distinct parallel system (involving the interstitial nucleus of Cajal) that effects vertical eye movements. Note the recent results of Kim et al. (2003; reviewed in chapter 3 by Taube) showing HD responses in the reference frame of a vertically oriented surface indicate that there is some plasticity in the responses of the HD network. In addition, rotational and translational motions are also independently processed and, as demonstrated by Glasauer in chapter 17, are sometimes inaccurately combined for navigation.

Distinct Multiple Brain Systems for Processing Head Orientation-Related Signals

The psychophysical studies reviewed in the chapter by Israël and Warren indicate that there are several brain systems detecting static head orientation, rotation angles, and movement dynamics. In one experiment, subjects were required to report the magnitude of passive angular displacements, and responses were made either during or after the movement. Interestingly, the reports during movements were less accurate, presumably because of interference between perception and simultaneous reporting. This suggests that perception and reporting share some common, limited neural computational substrates. Another type of disparity was observed between accuracy in gaze stabilization after passive rotations, and subjects' reports of angles rotated. This is interesting because the same vestibular signals are essential for both of these responses. Thus, even though only one angular displacement signal is transmitted from vestibular end organs to the brainstem nuclei, they diverge and are sent respectively to oculomotor and perceptual/ cognitive systems leading to these differences in accuracy. Such pathways could respectively originate in VO and other types of vestibular nucleus neurons.

The issue of multiple pathways for treating directional information is also reflected in the summary presented by Dudchenko et al. in chapter 11 of discordances between HD responses versus actual orientation behaviors. How are head direction signals exploited for orientation? One approach is to attempt to distinguish those behaviors that are concordant with head direction cell responses from those that are not. In chapter 10, Mizumori et al. pointed out differences among certain areas that contain HD cells. Their data indicate that laterodorsal thalamic (LD), striatal, and premotor cortical (PrCM) HD cells have distinctive differences from the LMN-AD-postsubiculum pathway in their responses in light and dark conditions, in reference frames used, and in correlations to behavior. It remains to be determined what are the criteria and mechanisms for the head direction signals of the various nuclei to be engaged for behavior. Such disparities are consistent with numerous studies showing multiple brain systems to be respectively specialized for different types of spatial behaviors. An often-cited example is that of the hippocampal system as involved in localizing goals on the basis of configurational cues, while the caudate nucleus would be necessary for approaches toward visible goals (Packard et al., 1989). These various systems appear to provide the bases for complementary spatial orientation strategies (Albertin et al., 2001).

As pointed out by Berthoz (2000), distinct brain pathways are respectively involved for processing static head orientation or the direction of movements (even though movement signals are likely to play a role in elaborating static head direction representations). In chapter 4, Zugaro and Wiener cited the cases of two rather different types of visual information that affect head direction cells: landmarks and optic field flow. Recall that optic flow concerns the apparent movement of the entire visual field in the direction opposite the head rotation. While this is technically considered an external cue, it is informative only about the velocity and distance of movements (and bears no direct information about absolute orientation). However, in chapter 15, Duffy et al. showed that vestibular and optic field flow information also informs heading responses in primate posterior cortex. The point here is that the latter concern the direction that the head is moving, rather than the orientation of the head, which is not necessarily facing in the direction of movement. These heading responses resemble those shown by Chen et al. (1994a,b; cited in the chapter by Stackman and Zugaro) in the rat parietal cortex (although here the animals were only tested moving nose forward). Duffy et al. discussed many brain areas that are likely substrates for processing rotational and directional information. For example, neurons in the parieto-insular vestibular cortex, discovered by of Grüsser (Guldin and Grüsser, 1998; cited in chapter 15), are sensitive to active rotations of the head in many directions, including those that combine the three orthogonal axes. The distinction between heading versus head direction is important for navigation, with heading indicating the displacement one has made regardless of viewing angle. In contrast, head direction would be more vital for deter-mining orientations at static positions on the basis of remembered views. Note that this type of reconstruction of one's position and orientation could require mental rotations if one is experiencing a familiar location from a novel viewpoint. Such processing would be expected to involve interactions between the head direction system, parietal cortex, and hippocampus.

On the other hand, processing of visual signals concerning landmarks is likely medi-ated via other pathways, such as the retinogeniculocortical route. Such signals would then enter the head direction system via areas like the retrosplenial cortex and postsubiculum. In chapter 10, Mizumori, et al. pointed out that signals could pass through the less well documented retinocollicular and posterior thalamic pathways. This would be responsible for polarizing directional responses relative to environmental cues in the visual back-ground. However the distinction between processing of optic field flow versus landmark cues was confounded by the results of Zugaro et al. (2003; chapter 4). Here we showed evidence that the head direction cell system can determine which (anchoring) cues are in the background on the basis of relative velocities of optic flow. During translational head movements, parallax makes these background objects appear to move more slowly across the retina. Thus, there must be some interaction between brain areas that detect apparent velocity and those that mark the bearing of visual landmark cues.

Landmark Familiarity and Memory in Polarizing Directional Responses

As the brain establishes directional responses when a rat enters an environment, there is apparently an interplay between parameters such as familiarity, cue stability, and disori-entation state, as evidenced by Knierim's observations of drift in directional responses after several minutes, slow drift, etc. To explain this, in chapter 8, Knierim proposes a compelling conceptual model including synaptic mechanisms; this remains to be experimentally tested. He indicated how Hebbian learning processes could be responsible for the stronger influences exerted by familiar visual cues. What are the mechanisms for this detection of familiarity? There also is the intriguing interplay between learned familiarity and the different responses of the network to 45° versus 180° cue rotations, which provide different levels of conflict between idiothetic and allothetic cues. Is higher cortical and hippocampal processing involved in this updating of the head direction system? For example, these inputs could reset the HD cell network to the previous polarity after arrival in a familiar environment from a new direction, or after it has been changed. Mizumori et al. (chapter 10) suggest that the retrosplenial cortex is the pivotal structure that sends a mnemonic signal to the rest of the HD system.

Experimental lesions of these respective structures could help better define their roles in familiarity detection and mnemonic signalling to the HD system. It would be interesting to observe the activity within, and interactions between, the hippocampal formation and the various structures of the HD system during the first few minutes in a novel environment, as the head direction cells become anchored to visual landmarks (Goodridge et al., 1998; cited in chapter 3). In order to distinguish among the various mechanisms for polarizing directional responses, experimental designs could exploit the fact that they operate on different timescales, with resetting in familiar environments occurring within 80 ms (Zugaro et al., 2003; cited in chapter 4) while drift and disorientation-related resetting can occur over the course of minutes (chapter 8).

The Influence of Maze Shape

Another issue evoked in several chapters, including those by Taube, Dudchenko et al., and Knierim, is the influence of the shape of the experimental maze on head direction responses. For example, several studies have shown that the contour of maze borders can influence head direction cells more strongly than distal environmental cues. For example in experimental mazes in the form of a square, rectangle, T, radial "sunburst", or spiral, this shape is a strong cue that can polarize the HD cell system, overpowering the influences of many salient cues in the room beyond the limits of the maze. The responses even follow the maze surface when rotated into the vertical plane (Kim et al., 2003; cited in chapter 3), defying stable distant visual cues. These observations counter the notion that head direction cells are simply a kind of internal compass, representing the orientation of the animal in a global maplike reference frame, dominated by background visual cues. Directional responses in hippocampal place cells (see Brunel and Muller's chapter 9) are also highly sensitive to the maze layout (when its shape is asymmetric or otherwise polarizing). In contrast to earlier work with place and head direction cells in high-walled apparatuses (Lever et al., 2002; Taube and Burton, 1995; Muller et al., 1987, cited in chapter

8), the studies cited above were performed on elevated mazes with only short walls surrounding them. Thus, in these cases, more distal room cues were visible but ignored despite the limited visual information about the geometry of the maze, which only included the rat's perspective view of the maze floor and low walls.

Considering the sparseness and complexity of the latter cues, it may be worthwhile to revive the concept of "action-space" in interpreting these results; that is, the spatial representation is polarized by the animal's activities in the arena. Thus, the brain may represent the environment in terms of the history of, or even the anticipation of, possible actions that may be taken there. Such a computation would be expected to take place over at least several minutes. This interpretation could apply to data in the blindfold and dark trials on Frohardt et al.'s circular maze (cited in chapter 11), where HD cells anchored directional responses relative to the point from which the rat enters the environment. Markus et al. (1995; reviewed in chapter 9) showed that the hippocampal place responses changed their directional properties after the rats shifted from a random foraging task to oriented running along a diamond pattern in the same environment. Note that in the 1995 study by Markus et al., the shift in activity occurred only a few minutes after the rat started running in the new pattern. Are the mechanisms for evaluating the possible actions of a given environment intrinsic to the hippocampus or other brain areas? Calton et al. (2003; cited in chapter 9) showed in ADN/Pos-lesioned rats evidence that hippocampal response directionality is independent of the head direction, and in fact the place cells had *greater* directional modulation than in control animals! Thus, action-space is computed outside the HD system. Lesion experiments could determine the pathways essential for processing information concerning the local geometry, or action-space, and its influence on head direction responses.

Reconciling Signals of Voluntary Motor Command, Motor Efferent Collateral and Proprioceptive Information for Spatial Orientation

It remains to be determined how and where in the brain motor-related signals are processed for spatial orientation, and how these signals articulate with the head direction system. Despite the fact that efferent collateral signals were first described in the 1950s, their neuroanatomical substrates have not yet been identified for locomotor displacements, although they are known for the oculomotor system. Processing executive motor command or efferent collateral signals is a complex task, since the amount of force exerted does not provide sufficient information to determine the magnitude of the displacement; it is also necessary to take into account how much resistance was encountered. For example, when walking on a slippery surface (or swimming against the current), the number of paces (or strokes) executed will not provide an accurate estimate of the distance covered. For the oculomotor system, this is not a problem since there is virtually no frictional drag for eye rotation movements. It is not yet possible to record neural signals corresponding to executive commands, efferent collaterals, and the ensemble of relevant proprioceptive signals. By training rats to be passively rotated while standing immobile, Zugaro et al. (2001; chapter 7) demonstrated that motor signals regulate peak firing of HD cells but do not alter tuning curve width or actual preferred direction. This suggests that motor state (i.e., free movement versus learned immobility) somehow gates the head direction signal, perhaps through a neuromodulatory pathway. Such a mechanism may be distinct from the weaker modulation of head direction cell activity in rapid versus slow velocity episodes in freely moving animals. This latter velocity modulation could result from velocity-related DTN signals. In chapter 7, Stackman and Zugaro reviewed recent experiments showing that optic field flow stimuli (generated by a rotating planetarium projector; Arleo et al., 2004; cited in chapter 7) can also influence AD HD cells. It would be interesting to see if peak firing rates of HD cells are dependent on the velocity of rotation of the projector.

Interesting recent results about proprioceptive processing concern the podokinetic system, which has yet to be studied in the rat. Mergner et al. (1993; cited in chapter 16 by Israël and Warren) found that the somatic receptors of the feet and legs transmit influential information concerning orientation. For example, in stationary, seated subjects, rotation of a platform on which the feet are resting induces sensations of trunk rotation as well as ocular nystagmus, a response more typically associated with head rotation. Israël and Warren suggest that podokinetic and vestibular information are responsible for the greater accuracy of estimates of angular displacements during active movements (Chance et al., 1998; cited in chapter 16). Such estimates are also more accurate when responses are made in reference to the frontward orientation of the body or to a visual reference cue. Furthermore, vestibular contributions to rotations were most accurately perceived in the simplest experimental conditions (when the head was rotated on the stationary upright trunk, with neither distracting visual targets nor trunk or leg movements). The authors found however, in general, estimates were better when the vestibular and proprioceptive systems were stimulated together. Mergner et al. (1993; see chapter 16) conclude "self-motion perception normally takes the visual scene as a reference, and vestibular input is simply used to verify the kinematic state of the scene; if the scene appears to be moving with respect to an earth-fixed reference frame, the visual signal is suppressed and perception is based on the vestibular signal."

Effects of Tight Restraint on Neural Orienting Systems

Another remaining mystery, possibly related to proprioceptive, vestibular, and motor signals, is the observation that most head direction cells stop firing when the rat is tightly restrained (Taube, et al., 1990; Taube, 1995; cited in chapter 7), even if it is passively reoriented into the preferred direction. Similar results were observed by Foster, et al. (1989; cited in chapter 7) with hippocampal place cells, which lost their initial place responses when the animal was returned to the firing field while under tight restraint. While the underlying mechanisms for this remain unclear, it has been shown that when tightly restrained rats are displaced passively in the light or dark, hippocampal cells still can show broad spatially selective responses (Gavrilov et al., 1998; cited in chapter 7). Furthermore, in hippocampal pyramidal cells showing spatially selective responses when the rat runs in only one direction in a running wheel, the activity drops to zero when the (unrestrained) animal stops running, but remains in the wheel (Czurkó et al., 1999; cited in chapter 7). This is not the case for head direction cells, which continue firing as the unrestrained animal remains immobile. One factor associated with this observation may be the close correlation of hippocampal theta (8 Hz) EEG with place cell activity and running. Is the cessation of HD cell firing during immobility (and perhaps even after vestibular lesions) related to the reduction of theta EEG activity? Perhaps firing rate is modulated by theta amplitude. While in freely moving rats there are no reports of hippocampal theta EEG modulation of head direction cells, studies in anesthetised animals have shown theta modulation in ADN (Albo et al., 2003; cited in chapters 2 and 13). However very few of the rhythmic ADN neurons showed high coherence with theta EEG, in contrast to those in the laterally adjacent anteroventral thalamic nucleus (AV). Note that AV receives hippocampal output projections, unlike ADN. This leads to the question whether we can characterize these adjacent nuclei as respectively belonging to two functionally distinct branches of the Papez circuit (chapter 13). As Bassett and Taube noted in chapter 5, the ascending pathway (DTN-LMN-AD-postsubiculum) would carry the head direction signal to the hippocampus, while hippocampal outputs to AV would then address signals back to cortical areas such as retrosplenial cortex, as well as to a descending pathway (AV—medial mammillary nucleus—ventral tegmental nucleus of Gudden). These would carry more intensely theta-modulated hippocampal output signals that are vital for certain types of learning (as discussed by Aggleton in chapter 13) and may provide a type of binding signal because of their synchronous rhythmic activity. This discussion ties in with Gray and McNaughton's (2000) theory of the hippocampal role in anxiety and schizophrenia, which involves activity in hippocampal output pathways (cited in chapters 2 and 13). In another viewpoint, Mizumori (chapter 10) proposes functional hypotheses concerning these hippocampal afferent versus efferent pathways that respectively code for focus of attention versus definition of behavioral responses. Such network interactions could provide the basis for the (provisional) rules that Knierim observed for the coupling of head direction cell and hippocampal place responses. Recall that in familiar environments, sudden but coherent shifts of head direction responses within the network correspond to the chaotic resetting (so-called "remapping") of hippocampal place responses. And, as noted above, familiarity signals could be signaled by the hippocampus to the head direction system, affording a stronger influence to environmental cues.

Brain Mechanisms for Navigation in Humans

The human brain contains all of the structures in which head direction and place cells have been recorded in the rat. The studies of Rolls (chapter 14) and Nishijo et al. (1997; cited in chapters 7 and 15) support the notion that these areas could also have comparable roles for orienting and navigation. Chapters 13 and 17 review functional imagery literature supporting such a functional homology. The studies of Duffy et al. (chapter 15) suggest that MSTd cortical neurons, which are selective for the direction of instantaneous self-movement, could also provide a neural basis for deriving the path of movements made prior to arriving at the current head direction. Furthermore, some MSTd neurons are particularly selective for the locations at which some of these movements occur. Duffy et al. propose that this is part of a system forming a dorsal limb of Papez's circuit (Papez 1937, cited in chapter 15), integrating limbic and posterior cingulate mechanisms serving the control of navigation and spatial orientation. A role for retrosplenial (i.e., posterior cingulate) cortex in navigation comes from functional imaging studies (Maguire 2001b; Burgess 2002; cited in chapter 13) involving large scale navigation, for instance, using film footage or virtual reality.

Aggleton (chapter 13) explained Burgess's (2002) proposal as follows: "the retrieval of spatial information, and hence spatial episodes, requires the setting of a particular viewpoint. This, in turn, depends on the representation of head direction and, hence, the input from the head direction system. The parietal cortex and retrosplenial cortices are given especial prominence in this model as they represent regions where there is an integration of different spatial systems (allocentric, egocentric, body orientation). As a consequence, information about current head direction makes it possible to translate allocentric representations into egocentric ones and vice versa (Burgess, 2002). This, in turn, helps the creation of distinctive episodes of information." It is important to note that only fractions of the cells in the respective structures of the HD system are actually sensitive to head direction. Perhaps the other cells are related to processing non-spatial memories since, as Aggleton notes, increased retrosplenial cortex activity is also found in neuroimagery studies of memory (Maguire 2001a; chapter 13), including studies of autobiographical event recall (Maguire 2001b; chapter 13).

Why Do So Many Brain Areas Have HD Cells?

This question may be more rigorously stated as follows: "What evolutionary advantage could arise from so many brain areas containing HD cells?" Nowhere near so many examples of essentially the same signal have been found in any sensory or motor system of the brain. There could be many reasons for this. For example, as previously alluded to, this may facilitate distinct entry points of self-movement versus visual landmark (and other) signals. The fact that many of these structures are interconnected suggests that this may provide stability and, in the case where only a fraction of sensory or motor signals are present, eventually permit substitution by other signal modalities. Mizumori, et al. (chapter 10) suggest that the coactivation of corresponding head direction cells in these multiple structures may provide a form of binding, a process implicated in the origins of conscious perception and emergence of holistic experience. This is consistent with Burgess's (2002; cited in chapter 13) suggestion that an important role for the head direction system in concert with the parietal cortex and hippocampus for mnemonic processing, where particular viewpoints (and the corresponding experience) serve as a key to the trace of episodic memory. This could be facilitated by the coherent activity within some or all of the many structures containing head direction cells.

Hopkins, Bassett and Taube, as well as Aggleton, have pointed out in their chapters that many mnemonic associated areas (such as the anteroventral thalamic nucleus, medial mammillary nucleus and habenula) have direct connections with areas containing head direction cells, and this may confer the latter with properties also related to navigation and memory. However, the properties of the nondirectional neurons in these structures remain poorly characterized even now, offering a promising and intriguing area of research. We may well discover other exciting cognition-correlated activity in these neurons. In particular the role of the cerebellum in directional processing as well as in other aspects of spatial orientation and navigation remains to be further investigated. What are the roles of the cerebellum, associated pontine areas, and the nucleus prepositus hypoglossi in the generation and maintenance of head direction signaling? One interesting point of convergence of chapters by Hopkins and by Glasauer concerns the mystery of the role of the cerebellum in head direction processing. The cerebellum is known to be involved in modulating the mathematical integration of vestibular acceleration signals for the vestibulo-ocular reflex and related adaptive processes. Thus, ascending signals through the vestibular nuclei-nucleus prepositus hypoglossi-DTN pathway benefit from cerebellar processing, although the exact nature of this remains to be elucidated. In chapter 2, Hopkins also showed a descending projection from the mammillary nuclei to a pontine region that projects to the cerebellum. If these arise from the lateral mammillary nuclei, and this pontine region projects to the same vestibulocerebellar region involved in head velocity integration, this might serve a functional role in this processing as a directional feedback signal. Alternatively, if these projections originate in the medial mammillary nucleus, the preceding arguments indicate that they would be more concerned with transmitting hippocampal output signals, perhaps with theta rhythmic modulation, and have a possible role in hippocampal-related learning processes.

Thus, there remain many avenues toward further advances in understanding how the brain elaborates and modulates neural activity related to spatial orientation. On an integrative level, it is of interest to determine how the multiple systems processing signals for head direction, trunk direction, heading, movement direction, and static position exercise their particular roles for spatial cognition and orienting behaviors, and how they interact and communicate with one another. We hope the work presented here will also inspire curiosity to drive future endeavors to discover other fundamental neural mechanisms of cognitive functions, and encourage the participation of specialists and students of the disciplines represented here, as well as others outside of the neurosciences and computational sciences.

References

Albertin SV, Mulder AB, Tabuchi E, Zugaro MB, Wiener SI (2000) Lesions of the medial shell of the nucleus accumbens impair rats in finding larger rewards, but spare reward-seeking behavior. Behav Brain Res 117: 173–183.

Berthoz A (2000) The Brain's Sense of Movement. Transl.: G Weiss, Cambridge, MA: Harvard University Press.

Gray JA, McNaughton N (2000) The Neuropsychology of Anxiety: An Enquiry into the Function of the Septo-Hippocampal System. Oxford: Oxford University Press.

Packard MG, Hirsh R, White NM (1989). Differential effects of fornix and caudate nucleus lesions on two radial maze tasks: evidence for multiple memory systems. J Neurosci 9: 1465–1472.

Contributors

John P. Aggleton
School of Psychology
Cardiff University, Cardiff
Wales, United Kingdom

Angelo Arleo
CNRS-Collège de France Laboratoire de Physiologie de la Perception et de l'Action
Paris, France

Joshua Bassett
Department of Psychological and Brain Sciences
Center for Cognitive Neuroscience, Dartmouth College
Hanover, New Hampshire

Alain Berthoz
CNRS-Collège de France Laboratoire de Physiologie de la Perception et de l'Action
Paris, France

Nicolas Brunel
CNRS-Université René Descartes
Paris, France

Paul A. Dudchenko
Department of Psychology
University of Stirling
Stirling, Scotland

Charles J. Duffy
Departments of Neurology, Neurobiology and Anatomy, Ophthalmology, Brain and
Cognitive Sciences
and The Center for Visual Science, The University of Rochester Medical Center
Rochester, New York

Michael T. Froehler
Departments of Neurology, Neurobiology and Anatomy, Ophthalmology, Brain and
Cognitive Sciences
and The Center for Visual Science, The University of Rochester Medical Center
Rochester, New York

Russell J. Frohardt
Department of Psychological and Brain Sciences
Dartmouth College
Hanover, New Hampshire

Wulfram Gerstner
Laboratory of Computational Neuroscience
Swiss Federal Institute of Technology Lausanne EPFL
Lausanne, Switzerland

Katherine M. Gill
Department of Psychology
University of Washington
Seattle, Washington

Stefan Glasauer
Center for Sensorimotor Research
Department of Neurology
Ludwig-Maximilians-University
Munich, Germany

Alex Guazzelli
Department of Psychology
University of Washington
Seattle, Washington

Halim Hicheur
CNRS-Collège de France Laboratoire de Physiologie de la Perception et de l'Action
Paris, France

David A. Hopkins
Department of Anatomy and Neurobiology
Dalhousie University
Halifax, Nova Scotia, Canada

James J. Knierim
Department of Neurobiology and Anatomy
W.M. Keck Center for the Neurobiology of Learning and Memory
University of Texas Medical School at Houston
Houston, Texas

Sheri J. Y. Mizumori
Department of Psychology
University of Washington
Seattle Washington

Gary M. Muir
Department of Psychological and Brain Sciences
Dartmouth College
Hanover, New Hampshire

Robert U. Muller
Department of Physiology and Pharmacology
SUNY Downstate Medical Center

Brooklyn, New York
and MRC Centre for Synaptic Plasticity
University of Bristol
Bristol, United Kingdom

William K. Page
Departments of Neurology, Neurobiology and Anatomy, Ophthalmology, Brain and
Cognitive Sciences
and The Center for Visual Science
University of Rochester Medical Center
Rochester, New York

Corey B. Puryear
Department of Psychology
University of Washington
Seattle, Washington

James B. Ranck Jr
Department of Physiology
SUNY Health Sciences Center, Brooklyn
Brooklyn, New York

Edmund T. Rolls
Department of Experimental Psychology
University of Oxford
Oxford, England

Françoise Schenk
Faculté des SSP, Institute of Psychology and Department of Physiology
Université de Lausanne
Lausanne, Switzerland

Patricia E. Sharp
Department of Psychology
Bowling Green State University
Bowling Green, Ohio

Robert W. Stackman
Department of Behavioral Neuroscience
Oregon Health and Science University
Portland, Oregon

Jeffrey S. Taube
Department of Psychological and Brain Sciences
Dartmouth College
Hanover, New Hampshire

David S. Touretzky
Computer Science Department and Center for the Neural Basis of Cognition
Carnegie Mellon University
Pittsburgh, Pennsylvania

Stéphane Vieilledent
CNRS-Collège de France Laboratoire de Physiologie de la Perception et de l'Action
Paris, France

William H. Warren
Department of Cognitive and Linguistic Sciences
Brown University
Providence, Rhode Island

Sidney I. Wiener
CNRS-Collège de France Laboratoire de Physiologie de la Perception et de l'Action
Paris, France

Michaël B. Zugaro
CNRS-Collège de France Laboratoire de Physiologie de la Perception et de l'Action
Paris, France

Index